P9-CRV-486

Molecular mechanisms
of atherosclerosis

Molecular mechanisms of atherosclerosis

Edited by

Joseph Loscalzo MD PhD

Wade Professor of Medicine and Chairman, Department of Medicine
Director, Whitaker Cardiovascular Institute
Boston University School of Medicine
Boston, MA

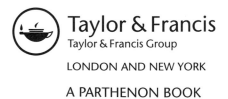
Taylor & Francis
Taylor & Francis Group

LONDON AND NEW YORK

A PARTHENON BOOK

First published in the United Kingdom in 2005
by Taylor & Francis,
an imprint of the Taylor & Francis Group,
2 Park Square, Milton Park
Abingdon, Oxon OX14 4RN, UK

Tel: +44 (0) 1235 828600
Fax: +44 (0) 1235 829000
Website: www.tandf.co.uk

British Library Cataloguing in Publication Data

Data available on application

Library of Congress Cataloging-in-Publication Data

Data available on application

ISBN 1-84214-243-7

Distributed in North and South America by

Taylor & Francis
2000 NW Corporate Blvd
Boca Raton, FL 33431, USA

Within Continental USA
Tel: 800 272 7737; Fax: 800 374 3401
Outside Continental USA
Tel: 561 994 0555; Fax: 561 361 6018
E-mail: orders@crcpress.com

Distributed in the rest of the world by
Thomson Publishing Services
Cheriton House
North Way
Andover, Hampshire SP10 5BE, UK
Tel: +44 (0) 1264 332424
E-mail: salesorder.tandf@thomsonpublishingservices.co.uk

Composition by Parthenon Publishing
Printed and bound by Scotprint, Haddington, UK

Contents

Contributors

Angeliki Chroni
Post-Doctoral Fellow
Molecular Genetics
Whitaker Cardiovascular Institute
Boston University School of Medicine
715 Albany Street, W509
Boston, MA 02118
USA

Lindsay A. Farrer PhD
Professor and Chief of Genetics Unit
Boston University School of Medicine
715 Albany Street, L320
Boston, MA 02118
USA

Jane E. Freedman MD
Associate Professor of Medicine and Pharmacology
Boston University School of Medicine
715 Albany Street, W507
Boston, MA 02118
USA

Haralambos Gavras MD
Professor of Medicine
Boston University School of Medicine
Chief, Hypertension Section
Whitaker Cardiovascular Institute
715 Albany Street, W508
Boston, MA 02118
USA

Caroline Attardo Genco PhD
Professor
Section of Infectious Diseases
Boston University School of Medicine
650 Albany Street, X637
Boston, MA 02118
USA

Frank C. Gibson III
Section of Infectious Diseases
Boston University School of Medicine
650 Albany Street, X637
Boston, MA 02118
USA

Naomi M. Hamburg MD
Fellow in Cardiology
Boston University School of Medicine
88 E. Newton Street, C818
Boston, MA 02118
USA

Diane E. Handy PhD
Associate Professor of Medicine
Boston University School of Medicine
Whitaker Cardiovascular Institute
715 Albany Street, W507
Boston, MA 02118
USA

Yasuo Ido
Boston University School of Medicine
715 Albany Street, X827
Boston, MA 02118
USA

Aran Kadar MD MPH TM
The Pulmonary Center
Boston University School of Medicine
715 Albany Street, R304
Boston, MA 02118
USA

Dimitris Kardassis
Professor of Biochemistry
Department of Biochemistry
Division of Basic Sciences
Institute of Molecular Biology and Biotechnology
University of Crete Medical School
71409 Haraklion
Crete

John F. Keaney Jr MD
Associate Professor of Medicine
Boston University School of Medicine
715 Albany Street, W601
Boston, MA 02118
USA

Kyriakos E. Kypreos
Molecular Genetics
Whitaker Cardiovascular Institute
Boston University School of Medicine
715 Albany Street, W509
Boston, MA 02118
USA

Jane A. Leopold MD
Assistant Professor of Medicine
Whitaker Cardiovascular Institute
Boston University School of Medicine
715 Albany Street, W507
Boston, MA 02118
USA

Joseph Loscalzo MD PhD
Wade Professor of Medicine and Chairman, Department
  of Medicine
Director, Whitaker Cardiovascular Institute
Boston University School of Medicine
715 Albany Street, W507
Boston, MA 02118
USA

Claudia Panzer
Boston Medical Center
88 E. Newton Street, E201
Boston, MA 02118
USA

Frederick L. Ruberg MD
Instructor in Medicine
Cardiology Division
Boston University School of Medicine
88 E. Newton Street, C818
Boston, MA 02118
USA

Neil Ruderman MD DPhil
Professor of Medicine
Boston University School of Medicine
715 Albany Street, X825
Boston, MA 02118
USA

Avrum Spira MD MSc
Assistant Professor of Medicine
Adjunct Assistant Professor of Bioinformatics
Department of Medicine
Boston University School of Medicine
715 Albany Street, R304
Boston, MA 02118
USA

Roland Stocker PhD
Center for Vascular Research
School of Medical Sciences, Faculty of Medicine
University of New South Wales
UNSW Sydney NSW 2052
Australia

Joseph A. Vita MD
Professor of Medicine
Boston University School of Medicine
88 E. Newton Street, C818
Boston, MA 02118
USA

Peter W.F. Wilson MD
Professor of Medicine
Program Director, General Clinical Research Center
Medical University of South Carolina
96 Jonathan Lucas Street
Suite 215, PO Box 250609
Charleston, SC 29425
USA

Diego F. Wyszynski MD MHS PhD
Assistant Professor of Medicine, Genetics Program
Department of Medicine
Boston University School of Medicine
Assistant Professor of Epidemiology
Boston University School of Public Health
715 Albany Street, L320
Boston, MA 02118
USA

Eleni E. Zanni
Assistant Professor Molecular Genetics
Whitaker Cardiovascular Institute
Boston University School of Medicine
715 Albany Street, W509
Boston, MA 02118
USA

Vassilis I. Zannis PhD
Chief, Molecular Genetics
Whitaker Cardiovascular Institute
Boston University School of Medicine
715 Albany Street, W509
Boston, MA 02118
USA

1

Introduction and overview

Joseph Loscalzo

The term 'atherosclerosis' is translated from the Greek for 'gruel', to describe the contents of the typical atheromatous plaque. Over the last century, atherosclerotic vascular disease has become and remains the major cause of morbidity and mortality in the western world. In 2000, the clinical expressions of atherothrombotic diseases were responsible for over 850 000 deaths in the United States, accounting for more than one-third of all deaths.[1] Importantly, atherosclerosis claims more lives than all types of cancer combined, with considerable economic costs to society. Although currently a problem largely in the developed world, the World Health Organization predicts that a worldwide epidemic of atherosclerotic vascular disease will evolve as developing countries acquire the proatherogenic habits of the western world.

Since the early pathological reports describing atherosclerotic lesions, and especially over the past 30 years, extraordinary advances have been made in our understanding of the molecular and cellular mechanisms of atherogenesis. These advances evolved in parallel with a growing understanding of vascular biology, hemostasis, and lipid metabolism. In this book we approach the problem of atherosclerosis from a mechanistic perspective, and do so in the context of contemporary knowledge of molecular and cellular pathobiology. We begin with an epidemiological overview of the problem of atherosclerotic vascular disease,

followed by a review of the genetics and genetic epidemiology of this complex trait. We turn next to specific chapter topics on each of four fundamental mechanisms common to all risk factors for atherosclerosis, namely, inflammation, oxidative stress, thrombosis, and endothelial dysfunction. Thereafter, we review the mechanisms underlying four common risk factors for atherogenesis: dyslipidemias, diabetes mellitus, hypertension and smoking. More recently proposed risk factors, hyperhomocysteinemia and infection, are then considered, followed by a discussion of rational molecular therapies to prevent and combat established atherothrombotic disease.

Taken together, these chapters offer a broad, contemporary review of the molecular and cellular mechanisms of atherothrombogenesis. Although not all-inclusive, the topics considered and the order of presentation were chosen to provide the reader with the information necessary to understand the complexity of the disease process. Armed with the information contained in this text, the reader should be able confidently to approach cutting-edge findings in the field with insight and foresight about their implications for disease diagnosis, prevention, and treatment.

Reference

1. National Vital Statistics Report 2002; 16:50.

2

The epidemiology of atherosclerotic disease

Peter W.F. Wilson

Introduction

Atherosclerotic disease is a source of great morbidity and mortality in North America and Europe. The clinical outcomes of coronary heart disease (CHD), cardiovascular disease (CVD), and cerebrovascular disease are largely attributable to the process of atherosclerosis. This disease develops relatively silently through late adolescence and early adulthood, and clinical sequelae are often not evident until after the age of 45 years. Newer methods of assessment now allow the detection of subclinical atherosclerotic disease in a variety of arterial beds. This chapter focuses on the development of clinical atherosclerotic outcomes on a population basis, and provides some information on the prevalence of subclinical disease across the adult age spectrum.

Burden of atherosclerotic disease

Cardiovascular disease is the leading cause of death in US adults, accounting for approximately 40% of deaths in men and 41% in women (Figure 2.1). Cancer ranks a distant second, followed by other conditions.[1] Rates for CVD mortality used to be higher, peaked in the USA during the 1970s, and have declined more than 30% since then. Multiple factors related to prevention and the care of patients with CVD appear to account for the decline (Figure 2.2).[2,3] The decrease in CVD deaths has been more consistent over the past decade for men than for women.

A slightly different situation has pertained for the occurrence of a first heart attack over the past two decades. The Atherosclerosis Risk in Communities (ARIC) study has been tracking the rate of CHD in four communities around the USA, and only a modest decline in non-fatal heart attack rates has occurred over the past 20 years. For the period 1987–1994, ARIC investigators reported that the highest CHD rates were observed in black men, with reported rates successively lower in white men, in black women, and in white women. These differences held for persons 35–74 years of age, emphasizing the increased risk for CHD in minority groups (Figure 2.3).[4] The large decline in CVD mortality, the mild decline in CHD morbidity, and the aging of the US population has led to an increased prevalence of CVD in the US that is highly related to age and sex. Although cardiovascular disease affects approximately 30% of men and women at age 50, the prevalence rises to approximately 75% by age 75. Cardiovascular disease is consistently more common in men than in women at all ages for adults 20–75 years who were included in the National Health and Nutrition Examination Survey (NHANES) III conducted from 1988 to 1994 (Figure 2.4).[1]

The lifetime risk of CHD is also highly related to sex and age. At age 40 years the Framingham men experienced a 49% risk of developing CHD (angina pectoris, myocardial infarction, or coronary heart disease death) prior to death. The lifetime incidence was lower for older persons who had never experienced CHD, and at age 70 years the lifetime risk for CHD in men was 35% (Figure 2.5). The lifetime risks for CHD in women were lower at each age in comparison to the men. Overall, the lifetime risk for CHD was approximately 40% in men and 30% in women.[5] In contrast, the lifetime risk for developing breast cancer in women is approximately 10%, a rate that is much lower than a woman's lifetime risk for CHD.

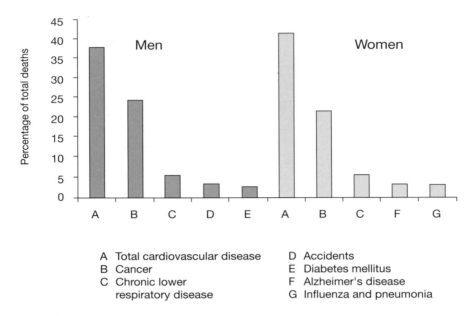

Figure 2.1   Leading causes of death for white men and women, USA 2000 (AHA Heart and Stroke Facts Book 2003)

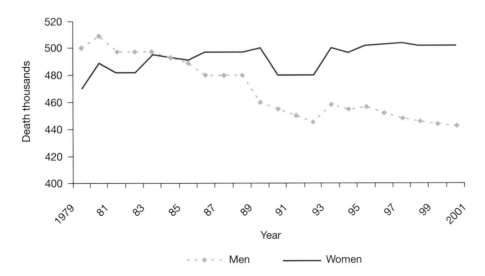

Figure 2.2   Cardiovascular disease mortality trends for men and women, USA 1979–2000 (AHA Heart and Stroke Facts Book 2003)

Coronary heart disease may manifest itself in several different ways. Angina pectoris is the most common first CHD event in women,[6] followed by myocardial infarction, and CHD death; sudden cardiac death is extremely uncommon in women.

Different patterns of first CHD events have been observed for men, with myocardial infarction being the most common first CHD event, followed by angina pectoris, and coronary death.[6] The frequency of sudden cardiac death has diminished considerably

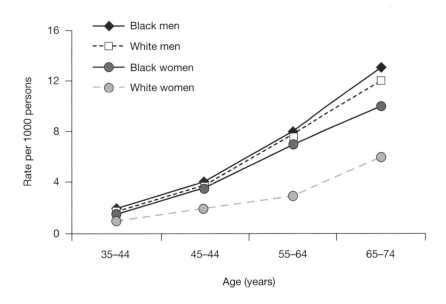

Figure 2.3 Annual rate of first heart attacks by age, sex and race, USA 1987–1994 (N Engl J Med 1998; 339:861)

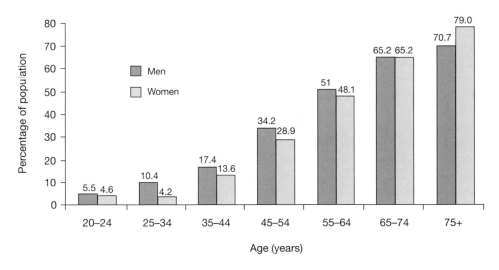

Figure 2.4 Prevalence of cardiovascular disease in Americans aged 20 and older by age and sex, USA 1988–1994 (NHANES III (1988–1994), CDC/NCHS; AHA Heart and Stroke Facts Book 2003)

in recent years, as identification of susceptible patients and appropriate medical care has improved greatly.[7–12] Importantly, after age 40, sudden cardiac death is most likely to be related to atherosclerotic disease.

Coronary heart disease in women

Coronary heart disease in women tends to occur after the menopause, and rates are significantly higher than

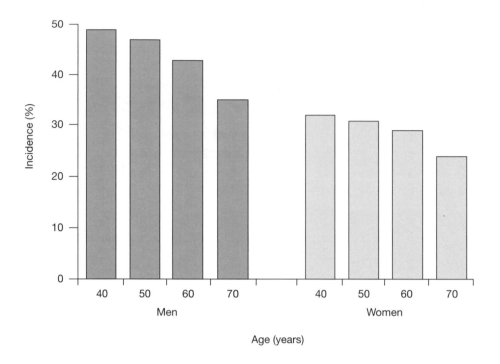

Figure 2.5   Lifetime risk of coronary heart disease – Framingham men and women (Lloyd-Jones, D et al. Lancet 1999)

for other common diseases of aging, including fractures, cerebrovascular disease, breast cancer, and uterine cancer. Decreased estrogen production after the menopause has been thought to be an important determinant of increased risk for CHD in older women. The majority of observational studies undertaken in the 1970s and 1980s showed consistently lower CHD rates in women who took postmenopausal estrogen.[13–15] Meta-analyses of observational studies estimated a 50% reduction in risk of a first heart attack with postmenopausal estrogens.[16]

Several randomized clinical trials have been undertaken to test the efficacy of estrogen as a cardioprotective agent in postmenopausal women. The trial results have not confirmed the observational study reports. For example, in the Heart and Estrogen/progestin Replacement Study (HERS) the overall relative risk for CHD in the clinical trial did not differ for women taking estrogen compared to women who did not take estrogen (Figure 2.6).[17] During the trial there was a trend over time towards more favorable effects of estrogen on CHD risk, and consistently unfavorable effects of estrogen on the risk of venous thromboembolism. It

was proposed that the effect of estrogen on CHD risk, was time dependent, with its use having an adverse effect on the risk of atherosclerotic disease early in the course of therapy, but a favorable effect that was evident only with a longer duration of treatment.

Unfavorable effects of combined estrogen–progestin therapy on CHD risk were observed in the Women's Health Initiative.[18,19] Risk reduction with estrogen replacement was observed for fractures and colon cancer, but increased risks for breast cancer, cardiovascular disease, blood clots, stroke, and heart attack were obtained. The authors concluded that the adverse risks of postmenopausal estrogen–progestin combination therapy outweighed the favorable effects, and that postmenopausal estrogen–progestins were not recommended to prevent CHD (Figure 2.7).

Atherosclerotic disease risk factors

There are several ways to consider coronary disease risk factors and risk factors for atherosclerosis. A common

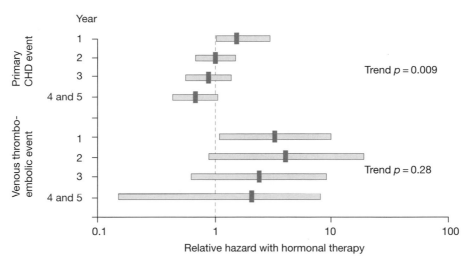

Figure 2.6 Heart and Estrogen/progestin Replacement Study (HERS) relative hazard for vascular events over 5 years of follow-up. CHD, coronary heart diseas (J Am Med Assoc 1998; 280:610)

Table 2.1 Coronary risk factors – initial coronary heart disease		
Definitely modifiable	*Potentially modifiable*	*Fixed*
Cholesterol	Lp(a)	Age
HDL-C	Oxidized lipids	Sex
Triglycerides	Hematologic	Family
Blood pressure	Glucose	
Cigarettes	intolerance	
Diabetes	LVH/LV mass	
Obesity		
Sedentary lifestyle		
Alcohol		

HDL-C, high-density lipoprotein cholesterol; Lp(a), lipoprotein (a); LVH, left ventricular hypertrophy

approach is to use groupings such as definitely modifiable, potentially modifiable, and fixed risk factors (Table 2.1). Cholesterol, blood pressure, cigarette smoking, lifestyle and behavioral factors are on the definitely modifiable list. The potentially modifiable risk factors usually include newer measurements that are being actively investigated as contributors to the greater risk of atherosclerotic disease. The scientific information for these factors is generally less certain than for the definitely modifiable factors. Finally, age,

sex, and family history have been considered fixed risk factors for CVD. Genetics may contribute to each of these groupings and alter CVD risk. For example, the genetic disorder familial hypercholesterolemia is now considered a definitely modifiable condition, and modern lipid-lowering therapy can reduce CVD risk in these individuals. Variations in lipoproteins and other metabolic factors may have a genetic basis and can augment the risk of atherosclerotic disease, especially when specific environmental or dietary conditions are present.

Another scheme to assess the development of atherosclerotic disease is shown in Figure 2.8. Using this approach, fundamental factors lead to the development of subclinical atherosclerotic disease, which is followed by an initial vascular disease event that may be followed by a variety of other CVD outcomes. As shown in the middle of Figure 2.8, environmental factors appear to be especially important for the development of subclinical disease, which can be assessed by techniques including imaging, ultrasound, and physiological devices such as ankle–brachial blood pressure measurements. At the bottom of Figure 2.8 are shown some of the mechanisms that are used to assess the initiation and development of atherosclerotic disease. For example, lipids, glucose, and homocysteine may foster the development of subclinical atherosclerotic disease; hematologic and inflammatory mechanisms may accelerate the progression of subclinical disease to definite

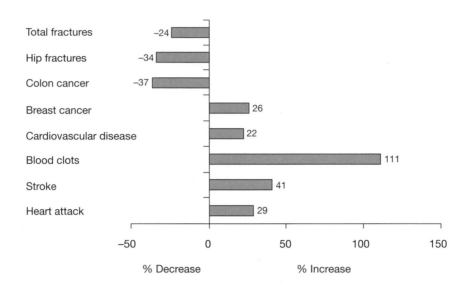

Figure 2.7   Health risks with combined hormone replacement therapy (HRT) Women's Health Initiative (J Am Med Assoc 2002; 288:321)

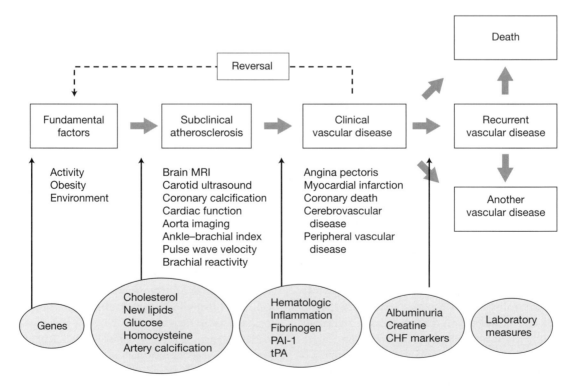

Figure 2.8   Vascular disease diagnoses, events, and investigations. PAI-1, plasminogen activator inhibitor-1; tPA, tissue-type plasminogen activator; CHF, congestive heart failure

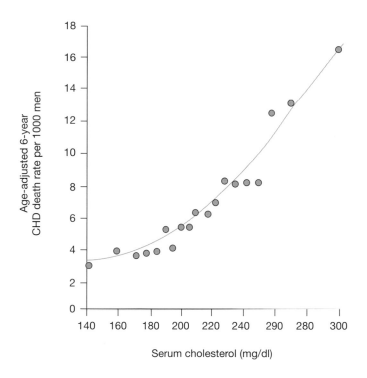

Figure 2.9   Cholesterol level and risk of coronary heart disease (CHD) death, Multiple Risk Factor Intervention Trial (MRFIT) screened population (Lancet 1986; 2:933)

clinical outcomes. The factors shown are only illustrative as the pathological processes are more complex. This schema highlights the different factors that may be important for progression from one phase of atherosclerosis to another.

Lipids

Higher levels of cholesterol are related to the development of CVD. In more than 300 000 middle-aged men screened for the Multiple Risk Factor Intervention Trial (MRFIT) higher cholesterol levels led to an increased risk of CHD death (Figure 2.9).[20] Using a cholesterol level of 200 mg/dl as the comparison, a level of 250 mg/dl led to a twofold risk of CVD death and a level of 300 mg/dl led to a threefold risk.[21]

High-density lipoprotein (HDL) cholesterol is a major fraction of cholesterol in the plasma and is an important determinant of risk for CHD and myocardial infarction, even when the total cholesterol level is known. In Framingham women the 12-year incidence of myocardial infarction was positively related to cho-

lesterol level and inversely to HDL cholesterol level (Figure 2.10).[22] At a total cholesterol level < 211 mg/dl the HDL cholesterol levels were inversely related to the risk of developing myocardial infarction in these women. Similar results were obtained for men and in other studies, helping to provide the rationale for cholesterol and HDL cholesterol screening to assess CVD risk.

A large variety of lipoprotein particles have been identified, and several techniques are available to assess their density, diameter, electrophoretic characteristics, and nuclear magnetic resonance properties. Initially the low-density lipoprotein (LDL) particles received the most attention, as apolipoprotein B is present in the LDL fraction. Research interest has spread to investigate the role of all particle groups, as newer methods have allowed rapid assessment of the numbers and concentrations of lipoprotein particles.[23–26] There are complex interrelations between the number of particles and some of the commonly measured lipids. For example, with increasing concentrations of triglycerides the percentage of smaller, denser LDL particles increases

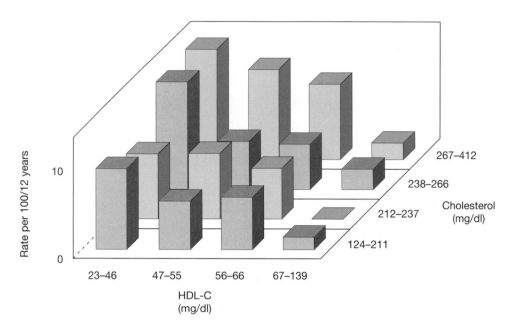

Figure 2.10 12-Year incidence of myocardial infarction in women in the Framingham study. HDL-C, high-density lipoprotein cholesterol (Arteriosclerosis 1988; 8:207)

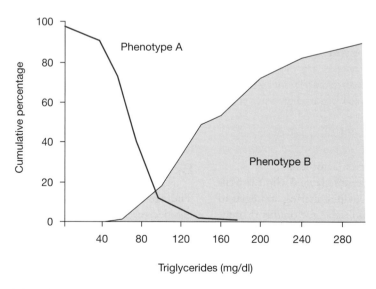

Figure 2.11 Cumulative distribution of adjusted triglyceride levels by low-density lipoprotein subclass phenotype (Circulation 1990; 82:495)

and the frequency of large, buoyant LDL particles decreases (Figure 2.11).[23] The smaller, denser LDL particles may be associated with greater risk, but the added usefulness of these measurements for the assess-

ment of cardiovascular disease risk in prospective studies is not certain at present.[27,28]

Lipoprotein (a) (Lp(a)) is an accepted determinant of CVD risk, and this particle includes an LDL moiety

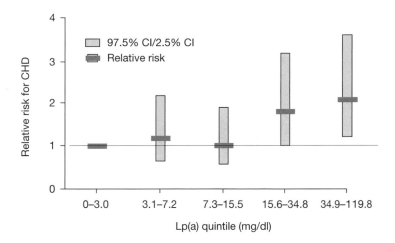

Figure 2.12   Lipoprotein (a) (Lp(a)) level and risk for coronary heart disease (CHD) in Lipid Research Clinics study of men 35–59 years with 7–10 years' follow-up (J Am Med Assoc 1994; 274:1002)

that is linked to a protein chain that bears homology to plasminogen. The length of the apo (a) protein varies and is heritable. A variety of methods have been undertaken to assay Lp(a),[29] but standardization has been difficult because the particle varies in composition from person to person.[30] Levels of Lp(a) are higher in Africans and African-Americans than in whites.[31] In African populations the particle concentrations follow a normal statistical distribution, but Lp(a) levels are lower and the distribution is skewed in whites. Lp(a) has generally been shown to be a CVD risk factor, especially at the higher concentrations (> 30 mg/dl) in whites (Figure 2.12).[32] Routine screening for Lp(a) levels has been recommended for persons with premature CVD that is not explained by conventional risk factor levels.[33,34]

Over the past two decades, several clinical trials have been undertaken with lipid-altering strategies to prevent CVD. Initial strategies focused on diet therapy, but several of the interventions were not effective, and lowering blood cholesterol by more than 10% was relatively uncommon.[21,35] Clinical trials with bile acid resins, nicotinic acid, and fibrates followed, with generally favorable results, but patient compliance with the regimens was problematic.[36–38] Often the degree of cholesterol and LDL cholesterol reduction was proportional to the decrease in coronary heart disease events observed over the course of the trial.

The advent of hydroxymethylglutaryl coenzyme A (HMGCoA) reductase inhibitors in the late 1980s led to an improved ability to reduce LDL cholesterol. A large number of diet and lipid therapy trials ensued, and favorable treatment effects on subclinical and clinical disease were observed for the coronary and carotid arteries, initial CHD events, recurrent CHD events, and stroke with a variety of regimens.[39–48] In general, more cholesterol-lowering has led to a greater reduction in risk of initial and recurrent CHD in these studies. The efficacy of cholesterol therapy in these trials has largely been premised upon the intention to treat, and not on the degree of cholesterol-lowering achieved or the ability to reach predefined target levels of cholesterol or LDL cholesterol.

Blood pressure

The age-adjusted prevalence of high blood pressure has decreased from the late 1970s to the 1990s for several ethnic groups in the USA. Throughout the interval, the non-Hispanic blacks have had higher rates of hypertension (> 140/90 mmHg) than whites or Hispanics; in all ethnic groups the prevalence of hypertension was higher in men than in women (Figure 2.13). In these surveys, many Americans were unaware that they had high blood pressure or were inadequately treated for the condition. As seen in Figure 2.14, approximately 50% of persons with high blood pressure were treated and only 15–34% were under control. A sizeable fraction, ranging from 27 to

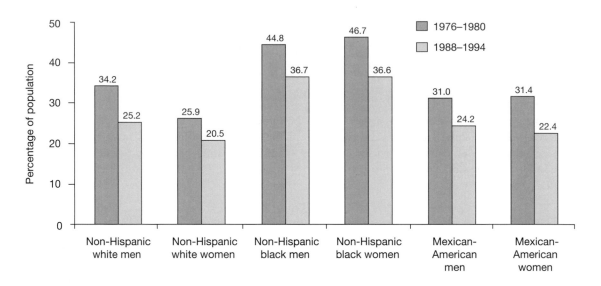

Figure 2.13 Age-adjusted prevalence trends for high blood pressure, age 20–74, by race/ethnicity, sex and survey, USA 1976–1980 and 1988–1994. Source: NHANES II (1976–1980) and NHANES III (1988–1994) CDC/NCHS. Data based on multiple measures of blood pressure (AHA Heart and Stroke Facts Book 2003)

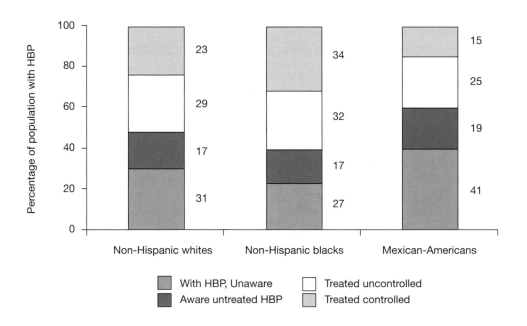

Figure 2.14 Extent of awareness, treatment and control of high blood pressure (HBP) by race/ethnicity, USA 1988–1994 (N Engl J Med 2001; 345:479–486)

41% of persons with high blood pressure, were unaware that they were affected.[49]

The risk of CVD is highly related to blood pressure level, and levels of systolic pressure are typically more highly associated with the development of CVD than levels of diastolic pressure. Systolic and diastolic hypertension generally confer a relative risk of 1.6 for CVD; for combined systolic and diastolic hypertension the relative risk is 2.0.[50,51] Pulse pressure is also related to cardiovascular disease outcomes, especially in older persons, as diastolic pressures are typically lower in the elderly than in middle age.[52]

Blood pressure levels that do not meet the criteria for hypertension increase the risk for a first major CVD event, and long-term comparisons have shown that the risk of CVD is increased in persons with high normal blood pressure (systolic pressure 130–139 mmHg with diastolic 85–89 mmHg). As high normal pressure level is a common condition, this level of blood pressure accounts for a sizeable fraction of CVD events, and on a population basis is nearly as important as hypertension itself.[53]

The overall effect of blood pressure on CVD death has been summarized in a review analysis of 61 prospective observational studies of blood pressure and mortality.[54] At age 40–69 years a difference of 20 mmHg in systolic pressure or 10 mmHg in diastolic pressure was related to approximately a twofold difference in death rate from ischemic heart disease.

A large number of clinical trials have been undertaken to lower blood pressure, and have demonstrated that CHD risk is reduced when diastolic and systolic blood pressure levels are lowered with diet or a variety of agents, although safety with some treatments has been an issue.[55–57] Research has recently concentrated on treatment in special groups, especially older persons and those with elevated systolic pressure. These trials have demonstrated efficacy in reducing vascular disease risk in the Systolic Hypertension in the Elderly Program (SHEP), the Systolic Hypertension in Europe Trial (Syst-Eur), and the Systolic Hypertension in China Trial (SYSt-China).[58–60]

The Antihypertensive and Lipid-Lowering Treatment to Prevent Heart Attack Trial (ALLHAT), a study with more than 40 000 US participants, tested the efficacy of several treatment modalities for elevated blood pressure in older Americans. This study found that thiazide diuretics were as effective as calcium

channel blockers and angiotensin-converting enzyme (ACE) inhibitors as initial therapy in the prevention of CVD risk.[61] The addition of a statin provided no additional benefit, but the difference in cholesterol levels between placebo users and those randomized to the active agent used was approximately 10% during the trial.[61,62] Different results were obtained in the combined blood pressure and lipid treatment arms from the Anglo-Scandinavian Cardiac Outcomes Trial (ASCOT), which used blood pressure medications and more potent statin therapy, which effected a difference in cholesterol levels that exceeded 40 mg/dl. In ASCOT, lower CVD risk was related to both the lipid and the blood pressure treatments.[46]

Nutrition and heart disease

Several dietary components are related to lipid levels and have been studied intensively over the past half century. One of the early reports was the Seven Countries Study, a long-term survey of men from Europe, North America, and Asia.[63] This investigation showed that dietary intake of cholesterol and saturated fat was related to greater cholesterol levels in the population, and long follow-up of this cohort confirms this observation.[64,65] Finland, the region with the highest mean levels of cholesterol in the 1970s, enacted countrywide programs to improve the diet, and cholesterol levels < 250 mg/dl had declined from 16% of the population to 3% by the 1990s.[66]

Cholesterol levels have diminished modestly in the US over the past two decades, and the average cholesterol in adults is approximately 204 mg/dl.[67] Lower consumption of fat is largely responsible for this change,[67] and switching from the usual American diet, which includes 35–41% of calories as fat, to an American Heart Association Step I diet with < 30% calories as fat, would be expected to change cholesterol levels by 15% from baseline.[68] Dietary cholesterol guidelines promulgated by expert committees[69] now recommend the consumption of a variety of foods, including fruits, vegetables, and grains, and that a healthy body weight, desirable cholesterol levels in the blood, and desirable blood pressure levels are all important.[69] Adult blood cholesterol levels < 200 mg/dl are becoming the aim, and approximately half of the population is not on target with these criteria. An aggressive goal of an LDL cholesterol < 100 mg/dl has been set for

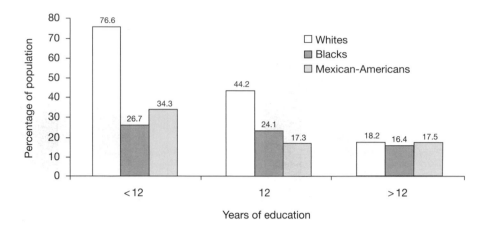

Figure 2.15   Age-adjusted prevalence trends for high blood pressure, age 20–74, by race/ethnicity, sex and survey, USA 1976–1980 and 1988–1994 (J Am Med Assoc 1999; 281:1006–1013)

persons with known CVD, and it has been estimated that only 18% of the candidates are on target.[70]

Increased oxidation has been proposed as an important contributor to atherosclerosis, and interest in nutrients that have antioxidant properties has increased.[71] Vitamins B, C, and E have been studied the most, and several observational studies have suggested that greater intake of these vitamins in regular food or as supplements had a favorable effect on cardiovascular risk,[72,73] but controlled clinical trials, recently in the setting of a 2×2 factorial trial with other antiatherosclerotic regimens, have generally not demonstrated reductions in risk.[40,74,75]

Greater alcohol intake has consistently been related to a reduced risk of coronary heart disease, and an intake in the range of more than two drinks per day in men and more than one drink a day in women appears to confer this reduced risk.[76–79] Favorable effects on HDL cholesterol levels are thought to be important in exerting this effect, as well as anti-inflammatory and antiplatelet effects. Greater alcohol intake is not without hazards, and a greater risk of gastrointestinal bleeding, hemorrhagic stroke, accidents, suicide, and cirrhosis may occur with increased intake.[80,81]

Smoking

The prevalence of cigarette smoking has declined in the US since the 1960s. Data from the National Health and Nutrition Examination Survey from 1988 to 1994 (NHANES III) showed that cigarette smoking rates were lowest among individuals with more than 12 years of education for white, black, and Mexican-American participants, but approximately 20% of adult Americans smoke cigarettes regularly (Figure 2.15). Higher smoking rates were present for those with less education, especially whites with less than 12 years of education.[82]

Cigarette smoking generally doubles the risk of CVD outcomes. Both regular and filter cigarettes have similar adverse effects on CHD risk.[83] Low-tar and low-nicotine cigarettes have shown no reduction in CVD risk compared with products that are higher in tar and nicotine.[84] Cessation of cigarette smoking was associated with a halved risk of CVD death in 1–2 years after quitting in men screened as part of the MRFIT study.[85]

Passive smoking has been related to an increased risk of CHD that is approximately 30% greater than the risk for non-smokers,[86] and it has also been reported that persons exposed to environmental smoke have increased intima medial thickness of their carotid arteries, an indication of subclinical arteriosclerosis, compared to non-smokers.[87]

Physical activity and fitness

Persons with a more active lifestyle are generally at lower risk of CVD. Early studies investigated occupations

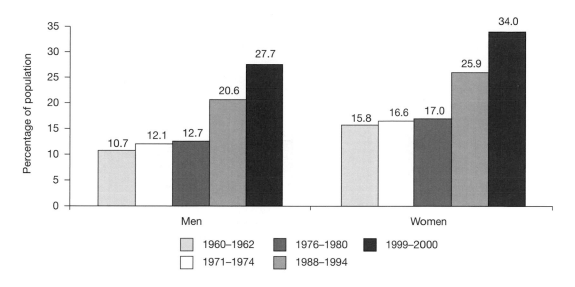

Figure 2.16 Age-adjusted prevalence of obesity, USA 1960–1962, 1971–1974, 1976–1980, 1988–1994 and 1999–2000. Obesity is defined as a BMI > 30.0 or higher (J Am Med Assoc 1999; 281:1006–1013)

and their risk for CVD, but more recent research has concentrated on leisure-time physical activity. A key report from the Harvard Alumni Study showed that greater exercise was inversely related to the risk of fatal and non-fatal myocardial infarction over an 8-year period.[88] This result and others showed that physical activity in middle-aged adults was important in reducing CVD risk.[89] There is an increased risk for sudden cardiac death during or following exercise in persons who generally perform little exercise, but adverse events are uncommon.[90,91] Current recommendations call for physical activity of 30 minutes a day at least five times a week.[92–94]

Greater fitness that has been documented by longer exercise treadmill times has been related to reduced risk for CVD in both men and women.[95] Persons in the lowest quintile of fitness experienced the highest CVD event rates, and even modest degrees of fitness were related to lower risk of CVD in these studies of middle-aged men and women.

Obesity

Excess adiposity has been defined by the World Health Organization and two general measures are used, the body mass index (BMI = body weight in kg divided by

height in m²) and abdominal girth (the greatest circumference of the abdomen when a subject is standing).[96] Using these measures, overweight is indicated by a BMI 25–29.9 kg/m² and obesity by a BMI > 30 kg/m². Increased abdominal adiposity is defined as > 90 cm for women and > 100 cm for men.

The prevalence of obesity has increased dramatically over the course of the past 30 years in the USA.[97] Data from US surveys show that the prevalence of obesity has risen from 10% to 27% in men, and from 16% to 34% in women from 1960 to 2000 (Figure 2.16). The prevalence of overweight has also increased correspondingly, and it is now estimated that over 50% of American adults are either overweight or obese.[1,96]

Obesity contributes to the development of several CVD risk factors, especially hypertension, diabetes mellitus, low HDL cholesterol, elevated triglycerides, and elevated levels of inflammatory markers. Weight gain during the adult years is highly related to the development of a greater risk factor burden, and this phenomenon has been observed with relatively modest weight increases in prospective studies such as the Framingham offspring investigation.[98] Obesity accounts for approximately 23% of CHD in men and 15% in women in long-term analyses of the Framingham data.[99]

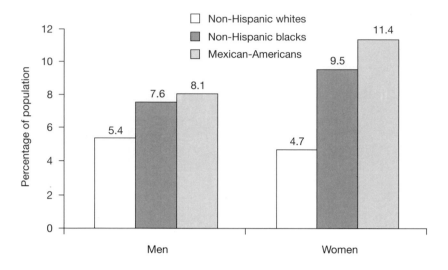

Figure 2.17   Age-adjusted prevalence of physician-diagnosed diabetes mellitus in Americans aged 20 and older by sex and race/ethnicity, USA 1988–1994 (Diabetes Care 1998; 21:518–524)

Diabetes mellitus and the metabolic syndrome

An increased prevalence of type 2 diabetes mellitus is following on the heels of the obesity epidemic in the US. The prevalence of type 2 diabetes mellitus rises with age in both sexes and at age 50 years approximately 4% of the population is affected. The lowest prevalence of type 2 diabetes mellitus is commonly observed in non-Hispanic whites, higher levels are seen in non-Hispanic blacks, and the highest levels have been reported for Mexican-Americans and Native Americans (Figure 2.17).[100]

The risk of CVD is increased twofold among younger men with type 2 diabetes mellitus, and varies according to the type of vascular complication. In Framingham, as well as in several other studies, even greater relative risks for CVD have been observed for younger women with type 2 diabetes mellitus (Figure 2.18).[101] Data from Finland have suggested that the risk for a heart attack in a person with diabetes is very similar to that in persons who have had a heart attack and are at risk for a subsequent heart attack. This result led to the concept of type 2 diabetes mellitus as a CHD risk equivalent, and emphasizes the need for aggressive treatment of risk factors in persons with type 2 diabetes mellitus to prevent CVD events.[102]

Cardiovascular risk reduction efforts have only recently targeted persons with type 2 diabetes mellitus, and lower thresholds for LDL cholesterol and blood pressure for such persons are now recommended.[103–105] The basis for these aggressive approaches came from subgroup analyses of treatment effects for blood pressure and lipid lowering in type 2 diabetics in randomized clinical trials. The efficacy of this approach has been published in a Danish trial using aggressive therapy for hyperglycemia, hypertension, dyslipidemia, and microalbuminuria in persons with type 2 diabetes mellitus.[106]

Data to support concerted glucose control as a CVD prevention strategy have obtained support from observational studies, and glucose and HBA_1C data from clinical trials have been impressive for the prevention of microvascular eye and kidney complications, but little added benefit has been shown for tight glucose control with current regimens for CVD prevention.[107–111] This issue is being addressed with large-scale multifactorial intervention trials in patients with type 2 diabetes mellitus.

Several CVD risk factors occur at a frequency greater than expected, and insulin resistance is thought to account for clustering of these traits, especially higher blood pressure, impaired fasting glucose, increased triglycerides, decreased HDL cholesterol,

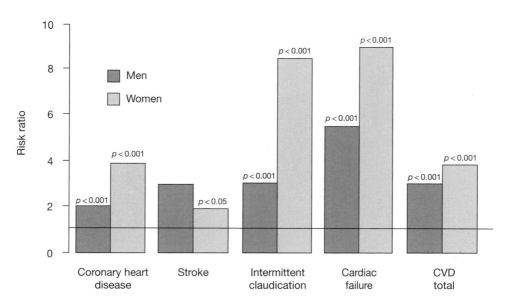

Figure 2.18 Diabetes and cardiovascular disease (CVD) risk in Framingham cohort aged 35–64 years–30-year follow-up (Am J Kidney Dis 1998; 32:S89–100)

Table 2.2 ATP III: the metabolic syndrome (from J Am Med Assoc 2001; 285:2486)	
Risk factor	*Definition*
Waist circumference	> 102 cm (> 40 in) men > 88 cm (> 35 in) women
Triglycerides	≥ 150 mg/dl
HDL-cholesterol	< 40 mg/dl men < 50 mg/dl women
Blood pressure	≥ 130/≥ 85 mmHg
Fasting glucose	> 110 mg/dl
HDL, high-density lipoprotein	

and greater abdominal adiposity. The presence of three or more of these five abnormalities has been named the metabolic syndrome, and some of the criteria are sex specific (Table 2.2).[103]

The metabolic syndrome is present in approximately 24% of American adults according to US survey data from the early 1990s, and the prevalence is highly related to age, ranging from 7% in those aged 20–29 years to 43% in those aged 60–69 years (Figure 2.19).[112] The presence of the metabolic syndrome in adults has been shown to confer an increased risk of diabetes mellitus, CHD, and CVD death.[113–115]

Inflammation

A variety of factors related to hematologic, endothelial, or inflammatory processes have been studied for their relation to CVD. Early studies investigated leukocyte count, and these were followed by fibrinogen determinations. In a meta-analysis the top third of fibrinogen levels led to a doubling of risk for initial and recurrent CVD events.[116] A European investigation assessed the relations between recurrent CHD and levels of fibrinogen, von Willebrand factor antigen, t-PA antigen, and C-reactive protein in persons with angina pectoris. Each of these markers was highly related to a greater risk of subsequent CHD in categorical analyses that used quintiles of each factor (Figure 2.20).[117] Subsequent research in a large number of studies has shown that inflammatory markers, especially C-reactive protein, are highly related to an increased risk of atherosclerotic events (Figure 2.21),[118] including initial and recurrent CVD, as well as stroke.[119–122] Measurement of inflammatory markers, specifically C-reactive protein, is now considered a reasonable adjunct to the major risk factors further to assess absolute risk for coronary disease primary prevention.[123]

Blood levels of the amino acid homocysteine have been been studied for their relation to CVD risk.

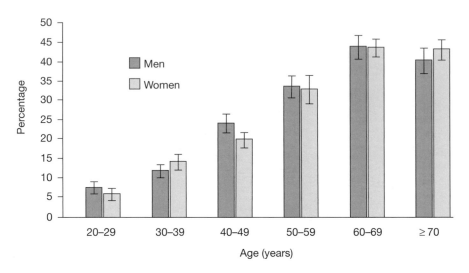

Figure 2.19 Age-specific prevalence of the metabolic syndrome in National Health and Nutrition Examination Survey (NHANES) III. Data presented as percentage (SE) (J Am Med Assoc 2002; 287:356–359)

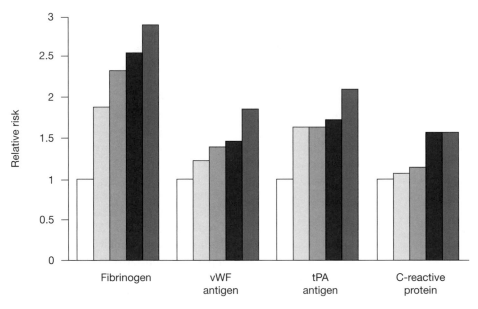

Figure 2.20 Relative risk of coronary heart disease events in patients with angina pectoris according to quintile of hemostatic factors. tPA, tissue-type plasminogen activator; vWF, von Willebrand factor (N Engl J Med 1995; 332:635)

Investigations in the early 1990s showed that a lower intake of B vitamins (folate, vitamin B_6, vitamin B_{12}) was related to greater concentrations of homocysteine.[124] Persons with higher homocysteine levels experienced a greater risk for CVD, and the results were stronger in the earlier reports than in more recent investigations (Figure 2.22).[125,126] Folate fortification of cereals and grains was undertaken in the US during the late 1990s and has appeared to reduce the frequency of elevated homocysteine levels in the free-living population.[127] Additional folate intake from supplementary vitamins and multivitamins may be

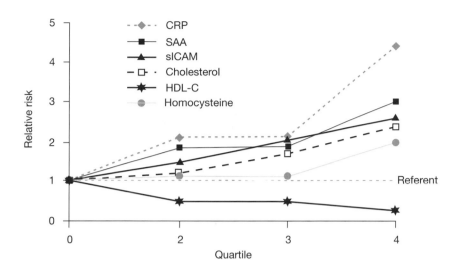

Figure 2.21 Inflammation markers and cardiovascular disease, Women's Health Study. CRP, C-reactive protein; SAA, serum amyloid A; sICAM, soluble intercellular adhesion molecule type 1; HDL-C, high-density lipoprotein cholesterol (N Engl J Med 2000; 342:836)

contributing to a reduced importance for homocysteine as a CVD risk factor.

Homocysteine may be an important contributor to greater CVD risk in specific situations. Extremely high homocysteine levels despite folate supplementation are commonly observed in persons with impaired kidney function, and may contribute to the accelerated atherosclerosis observed with this condition.[128] Clinical trials are under way to test the utility of folate supplementation to reduce atherosclerosis in patients with reduced kidney function.[129]

Genetics

Genetic abnormalities and variants in common genes contribute to the risk of atherosclerotic disease, and research is very active in this field.[130,131] Time-honored diseases such as familial hypercholesterolemia have been shown to have several potential causes and, taken together, probably account for approximately 5% of the case burden of persons with myocardial infarction.[132] The different alleles of apolipoprotein E have been related to cholesterol and triglyceride levels in young adults, the risk of cardiovascular disease in middle age, and dementia in older age.[133–135] The apolipoprotein E4 allele is present in approximately

24% of the population, and a relative risk for CHD of 1.5 has led to the realization that this gene variant accounts for approximately 10–15% of coronary heart disease.[134,136] Furthermore, the different alleles of the apolipoprotein E gene may affect responses to diet and lipid-altering medications.[137,138] Variants of several other genes, including the angiotensin-converting enzyme,[139] lipoprotein (a),[30] cholesterol ester transfer protein,[140] hepatic lipase,[141] and methylene tetrahydrofolate reductase (MTHFR) (related to folate and homocysteine metabolism),[142] are examples of candidate genes that have been studied for their relation to metabolic factors and CVD risk, and the list of candidates is growing rapidly. Gene–environment effects appear to be operative in the case of apolipoprotein E and MTHFR. Several observational studies have undertaken large-scale genome efforts to screen for relations between genetic markers and the presence of a variety of cardiovascular phenotypes, such as abnormal cholesterol levels, hypertension, and other risk factors.[143] This research typically involves the use of anonymous markers every 5–10 centimorgans (cM) along the human chromosome, and includes 300 or more genetic tests for each individual. Positive results are then used to perform fine mapping and further genetic testing in an effort to identify genes that are responsible for the different phenotypes.

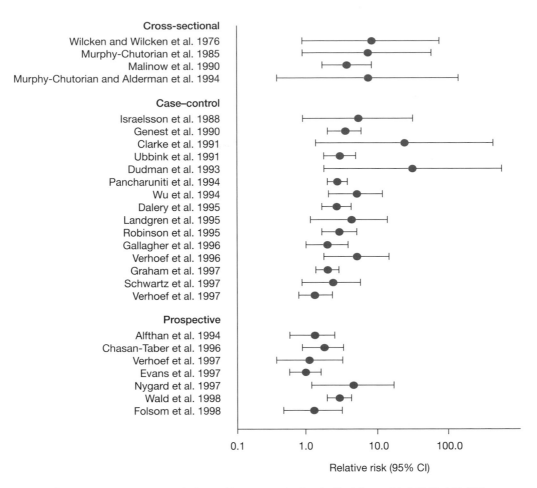

Figure 2.22   Coronary heart disease and elevated homocysteine levels (Arch Intern Med 2000; 160:422)

Subclinical cardiovascular disease

Atherosclerosis develops and progresses at different rates in the vasculature. The aorta is the region most likely to develop early atherosclerosis, and fatty streaks are common during adolescence, as noted in earlier studies of war victims and recent investigations from the Premature Development of Atherosclerosis in Youth (PDAY) study.[144,145] Early adulthood often leads to fibrous plaque formation and calcification of the aorta, especially in the arch and distally near the bifurcation into the iliac arteries. This calcification is equally common in men and women at age 50, and the severity of the calcification on radiographs has

been shown to predict the occurrence of cardio-vascular disease events over and above traditional risk factors.[146]

Modern techniques can provide assessment of sub-clinical vascular disease in smaller arteries. The carotid arteries have been studied with B-mode ultrasound, and more recently with magnetic resonance imaging (MRI). Greater carotid stenosis in older persons has correlated with the burden of smoking, blood pressure, and cholesterol during the adult years,[147] and increased intima medial thickening of the carotid arteries in the elderly has been shown to be predictive of the subsequent development of cardiovascular disease.[148] The usefulness of this testing is limited by the need for accurate measurements and trained sonographers.

Over the past few years scanning of the coronary arteries for the presence of calcification has been proposed as a useful strategy to identify persons at high risk for the development of clinical cardiovascular disease.[149,150] Data are limited at present, but large investigations such as the Multi-Ethnic Study of Atherosclerosis should help to provide a critical assessment of the added usefulness of these newer screening modalities in non-selected population cohorts.[151]

Peripheral arterial disease

Peripheral arterial disease (PAD) in the lower limbs leads to partial blockage of the large arteries, vascular bruits, and diminution of arterial blood flow. The disease may be recognized by eliciting a history of intermittent claudication, and diabetes mellitus, cigarette smoking, and blood pressure level have been especially important determinants.[152,153] Newer diagnostic methods include measurement of the blood pressure in the arm and at the ankle with a Doppler device, using an ankle–brachial index (ABI) of < 0.90 as diagnostic of PAD.[154] The PAD Awareness, Risk, and Treatment: New Resources for Survival (PARTNERS) study surveyed physicians' offices and included more than 6900 patients over 70 or 50–69 years with a smoking or diabetes history. In 2001, this group reported the prevalence of PAD and CVD as 13% PAD only, 16% PAD and CVD, 24% CVD only, and 47% no PAD or CVD.[155] Classic claudication was present in only 11% of those affected by PAD in this study, and it was recommended that ABI determinations should be performed more often on high-risk patients.

Cerebrovascular disease

The topic of cerebrovascular disease is quite large, and its mention here is just to note the similarities and differences for atherosclerotic risk factors that underlie CVD versus cerebrovascular disease. Approximately 60% of strokes in the USA are thrombotic, and age, previous vascular disease, blood pressure, cigarette smoking, and diabetes are probably the most important determinants of risk for cerebrovascular disease, noting that lipids have not been considered to play an important role.[156] Hemorrhagic cerebrovascular disease is particularly related to vascular malformations, bleeding tendencies, age, trauma, and blood pressure. On the other hand, atrial fibrillation, mitral valve disease, and diseases of the heart and aortic arch appear to increase the risk of thrombotic cerebrovascular disease.[157,158]

Renal disease

Proteinuria was noted in the 1980s to be related to an increased risk of CVD,[159] and more recent research has focused on microalbuminuria (> 30 mg/g urinary creatinine) as a marker of renal impairment in persons with hypertension or diabetes mellitus. Modest decrements in estimated glomerular filtration rate and the presence of microalbuminuria have been shown to be important predictors of a decline in renal function and in the development of CVD.[160,161] Assessment of albumin excretion is now recommended at regular intervals for persons with diabetes mellitus or hypertension.

Long-term treatment of hypertension and type 2 diabetes mellitus has led to extension of life, but chronic kidney failure may occur. These two diseases are now the most common diagnoses for persons who need to start chronic dialysis.[162] Once renal failure has developed the prognosis is quite poor. Atherosclerosis appears to enter an accelerated phase, and death from CVD or from cardiac failure is quite common. New guidelines for the aggressive treatment of blood pressure and lipids have been developed for these patients, and an American Heart Association group of experts has recommended that chronic kidney failure itself be considered a heart disease risk factor.[163]

Multivariable CHD risk estimation

Risk for cardiovascular disease events can be estimated with multivariable prediction equations using a score sheet, pocket calculator, or computer. The variables age, systolic blood pressure, smoking, cholesterol, HDL cholesterol, and diabetes mellitus are commonly used to estimate risk for initial CHD events, employing separate equations for men and women. This approach has been validated in the US across several observational studies.[164,165] Estimation of CHD risk is generally valid for middle-class, white populations in North America and Europe, where risk factors and heart disease rates approximate the experience of studies such as Framingham that provided the estimates. Overestimates of CHD risk may be obtained in other locales, especially where CHD risk is low, such as in Spain or Hawaii.[165,166]

Using a slightly different set of variables, equations that estimate CHD risk have been developed in Germany to predict initial CHD events in men.[167] European investigators from several countries have also developed algorithms to estimate the risk of CHD disease mortality.[168] For persons with type 2 diabetes mellitus, British investigators have developed a CHD risk estimating equation, and this approach includes factoring in levels of glycosylated hemoglobin and the duration of diabetes mellitus.[169]

Estimating CHD risk can help clinicians match the estimated risk of CHD with the aggressiveness of risk factor management. Separate risk estimating equations have been developed for the prediction of stroke, intermittent claudication, and the individual components of coronary heart disease.[152,156,170]

Estimation of CHD risk with multivariable equations is a dynamic process, and new information is constantly being evaluated as it may change the approach. It is important to assess and whether it improves the overall prediction of CHD within a population. Accuracy and precision of the new measurement, standardization of the technique, low correlation with existing predictive variables, validation in other observational studies, and biological relevance are examples of features that need to be considered prior to the inclusion of newer variables in risk-estimating approaches.[171,172]

References

1. American Heart Association. Heart disease and stroke statistics – 2003 Update. Dallas, TX: American Heart Association, 2002.
2. Guidry UC, Evans JC, Larson MG et al. Temporal trends in event rates after Q-wave myocardial infarction: the Framingham Heart Study. Circulation 1999; 100:2054–2059.
3. McGovern PG, Pankow JS, Shahar E et al. Recent trends in acute coronary heart disease – mortality, morbidity, medical care, and risk factors. The Minnesota Heart Survey Investigators. N Engl J Med 1996; 334:884–890.
4. Rosamond WD, Chambless LE, Folsom AR et al. Trends in the incidence of myocardial infarction and in mortality due to coronary heart disease, 1987 to 1994. N Engl J Med 1998; 339:861–867.
5. Lloyd-Jones DM, Larson MG, Beiser A et al. Lifetime risk of developing coronary heart disease. Lancet 1999; 353:89–92.
6. Lerner DJ, Kannel WB. Patterns of coronary heart disease morbidity and mortality in the sexes: a 26-year follow-up of the Framingham population. Am Heart J 1986; 111:383–390.
7. Naghavi M, Libby P, Falk E et al. From vulnerable plaque to vulnerable patient: a call for new definitions and risk assessment strategies: Part II. Circulation 2003; 108:1772–1778.
8. Maron BJ. Sudden death in young athletes. N Engl J Med 2003; 349:1064–1075.
9. Maron BJ. Contemporary considerations for risk stratification, sudden death and prevention in hypertrophic cardiomyopathy. Heart 2003; 89:977–978.
10. Priori SG, Aliot E, Blomstrom-Lundqvist C et al. Update of the guidelines on sudden cardiac death of the European Society of Cardiology. Eur Heart J 2003; 24:13–15.
11. Maron BJ, Shirani J, Poliac LC et al. Sudden death in young competitive athletes: clinical, demographic, and pathological profiles. J Am Med Assoc 1996; 276:199–204.
12. Maron BJ. Hypertrophic cardiomyopathy: a systematic review. J Am Med Assoc 2002; 287:1308–1320.
13. Wilson PW, Garrison RJ, Castelli WP. Postmenopausal estrogen use, cigarette smoking, and cardiovascular morbidity in women over 50. The Framingham Study. N Engl J Med 1985; 313:1038–1043.
14. Stampfer MJ, Willett WC, Colditz GA et al. A prospective study of postmenopausal estrogen therapy and coronary heart disease. N Engl J Med 1985; 313:1044–1049.
15. Bush TL, Cowan LD, Barrett-Connor EL et al. Estrogen use and all-cause mortality. J Am Med Assoc 1983; 249:903–906.
16. Grady D, Rubin SM, Petitti DB et al. Hormone therapy to prevent disease and prolong life in postmenopausal women. Ann Intern Med 1992; 117:1016–1037.
17. Hulley S, Grady D, Bush T et al. Randomized trial of estrogen plus progestin for secondary prevention of coronary heart disease in postmenopausal women. Heart and Estrogen/progestin Replacement Study (HERS) Research Group. J Am Med Assoc 1998; 280:605–613.
18. Grodstein F, Stampfer MJ, Manson JE et al. Postmenopausal estrogen and progestin use and the risk of cardiovascular disease. N Engl J Med 1996; 335:453–461.
19. Rossouw JE, Anderson GL, Prentice RL et al. Risks and benefits of estrogen plus progestin in healthy post-

menopausal women: principal results from the Women's Health Initiative randomized controlled trial. J Am Med Assoc 2002; 288:321–333.

20. Martin MJ, Hulley SB. Serum cholesterol, blood pressure, and mortality: implications from a cohort of 361 662 men. Lancet 1986; 2:933–936.

21. Gotto AM Jr, LaRosa JC, Hunninghake D et al. The cholesterol facts: a summary of the evidence relating dietary fats, serum cholesterol, and coronary heart disease: a joint statement by the American Heart Association and the National Heart, Lung and Blood Institute. Circulation 1990; 81:1721–1733.

22. Abbott RD, Wilson PW, Kannel WB et al. High density lipoprotein cholesterol, total cholesterol screening, and myocardial infarction. The Framingham Study. Arteriosclerosis 1988; 8:207–211.

23. Austin MA, King MC, Vranizan KM et al. Atherogenic lipoprotein phenotype. A proposed genetic marker for coronary heart disease risk. Circulation 1990; 82:495–506.

24. Otvos JD, Jeyarajah EJ, Bennett DW et al. Development of a proton nuclear magnetic resonance spectroscopic method for determining plasma lipoprotein concentrations and subspecies distributions from a single, rapid measurement. Clin Chem 1992; 38:1632–1638.

25. Reaven GM, Abbasi F, Bernhart S et al. Insulin resistance, dietary cholesterol, and cholesterol concentration in postmenopausal women. Metabolism 2001; 50:594–597.

26. Campos H, McNamara JR, Wilson PWF et al. Differences in low density lipoprotein subfractions and apolipoproteins in premenopausal and postmenopausal women. J Clin Endocrinol Metab 1988; 67:30–35.

27. Gardner CD, Fortmann SP, Krauss RM. Association of small low-density lipoprotein particles with the incidence of coronary artery disease in men and women. J Am Med Assoc 1996; 276:875–881.

28. Lamarche B, St Pierre AC, Ruel IL et al. A prospective, population-based study of low density lipoprotein particle size as a risk factor for ischemic heart disease in men. Can J Cardiol 2001; 17:859–865.

29. Marcovina SM, Albers JJ, Scanu AM et al. Use of a reference material proposed by the International Federation of Clinical Chemistry and Laboratory Medicine to evaluate analytical methods for the determination of plasma lipoprotein(a). Clin Chem 2000; 46:1956–1967.

30. Marcovina SM, Hegele RA, Koschinsky ML. Lipoprotein(a) and coronary heart disease risk. Curr Cardiol Rep 1999; 1:105–111.

31. Gidding SS, Liu K, Bild DE et al. Prevalence and identification of abnormal lipoprotein levels in a biracial population aged 23 to 35 years (the CARDIA study). The Coronary Artery Risk Development in Young Adults Study. Am J Cardiol 1996; 78:304–308.

32. Schaefer EJ, Lamon-Fava S, Jenner JL et al. Lipoprotein(a) levels and risk of coronary heart disease in men: the Lipid Research Clinics Coronary Primary Prevention Trial. J Am Med Assoc 1994; 271:999–1003.

33. Scanu AM. Lp(a) lipoprotein – coping with heterogeneity. N Engl J Med 2003; 349:2089–2090.

34. Scanu AM. Lipoprotein(a) and the atherothrombotic process: mechanistic insights and clinical implications. Curr Atheroscler Rep 2003; 5:106–113.

35. Multiple Risk Factor Intervention Trial Research Group. MRFIT: risk factor changes and mortality results. J Am Med Assoc 1982; 248:1465–1477.

36. Lipid Research Clinics Program. The Lipid Research Clinics Coronary Primary Prevention Trial results, I: reduction in incidence of coronary heart disease. J Am Med Assoc 1984; 251:351–364.

37. Lipid Research Clinics Program. The Lipid Research Clinics Coronary Primary Prevention Trial results, II. The relationship of reduction in incidence of CHD and cholesterol lowering. J Am Med Assoc 1984; 251:365–374.

38. Canner PL, Berge KG, Wenger NK. Fifteen year mortality in Coronary Drug Project patients: long-term benefit with niacin. J Am Coll Cardiol 1986; 8:1245–1255.

39. Blankenhorn DH, Nessim SA, Johnson RL et al. Beneficial effects of combined colestipol–niacin therapy on coronary atherosclerosis and coronary venous bypass grafts. J Am Med Assoc 1987; 257:3233–3240.

40. Brown BG, Zhao XQ, Chait A et al. Simvastatin and niacin, antioxidant vitamins, or the combination for the prevention of coronary disease. N Engl J Med 2001; 345:1583–1592.

41. Shepherd J, Cobbe SM, Ford I et al. Prevention of coronary heart disease with pravastatin in men with hypercholesterolemia. West of Scotland Coronary Prevention Study Group. N Engl J Med 1995; 333:1301–1307.

42. Frick MH, Elo O, Haapa K et al. Helsinki Heart Study: primary-prevention trial with gemfibrozil in middle-aged men with dyslipidemia. Safety of treatment, changes in risk factors, and incidence of coronary heart disease. N Engl J Med 1987; 317:1237–1245.

43. The 4S Group. Randomised trial of cholesterol lowering in 4444 patients with coronary heart disease: the Scandinavian Simvastatin Survival Study (4S). Lancet 1994; 344:1383–1389.

44. Kreger BE, Kannel WB, Cupples LA. Electrocardiographic precursors of sudden unexpected death: The Framingham Study. Circulation 1987; 75(Suppl 2):22–24.

45. Rubins HB, Robins SJ, Collins D et al. Gemfibrozil for the secondary prevention of coronary heart disease in men with low levels of high-density lipoprotein cholesterol. Veterans Affairs High-Density Lipoprotein Cholesterol Intervention Trial Study Group. N Engl J Med 1999; 341:410–418.

46. Sever PS, Dahlof B, Poulter NR et al. Prevention of coronary and stroke events with atorvastatin in hypertensive patients who have average or lower-than-average cholesterol concentrations, in the Anglo-Scandinavian Cardiac Outcomes Trial – Lipid Lowering Arm (ASCOT-LLA): a multicentre randomised controlled trial. Lancet 2003; 361:1149–1158.

47. MRC/BHF Heart Protection Study of cholesterol lowering with simvastatin in 20 536 high-risk individuals: a randomised placebo-controlled trial. Lancet 2002; 360:7–22.

48. Shepherd J, Blauw GJ, Murphy MB et al. Pravastatin in elderly individuals at risk of vascular disease (PROSPER): a randomised controlled trial. Lancet 2002; 360:1623–1630.

49. Hyman DJ, Pavlik VN. Characteristics of patients with uncontrolled hypertension in the United States. N Engl J Med 2001; 345:479–486.

50. Basile JN. The importance of systolic blood pressure control and cardiovascular disease prevention. Curr Treat Options Cardiovasc Med 2003; 5:271–277.

51. Kannel WB. Elevated systolic blood pressure as a cardiovascular risk factor. Am J Cardiol 2000; 85:251–255.

52. Franklin SS, Larson MG, Khan SA et al. Does the relation of blood pressure to coronary heart disease risk change with aging? The Framingham Heart Study. Circulation 2001; 103:1245–1249.

53. Vasan RS, Larson MG, Leip EP et al. Impact of high-normal blood pressure on the risk of cardiovascular disease. N Engl J Med 2001; 345:1291–1297.

54. Lewington S, Clarke R, Qizilbash N et al. Age-specific relevance of usual blood pressure to vascular mortality: a meta-analysis of individual data for one million adults in 61 prospective studies. Lancet 2002; 360:1903–1913.

55. Pahor M, Psaty BM, Alderman MH et al. Therapeutic benefits of ACE inhibitors and other antihypertensive drugs in patients with type 2 diabetes. Diabetes Care 2000; 23:888–892.

56. Sacks FM, Svetkey LP, Vollmer WM et al. Effects on blood pressure of reduced dietary sodium and the Dietary Approaches to Stop Hypertension (DASH) diet. DASH–Sodium Collaborative Research Group. N Engl J Med 2001; 344:3–10.

57. Furberg CD, Psaty BM, Meyer JV. Nifedipine. Dose-related increase in mortality in patients with coronary heart disease. Circulation 1995; 92:1326–1331.

58. Systolic Hypertension in the Elderly Program Cooperative Research Group. Prevention of stroke by antihypertensive drug treatment in older persons with isolated systolic hypertension: final results of the Systolic Hypertension in the Elderly Program (SHEP). J Am Med Assoc 1991; 265:3255–3264.

59. Staessen JA, Fagard R, Thijs L et al. Randomised double-blind comparison of placebo and active treatment for older patients with isolated systolic hypertension. The Systolic Hypertension in Europe (Syst-Eur) Trial Investigators. Lancet 1997; 350:757–764.

60. Wang JG, Staessen JA, Gong L et al. Chinese trial on isolated systolic hypertension in the elderly. Systolic Hypertension in China (Syst-China) Collaborative Group. Arch Intern Med 2000; 160:211–220.

61. ALLHAT officers and coordinators for the ALLHAT Collaborative Research Group. Major outcomes in high-risk hypertensive patients randomized to angiotensin-converting enzyme inhibitor or calcium channel blocker vs diuretic: the Antihypertensive and Lipid-Lowering Treatment to Prevent Heart Attack Trial (ALLHAT). J Am Med Assoc 2002; 288:2981–2997.

62. Major cardiovascular events in hypertensive patients randomized to doxazosin vs chlorthalidone: the antihypertensive and lipid-lowering treatment to prevent heart attack trial (ALLHAT). ALLHAT Collaborative Research Group. J Am Med Assoc 2000; 283:1967–1975.

63. Keys A, Menotti A, Aravanis C. The Seven Countries Study: 2289 deaths in 15 years. Prev Med 1984;13:141–154.

64. Keys A, Karvonen JM, Punsar S. HDL serum cholesterol and 24-year mortality of men in Finland. Int J Epidemiol 1984; 13:428–435.

65. Verschuren WM, Jacobs DR, Bloemberg BP et al. Serum total cholesterol and long-term coronary heart disease mortality in different cultures. Twenty-five-year follow-up of the Seven Countries Study. J Am Med Assoc 1995; 274:131–136.

66. Jousilahti P, Vartiainen E, Pekkanen J et al. Serum cholesterol distribution and coronary heart disease risk: observations and predictions among middle-aged population in eastern Finland. Circulation 1998; 97:1087–1094.

67. Lichtenstein AH, Kennedy E, Barrier P et al. Dietary fat consumption and health. Nutr Rev 1998; 56:S3–19.

68. Schaefer EJ, Lamon-Fava S, Ausman LM et al. Individual variability in lipoprotein cholesterol response to National Cholesterol Education Program Step 2 diets. Am J Clin Nutr 1997; 65:823–830.

69. Krauss RM, Eckel RH, Howard B et al. AHA Dietary Guidelines: revision 2000: a statement for healthcare professionals from the Nutrition Committee of the American Heart Association. Circulation 2000; 102:2284–2299.

70. Pearson TA, Laurora I, Chu H et al. The lipid treatment assessment project (L-TAP): a multicenter survey to evaluate the percentages of dyslipidemic patients receiving lipid-lowering therapy and achieving low-density lipoprotein cholesterol goals. Arch Intern Med 2000; 160:459–467.

71. Steinberg D, Parthasarathy S, Carew TE et al. Beyond cholesterol: modifications of low-density lipoproteins that increase its atherogenicity. N Engl J Med 1989; 320:915–924.

72. Rimm EB, Stampfer MJ, Ascherio A et al. Vitamin E consumption and the risk of coronary heart disease in men. N Engl J Med 1993; 328:1450–1456.

73. Stampfer MJ, Hennekens CH, Manson JE et al. Vitamin E consumption and risk of coronary heart disease in women. N Engl J Med 1993; 328:1444–1449.

74. Yusuf S, Dagenais G, Pogue J et al. Vitamin E supplementation and cardiovascular events in high-risk patients. The Heart Outcomes Prevention Evaluation Study Investigators. N Engl J Med 2000; 342:154–160.

75. MRC/BHF Heart Protection Study of antioxidant vitamin supplementation in 20 536 high-risk individuals: a ran-

domised placebo-controlled trial. Lancet 2002; 360:23–33.

76. Kannel WB, Ellison RC. Alcohol and coronary heart disease: the evidence for a protective effect. Clin Chim Acta 1996; 246:59–76.

77. Klatsky AL. Alcohol, coronary disease, and hypertension. Annu Rev Med 1996; 47:149–160.

78. Shaper AG. Alcohol and coronary heart disease. Eur Heart J 1995; 16:1760–1764.

79. Rimm EB, Willett WC, Hu FB et al. Folate and vitamin B6 from diet and supplements in relation to risk of coronary heart disease among women. J Am Med Assoc 1998; 279:359–364.

80. Ellison RC. Cheers! Epidemiology 1990; 1:337–339.

81. Boffetta P, Garfinkel L. Alcohol drinking and mortality among men enrolled in an American Cancer Society Prospective Study. Epidemiology 1990; 1:342–348.

82. Winkleby MA, Robinson TN, Sundquist J et al. Ethnic variation in cardiovascular disease risk factors among children and young adults: findings from the Third National Health and Nutrition Examination Survey, 1988–1994. J Am Med Assoc 1999; 281:1006–1013.

83. Castelli WP, Garrison RJ, Dawber TR et al. The filter cigarette and coronary heart disease: the Framingham Study. Lancet 1981; 2:109–113.

84. Palmer JR, Rosenberg L, Shapiro S. 'Low yield' cigarettes and the risk of nonfatal myocardial infarction in women. N Engl J Med 1989; 320:1569–1573.

85. Ockene JK, Kuller LH, Svendsen KH et al. The relationship of smoking cessation to coronary heart disease and lung cancer in the Multiple Risk Factor Intervention Trial (MRFIT). Am J Public Health 1990; 80:954–958.

86. Steenland K. Passive smoking and the risk of heart disease. J Am Med Assoc 1992; 267:94–99.

87. Howard G Burke GL Szklo M et al. Active and passive smoking are associated with increased carotid wall thickness. The Atherosclerosis Risk in Communities Study. Arch Intern Med 1994; 154:1277–1282.

88. Paffenbarger RS Jr, Hyde RT, Wing AL et al. Physical activity, all-cause mortality, and longevity of college alumni. N Engl J Med 1986; 314:605–613.

89. Paffenbarger RS Jr, Hyde RT, Wing AL et al. The association of changes in physical-activity level and other lifestyle characteristics with mortality among men. N Engl J Med 1993; 328:538–545.

90. Mittleman MA, Maclure M, Tofler GH et al. Triggering of acute myocardial infarction by heavy physical exertion. Protection against triggering by regular exertion. Determinants of Myocardial Infarction Onset Study Investigators. N Engl J Med 1993; 329:1677–1683.

91. Mittleman MA, Siscovick DS. Physical exertion as a trigger of myocardial infarction and sudden cardiac death. Cardiol Clin 1996; 14:263–270.

92. Thompson PD, Buchner D, Pina IL et al. Exercise and physical activity in the prevention and treatment of atherosclerotic cardiovascular disease: a statement from the council on clinical cardiology (subcommittee on exercise, rehabilitation, and prevention) and the council on nutrition, physical activity, and metabolism (subcommittee on physical activity). Arterioscler Thromb Vasc Biol 2003; 23:E42–E49.

93. Thompson PD, Lim V. Physical activity in the prevention of atherosclerotic coronary heart disease. Curr Treat Options Cardiovasc Med 2003; 5:279–285.

94. Thompson PD. Exercise and physical activity in the prevention and treatment of atherosclerotic cardiovascular disease. Arterioscler Thromb Vasc Biol 2003; 23:1319–1321.

95. Blair SN, Kampert JB, Kohl HW III et al. Influences of cardiorespiratory fitness and other precursors on cardiovascular disease and all-cause mortality in men and women. J Am Med Assoc 1996; 276:205–210.

96. Expert Panel. Clinical guidelines on the identification, evaluation, and treatment of overweight and obesity in adults. [1]. Bethesda, MD: Public Health Service, NIH, NHLBI. 1998.

97. Mokdad AH, Serdula MK, Dietz WH et al. The spread of the obesity epidemic in the United States, 1991–1998. J Am Med Assoc 1999; 282:1519–1522.

98. Wilson PW, Kannel WB, Silbershatz H et al. Clustering of metabolic factors and coronary heart disease. Arch Intern Med 1999; 159:1104–1109.

99. Wilson PW, D'Agostino RB, Sullivan L et al. Overweight and obesity as determinants of cardiovascular risk: the Framingham experience. Arch Intern Med 2002; 162:1867–1872.

100. Harris MI, Flegal KM, Cowie CC et al. Prevalence of diabetes, impaired fasting glucose, and impaired glucose tolerance in US adults. The Third National Health and Nutrition Examination Survey, 1988–1994. Diabetes Care 1998; 21:518–524.

101. Wilson PW. Diabetes mellitus and coronary heart disease. Am J Kidney Dis 1998; 32:S89–100.

102. Haffner SM, Lehto S, Ronnemaa T et al. Mortality from coronary heart disease in subjects with type 2 diabetes and in nondiabetic subjects with and without prior myocardial infarction. N Engl J Med 1998; 339:229–234.

103. Executive Summary of The Third Report of the National Cholesterol Education Program (NCEP) Expert Panel on Detection, Evaluation, and Treatment of High Blood Cholesterol in Adults (Adult Treatment Panel III). J Am Med Assoc 2001; 285:2486–2497.

104. Haffner SM. Management of dyslipidemia in adults with diabetes. Diabetes Care 1998; 21:160–178.

105. Sowers JR, Epstein M, Frohlich ED. Diabetes, hypertension, and cardiovascular disease: an update. Hypertension 2001; 37:1053–1059.

106. Gaede P, Vedel P, Larsen N et al. Multifactorial intervention and cardiovascular disease in patients with type 2 diabetes. N Engl J Med 2003; 348:383–393.

107. Diabetes Control and Complications Trial Research Group. The effect of intensive treatment of diabetes on the

development and progression of long-term complications in insulin-dependent diabetes mellitus. The Diabetes Control and Complications Trial Research Group. N Engl J Med 1993; 329:977–986.

108. Singer DE, Nathan DM, Anderson KM et al. Association of HbA1c with prevalent cardiovascular disease in the original cohort of the Framingham Heart Study. Diabetes 1992; 41:202–208.

109. Kuusisto J, Mykkanen L, Pyorala K et al. NIDDM and its metabolic control predict coronary heart disease in elderly subjects. Diabetes 1994; 43:960–967.

110. Turner RC. The UK Prospective Diabetes Study. A review. Diabetes Care 1998; 21(Suppl 3):C35-C38.

111. Turner RC, Cull CA, Frighi V et al. Glycemic control with diet, sulfonylurea, metformin, or insulin in patients with type 2 diabetes mellitus: progressive requirement for multiple therapies (UKPDS 49). UK Prospective Diabetes Study (UKPDS) Group. J Am Med Assoc 1999; 281:2005–2012.

112. Ford ES, Giles WH, Dietz WH. Prevalence of the metabolic syndrome among US adults: findings from the third National Health and Nutrition Examination Survey. J Am Med Assoc 2002; 287:356–359.

113. Isomaa B, Almgren P, Tuomi T et al. Cardiovascular morbidity and mortality associated with the metabolic syndrome. Diabetes Care 2001; 24:683–689.

114. Lakka HM, Laaksonen DE, Lakka TA et al. The metabolic syndrome and total and cardiovascular disease mortality in middle-aged men. J Am Med Assoc 2002; 288:2709–2716.

115. Sattar N, Gaw A, Scherbakova O et al. Metabolic syndrome with and without C-reactive protein as a predictor of coronary heart disease and diabetes in the West of Scotland Coronary Prevention Study. Circulation 2003; 108:414–419.

116. Danesh J, Collins R, Appleby P et al. Association of fibrinogen, C-reactive protein, albumin, or leukocyte count with coronary heart disease: meta-analyses of prospective studies. J Am Med Assoc 1998; 279:1477–1482.

117. Thompson SG, Kienast J, Pyke SD et al. Hemostatic factors and the risk of myocardial infarction or sudden death in patients with angina pectoris. European Concerted Action on Thrombosis and Disabilities Angina Pectoris Study Group. N Engl J Med 1995; 332:635–641.

118. Ridker PM, Hennekens CH, Buring JE et al. C-reactive protein and other markers of inflammation in the prediction of cardiovascular disease in women. N Engl J Med 2000; 342:836–843.

119. Ridker PM, Cushman M, Stampfer MJ et al. Plasma concentration of C-reactive protein and risk of developing peripheral vascular disease. Circulation 1998; 97:425–428.

120. Ridker PM, Glynn RJ, Hennekens CH. C-reactive protein adds to the predictive value of total and HDL cholesterol in determining risk of first myocardial infarction. Circulation 1998; 97:2007–2011.

121. Ridker PM, Rifai N, Rose L et al. Comparison of C-reactive protein and low-density lipoprotein cholesterol levels in the prediction of first cardiovascular events. N Engl J Med 2002; 347:1557–1565.

122. Rost NS, Wolf PA, Kase CS et al. Plasma concentration of C-reactive protein and risk of ischemic stroke and transient ischemic attack: the Framingham Study. Stroke 2001; 32:2575–2579.

123. Pearson TA, Mensah GA, Alexander RW et al. Markers of inflammation and cardiovascular disease: application to clinical and public health practice: a statement for healthcare professionals from the Centers for Disease Control and Prevention and the American Heart Association. Circulation 2003; 107:499–511.

124. Nathan DM, Singer DE, Hurxthal K et al. The clinical information value of the glycosylated hemoglobin assay. N Engl J Med 1984; 310:341–346.

125. Christen WG, Ajani UA, Glynn RJ et al. Blood levels of homocysteine and increased risks of cardiovascular disease: causal or casual? Arch Intern Med 2000; 160:422–434.

126. Homocysteine Studies Collaboration. Homocysteine and risk of ischemic heart disease and stroke: a meta-analysis. J Am Med Assoc 2002; 288:2015–2022.

127. Jacques PF, Selhub J, Bostom AG et al. The effect of folic acid fortification on plasma folate and total homocysteine concentrations. N Engl J Med 1999; 340:1449–1454.

128. Bostom AG, Gohh RY, Liaugaudas G et al. Prevalence of mild fasting hyperhomocysteinemia in renal transplant versus coronary artery disease patients after fortification of cereal grain flour with folic acid. Atherosclerosis 1999; 145:221–224.

129. Bostom AG, Selhub J, Jacques PF et al. Power shortage: clinical trials testing the 'homocysteine hypothesis' against a background of folic acid-fortified cereal grain flour. Ann Intern Med 2001; 135:133–137.

130. Nabel EG. Cardiovascular disease. N Engl J Med 2003; 349:60–72.

131. Breslow JL. Genetic markers for coronary heart disease. Clin Cardiol 2001; 24:2–7.

132. Goldstein JL, Hazzard WR, Schrott HG et al. Hyperlipidemia in coronary heart disease I. Lipid levels in 500 survivors of myocardial infarction. J Clin Invest 1973; 52:1533–1543.

133. Dallongeville J, Lussier-Cacan S, Davignon J. Modulation of plasma triglyceride levels by apoE phenotype: a meta-analysis. J Lipid Res 1992; 33:447–454.

134. Wilson PW, Myers RH, Larson MG et al. Apolipoprotein E alleles, dyslipidemia, and coronary heart disease. The Framingham Offspring Study. J Am Med Assoc 1994; 272:1666–1671.

135. Corder EH, Saunders AM, Strittmatter WJ et al. Gene dose of apolipoprotein E type 4 allele and the risk of Alzheimer's disease on late onset families. Science 1993; 261:921–923.

136. Luc G, Bard J-M, Arveiler D et al. Impact of apolipoprotein E polymorphism on lipoproteins and risk of myocar-

dial infarction: the ECTIM Study. Arterioscler Thromb 1994; 14:1412–1419.

137. Lopez-Miranda J, Ordovas JM, Mata P et al. Effect of apolipoprotein E phenotype on diet-induced lowering of plasma low density lipoprotein cholesterol. J Lipid Res 1994; 35:1965–1975.

138. Mooser V, Helbecque N, Miklossy J et al. Interactions between apolipoprotein E and apolipoprotein(a) in patients with late-onset Alzheimer disease. Ann Intern Med 2000; 132:533–537.

139. Cambien F, Poirier O, Lecer L et al. Deletion polymorphism in the gene for angiotensin-converting enzyme is a potent risk factor for myocardial infarction. Nature 1993; 359:641–644.

140. Zhong S, Sharp DS, Grove JS et al. Increased coronary heart disease in Japanese-American men with mutation in the cholesteryl ester transfer protein gene despite increased HDL levels. J Clin Invest 1996; 97:2917–2923.

141. Despres JP, Couillard C, Gagnon J et al. Race, visceral adipose tissue, plasma lipids, and lipoprotein lipase activity in men and women: the Health, Risk Factors, Exercise Training, and Genetics (HERITAGE) family study. Arterioscler Thromb Vasc Biol 2000; 20:1932–1938.

142. Klerk M, Verhoef P, Clarke R et al. MTHFR 677C—>T polymorphism and risk of coronary heart disease: a meta-analysis. J Am Med Assoc 2002; 288:2023–2031.

143. Shearman AM, Ordovas JM, Cupples LA et al. Evidence for a gene influencing the TG/HDL-C ratio on chromosome 7q32.3-qter: a genome-wide scan in the Framingham Study. Hum Mol Genet 2000; 9:1315–1320.

144. Relationship of atherosclerosis in young men to serum lipoprotein cholesterol concentrations and smoking. A preliminary report from the Pathobiological Determinants of Atherosclerosis in Youth (PDAY) Research Group. J Am Med Assoc 1990; 264:3018–3024.

145. McGill HC, McMahan CA, Herderick EE et al. Effects of coronary heart disease risk factors on atherosclerosis of selected regions of the aorta and right coronary artery. PDAY Research Group. Pathobiological Determinants of Atherosclerosis in Youth. Arterioscler Thromb Vasc Biol 2000; 20:836–845.

146. Wilson PW, Kauppila LI, O'Donnell CJ et al. Abdominal aortic calcific deposits are an important predictor of vascular morbidity and mortality. Circulation 2001; 103:1529–1534.

147. Wilson PWF, Hoeg JM, D'Agostino RB et al. Cumulative effects of high cholesterol levels, high blood pressure, and cigarette smoking on carotid stenosis. N Engl J Med 1997; 337:516–522.

148. O'Leary DH, Polak JF, Kronmal RA et al. Carotid-artery intima and media thickness as a risk factor for myocardial infarction and stroke in older adults. Cardiovascular Health Study Collaborative Research Group. N Engl J Med 1999; 340:14–22.

149. Raggi P, Callister TQ, Cooil B et al. Identification of patients at increased risk of first unheralded acute myocar-

dial infarction by electron-beam computed tomography. Circulation 2000; 101:850–855.

150. Raggi P, Cooil B, Callister TQ. Use of electron beam tomography data to develop models for prediction of hard coronary events. Am Heart J 2001; 141:375–382.

151. Bild DE, Bluemke DA, Burke GL et al. Multi-ethnic study of atherosclerosis: objectives and design. Am J Epidemiol 2002; 156:871-881.

152. Murabito JM, D'Agostino RB, Silbershatz H et al. Intermittent claudication: a risk profile from the Framingham Heart Study. Circulation 1997; 96:44–49.

153. Murabito JM, Evans JC, Nieto K et al. Prevalence and clinical correlates of peripheral arterial disease in the Framingham Offspring Study. Am Heart J 2002; 143:961–965.

154. Criqui MH, Langer RD, Fronek A et al. Mortality over a period of 10 years in patients with peripheral arterial disease. N Engl J Med 1992; 326:381–386.

155. Hirsch AT, Criqui MH, Treat-Jacobson D et al. Peripheral arterial disease detection, awareness, and treatment in primary care. J Am Med Assoc 2001; 286:1317–1324.

156. Wolf PA, D'Agostino RB, Belanger AJ et al. Probability of stroke: a risk profile from the Framingham Study. Stroke 1991; 3:312–318.

157. Benjamin EJ, Plehn JF, D'Agostino RB et al. Mitral annular calcification and the risk of stroke in an elderly cohort. N Engl J Med 1992; 327:374–379.

158. Benjamin EJ, Wolf PA, D'Agostino RB et al. Impact of atrial fibrillation on the risk of death: the Framingham Heart Study. Circulation 1998; 98:946–952.

159. Kannel WB, Stampfer MJ, Castelli WP et al. The prognostic significance of proteinuria: the Framingham Study. Am Heart J 1984; 108:1347–1352.

160. Culleton BF, Larson MG, Wilson PW et al. Cardiovascular disease and mortality in a community-based cohort with mild renal insufficiency. Kidney Int 1999; 56:2214–2219.

161. Tight blood pressure control and risk of macrovascular and microvascular complications in type 2 diabetes: UKPDS 38. UK Prospective Diabetes Study Group. Br Med J 1998; 317:703–713.

162. Levey AS, Beto JA, Coronado BE et al. Controlling the epidemic of cardiovascular disease in chronic renal disease: what do we know? What do we need to learn? Where do we go from here? Am J Kidney Dis 1998; 32:853–906.

163. Szabo A, Sallay P, Tausz I. The serum hormone levels, phosphate complex concentrations and enzyme activities in haemodialysed and kidney-transplanted children. Acta Paediatr Hung 1990; 30:73–88.

164. Wilson PW, D'Agostino RB, Levy D et al. Prediction of coronary heart disease using risk factor categories. Circulation 1998; 97:1837–1847.

165. D'Agostino RB Sr, Grundy S, Sullivan LM et al. Validation of the Framingham coronary heart disease prediction scores: results of a multiple ethnic groups investigation. J Am Med Assoc 2001; 286:180–187.

166. Marrugat J, Solanas P, D'Agostino R et al. Coronary risk estimation in Spain using a calibrated Framingham function. Rev Esp Cardiol 2003; 56:253–261.

167. Assmann G, Cullen P, Schulte H. Simple scoring scheme for calculating the risk of acute coronary events based on the 10-year follow-up of the prospective cardiovascular Munster (PROCAM) study. Circulation 2002; 105:310–315.

168. Conroy RM, Pyorala K, Fitzgerald AP et al. Estimation of ten-year risk of fatal cardiovascular disease in Europe: the SCORE project. Eur Heart J 2003; 24:987–1003.

169. Stevens RJ, Kothari V, Adler AI et al. The UKPDS risk engine: a model for the risk of coronary heart disease in type II diabetes (UKPDS 56). Clin Sci (London) 2001; 101:671–679.

170. Anderson KM, Odell PM, Wilson PWF et al. Cardiovascular disease risk profiles. Am Heart J 1991; 121:293–298.

171. Wilson PW. Metabolic risk factors for coronary heart disease: current and future prospects. Curr Opin Cardiol 1999; 14:176–185.

172. Mosca L. C-reactive protein – to screen or not to screen? N Engl J Med 2002; 347:1615–1617.

3

Genetics of atherosclerosis in humans

Diego F. Wyszynski, Lindsay A. Farrer

The recent completion of a high-quality, comprehensive sequence of the human genome has fostered the search for the genetic component of most human diseases. Since Avery, McCloud, and McCarty demonstrated 60 years ago that DNA is the genetic material[1] and the double-helical antiparallel, complementary nature of DNA was discovered by James Watson and Francis Crick several years later,[2] genetics has become an integral part of our lives. Interwoven advances in genetics, comparative genomics, high-throughput biochemistry, and bioinformatics are providing biologists with a markedly improved repertoire of research tools that will allow the functioning of organisms in health and disease to be analyzed and comprehended at an unprecedented level of molecular detail.[3] As of 12 February 2004, 11 283 Mendelian conditions have been mapped to a particular chromosomal location (OMIM, 2004), and nearly 1500 genes associated with disease have been identified. GeneTests (www.genetests.org) lists more than 1030 diseases for which there are molecular tests, 690 of which are clinically available.

The tremendous success in identifying genes responsible for Mendelian traits has not been followed, however, by similar successes in the identification of genes responsible for complex diseases or for variations in quantitative traits. Despite more than 1300 National Institutes of Health (NIH)-funded studies of complex genetic disease (Computer Retrieval Information on Scientific Projects; http://crisp.cit.nih.gov/) and numerous reports on at least 166 genes, as few as 10–50 causative polymorphisms for complex diseases have thus far been identified in humans.[4–6]

Atherosclerosis is a complex chronic inflammatory disease of the large and medium arteries that is most often associated with hyperlipidemia and/or several other risk factors.[7] Myocardial infarction and stroke,

the principal causes of death in western society, result largely from atherosclerosis.[8] Genetic factors contribute importantly to atherosclerosis in human populations, with a heritability estimated to be approximately 50%. Although there has been considerable success in identifying genes for rare disorders associated with atherosclerosis, the understanding of genes involved in the common forms is largely incomplete.[9] The modes of inheritance of atherosclerosis are, if these rarer monogenic disorders are excluded, complex and multifactorial, i.e. the disease phenotype is a consequence of interactions between genetic and environmental factors. Although atherosclerosis aggregates in some families, it does not segregate in Mendelian fashion. This observation predicts that individual alleles are neither necessary nor sufficient to cause the phenotype; thus, atherosclerosis alleles may be prevalent in the non-diseased population, and a high proportion of individuals possessing the inherited susceptibility do not manifest disease, presumably because they lack sufficient liability (e.g. other genes and environmental exposures).

One approach to the study of the genetics of atherosclerosis is to dissect the genetic basis of constituent *endophenotypes* known to have a strong genetic component.[10] Table 3.1 lists six atherosclerosis endophenotypes with appreciable heritability. Studies have indicated that lipid levels are substantially heritable. Point estimates of heritability for total cholesterol, HDL cholesterol (HDL-C), and plasma triglycerides (TG) range from 42% to 65%, 45% to 83%, and 37% to 75%, respectively, with twin studies providing higher point estimates.[11–14] At least half of the normal variation in low-density lipoprotein cholesterol (LDL-C) concentration is due to genetic factors.[15,16] Several segregation analyses have suggested major genes for lipid traits.[17–19] The San

Table 3.1   Genetic factors associated with atherosclerosis and coronary heart disease (modified from Lusis[95])

Elevated levels of LDL	Associations demonstrated in epidemiological studies and supported by studies of genetic disorders and animal models. Clinical trials have shown benefits of cholesterol reduction[96]
Reduced levels of HDL	Associations demonstrated by numerous epidemiological studies and supported by studies of genetic diseases and animal models[97]
Elevated levels of lipoprotein (a)	Associations observed in many, but not all, epidemiological studies. Animal studies have been contradictory[98]
Elevated blood pressure	Associations observed in epidemiological studies. Clinical trials have demonstrated benefits of blood pressure reduction, with particularly strong effects on stroke[96,99]
Elevated levels of homocysteine	Associations have been observed in epidemiological studies and studies of homocystinuria, which result in severe occlusive vascular disease[100]
Metabolic syndrome	This cluster of metabolic disturbances, with insulin resistance as a central feature, is strongly associated with coronary heart disease[101]

LDL, low-density lipoprotein; HDL, high-density lipoprotein

Antonio Heart Study reported segregation analysis evidence of a major gene for HDL-C, but concluded that this locus was not any of the following major candidate loci: apoA-I/apoC-III, apoB, hepatic lipase, lipoprotein lipase, LDL receptor, or apoE.[20] Similarly, data from the National Heart, Lung, and Blood Institute (NHLBI) Family Heart Study (FHS) show a major gene effect for mild elevation in LDL-C that is not attributable to the LDL receptor, apoE, or the cholesterol 7-hydroxylase genes.[21] These studies indicate that whole genome scans may reveal new major loci underlying quantitative lipid traits[13]. Table 3.2 lists some of the genes that have been associated with atherosclerosis, sorted by physiological mechanism (lipid metabolism, renin–angiotensin, homocysteine metabolism, thrombosis, leukocyte adhesion). This chapter will review the literature on the efforts towards the identification of genetic factors that increase susceptibility to three of these traits: elevated LDL, low HDL, and metabolic syndrome.

Elevated levels of LDL

Clinical familial hypercholesterolemia (FH) is defined as a very high (twice normal) LDL cholesterol level, with clear bimodality within families.[11] The ranges of serum cholesterol and LDL cholesterol are, respectively

in mg/dl, 250–450 and 200–400 in heterozygotes, > 500 and > 450 in affected homozygotes, and 150–250 and 75–175 in unaffected homozygotes, with some positive correlation with age.[22,23] Tendon xanthomas and corneal arcus are diagnostic for this condition but are often absent, especially at young ages.[13] Three genetic loci have been implicated in this clinical disorder: the LDL receptor gene (LDLR), whose loss of activity may lead to autosomal dominant FH or to autosomal recessive hypercholesterolemia, or ARH;[24,25] the apolipoprotein B-100 gene, whose impaired function may result in familial ligand-defective apoB-100, or FDB;[26] and two ABC transporters, ABCG5 and ABCG8, whose loss of function has been associated with the rare autosomal recessive disorder sitosterolemia.[25,27]

FH patients who are heterozygous for the LDLR defect produce one-half the normal number of LDLR, and on average they have a 2.5-fold elevation in the number of LDL particles in plasma.[28] The incidence of heterozygous FH is at least 1 in 500 people in all populations so far studied, making this disorder one of the most common monogenic diseases. It is the most frequent cause of premature coronary heart disease resulting from a single gene defect, and accounts for 5% of heart attacks in patients 60 years of age or less. The rare FH homozygotes (1 in 1 million) have LDL

Table 3.2 Genes associated with cardiovascular atherosclerosis (modified from Stavljenić-Rukavina A, eJIFCC 2004; 14:http://www.ifcc.org/ejifcc/vol14no2/140206200305n.htm.)[102]

Gene	Chromosomal location	Function/Phenotypic traits
1. Lipid metabolism		
Apolipoprotein B (apoB)	2p	Component of plasma lipoproteins, particularly LDL; mediates binding to LDL receptor
tHR 71-Ile		Possibly associated with increased plasma LDL cholesterol and apoB levels; arg-3531-cys LDL receptor binding defect appears to segregate with Thr allele
Arg-3500-Gln		Disorder of hypercholesterolemia known as familial defective apoB-100, due to reduced binding to LDL receptor
Apolipoprotein CIII (apoCIII)	11q	Component of plasma proteins
T(625)del, C(482)T, T(455)C, C3175G (Sst)I, C1100T, T3206G		Increased plasma triglyceride levels
Apolipoprotein E (apoE)	19q	Component of plasma proteins; mediates binding to the LDL and remnant (apoE) receptors
e3/e2, e4		Interindividual variation in plasma total and LDL cholesterol levels, atherosclerotic progression
Cholesteryl ester transfer protein (CETP)	16q	Reverse cholesterol transport pathway; possible proatherogenic role in presence of dyslipidemia
Ile-405-Val, Asp-442-Gly		Increased plasma HDL-C and apoA-I levels
Lipoprotein lipase (LPL)	8p	Hydrolysis of plasma triglycerides
T(93)G		Increased LPL promoter activity, reduced plasma triglycerides
T(39)C		Reduced LPL promoter activity
Asp9-Asn		Increased plasma triglycerides, increased atherosclerotic progression
Asn-291-Ser		Reduced plasma HDL-C, increased triglyceride levels
Ser-447-Ter		Increased plasma HDL-C, reduced plasma triglyceride levels; possible impact on responsiveness to blockers
PON	7q	HDL-associated enzyme known to hydrolyze organophosphate poisons; possible contribution to HDL's protective capacity against LDL oxidation
Gln-192-Arg		Increased enzymatic activity; *in vitro*, reduced protection against lipid peroxidation
2. Renin–angiotensin system		
Angiotensin-converting enzyme (ACE)	17q	Proteolyzes angiotensin I to produce angiotensin II
Alu element insertion/ deletion in intron 16		Increased plasma ACE levels; mixed evidence of association with myocardial infarction
Angiotensin II receptor type 1 (ATIIR1)	3q	One of two receptors for angiotensin II, particularly in vascular smooth muscle cells
A1166C		Hypertension; possible synergism with ACE, conferring risk of myocardial infarction
Angiotensinogen (AGT)	1q	Substrate for renin, yielding angiotensin I
Met-235-Thr		Increased plasma AGT levels; hypertension

Continued

Table 3.2 Continued

Gene	Chromosomal location	Function/Phenotypic traits
3. Homocysteine metabolism		
Cystathionine-synthase (CBS)	21q	Transulfuration pathway, converting homocysteine to cystathionine, with pyridoxine as cofactor
Ala-114-Va,		
Ile-278-Thr,		Pyridoxine-responsive homocystinuria
Arg-125-Gln,		
glu131asp,		Pyridoxine-unresponsive homocystinuria
Gly-307-Ser		
68-bp insertion		Linkage disequilibrium with 278thr
Methylene tetrahydrofolate reductase (MTHFR)	1p	Remethylation pathway, generating the 5-methyltetrahydrofolate that serves as the methyl group donor
C677T (Ala/Val)		Associated with hyperhomocysteinemia given low dietary folate; increased risk for deep-vein thrombosis in carriers of factor V Leiden
C692T		Absence of enzyme activity
4. Thrombosis		
Glycoprotein IIIa (GPIIIa)	17q	Component of GPIIb/IIIa platelet adhesion receptor, binding fibrinogen, fibronectin, and von Willebrand factor
Leu-33-Pro		Interindividual variation in platelet adhesion and/or adhesion; mixed evidence of association with risk of coronary thrombosis
Fibrinogen	4q	Determinant of plasma viscosity, cofactor for platelet aggregation, precursor of fibrin (component of plaques)
chain G(455)A		Increased plasma fibrinogen levels and progression of atherosclerosis
Factor V	1q	Activated form is procoagulant cofactor in prothrombin activation, inactivated through cleavage by activated protein C
Arg-506-Gln (Leiden mutation)		Resistance to activated protein C; hypercoagulability
5. Leukocyte adhesion		
Endothelial leukocyte adhesion molecule-1 (ELAM)	1q	Adhesion of leukocytes to activated arterial endothelium; also known as E-selectin
G98T,		
Ser-128-Arg,		Increased risk for severe atherosclerosis
Leu-554-Phe		

LDL, low-density lipoprotein; HDL, high-density lipoprotein; HDL-C, HDL cholesterol

levels that are 6–10-times above normal. These individuals have virulent coronary atherosclerosis, often dying from heart attacks in childhood.[29] Heterozygous FDB is common in Europeans (1 per 1000). The syndrome is similar to heterozygous FH, although not as severe. The rare FDB homozygotes have higher levels of LDL than the FDB heterozygotes. Young adults and children with ARH exhibit severe hypercholesterolemia, premature coronary heart disease, and massive deposits of LDL-derived cholesterol in the skin.[28] Isotopic tracer studies show that these individuals, like FH homozygotes, have a severe defect in the removal of LDL from plasma.[30] Yet Garcia and colleagues[25] showed that LDLR activity in cultured fibroblasts from ARH patients is almost normal.

Three independent linkage studies, by Ott and colleagues,[31] Berg and Heiberg,[32] and Elston and colleagues,[33] strongly suggested a loose linkage between familial hypercholesterolemia and the third component of complement; C3 has been mapped to chromosome 19 by somatic cell hybridization. Donald and colleagues[34] presented further data on HC–C3 linkage, bringing the combined male–female LOD (logarithms of odds) score to a maximum of 3.79 at θ 0.25. C3 and FHC are about 20 cM apart; APOE and C3 are about 15 cM apart. FHC is not closely linked to APOE, suggesting that these two loci are on opposite sides of C3. The LDLR gene was regionalized to 19p13.1–p13.3 by in situ hybridization.[35] Judging by the sequence of loci suggested by linkage data (pter–FHC–C3–APOE/APOC2), the location of FHC (LDLR) is probably 19p13.2–p13.12, and that of C3 19p13.2–p13.11. Leppert and colleagues[36] found tight linkage between an RFLP of the LDL receptor gene and dominantly inherited hypercholesterolemia; specifically, no exception to cosegregation was found between the high-LDL-C phenotype and a unique allele at the LDLR locus. The maximum LOD score was 7.52 at $\theta = 0$.

Over 600 mutations are described for the LDL receptor.[29] Despite this large number, mutations have not been identified in up to 30% of all persons with FH. Haddad and colleagues[37] were able to find specific mutations in only 19 of 47 probands with clinical FH. Linkage to the LDL receptor was found in an additional four of five families large enough to test for linkage. Deletion of gly197 is the most prevalent LDL receptor mutation causing familial hypercholesterolemia in Ashkenazi Jewish individuals. Studying index cases from Israel, South Africa, Russia, The Netherlands, and the United States, Durst and colleagues[38] found that all traced their ancestry to Lithuania. A highly conserved haplotype was identified in chromosomes carrying this deletion, suggesting a common founder. When two methods were used for analysis of linkage disequilibrium between flanking polymorphic markers and the disease locus and for the study of the decay of LDL receptor over time, the estimated age of the deletion was found to be 20 ± 7 generations, so that the most recent common ancestor of the mutation-bearing chromosomes would date to the 14th century. This corresponds with the founding of the Jewish community of Lithuania (AD 1338), as well as with the great demographic expansion of Ashkenazi

Jews in eastern Europe that followed this settlement. Durst and colleagues[38] could find no evidence supporting a selective evolutionary metabolic advantage. Therefore, the founder effect in a rapidly expanding population from a limited number of families remains a simple, parsimonious hypothesis explaining the spread of this mutation in Ashkenazi Jews.

Broeckel and colleagues[39] identified 513 western European families with at least two members that had been affected at 59 years or younger with myocardial infarction (MI) and/or severe premature coronary artery disease (CAD), corresponding to a total of 1406 individuals. They analyzed known risk factors as quantitative traits (concentrations of HDL-C, LDL-C, lipoprotein (a) (Lp(a) and triglycerides) and qualitative traits (diabetes mellitus type 2, hypercholesterolemia, and systolic and diastolic arterial hypertension). A total genome scan was carried out with 394 microsatellite markers at an average marker distance of 10 cM. They found suggestive linkage for LDL-C concentrations on chromosomes 17 (89 cM) and 14 (35 cM), with LOD scores of 2.29 and 1.5, respectively.

Coon and colleagues[40] performed a genome scan for LDL-C concentration in white subjects who were ascertained through the NHLBI Family Heart Study (FHS). The NIH Mammalian Genotyping Service (Marshfield, WI) genotyped 401 autosomal markers spaced at approximate 10-cM intervals. Additional FHS families were genotyped by the FHS Molecular Laboratory at the University of Utah for 243 markers; 645 subjects were typed in both laboratories, so that a combined map of the 644 markers from the two screening sets (average distance of 5.46 cM) could be produced. Analyses were done on 2799 genotyped subjects in 500 families where at least two genotyped persons in the family had measured LDL-C levels (average number of genotyped family members = 5.95). The variance components method was used, as implemented in GeneHunter. Prior to analysis, each phenotype was adjusted, within sex, for age, age squared, body mass index, waist–hip ratio, alcohol, smoking, medication status for diabetes and hypertension, estrogen use, and field center location. Linkage analyses were performed, first excluding 305 subjects on lipid-lowering medications, then again including the data from these subjects. The highest peak was on chromosome 11 at 56.3–56.4 cM, with a maximum LOD score of 3.72. Two genome scans of lipid traits in other populations have found peaks in this region. Other scores at or above 1.9 occurred on chromosomes 5 (LOD = 1.89 at 1.6 cM), 10 (LOD = 2.47 at 127.1 cM), 17 (LOD = 2.33 at 116.3 cM), and 21 (LOD = 2.74 at 45.2 cM). In a similar study, Austin and colleagues carried out a whole-genome scan for linkage to LDL size and triglyceride levels in 26 kindreds with familial hypertriglyceridemia (FHTG).[41] LDL size was estimated using gradient gel electrophoresis, and genotyping was performed for 355 autosomal markers with an average heterozygosity of 76% and an average spacing of 10.2 cM. Using variance components linkage analysis, one possible linkage was found for LDL size (LOD = 2.1) on chromosome 6, peak at 140 cM distal to marker F13A1 (closest marker D6S2436). With adjustment for TG and/or HDL-C the LOD scores were reduced, but remained in exactly the same location. For TG, LOD scores of 2.56 and 2.44 were observed at two locations on chromosome 15, with peaks at 29 and 61 cM distal to marker D15S822 (closest markers D15S643 and D15S211, respectively). These peaks were retained with adjustment for LDL size and/or HDL-C.

FH, FDB, and ARH are currently underdiagnosed throughout the world, and many of those who have been diagnosed with any one of these disorders are not adequately treated.[42,43] The statin drugs have greatly increased physicians' ability to control high levels of LDL-C, yet not all patients respond equally to treatment. The existence of other loci that cause elevated LDL-C similar to FH and FDB may elucidate other disease mechanisms for which new, effective drugs could be developed. Such drugs could not only help to target the defects of this new locus, but also might be used as therapy for other genetic cholesterol disorders, such as FH, FDB, ARH, familial combined hyperlipidemia, and polygenic hypercholesterolemia.

Reduced levels of HDL

Low plasma HDL-C concentration is a major risk factor for cardiovascular disease, especially coronary heart disease (CHD), which remains the largest source of morbidity and mortality in the United States and other industrialized countries. Recent studies show that HDL particles influence the atherosclerotic process in many ways, including by reducing oxidation of LDL particles

and inhibiting various coagulation pathways; but it is their role in the reverse cholesterol transport pathway that is believed to be most important. During reverse cholesterol transport, HDL particles remove cholesterol from peripheral tissues and transport it to the liver for either repackaging or excretion through the bile.[44] This process depends on many enzymes to move the cholesterol molecules from the peripheral tissues to the liver. Despite the large number of control points involved in the movement of cholesterol by HDL particles, relatively few environmental predictors have been identified from large prospective studies. Plasma levels of HDL-C, like many quantitative risk factors for complex disease, have been extensively characterized through epidemiological, family, and association studies, which have demonstrated a strong genetic component and have provided clues about which subphenotypes may be most closely related to disease risk.[45] Heritabilities of total HDL-C have been estimated to be 0.20–0.61.[11,15,16,20,45–52]

Segregation analyses in randomly ascertained samples suggest the presence of a major gene for HDL-C levels;[17,20,53] however, recent studies investigating the roles of candidate genes, such as those for angiotensin-converting enzyme, hepatic lipase, lipoprotein lipase, cholesterol ester transfer protein, and apolipoproteins AI, AII, CIII, and B, in the control of HDL-C levels have produced mixed results, with some studies finding effects of these genes on HDL-C and others either failing to find associations with the same polymorphisms or excluding linkage of HDL-C levels to these regions.[20,45,54–67] As HDL-C levels are likely to be controlled by the actions of several genes, a number of these candidate loci may yet be shown to be involved in HDL-C regulation; however, none of them has emerged as a clear contender for the major gene for HDL-C levels that has been predicted by segregation analyses. It may be that the candidate polymorphisms currently being studied are not themselves functional, but show an imperfect association with HDL-C levels because they are in linkage disequilibrium with functional polymorphisms.[45] Another alternative is that the major genetic determinants of HDL-C levels are unknown loci yet to be identified. Both of these possibilities are best explored through linkage analyses with highly polymorphic markers, a method that is not dependent on either specification of known candidates or linkage disequilibrium between markers and functional polymorphisms.[45]

A recently identified genetic risk factor for low HDL-C levels in some populations is the apolipoprotein A-I$_{Milano}$ (apoA-I$_M$) mutation. Described in a family originating from Limone sul Garda in northern Italy,[68] this apoA-I variant shows a single amino acid substitution, arginine 173 to cysteine, that leads to the formation of homodimers (A-I$_M$/A-I$_M$) and heterodimers with apoA-II (A-I$_M$/A-II).[69] All carriers are heterozygous for the mutation[70] and share a lipoprotein disorder characterized by very low plasma levels of HDL-C with moderate hypertriglyceridemia.[71] Sirtori and colleagues[72] compared 21 A-I$_M$ carriers with age- and sex-matched control subjects from the same kindred and with two series of matched subjects with primary hypoalphalipoproteinemia (HA). Structural changes in the carotid arteries were defined as the intima-media thickness (IMT) measured by B-mode ultrasound. HA subjects showed significant thickening of the carotids (average IMT 0.86 ± 0.25 and 0.88 ± 0.29 mm, respectively) compared with control subjects (average IMT 0.64 ± 0.12 mm); the apoA-I$_M$ carriers instead showed normal arterial thickness (average IMT 0.63 ± 0.10 mm). Moreover, a significantly higher prevalence of atherosclerotic plaques was found in patients and blood donors with HA (both 57%) than in apoA-I$_M$ carriers (33%) and control subjects (21%). Echocardiographic findings and maximal treadmill ECG did not differ significantly between apoA-I$_M$ carriers and control subjects, apart from a slight increase in left ventricular end-diastolic dimension in the carriers. The authors concluded that carriers of the apoA-I$_M$ mutant do not show structural changes in the arteries and heart, thus exerting some cardiovascular protective effect, in contrast to HA subjects, who are characterized by a marked increase in carotid IMT and an increased prevalence of atherosclerotic plaques.

There is evidence that HA is caused in some families by mutation in the *ABC*1 gene, which is also the site of mutations causing Tangier disease. Hypoalphalipoproteinemia is observed with mutations in the apolipoprotein A1 gene (*APOA*1), which maps to 11q23.3. A possibly distinct form of primary HA has been thought to map to the same region, 11q23.3 (HDLD3). Duggirala and colleagues[73] conducted a genome-wide scan for susceptibility genes influencing plasma triglyceride (TG) levels in a Mexican-American population. They used both phenotypic and genotypic data from 418 individuals distributed across 27 low-income, extended Mexican-American families.

Shearman and colleagues[74] carried out a 10 cM genome-wide scan for log(TG) level and log(TG/HDL-C) for the largest 332 extended families of the Framingham Heart Study (1702 genotyped individuals). The highest multipoint variance component LOD scores obtained for both log(TG) and log(TG/HDL-C) were on chromosome 7 (at 155 cM), where the results for the two phenotypes were 1.8 and 2.5, respectively. The 7q32.3–qter region contains several candidate genes. Four other regions with multipoint LOD scores > 1 were identified on chromosome 3 (LOD score for log(TG/HDL-C) = 1.8 at 140 cM), chromosome 11 (LOD score for log(TG/HDL-C) = 1.1 at 125 cM), chromosome 16 (LOD score for log(TG) = 1.5 at 70 cM, LOD score for log(TG/HDL-C) = 1.1 at 75 cM) and chromosome 20 (LOD score for log(TG/HDL-C) = 1.7 at 35 cM, LOD score for log(TG) = 1.3 at 40 cM).

Klos and colleagues[75] reported the results of genome-wide linkage analyses to identify chromosomal regions that influence interindividual variation in plasma lipid and apolipoprotein levels of subjects participating in the Rochester (Minnesota) Heart Study. Evidence suggestive of a quantitative trait locus (QTL) near marker D17S928 at the end of the long arm of chromosome 17 (LOD score 2.48) that influences plasma total-C/HDL-C variation was observed. Additional tentative evidence of a QTL influencing variation in total-C/HDL-C was found on chromosome 5q near the marker D5S408 (LOD score 1.57). Peacock and colleagues[76] conducted a genome-wide linkage scan for QTL influencing HDL-C concentration in a sample of 1027 whites from 101 families participating in the NHLBI Family Heart Study. To maximize the relative contributions of genetic components of variance to the total variance of HDL-C, the HDL-C phenotype was adjusted for age,[2] body mass index, and Family Heart Study field center, and standardized HDL-C residuals were created separately for men and women. All analyses were completed by the variance components method, as implemented in the program GeneHunter using 383 anonymous markers typed at the NHLBI Mammalian Genotyping Service in Marshfield, WI. Evidence for linkage of residual HDL-C was detected near marker D5S1470 at location 39.9 cM from the p-terminal of chromosome 5 (LOD = 3.64). A suggestive linkage was detected near marker D13S1493 at location 27.5 cM on chromosome 13 (LOD = 2.36). The authors concluded that at least one genomic region is likely to harbor a gene that influences interindividual variation in HDL-C. Elbein and Hasstedt[14] performed a 10-cM genome scan using 440 markers in 379 members of 19 multiplex families ascertained for two diabetic siblings (screening study). They then extended findings for three regions with initial LOD scores > 1.5 to an additional 23 families, for a total of 576 genotyped individuals (extended study). Suggestive evidence of a QTL for HDL was found on chromosomes 1 (16–49 cM, LOD score 2.17; 190–210 cM, LOD score: 1.49), 2 (277–285 cM, LOD score 2.31), and 13 (33–49, LOD score 2.01). Using a multipoint variance components linkage approach, Arya and colleagues[77] found strong evidence of linkage of a QTL for HDL-C level to a genetic location between markers D9S925 and D9S741 on chromosome 9p in Mexican-Americans (HDLC1). By another genome-wide scan for genes predisposing to low HDL-C in 25 well-defined Finnish families that had been ascertained for familial low HDL-C and premature coronary heart disease, Soro and colleagues[78] found evidence for linkage between the low HDL-C trait and a locus on 8q23 (HDLC2). Evidence for linkage also emerged for loci on 16q24.1–q24.2 and 20q13.11, the latter representing a characterized region for type 2 diabetes (NIDDM3). Low HDL-C is a common feature in type 2 diabetes. Pajukanta and colleagues[79] confirmed a locus for low serum HDL-C (HDLC3) on 16q24.1.

Arking and colleagues[80] were interested in determining whether an allele of the gene KLOTHO, termed 'KL-VS', influences atherosclerotic risk in humans. They performed cross-sectional studies to assess the association between this allele and occult coronary artery disease (CAD) in two independent samples of apparently healthy siblings of individuals with early-onset (age < 60 years) CAD (SIBS-I ($n = 520$) and SIBS-II ($n = 436$)). Occult CAD was defined as the occurrence of a reversible perfusion defect during exercise thallium scintigraphy and/or as an abnormal result of an exercise electrocardiogram (SIBS-I, $n = 97$; SIBS-II, $n = 56$). In SIBS-I, the KL-VS allele conferred a relative odds of 1.90 (95% CI 1.21–2.98) for occult CAD, after adjusting for familial intraclass correlations ($p < 0.005$). Logistic regression modeling, incorporating known CAD risk factors, demonstrated that the KL-VS allele is an independent risk factor ($p < 0.019$) and that the imposed risk of KL-VS allele status is influenced by modifiable risk factors. Hypertension ($p < 0.022$) and increasing HDL-C levels ($p < 0.022$), respectively, mask or reduce the risk conferred by the KL-VS allele, whereas current smoking ($p < 0.004$) increases the risk. The authors concluded that these results demonstrate that the KL-VS allele is an independent risk factor for occult CAD in the two independent high-risk samples. Furthermore, they showed that modifiable risk factors, including hypertension, smoking status, and HDL-C level, appear to influence the risk imposed by this allele.

Wang and colleagues[81] described an autosomal dominant form of CAD/MI (or adCAD1) that is caused by the deletion of seven amino acids in the myocyte enhancer factor-2 (MEF2A). The deletion disrupts nuclear localization of MEF2A, reduces MEF2A-mediated transcription activation, and abolishes synergistic activation by MEF2A and by the transcription factor GATA-1 through a dominant-negative mechanism. The MEF2A protein demonstrates strong expression in the endothelium of coronary arteries. The identification of a pathogenic gene for a familial vascular disease with features of CAD may prove to be important for a better understanding of the pathogenesis of CAD/MI.

Metabolic syndrome

The metabolic syndrome is a clustering of several metabolic aberrations[82–84] associated with a markedly increased risk for cardiovascular disease and type 2 diabetes mellitus.[85–87] The most commonly identified components of the metabolic syndrome are abdominal obesity, atherogenic dyslipidemia[88] (elevated plasma triglycerides, low levels of HDL-C and small LDL particles), insulin resistance, and elevated blood pressure. These features can occur in various degrees and different combinations within individuals, so that the condition is clinically heterogeneous. Recently, the National Cholesterol Education Program (NCEP) Expert Panel on Detection, Evaluation, and Treatment of High Blood Cholesterol in Adults, Adult Treatment Panel III (ATP-III) published criteria for a clinical diagnosis of the metabolic syndrome (http://www.nhlbi.nih.gov/guidelines/cholesterol/index.htm). In adults, this diagnosis requires three or more of the following: waist circumference ≥ 102 (M)/88 (F) cm, serum triglycerides > 150 mg/dl, serum HDL-C < 40 (M)/50 (F) mg/dl, systolic blood pressure (SBP) > 130 mmHg or diastolic blood pressure ≥ 85 mmHg, and fasting plasma glucose ≥ 110 mg/dl.

The metabolic syndrome is highly prevalent in the United States. Applying the ATP-III criteria to the National Health and Nutrition Examination Survey (NHANES) III database (1988–1994), Ford et al.[89] showed that the unadjusted and age-adjusted prevalence of metabolic syndrome was particularly high, i.e. 21.8% and 23.7%, respectively. The prevalence increased from 6.7% among participants aged 20–29 years to 43.5% in the age group 60–69 years and 42.0% in those over 70. In the NHANES III population, the prevalence of the metabolic syndrome increased strikingly with body mass index (BMI), ranging from 4.6% in normal weight, 22.4% in overweight, to 59.6% in obese men.[90]

The mechanism underlying the development of the metabolic syndrome is incompletely understood. Insulin resistance is largely considered to be a hallmark for this condition and is closely associated with the accumulation of lipids in the liver and muscle, atherogenic dyslipidemia, and visceral adiposity;[82] however, it is not known which, if any, of these features precedes the others.

There is strong evidence that metabolic syndrome has a genetic component,[91,92] and elucidation of the genetic defects predisposing to metabolic syndrome should allow identification of the initiating components or critical pathways involved in this syndrome. At present, it is not known which and how many genes are involved in the pathogenesis of metabolic syndrome. It is possible that single gene defects may suffice to trigger the development of the disease and lead to its full-blown clinical expression, as exemplified by monogenic forms of lipodystrophy.[93] Alternatively, it is also possible – and perhaps more likely – that a variety of gene variants act in concert with specific environmental factors (such as physical inactivity and excess caloric intake) to facilitate the development of the syndrome. Identification of susceptibility genes for

metabolic syndrome has been difficult, owing partly to the heterogeneity of this disorder, the limited access to large collections of biological samples from well-phenotyped individuals and families, and the importance of gene–environment interactions in the pathogenesis of this condition.

In 2003, 12 teams of investigators constituted a group which analyzed phenotypes related to metabolic syndrome, making use of the available longitudinal measurements from the family component of the Framingham Heart Study or the simulated data, as distributed by Genetic Analysis Workshop 13.[94] Body mass index, obesity, lipid abnormalities, glucose, or combinations of these traits were analyzed. A wide variety of approaches were taken to construct phenotypes from the longitudinal measurements, including considering single or multiple cross-sectional time points, single ages, minimum values, maximum values, means, other lifetime values, ever/never dichotomy, or age at onset of some threshold value. Approaches also differed in the family structures utilized (sibling pairs to full extended pedigrees), the genetic data considered (two-point or multipoint), and the statistics calculated (model-free and parametric), and led to a diverse set of analyses being performed. Inferences were made about heritability, and attempts were made to map underlying genes. Over 40 genome-wide linkage analyses were conducted. Despite the broad range of approaches, several regions of the genome were repeatedly identified across multiple analyses. Table 3.3 illustrates regions that were identified by a single group with a signal equivalent to a LOD score of at least 3.0.

Conclusion

It is an exciting time in the study of atherosclerosis: in the past decade we have learned a lot about the endophenotypes underlying these diseases, yet the excitement is not over, as we realize that most challenging issues have still to be addressed. Development will come from novel studies that will be able to assess the function of mutant proteins in preparations that are more closely related to the physiological environment in which these proteins are distributed, and the development of transgenic models in animal species that have an action potential more closely related to that present in humans. These more physiological

Table 3.3 Chromosomal areas with markers reaching a LOD score > 3.0, with supporting evidence from other studies (from Goldin and colleagues[94])

Location	LOD Score	Distance from pter (in cm)	Interval	Phenotype	Method	Software
Chromosome 2						
North et al.[103]	3.4	151	129–158	HDL exam 11	MPT- VC	SOLAR
Martin et al.[104]	2.6	150		HDL	MPT- VC	SOLAR
North et al.[103]	1.1	122		HDL exam 20	MPT- VC	SOLAR
Moslehi et al.[105]	1.0	167		BMI	MPT- sib-pair -nonpar	SAGE
McQueen et al.[106]	1.7	179		Glucose	MPT- VC	SOLAR
Stein et al.[107]	1.6	180.6		MS	MPT- sib-pair -nonpar	Mx
Chromosome 11						
Moslehi et al.[105]	3.0	143.1	134–end	BMI	mpt.sib-pair.nonpar	SAGE
Engelman et al.[108]	1.4	134.1		overweight	2PT- sib-pair -nonpar	SAGE
Horne et al.[109]	1.6	161.7		Low TG : HDL	2PT-.par	LINKAGE
Horne et al.[109]	1.1	161.7		Low TG : HDL	MPT-MCMC-par	MCLINK
Strug et al.[110]	2.1	131		mean gain BMI	2PT- VC	SOLAR
Chromosome 16						
Geller et al.[111]	3.2	76	52–83	BMI	MPT- VC	SOLAR
Geller et al.[111]	2.8	78.56		BMI	MPT- VC	MERLIN
Geller et al.[111]	2.5	63.74		BMI	MPT- Reg	MERLIN
McQueen et al.[106]	1.3	75		BMI	MPT- VC	SOLAR
Engelman et al.[108]	1.2	63.7		Overweight survival	2PT- sib-pair- nonpar	SAGE
Li et al.[112]	2.9	46		mean BMI (4 time pts)	MPT- VC	SOLAR
Cheng et al.[113]	~1.1	~70		mean BMI (3 exams)	MPT- VC	SOLAR
Chromosome 19						
Moslehi et al.[105]	3.3	86.4	NA(2PT)	BMI	2PT-sib-pair -nonpar	SAGE
Moslehi et al.[105]	1.8	86.4		BMI	MPT-sib-pair- nonpar	SAGE
Engelman et al.[108]	1.0	86.4		Obese- survival	2PT-sib-pair-nonpar	SAGE
Martin et al.[104]	1.0	80		HDL	MPT- VC	SOLAR
Chromosome 22						
Horne et al.[109]	3.4	20.9	NA(2PT)	Low TG : HDL	2PT- par	LINKAGE
North et al.[103]	1.4	19		HDL exam 15	MPT- VC	SOLAR
Horne et al.[109]	1.3	20.9		Low TG : HDL	2PT- VC	SOLAR
Horne et al.[109]	1.0	20.9		Low TG : HDL	MPT- MCMC-par	MCLINK

HDL, high-density lipoprotein; BMI, body mass index; TG, triglyceride; MS, metabolic syndrome; MPT, multipoint linkage analysis; 2PT, two-point linkage analysis; VC, variance components; Reg, regression; nonpar, non-parametric linkage analysis; par, parametric linkage analysis

models will be useful not only to characterize individual mutations, but also to elucidate the effect of mutations. Also, both environmental determinants and underlying genetic susceptibility are undoubtedly involved in atherosclerosis. However, determining the relative contributions of environmental and genetic factors of complex diseases is difficult. Adding to the

difficulty is the possibility of gene–environment interaction in the expression of these traits. That is, the genetic contribution to a disease may vary according to a person's level of environmental exposure, and conversely, environmental exposure may have different effects depending on one's genetic background. Valuable insights into the causation of complex diseases will come as we learn to dissect these complicated gene–environment relationships. It is expected that the results of these future studies will provide novel therapeutic strategies for patients that will eventually encompass gene therapy.

References

1. Avery OT, MacLeod CM, McCarty M. Studies on the chemical nature of the substance inducing transformation of pneumococcal types: induction of transformation by a desoxyribonucleic acid fraction isolated from Pneumoccus type III. J Exp Med 1944; 79:137–158.

2. Watson JD, Crick FHC. A structure for deoxyribose nucleic acid. Nature 1953; 171:737–738.

3. Collins FS, Green ED, Guttmacher AE et al. A vision for the future of genomics research. Nature 2003; 422:835–847.

4. Ioannidis JP, Trikalinos TA, Ntzani EE et al. Genetic associations in large versus small studies: an empirical assessment. Lancet 2003; 361:567–571.

5. Lohmueller KE, Pearce CL, Pike M et al. Meta-analysis of genetic association studies supports a contribution of common variants to susceptibility to common disease. Nature Genet 2003; 33:177–182.

6. Page GP, George V, Go RC et al. 'Are we there yet?': Deciding when one has demonstrated specific genetic causation in complex diseases and quantitative traits. Am J Hum Genet 2003; 73:711–719.

7. VanderLaan PA, Reardon CA, Getz GS. Site specificity of atherosclerosis. Site-selective responses to atherosclerotic modulators. Arterioscler Thromb Vasc Biol 2004; 24:11–22.

8. Hodgin JB, Maeda N. Minireview: estrogen and mouse models of atherosclerosis. Endocrinology 2002; 143:4495–4501.

9. Allayee H, Ghazalpour A, Lusis AJ. Using mice to dissect genetic factors in atherosclerosis. Arterioscler Thromb Vasc Biol 2003; 23:1501–1509.

10. Farrer LA. Collection of clinical and epidemiological data for linkage studies. In: Current protocols in human genetics. New York: Greene Publishing, 2004; (Suppl 40): 1.1.1–1.1.17.

11. Hunt SC, Hasstedt SJ, Kuida H et al. Genetic heritability and common environmental components of resting and stressed blood pressures, lipids, and body mass index in Utah pedigrees and twins. Am J Epidemiol 1989; 129:625–638.

12. Perusse L, Rice T, Despres JP et al. Familial resemblance of plasma lipids, lipoproteins and postheparin lipoprotein and hepatic lipases in the HERITAGE Family Study. Arterioscler Thromb Vasc Biol 1997; 17:3263–3269.

13. Coon H, Leppert MF, Eckfeldt JH et al. Genome-wide linkage analysis of lipids in the Hypertension Genetic Epidemiology Network (HyperGEN) blood pressure study. Arterioscler Thromb Vasc Biol 2001; 21:1969–1974.

14. Elbein SC, Hasstedt SJ. Quantitative trait linkage analysis of lipid-related traits in familial type 2 diabetes: evidence for linkage of triglyceride levels to chromosome 19q. Diabetes 2002; 51:528–535.

15. Austin MA, King MC, Bawol RD et al. Risk factors for coronary heart disease in adult female twins: genetic heritability and shared environmental influences. Am J Epidemiol 1987; 125:308–318.

16. Rice T, Vogler GP, Perry TS et al. Familial aggregation of lipids and lipoproteins in families ascertained through random and nonrandom probands in the Iowa Lipid Research Clinics Family Study. Hum Hered 1991; 41:107–121.

17. Friedlander Y, Kark JD, Stein Y. Complex segregation analysis of low levels of plasma high-density lipoprotein cholesterol in a sample of nuclear families in Jerusalem. Genet Epidemiol 1986; 3:285–297.

18. Williams RR, Hunt SC, Hopkins PN et al. Genetic basis of familial dyslipidemia and hypertension: 15-year results from Utah. Am J Hypertens 1993; 6:319S–327S.

19. Cupples LA, Myers RH. Segregation analysis for high density lipoprotein in the Berkeley data. Genet Epidemiol 1993; 10:629–634.

20. Mahaney MC, Blangero J, Rainwater DL et al. A major locus influencing plasma high-density lipoprotein cholesterol levels in the San Antonio Family Heart Study: segregation and linkage analyses. Arterioscler Thromb Vasc Biol 1995; 15:1730–1739.

21. Coon H, Leppert MF, Province MA et al. Evidence for a major gene unlinked to the LDL receptor accounting for mild elevation in LDL cholesterol: the NHLBI Family Heart Study. Ann Hum Genet 1998; 63:401–412.

22. Khachadurian AK. The inheritance of essential familial hypercholesterolemia. Am J Med 1964; 37:402–407.

23. Kwiterovich PO Jr, Fredrickson DS, Levy RI. Familial hypercholesterolemia (one form of familial type II hyperlipoproteinemia): a study of its biochemical, genetic, and clinical presentation in childhood. J Clin Invest 1974; 53:1237–1349.

24. Goldstein JL, Schrott HG, Hazzard WR et al. Hyperlipidemia in coronary heart disease, II: Genetic analysis of lipid levels in 176 families and delineation of a new inherited disorder, combined hyperlipidemia. J Clin Invest 1973; 52:1544–1568.

25. Garcia CK, Wilund K, Arca M et al. Autosomal recessive hypercholesterolemia caused by mutations in a putative LDL receptor adaptor protein. Science 2001; 292:1394–1398.

26. Innerarity TL, Weisgraber KH, Arnold KS et al. Familial defective apolipoprotein B-100: low density lipoproteins with abnormal receptor binding. Proc Natl Acad Sci USA 1987; 84:6919–6923.

27. Lee MH, Lu K, Hazard S et al. Identification of a gene, ABCG5, important in the regulation of dietary cholesterol absorption. Nature Genet 2001; 27:79–83.

28. Goldstein JL, Brown MS. Molecular medicine. The cholesterol quartet. Science 2001; 292:1310–1312.

29. Goldstein JL, Hobbs HH, Brown MS. In: Scriver CR, Beaudet AL, Sly WS et al, eds. The metabolic and molecular bases of inherited disease. New York: McGraw-Hill, 2001; Ch120.

30. Zuliani G, Arca M, Signore A et al. Characterization of a new form of inherited hypercholesterolemia: familial recessive hypercholesterolemia. Arterioscler Thromb Vasc Biol 1999; 19:802–809.

31. Ott J, Schrott HG, Goldstein JL et al. Linkage studies in a large kindred with familial hypercholesterolemia. Am J Hum Genet 1974; 26:598–603.

32. Berg K, Heiberg A. Linkage studies on familial hyperlipoproteinemia with xanthomatosis: normal lipoprotein markers and the C3 polymorphism. Cytogenet Cell Genet 1976; 16:266–270.

33. Elston RC, Namboodiri KK, Go RCP et al. Probable linkage between essential familial hypercholesterolemia and third complement component (C3). Cytogenet Cell Genet 1976; 16:294–297.

34. Donald JA, Humphries SE, Tippett P et al. Linkage relationships of familial hypercholesterolemia and chromosome 19 markers. Cytogenet Cell Genet 1984; 37:452.

35. Lindgren V, Luskey KL, Russell DW, Francke U. Human genes involved in cholesterol metabolism: chromosomal mapping of the loci for the low density lipoprotein receptor and 3-hydroxy-3-methylglutaryl-coenzyme A reductase with cDNA probes. Proc Natl Acad Sci USA 1985; 82:8567–8571.

36. Leppert MF, Hasstedt SJ, Holm T et al. A DNA probe for the LDL receptor gene is tightly linked to hypercholesterolemia in a pedigree with early coronary disease. Am J Hum Genet 1986; 39:300–306.

37. Haddad L, Day INM, Hunt S et al. Evidence for a third genetic locus causing familial hypercholesterolemia: a non-LDLr, non-apoB kindred. J Lipid Res 1999; 40:1113–1122.

38. Durst R, Colombo R, Shpitzen S et al. Recent origin and spread of a common Lithuanian mutation, G197del LDLR, causing familial hypercholesterolemia: positive selection is not always necessary to account for disease incidence among Ashkenazi Jews. Am J Hum Genet 2001; 68:1172–1188.

39. Broeckel U, Hengstenberg C, Mayer B et al. A comprehensive linkage analysis for myocardial infarction and its related risk factors. Nature Genet 2002; 30:210–214.

40. Coon H, Eckfeldt JH, Leppert MF et al. A genome-wide screen reveals evidence for a locus on chromosome 11 influencing variation in LDL cholesterol in the NHLBI Family Heart Study. Hum Genet 2002; 111:263–269.

41. Austin MA, Edwards KL, Monks SA et al. Genome-wide scan for quantitative trait loci influencing LDL size and plasma triglyceride in familial hypertriglyceridemia. J Lipid Res 2003; 44:2161–2168.

42. Williams RR, Schumacher MC, Barlow GK et al. Documented need for more effective diagnosis and treatment of familial hypercholesterolemia according to data from 502 heterozygotes in Utah. Am J Cardiol 1993; 72:18D–24D.

43. World Health Organization. Familial Hypercholesterolaemia (FH). Report of a WHO Consultation. Geneva: World Health Organization, 1998.

44. Tall AR. An overview of reverse cholesterol transport. Eur Heart J 1998; 19:A31–A35.

45. Almasy L, Hixson JE, Rainwater DL et al. Human pedigree-based quantitative-trait-locus mapping: localization of two genes influencing HDL-cholesterol metabolism. Am J Hum Genet 1999; 64:1686–1693.

46. Rao DC, Laskarzewski PM, Morrison JA et al. The Cincinnati Lipid Research Clinic family study: cultural and biological determinants of lipids and lipoprotein concentrations. Am J Hum Genet 1982; 34:888–903.

47. Whitfield JB, Martin NG. Plasma lipids in twins: environmental and genetic influences. Atherosclerosis 1983; 48:265-77.

48. Namboodiri KK, Kaplan EB, Heuch I et al. The Collaborative Lipid Research Clinics Family Study: biological and cultural determinants of familial resemblance for plasma lipids and lipoproteins. Genet Epidemiol 1985; 2:227–254.

49. Hamsten A, Iselius L, Dahlen G et al. Genetic and cultural inheritance of serum lipids, low and high density lipoprotein cholesterol and serum apolipoproteins A-I, A-II, and B. Atherosclerosis 1986; 60:199–208.

50. Bucher KD, Friedlander Y, Kaplan EB et al. Biological and cultural sources of familial resemblance in plasma lipids: a comparison between North America and Israel – the Lipid Research Clinics Program. Genet Epidemiol 1988; 5:17–33.

51. O'Connell DL, Heller RF, Roberts DCK et al. Twin study of genetic and environmental effects on lipid levels. Genet Epidemiol 1988; 5:323–341.

52. Heller DA, de Faire U, Pedersen NL et al. Genetic and environmental influences on serum lipid levels in twins. N Engl J Med 1993; 328:1150–1156.

53. Hasstedt SJ, Ash KO, Williams RR. A re-examination of major locus hypotheses for high density lipoprotein cholesterol level using 2 170 persons screened in 55 Utah pedigrees. Am J Med Genet 1986; 24:57–67.

54. Amos CI, Elston RC, Srinivasan SR et al. Linkage and segregation analyses of apolipoproteins A1 and B, and lipoprotein cholesterol levels in a large pedigree with excess coronary heart disease: the Bogalusa Heart Study. Genet Epidemiol 1987; 4:115–128.

55. Cohen JC, Wang Z, Grundy SM et al. Variation at the hepatic lipase and apolipoprotein AI/CIII/AIV loci is a major cause of genetically determined variation in plasma HDL cholesterol levels. J Clin Invest 1994; 94:2377–2384.

56. Gerdes C, Gerdes LU, Hansen PS et al. Polymorphisms in the lipoprotein lipase gene and their associations with plasma lipid concentrations in 40-year-old Danish men. Circulation 1995; 92:1765–1769.

57. Jemaa R, Fumeron F, Poirier O et al. Lipoprotein lipase gene polymorphisms: associations with myocardial infarction and lipoprotein levels, the ECTIM study: Étude Cas Temoin sur l'Infarctus du Myocarde. J Lipid Res 1995; 36:2141–2146.

58. Mattu RK, Needham EW, Galton DJ et al. A DNA variant at the angiotensin-converting enzyme gene locus associates

with coronary artery disease in the Caerphilly Heart Study. Circulation 1995; 91:270–274.

59. Minnich A, DeLangavant G, Lavigne J et al. GA substitution at position -75 of the apolipoprotein A-I gene promoter: evidence against a direct effect on HDL cholesterol levels. Arterioscler Thromb Vasc Biol 1995; 15:1740–1745.

60. Turner PR, Talmud PJ, Visvikis S et al. DNA polymorphisms of the apoprotein B gene are associated with altered plasma lipoprotein concentrations but not with perceived risk of cardiovascular disease: European Atherosclerosis Research Study. Atherosclerosis 1995; 116:221–234.

61. Dupuy-Gorce AM, Desmarais E, Vigneron S et al. DNA polymorphisms in linkage disequilibrium at the 3' end of the human APO AII gene: relationships with lipids, apolipoproteins and coronary heart disease. Clin Genet 1996; 50:191–198.

62. Kamboh MI, Aston CE, Nestlerode CM et al. Haplotype analysis of two APOA1/MspI polymorphisms in relation to plasma levels of apo A-I and HDL-cholesterol. Atherosclerosis 1996; 127:255–262.

63. McPherson R, Grundy SM, Guerra R et al. Allelic variation in the gene encoding the cholesteryl ester transfer protein is associated with variation in the plasma concentrations of cholesteryl ester transfer protein. J Lipid Res 1996; 37:1743–1748.

64. Guerra R, Wang J, Grundy SM et al. A hepatic lipase (LIPC) allele associated with high plasma concentrations of high density lipoprotein cholesterol. Proc Natl Acad Sci USA 1997; 94:4532–4537.

65. Bruce C, Sharp DS, Tall AR. Relationship of HDL and coronary heart disease to a common amino acid polymorphism in the cholesteryl ester transfer protein in men with and without hypertriglyceridemia. J Lipid Res 1998; 39:1071–1078.

66. Devlin CM, Prenger VL, Miller M. Linkage of the apo CIII microsatellite with isolated low high-density lipoprotein cholesterol. Hum Genet 1998; 102:273–281.

67. Kastelein JJ, Groenemeyer BE, Hallman DM et al. The Asn9 variant of lipoprotein lipase is associated with the -93G promoter mutation and an increased risk of coronary artery disease: The Regress Study Group. Clin Genet 1998; 53:27–33.

68. Franceschini G, Sirtori CR, Capurso A et al. A-I$_{Milano}$ apoprotein: decreased high density lipoprotein cholesterol levels with significant lipoprotein modifications and without clinical atherosclerosis in an Italian family. J Clin Invest 1980; 66:892–900.

69. Weisgraber KH, Rall SC Jr, Bersot TP et al. Apolipoprotein AI$_{Milano}$: detection of normal AI in affected subjects and evidence for a cysteine for arginine substitution in the variant AI. J Biol Chem 1983; 258:2508–2513.

70. Gualandri V, Franceschini G, Sirtori CR et al. A-I$_{Milano}$ apoprotein: identification of the complete kindred and evidence of a dominant genetic transmission. Am J Hum Genet 1985; 37:1083–1097.

71. Franceschini G, Sirtori CR, Bosisio E et al. Relationship of the phenotypic expression of the A-I$_{Milano}$ apoprotein with plasma lipid and lipoprotein patterns. Atherosclerosis 1985; 58:159–174.

72. Sirtori CR, Calabresi L, Franceschini G et al. Cardiovascular status of carriers of the apolipoprotein A-I$_{(Milano)}$ mutant: the Limone sul Garda study. Circulation 2001; 103:1949–1954.

73. Duggirala R, Blangero J, Almasy L et al. A major susceptibility locus influencing plasma triglyceride concentrations is located on chromosome 15q in Mexican Americans. Am J Hum Genet 2000; 66:1237–1245.

74. Shearman AM, Ordovas JM, Cupples LA et al. Evidence for a gene influencing the TG/HDL-C ratio on chromosome 7q32.3-qter: a genome-wide scan in the Framingham study. Hum Mol Genet 2000; 9:1315–1320.

75. Klos KL, Kardia SL, Ferrell RE et al. Genome-wide linkage analysis reveals evidence of multiple regions that influence variation in plasma lipid and apolipoprotein levels associated with risk of coronary heart disease. Arterioscler Thromb Vasc Biol 2001; 21:971–978.

76. Peacock JM, Arnett DK, Atwood LD et al. Genome scan for quantitative trait loci linked to high-density lipoprotein cholesterol: the NHLBI Family Heart Study. Arterioscler Thromb Vasc Biol 2001; 21:1823–1828.

77. Arya R, Duggirala R, Almasy L et al. Linkage of high-density lipoprotein-cholesterol concentrations to a locus on chromosome 9p in Mexican Americans. Nature Genet 2002; 30:102–105.

78. Soro A, Pajukanta P, Lilja HE et al. Genomes scans provide evidence for low-HDL-C loci on chromosomes 8q23, 16q24.1-24.2, and 20q13.11 in Finnish families. Am J Hum Genet 2002; 70:1333–1340.

79. Pajukanta P, Allayee H, Krass KL et al. Combined analysis of genome scans of Dutch and Finnish families reveals a susceptibility locus for high-density lipoprotein cholesterol on chromosome 16q. Am J Hum Genet 2003; 72:903–917.

80. Arking DE, Becker DM, Yanek LR et al. KLOTHO allele status and the risk of early-onset occult coronary artery disease. Am J Hum Genet 2003; 72:1154–1161.

81. Wang L, Fan C, Topol SE et al. Mutation of MEF2A in an inherited disorder with features of coronary artery disease. Science 2003; 302:1578–1581.

82. DeFronzo RA, Ferrannini E. Insulin resistance. A multifaceted syndrome responsible for NIDDM, obesity, hypertension, dyslipidemia, and atherosclerotic cardiovascular disease. Diabetes Care 1991; 14:173–194.

83. Reaven GM. Banting lecture 1988. Role of insulin resistance in human disease. Diabetes 1988; 37:1595–1607.

84. Rantala AO, Kauma H, Lilja M et al. Prevalence of the metabolic syndrome in drug-treated hypertensive patients and control subjects. J Intern Med 1999; 245:163–174.

85. Lakka HM, Laaksonen DE, Lakka TA et al. The metabolic syndrome and total and cardiovascular disease mortality in middle-aged men. J Am Med Assoc 2002; 288:2709–2716.

86. Ridker PM, Buring JE, Cook NR et al. C-reactive protein, the metabolic syndrome, and risk of incident cardiovascular events: an 8-year follow-up of 14719 initially healthy American women. Circulation 2003; 107:391–397.

87. Sattar N, Gaw A, Scherbakova O et al. Metabolic syndrome with and without C-reactive protein as a predictor of coronary heart disease and diabetes in the West of Scotland Coronary Prevention Study. Circulation 2003; 108:414–419.

88. Grundy SM. Hypertriglyceridemia, atherogenic dyslipidemia, and the metabolic syndrome. Am J Cardiol 1998; 81:18B–25B.

89. Ford ES, Giles WH, Dietz WH. Prevalence of the metabolic syndrome among US adults: findings from the third National Health and Nutrition Examination Survey. J Am Med Assoc 2002; 287:356–359.

90. Park YW, Zhu S, Palaniappan L et al. The metabolic syndrome: prevalence and associated risk factor findings in the US population from the Third National Health and Nutrition Examination Survey, 1988–1994. Arch Intern Med 2003; 163:427–436.

91. Liese AD, Mayer-Davis EJ, Tyroler HA et al. Familial components of the multiple metabolic syndrome: the ARIC study. Diabetologia 1997; 40:963–970.

92. Hong Y, Pedersen NL, Brismar K et al. Genetic and environmental architecture of the features of the insulin-resistance syndrome. Am J Hum Genet 1997; 60:143–152.

93. Agarwal AK, Arioglu E, De Almeida S et al. AGPAT2 is mutated in congenital generalized lipodystrophy linked to chromosome 9q34. Nature Genet 2002; 31:21–23.

94. Goldin LR, Camp NJ, Keen KJ et al. Analysis of metabolic syndrome phenotypes in Framingham Heart Study families from Genetic Analysis Workshop 13. Genet Epidemiol 2003; 25:S78–S89.

95. Lusis AJ. Atherosclerosis. Nature 2000; 407:233–241.

96. Assmann G, Cullen P, Jossa F et al. Coronary heart disease: reducing the risk: the scientific background to primary and secondary prevention of coronary heart disease. A worldwide view. International Task force for the Prevention of Coronary Heart disease. Arterioscler Thromb Vasc Biol 1999; 19:1819–1824.

97. Gordon DJ, Rifkind BM. High-density lipoprotein – the clinical implications of recent studies. N Engl J Med 1989; 321:1311–1316.

98. Kronenberg F, Kronenberg MF, Kiechl S et al. Role of lipoprotein(a) and apolipoprotein(a) phenotype in atherogenesis: prospective results from the Bruneck study. Circulation 1999; 100:1154–1160.

99. Luft FC. Molecular genetics of human hypertension. J Hypertens 1998; 16:1871–1878.

100. Gerhard GT, Duell PB. Homocysteine and atherosclerosis. Curr Opin Lipidol 1999; 10:417–428.

101. Lusis A, Weinreb A, Drake TA. Genetics of atherosclerosis In: Topol EJ, ed. Textbook of cardiovascular medicine. Philadelphia: Lippincott-Raven, 1998: 2389–2413.

102. Stavljenić-Rukavina A. Electr J Int Fed Clin Chem Lab Med 2003; 14:
http://www.ifcc.org/ejifcc/vol14no2/140206200305n.htm.

103. North KE, Martin LJ, Dyer T et al. HDL cholesterol in females in the Framingham Study is linked to a region of chromosome 2q. BMC Genet 2003; 4(Suppl 1):S98.

104. Martin LJ, North KE, Dyer T et al. 2003. Phenotypic, genetic, and genome-wide structure of the metabolic syndrome. BMC Genet 2003; 4(Suppl 1):S95.

105. Moslehi R, Goldstein AM, Beerman M et al. A genome-wide linkage scan for body mass index on Framingham Heart Study families. BMC Genet 2003; 4(Suppl 1):S97.

106. McQueen MB, Bertram L, Rimm EB et al. A QTL genome scan of the metabolic syndrome and its component traits. BMC Genet 2003; 4(Suppl 1):S96.

107. Stein CM, Song Y, Elston RC et al. Structural equation model-based genome scan for metabolic syndrome. BMC Genet 2003; 4(Suppl 1):S99.

108. Engelman CD, Brady HL, Baron AE et al. Comparison between two analytic strategies to detect linkage to obesity with genetically determined age of onset: The Framingham Heart Study. BMC Genet 2003; 4(Suppl 1):S90.

109. Horne BD, Malhotra A, Camp NJ. Comparison of linkage analysis methods for genome-wide scanning of extended pedigrees, with application to the TG/HDL ratio in the Framingham Heart Study. BMC Genet 2003; 4(Suppl 1):S93.

110. Strug L, Sun L, Corey M. The genetics of cross-sectional and longitudinal BMI. BMC Genet 2003; 4(Suppl 1):S14.

111. Geller F, Dempfle A, Gorg T. Genome scan for BMI and height in the Framingham Heart Study. BMC Genet 2003; 4(Suppl 1):S91.

112. Li X, Wang D, Yang K et al. Comparisons of genome-wide linkage analysis between cross-sectional and longitudinal traits for BMI and total cholesterol in a subsample of the Framingham Heart Study. BMC Genet 2003; 4(Suppl 1):S35.

113. Cheng R, Park N, Hodge SE, Juo S-HH. Comparing two methods to perform linkage analysis of longitudinal family data from the Framingham Family Study. BMC Genet 2003; 4(Suppl 1):S20.

GLOSSARY

Affected sib pair (ASP) analysis A form of non-parametric linkage analysis based on measuring haplotype sharing by siblings who both have the same disease.

Allele One of two or more alternative forms of a given gene.

Association (genetic) The non-random occurrence of a disease or trait and a particular allele or genotype.

Candidate gene A gene whose protein product suggests that it could be involved in the etiology of a particular disease or trait.

CentiMorgan (cM) The unit of genetic distance. Loci 1 cM apart have a 1% probability of recombination during meiosis.

Genetic marker A segment of DNA with an identifiable physical location on a chromosome with varying alleles whose inheritance can be followed. Often referred to simply as a marker.

Genome scan Evaluation of linkage using a panel of several hundred polymorphic markers, distributed across the entire genome.

Genotype Genetic constitution of an individual. Often used to refer to the combination of alleles at any given locus.

Heredity The passing of a trait such as eye color from parent to child. A person 'inherits' these traits through the genes.

Hereditary Transmitted or capable of being transmitted genetically from parent to offspring.

Linkage The association of genes or markers that lie near each other on a chromosome. Linked genes or markers tend to be inherited together.

Linkage analysis A method to identify whether or not alleles from two loci segregate together in families.

Linkage disequilibrium Non-random association of alleles at different loci in a population.

Locus (plural, loci) The position that a gene occupies on a chromosome or within a segment of DNA.

LOD score (log of the odds of linkage or z) A statistical estimate of whether two loci are likely to lie near each other on a chromosome and are therefore likely to be inherited together. A LOD score of 3.0 (odds of 1000 : 1 in favor) or more has been traditionally considered strong evidence in favor of linkage. One that is −2 or less is evidence against linkage.

Non-parametric linkage analysis Several statistical methods of linkage analysis have been developed that do not require specification of a genetic model for a trait locus. The most common approach one will encounter in the literature is the affected sib pair method (ASP).

Quantitative trait locus (QTL) A locus important in determining the phenotype of a continuous character.

Recombination fraction (or θ) For a given pair of loci, the proportion of meioses in which two loci are separated by recombination. Usually signified as θ, values vary between 0 and 0.5.

Restriction fragment length polymorphism (RFLP) Genetic variation at the site where a restriction enzyme cuts a piece of DNA. Such variants affect the size of the resulting fragments.

Susceptibility locus Gene that contributes (or is thought to contribute) to the risk of disease, but which may be neither a necessary nor a sufficient cause of disease.

4

Inflammation and atherothrombosis

Frederick L. Ruberg, Joseph Loscalzo

Higher prevalence rates of tobacco use, hypertension, and dyslipidemia are currently being observed in the developing world, and, concurrently, morbidity and mortality from atherosclerotic disease are also increasing.[1] Previously conceived as a 'natural' degenerative process of aging because of its higher prevalence with advancing age, our understanding of atherosclerosis now holds it to be a pathologic malady that occurs in the context of chronic vascular injury. The body's response to injury is inflammation, and decades of research into the pathogenesis of atherosclerosis have ultimately converged upon a unifying model of chronic inflammation that now serves as our present paradigm of understanding of this disease. Through the prism of inflammation, one may begin to understand more fundamental mechanisms that contribute to the development of atherosclerosis and the causal relationship of various traditional and emerging risk factors. A more rigorous understanding of the molecular mechanisms of vascular wall inflammation will undoubtedly yield new pharmacologic targets that might retard or halt development of the atheroma. Moreover, indices of inflammation that associate with atherosclerosis may predict future morbid or mortal events and response to therapy. This chapter will review the fundamental molecular mechanisms of inflammation as they pertain to atherosclerosis, and thoroughly explore the mounting evidence, both laboratory and clinical, that underlies this model.

Basic mechanisms of inflammation

Inflammation is itself an adaptive, homeostatic mechanism that has evolved as a protective response to cellular injury. Tissue injury – for example infarction, trauma, or infection – initiates a cascade of interactions that constitute the process of inflammation. Central to this mechanism are the circulating leukocytes of the immune system, including monocytes, polymorphonuclear neutrophils (PMN), and B and T lymphocytes. These cells interact with one another and with vascular endothelial cells (EC) via a vast array of surface receptors and released signaling molecules (inflammatory cytokines). The ultimate purpose of the inflammatory response is to sequester and remove the offending substrate and, allow normal, healthy tissue to replace it.

Chronic inflammation specifically involves circulating monocytes (which differentiate into tissue macrophages) and T lymphocytes that are recruited to the site of injury. It is this model of chronic vascular inflammation that has been applied to atherosclerosis and which now shapes our understanding of this disease. Atherosclerosis has long been associated with elevated cholesterol levels, and histologic evaluation of atheromata supported the notion that central to this disease is the accumulation of lipid within the vessel wall.[2] Early animal models of atherosclerosis showed the adherence of leukocytes to the endothelium following exposure to a high-cholesterol diet, suggesting the potential contribution of these inflammatory cells to the development of the atheroma.[3]

Concurrently, advances in our understanding of the fundamental mechanisms of inflammation facilitated the application of these observations to atherosclerosis. At the interface between circulating blood cells and the vessel wall lies the endothelium, a specialized and responsive layer of cells that not only serves a barrier function but is a fundamental participant in the cell–cell signaling interactions that initiate inflammation. The EC mediates adherence and transmigration (diapadesis) of leukocytes from the circulation to the site of injury. EC activation, the mechanisms of which are detailed below, results in the presentation of adhesion molecules on the luminal surface that support leukocyte adhesion.[4] Expression of these molecules occurs both constitutively and inducibly, and is regulated at the level of transcription by nuclear factor κ-B (NFκB).[5] Families of adhesion molecules and their relevant constituents include selectins (E-selectin, P-selectin), integrins (heterodimeric molecules such as vitronectin or $\alpha_v\beta_3$, MAC-1 or $\alpha_M\beta_2$, and GP IIb/IIIa or $\alpha_{2b}\beta_3$), and immunoglobulin superfamily members (intracellular adhesion molecule-1 or ICAM-1, and vascular cell adhesion molecule-1 or VCAM-1).[6] Leukocytes bind to these molecules via specific counter-receptors that mediate rolling, firm adherence, and diapadesis. Endothelial cell activation, and hence the expression of these molecules and the recruitment of leukocytes, occurs under a variety of conditions, including (in part) exposure to specific mediators, including tumor necrosis factor-α (TNF-α), interleukin-1β (IL-1β), and endotoxin, or to substances that directly alter the redox balance of the EC (oxidant stress).[7] Oxidant stress, or the process by which the protective antioxidant mechanisms of the EC are overwhelmed by exposure to oxidant radicals, is another means of EC activation to be discussed briefly below, and is the subject of another chapter of this book.

Under basal circumstances the EC does not express adhesion molecules at significant surface densities; however, upon stimulation these molecules are presented and mediate EC–leukocyte interactions. The process by which leukocytes demarginate and adhere to the EC has been well defined and follows a sequence of specific interactions. Leukocyte rolling is thought to be mediated (in part) by interactions between EC-expressed E-selectin and leukocyte-expressed E-selectin ligand-1 (ESL-1), whereas firm adhesion is probably mediated by EC-expressed ICAM-1 and VCAM-1 binding to leukocyte-expressed MAC-1 and other α_4- and α_D-integrins, respectively.[7] Once adherent, leukocytes are induced to transmigrate through the endothelial cell layer following local exposure to chemotactic mediators, including macrophage chemoattractant protein-1 (MCP-1). In the setting of vascular wall inflammation, these transmigrated leukocytes then participate in further cell–cell signaling through

cytokine release and direct ligand-mediated interactions. In atherosclerosis, following transmigration, leukocytes are activated through these interactions and serve to regulate the progression and/or dissolution of the atheroma, as well as recruiting more inflammatory cells into the lesion.[8]

In addition to its mediation of inflammatory cell recruitment, the EC also presents a non-thrombogenic surface to circulating blood that facilitates laminar flow. Through the carefully orchestrated release and expression of pro- and anticoagulant substances, the EC plays a central role in the regulation of hemostasis. Indeed, the presence of thrombosis or dysregulated hemostasis in the setting of atherosclerosis (atherothrombosis) is predicated upon endothelial cell dysfunction and activation, yielding acute vascular syndromes.[6]

Endothelial cell function is measured by its state of activation and its ability to synthesize and release nitric oxide (NO•) and prostacyclin (PGI$_2$), two critical regulators of vascular tone and platelet activation, aggregation, and adhesion.[9] Endothelial cell dysfunction in the setting of atherosclerotic lesions is a universally accepted phenomenon, and is known to contribute to both the initiation and the propagation of disease.[10] Recent studies support the concept that the level of EC oxidant stress determines the 'health' of the endothelial cell and regulates both gene expression and NO• production. Oxidant stress involves exposure of the EC to toxic oxidant radicals, including hydrogen peroxide (H$_2$O$_2$) and superoxide (•O$_2^-$), that react with and inactivate key cellular proteins and lipids. Oxidant radicals are generated through normal mitochondrial respiration, but are also liberated by cytosolic enzymes, including NAD(P)H oxidase and (under pathologic conditions) nitric oxide synthase (eNOS), or through exposure to various toxins. EC synthesize endogenous antioxidants, including glutathione (GSH/GSSG), that oppose oxidant stress and serve to rectify the normal redox balance of the EC. Dysregulation of key cellular enzymes that are responsible for glutathione disulfide reduction or utilization, including glucose-6-phosphate dehydrogenase (G6PD) and glutathione peroxidase (GPx), can also result in endothelial dysfunction. Plasma antioxidants, including GPx-3 and paraoxonase, also counter EC oxidant stress.[9] As outlined below and in other chapters, mechanisms of inflammation are intricately linked to mechanisms of oxidant stress.

Lesion initiation and triggers of inflammation

Hypercholesterolemia has long been associated with the development and progression of atherosclerosis. Early histolopathologic studies of young adults who died of traumatic (i.e. non-cardiovascular) causes demonstrated infiltration and deposition of lipid in the subintima, forming a preatherosclerotic lesion that became known as the fatty streak.[11] The atherosclerotic lesion itself was characterized by a lipid core with a dense fibrous adluminal layer (cap) that progressively enlarged, reduced vessel luminal diameter, and as a result impaired blood flow. Although early lipid infiltration suggested subsequent progression to the established atheroma, the mechanism leading from one stage to the next was not defined.

The histologic observation of chronic inflammatory cells, including macrophages and T lymphocytes, within the substance of the atheroma provided the first suggestion of a link between the fatty streak and the established atheroma. Animal studies demonstrating that a high-lipid diet can induce localization of inflammatory cells to the endothelium in the absence of a clear atherosclerotic lesion, provided further support

for this causal association between inflammation and the development of atherosclerosis.[3] Coincidentally with advances in the understanding of mechanisms of inflammation, including in part the discovery of the cell adhesion molecules described above, studies of atherosclerosis progressed beyond light microscopy and histopathology and into molecular biology. It is in this realm that the inflammatory hypothesis has garnered significant support.

It is now clear that inflammatory cells bind EC in the setting of hyperlipidemia owing to abnormal EC activation and expression of adhesion molecules that recruit the leukocytes into the subintima (Figure 4.1). Cholesterol feeding results in the upregulation of VCAM-1 and ICAM-1 synthesis and expression, as well as of both E- and P-selectin.[12,13] Hyperlipidemia and the subintimal deposition of lipid seems to be the underlying trigger that promotes EC dysfunction and activation in atherosclerosis, a theory supported not only by the observational histological evidence presented above, but also by rigorous mechanistic studies. Concurrent with abnormal expression of adhesion molecules, additional perturbations in EC homeostasis are observed in hyperlipidemia, including abnormal NO• production and dysregulated release of hemostatic

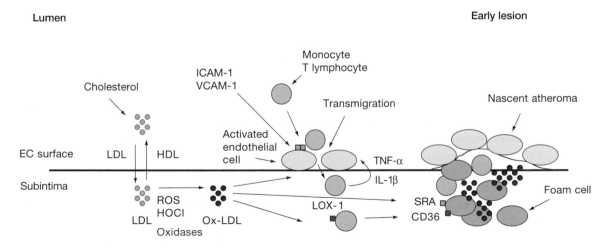

Figure 4.1 Initiation of the atherosclerotic lesion. Low-density lipoprotein (LDL) cholesterol particles diffuse into the subintima, where they are trapped. Oxidative modification of LDL to Ox-LDL occurs following reactions with reactive oxygen species (ROS), hypochlorous acid (HOCl), or cellular oxidases. Ox-LDL stimulates endothelial cell (EC) activation and macrophage uptake of lipid via stimulation of LOX-1 and upregulation of CD36 and SRA to form foam cells. Activated EC express adhesion molecules such as vascular cell adhesion molecule-1 (VCAM-1) and intracellular adhesion molecule-1 (ICAM-1), which recruit circulating macrophages and T lymphocytes into the subintima. Macrophages produce inflammatory cytokines such as tumor necrosis factor-α (TNF-α) and interleukin-1β (IL-1β), which further activate EC. HDL, high-density lipoprotein

substances, including decreased tissue plasminogen activator (tPA) and increased plasminogen activator inhibitor-1 (PAI-1).[14]

EC activation is a clear hallmark of early and advanced atherosclerosis, and although the mechanism by which the EC becomes activated is currently the subject of intense investigation, the association between EC activation and inflammation is now firmly established. Low-density lipoprotein (LDL) cholesterol particles diffuse through the EC luminal membrane and, if not metabolized within the cell, pass into the subintima, where they become trapped. Reverse transport from the subintima back into the circulation is mediated by high-density lipoprotein (HDL) particles, providing a means by which pathologic lipid deposition can be diminished. Once trapped in the subintima, the LDL particle is modified by oxidation, yielding oxidized apoprotein side chains, lipid hydroperoxides, and lysophospholipids, termed minimally modified or oxidized LDL (ox-LDL).[15] LDL oxidation may occur through a variety of reactions with substances such as metal ions, reactive nitrogen species, reactive oxygen species, macrophage oxidase enzymes (such as myeloperoxidase or phosphoplipase A_2), or leukocyte-derived hypochlorous acid (HOCl).[16] LDL oxidation appears to be a fundamental event in the development of the atherosclerotic lesion and the initiation of the inflammatory cascade. Ox-LDL can induce inflammatory cytokines, such as IL-1β and TNF-α, from tissue macrophages and T lymphocytes that are present in the vessel wall. Both directly and indirectly, ox-LDL pathologically alters the redox balance of the EC to contribute to the activated phenotype. Oxidized LDL also stimulates vascular smooth muscle cell (VSMC) migration from the vessel media via stimulation of the VSMC ox-LDL receptor-1 (LOX-1). LOX-1 engagement triggers macrophage accumulation of lipid to form the 'foam' cell noted on lesion histology, via the induction of scavenger receptor A (SRA) and CD-36, and supports the production of extracellular matrix proteins that form the fibrous cap of the lesion.[8]

Lesion propagation

Endothelial cell oxidant stress induced by the presence of oxidized LDL in the subintima probably then induces abnormal levels of adhesion molecule expression through the induction of NFκB and genes under its transcriptional control, including VCAM-1 and ICAM-1.[17] Coincidentally, the bioavailable levels of nitric oxide are also reduced, either through oxidative modification or through dysregulated synthesis of NO• by eNOS. Indeed, eNOS can become uncoupled in the setting of substrate deprivation that may occur in atherosclerosis (specifically, decreased levels of tetrahydrobiopterin or BH_4, or NADPH, or decreased L-arginine availability), to produce superoxide rather than nitric oxide. Both mechanisms probably participate in the reduction of bioavailable NO• resulting in the abnormalities of vascular tone and platelet function observed in atherosclerosis.[18] Indeed, if eNOS can be coaxed to produce more NO• (in overexpression models), NFκB activation can be inhibited.[19] Furthermore, perhaps shedding light upon the observation that atherosclerosis tends to occur at branch points in vessels where flow is turbulent, shear stress-response elements have been defined in antioxidant genes such as superoxide dismutase (SOD) which, when downregulated, may accentuate EC dysfunction.[20] Endothelial cell activation may be potentiated through the action of protease-activated receptors (PAR), G-protein coupled membrane proteins that can also induce NFκB when stimulated.[21]

Once adherent, monocytes and T lymphocytes transmigrate through the EC layer into the subintima following exposure to cytokines, including MCP-1 (Figure 4.2). Double-transgenic apo E-null mice also lacking the genes for either MCP-1 or its receptor CCR2 demonstrate atherosclerotic lesions with fewer infiltrated monocytes.[22] Other potential mediators of leukocyte transmigration include interleukin-8 (IL-8) and interferon-γ (IFN-γ).[23] Eotaxin may induce eosinophil infiltration into atherosclerotic lesions and promote subsequent mast cell differentiation.[24] Following transmigration, leukocytes then become activated. Specifically, monocytes morphologically transform into macrophages and express surface receptors that foster the phagocytosis of the deposited lipid. As with EC activation, the presence of ox-LDL participates in the upregulation of the macrophage surface scavenger receptors SRA and CD36 that bind ox-LDL and ultimately result in endocytosis. These proteins are under the transcriptional control of the peroxisome proliferator-activated receptor-γ (PPAR-γ).[25] Via SRA

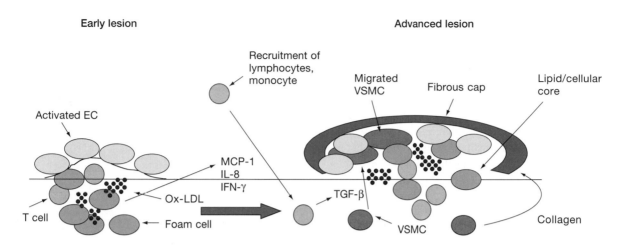

Figure 4.2 Propagation of the atherosclerotic lesion. Inflammatory cells are recruited into the developing plaque by the expression of chemotactic factors such as interleukin-8 (IL-8), interferon-γ (IFN-γ), and macrophage chemoattractant protein-1 (MCP-1). Vascular smooth muscle cells (VSMC) migrate from the media to the intima following stimulation by transforming growth factor-β (TGF-β). VSMC produce collagen, which forms the substance of the fibrous cap of the mature lesion. The interior of the lesion is populated predominantly by lipid-laden macrophages (foam cells) and cholesteryl ester. EC, endothelial cell; Ox-LDL, oxidized low-density lipoprotein

and CD36, macrophages accumulate significant cholesterol such that, morphologically, these cells appear riddled with lipid inclusion droplets, and hence are termed 'foam' cells, known to characterize the early atherosclerotic lesion. Cholesterol efflux from macrophages (a homeostatic response to pathologic lipid accumulation) occurs concurrently, mediated in part by another PPAR-γ regulated protein, ATP binding cassette transporter A1 (ABCA1).[26] Lipid accumulation supports the macrophage expression of cytokines such as IL-1β and TNF-α, that results in further EC activation and VSMC production of matrix proteins. Additional chemokines, including granulocyte–macrophage colony-stimulating factor-1 (GMCSF-1) and macrophage colony-stimulating factor-1 (MCSF-1), also support macrophage expression of SRA.[27] LDL deposition and oxidation is countered by HDL, both through reverse cholesterol transport and through antioxidant mechanisms conferred by the HDL particle.[28] HDL itself complexes with plasma antioxidant enzymes, including paraoxonase, platelet-activating factor acetylhydrolase, and lecithin–cholesterol acyltransferase, which, when delivered to the subintima, may counter LDL oxidation and promote atheroprotection.[29,30] The statin class of drugs, which block cholesterol synthesis through inhibition of 3-hydroxy-3-

methylglutaryl co-enzyme-A (HMG Co-A) reductase, are thought to reduce mortality through both LDL lowering and pleiotropic anti-inflammatory benefits, as described below.

The vulnerable plaque and lesion disruption

Inflammatory cytokines produced by macrophages and T lymphocytes stimulate the smooth muscle cells of the media to proliferate, migrate toward the vessel lumen, and produce extracellular matrix proteins such as collagen and fibronectin. As the lesion develops, the central core, consisting of deposited lipid (mostly esterified cholesterol) and both viable and necrotic inflammatory cells, is covered by a thick fibrous cap composed of migrated VSMC and extracellular matrix. As the lesion grows adluminally, the vessel lumen shrinks and blood flow is compromised, especially under conditions of increased demand, producing clinical ischemic syndromes. The classic view that this relentless process occurs at a rather glacial pace has recently been challenged. Evidence now suggests that lesion progression occurs in bursts, prompted by physical disruption of the fibrous cap of the plaque.[8]

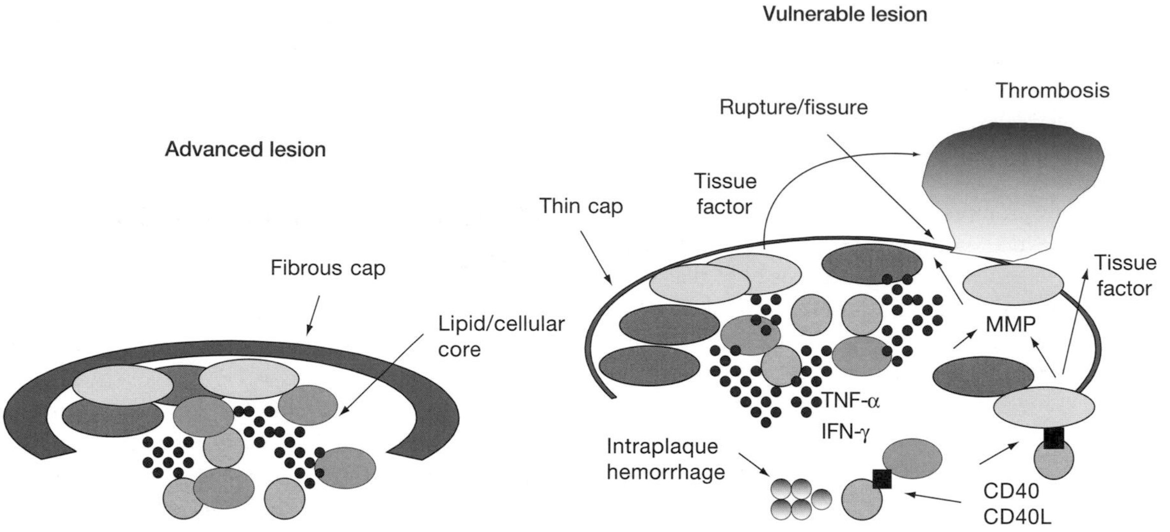

Figure 4.3 The vulnerable lesion. A thin fibrous cap marked by areas of fissure/rupture typifies the vulnerable plaque. Cap degradation by matrix metalloproteinases (MMP) and inhibition of collagen synthesis by interferon-γ (IFN-γ) are in part responsible for the loss of cap integrity. Signaling interactions between CD40- and CD40L-expressing cells result in MMP, cytokine, and tissue factor (TF) expression. Cap degradation exposes the thrombotic core of the lesion to circulating blood, fostering the development of a superimposed thrombus. Intraplaque hemorrhage from vasa vasorum rupture may also contribute to plaque vulnerability. TNF-α, tumor necrosis factor-α

The fibrous cap of the atheroma separates the subendothelial lipid-dense core of the lesion from circulating blood and, presents a non-thrombogenic surface that permits flow. Fissure or rupture of the plaque allows blood to contact the highly thrombogenic subendothelium, permitting thrombus development (atherothrombosis; Figure 4.3). Clinically manifest as acute coronary syndromes (ACS), the degree of luminal occlusion by the thrombus results in a definable clinical syndrome forming a continuum in the coronary circulation from unstable angina to non-ST segment elevation myocardial infarction (NSTEMI) to STEMI. Previously in ACS, an atherosclerotic lesion was conceptualized as an isolated plaque that could support thrombosis (culprit lesion). A consensus has now developed defining a broader sense of vulnerability to acute coronary events, and, a vulnerable plaque is now defined as one that is thrombosis prone but which occurs in the context of a vulnerable patient with other vulnerable plaques and pathologic dispositions toward the development of ACS.[31] These predisposing factors include hypercoagulability, at both the local and the systemic level, and systemic inflammation.

Histologically, a vulnerable plaque is characterized by a thin cap with a large lipid core, and/or evidence of active inflammation (large T-cell or macrophage infiltrates) or cap dissolution. Such lesions are prone to intraplaque hemorrhage or luminal thrombus following further disruption of the fibrous cap.[32]

The molecular cues that prompt a previously stable developing lesion with a thick fibrous cap to become vulnerable are the subject of intensive research. Whereas a clearly defined mechanism remains elusive, a number of clinical and laboratory observations have provided significant insight. Specific collagenases or cap degrading enzymes, matrix metalloproteinases (MMP), that have a defined role in normal vascular remodeling, have been identified in atherosclerotic lesions and implicated in cap degradation.[33] These enzymes are probably produced by the EC and VSMC following stimulation with the inflammatory cytokines TNF-α, IL-1β, and IL-18.[34] Concurrently, VSMC production of collagen is reduced, following exposure to the cytokine IFN-γ. Other matrix degrading enzymes, including neutrophil elastase[35] and cathepsin S,[36] may also be important in cap erosion. Signaling interactions between macrophages and lymphocytes also contribute to plaque destabilization. CD40 and CD40 ligand (CD40L or CD154) are surface proteins coexpressed by macrophages, activated T cells, EC, and VSMC (platelets express CD40L).[37] CD40/CD40L interactions represent key signaling events that operate at the interface between inflammation and thrombosis. Engagement prompts expression of IFN-γ and MMP (specifically MMP isoforms 1, 8, and 13) that facilitate cap dissolution, as well as tissue factor (TF) that initiates thrombogenesis upon exposure to circulating factor VII. Interruption of CD40/CD40L signaling in a mouse model of atherosclerosis drastically reduced lesion progression and new lesion formation.[38] Although the trigger that initiates CD40 expression is unknown, a potential culprit may be ox-LDL.[39] Elevated lipoprotein levels have been associated with increased expression of monocyte CD40 and platelet CD40L. Endothelial cell CD40 engagement induces oxidant stress and, as such, reduces bioavailable NO$^\bullet$ and activates the expression of adhesion molecules.[40] Furthermore, CD40L engagement can induce the expression of MCP-1, IL-1, IL-6, and TNF-α, highlighting the important role of this signaling pathway in both plaque progression and destabilization.[21] Finally, released soluble CD40L (sCD40L) liberated from activated platelets has emerged as a potentially useful biomarker in the prediction of adverse cardiac events (see below).

These mechanisms probably contribute to either superficial erosion or frank rupture of the overlying fibrous cap, resulting in a thrombotic event. Not all atherothrombotic events are clinically manifest, as antithrombotic mechanisms and/or collateral vessel growth and recruitment may limit the hemodynamic consequences of the acute event. Organization of the thrombus may result in an acute acceleration of the inflammatory process, and it is by this means that a plaque may dramatically increase in size over a short period of time. Additionally, intraplaque hemorrhage also probably contributes to rapid plaque expansion. Plaque neovascularization via proliferation of the vasa vasorum has been observed, and consequently, intraplaque rupture of these microvessels may lead to focal hemorrhage.[41] In support of this hypothesis, a histopathologic study demonstrating the presence of glycophorin A (a specific erythrocyte surface protein) within the lipid core of advanced human atherosclerotic lesions has recently been published. These data suggest that intraplaque hemorrhage may result in the accumulation of free cholesterol from the extravasated erythrocyte membranes, prompting rapid plaque expansion and, potentially, destabilization.[42]

Additional triggers of lesion formation

Through the context of inflammation, other conventional and non-conventional risk factors for the development of atherosclerosis may be better understood. Elevated levels of lipoprotein (a) (Lp(a)), a plasma lipoprotein similar to LDL but composed of apoprotein B100 and apoprotein (a), have been associated with the accelerated development and progression of atherosclerosis. Although the mechanism by which Lp(a) promotes atherosclerosis remains controversial, Lp(a) may contribute to VSMC proliferation by inhibition of transforming growth factor-β (TGF-β) (an inhibitor of VSMC proliferation), promote endothelial dysfunction, and potentiate thrombosis.[14] Furthermore, a potential link between Lp(a) and inflammation has been suggested by the observation that Lp(a) can stimulate cultured macrophages to produce the proinflammatory cytokine IL-8.[43] Numerous studies have noted an epidemiological association between Lp(a) and the development of atherosclerotic disease, including a recently published trial of elderly patients that demonstrated a proportional increase in the incidence of stroke, death from vascular disease, or death from any cause in men with Lp(a) levels as low as 8.2 mg/dl.[44]

Hypertension promotes EC and VSMC oxidant stress, in large part through the action of angiotensin II (AII), and as such contributes to the inflammatory milieu of the atherosclerotic lesion. AII induces NAD(P)H oxidase activity and elicits the production of superoxide.[45] Perhaps through this mechanism, AII can induce VCAM expression in EC, as well as MCP-1 and IL-6 expression.[46]

Diabetes mellitus, obesity, and dyslipidemia (the metabolic syndrome) often coassociate as risk factors for atherosclerosis. Hyperglycemia (and/or hyperinsulinemia) results in the non-enzymatic glycation and oxidation of proteins, termed advanced glycation endproducts (AGE), that bind a specific EC receptor

(RAGE, or receptor for AGE). RAGE engagement results in the activation of different signal transduction pathway mechanisms, including p21^{ras}, erk 1/2 kinase, and NFκB, promoting EC activation, adhesion molecule expression, and inflammation.[47] Reduced bioavailable NO$^\bullet$ has also been observed in diabetic patients, perhaps resulting from enhanced superoxide production by NAD(P)H oxidase and eNOS uncoupling, as well as eNOS inhibition by asymmetric dimethylarginine (ADMA).[48] In obese individuals at risk for atherosclerosis, adipocytes can synthesize the inflammatory cytokines TNF-α and IL-6, a finding that associates with insulin resistance.[49]

Finally, a link between chronic infection and vascular inflammation leading to atherosclerosis has also been explored. Extravascular infection and the production of inflammatory cytokines have been associated with endothelial cell dysfunction. Furthermore, induction of an autoimmune response that may support vascular inflammation following vascular infection with *Chlamydia pneumoniae* and *Helicobacter pylori* has been suggested. Autoantibodies to microbial heat-shock proteins have been demonstrated that can activate EC, macrophages, and VSMC.[50] Endothelial cell toll-like receptors (TLR), which recognize bacterial pathogens, may also be involved in EC activation and the induction of inflammation.[51] To date, clinical studies have produced inconsistent results, including the recent publication of two large clinical trials of azithromycin that failed to demonstrate a secondary prevention benefit in patients with known coronary atherosclerosis with either short- or long-term (5 days and 3 months, respectively) treatment.[52,53] The relationship of infection to atherosclerosis is discussed elsewhere in this book.

Serologic assessments of inflammation

The medical care of patients with known atherosclerotic disease, or those at risk for atherosclerotic disease, would be dramatically simplified if adverse events could be predicted non-invasively. Although various imaging modalities have been developed to permit a non-invasive means to characterize plaques, none has yet emerged as superior to invasive cardiac

Table 4.1 Potential serologic biomarkers of inflammation

C-reactive protein
Soluble CD40-ligand
Soluble cell adhesion molecules
    ICAM-1
    VCAM-1
    E-selectin
Leukocyte-derived enzymes
    Myeloperoxidase
    Lipoprotein-associated phospholipase A$_2$
    Secretory phospholipase A$_2$ type II
    Matrix metalloproteinases
Endothelial progenitor cells

ICAM-1, intracellular adhesion molecule-1; VCAM-1, vascular cell adhesion molecule-1

catheterization in the assessment of lesion stenosis or overall plaque burden (magnetic resonance (MR) angiography and ultrasonography are established in peripheral vascular disease). Moreover, no technique, not even catheterization, can reliably predict which lesions will ultimately become vulnerable and result in a morbid or mortal event. Therefore, considerable attention has been paid to measurable serum biomarkers and their potential to predict cardiovascular events (Table 4.1). Cholesterol level is perhaps the most important predictor for the development and progression of atherosclerosis and, if followed longitudinally, can reflect response to directed therapy with the proportionate reduction in risk. Numerous large prospective trials have demonstrated a reduction in the incidence of adverse cardiovascular endpoints with lipid-lowering therapy in patients at risk for or with known atherosclerotic disease. But with the advent of our current understanding of vascular inflammation in atherosclerosis, investigators began measuring systemic markers of inflammation and associating levels with the development of cardiovascular events. Virtually every component in the inflammatory cascade has been studied (to varying degrees), and many associate strongly and independently with the development of atherosclerosis. Moreover, as with lipid levels, some of these markers have been shown to respond to conventional therapy for atherosclerosis, and connote a reduction in risk.

C-reactive protein (CRP)

There is now a wealth of observational, prospective, and basic scientific data associating the acute-phase reactant C-reactive protein (CRP) with the development of atherosclerosis and adverse events. In fact, CRP may ultimately prove to be a more robust predictor of cardiovascular events than LDL cholesterol.[54] Studies now suggest that a serum high-sensitivity CRP (hsCRP) assay concentration in excess of 3 mg/l corresponds to a high risk for vascular events[55]. CRP may even predict the development of type 2 diabetes, hypertension, or vascular disease in patients without known disease.[16,56] CRP was initially thought to reflect the overall systemic inflammatory state, and is utilized by medical specialties to assess localized or systemic infection and autoimmune activation. As with LDL cholesterol, however, there is accumulating evidence supporting the role of CRP as a participant, rather than simply a bystander, in the development of atherosclerotic disease.[21]

Evidence supporting CRP as an effector in the development of atherosclerosis is derived predominantly from *in vitro* studies. EC exposed to recombinant CRP downregulate eNOS transcription, with a resultant reduction in bioavailable NO$^\bullet$.[57] Perhaps through modulation of the EC redox state, CRP can upregulate EC adhesion molecule expression, stimulate endothelin (ET-1), IL-6, and MCP-1 release, and thus alter vascular tone and facilitate macrophage LDL uptake.[58] EC activation in the setting of CRP and hyperglycemia is augmented, suggesting a possible link between diabetes and the development of vascular disease.[59] Finally, CRP also has deleterious effects upon VSMC, in that upregulation of angiotensin II receptor type I has been noted, with associated increased cell migration, proliferation, and ROS production.[60]

Clinically, CRP is an attractive biomarker to measure for numerous reasons. Unlike inflammatory cytokines, it has a relatively long half-life with no identified circadian variation. Furthermore, it is easily measured by commercially available high-sensitivity assays and is stable after freezing and thawing. CRP has consistently and reproducibly been associated with prediction of cardiovascular risk in a wide variety of patients encompassing more than a dozen population-based clinical trials.[16] Its ability to predict first myocardial infarctions, stroke, or peripheral vascular events,

has propelled CRP to the forefront of clinical biomarkers. CRP level adds additional prognostic information to the Framingham risk score, and even predicts adverse vascular events in the absence of hyperlipidemia.[61]

Again, similar to LDL, CRP can be followed with therapy, demonstrating a reduction in levels that is associated with a reduction in the risk of events. As previously mentioned, statin therapy significantly reduces the risk of death, myocardial infarction, and stroke in patients with or without known disease; however, this benefit may transcend its intended role of lipid lowering, in that reduction in risk has been observed even in patients with minimal change in LDL levels.[62] CRP may provide a window into the risk profile of such patients. Clinically, the anti-inflammatory role of statins is forged by the observation that CRP levels fall with statin therapy in a manner coincidental with reduction in risk. Short-term (16 weeks) statin therapy given to patients with ACS can reduce CRP,[63] and long-term statin use and CRP level reduction have been associated in numerous large, prospective clinical databases. Whereas CRP and LDL levels vary independently, both fall with statin therapy and both independently reflect risk reduction. Moreover, a reduction of CRP levels with statin therapy may predict cardiovascular risk even in individuals with normal lipid levels.[16] It is in this population of relatively low-risk individuals that CRP may provide the most clinically useful information. Therefore, CRP may soon emerge as a widely utilized screening tool, in conjunction with lipoprotein levels, to assess patients at risk for cardiovascular disease.

CD40 ligand (CD40L)

The significant experimental evidence linking CD40 and CD40L interactions with atherosclerosis has prompted a number of clinical studies to examine the potential association between CD40L and vascular disease. Rather than its membrane form, serum soluble CD40L (sCD40L) is probably derived from activated platelets or T lymphocytes, and has been associated with the development of cardiovascular events in a number of different patient populations.[64] Among patients with known coronary atherosclerosis, sCD40L was shown to be elevated with both stable and unstable anginal syndromes, with levels correlating to risk of death or myocardial infarction.[65] Following percutaneous coronary intervention (PCI), preprocedural level of sCD40L predicts restenosis event rates and identifies a subset of patients most likely to benefit from GPIIb/IIIa receptor blockade.[66] Elevated levels of sCD40L have been associated with diabetes mellitus independently of other conventional risk factors for atherosclerosis, including CRP. Moreover, as with CRP and LDL cholesterol, therapy intended to reduce glucose levels (troglitazone) also resulted in a reduction in sCD40L level, suggesting the utility of sCD40L as a potential measure by which therapy can be adjusted.[67] The potential application of this class of agents (the thiazolidinediones) to the treatment of vascular disease will be expanded below.

Adhesion molecules

The measurement of soluble EC adhesion molecules is a logical extension of the inflammatory hypothesis of atherosclerosis. Soluble VCAM-1, ICAM-1, and E-selectin have attracted particular attention, as all have been associated to varying degrees with adverse cardiovascular events in patients with atherosclerosis and without known disease.[68] None, however, has emerged as clinically relevant in the management of patients, despite early promise. A notable exception may prove to be soluble ICAM-1, as more consistent and robust demonstrated associations have been noted with not only coronary atherosclerosis but also peripheral vascular disease.[69] Debate continues over the mechanism by which soluble forms of the molecules are released into the circulation, reach steady state, and are metabolized.

Leukocyte enzymes/cytokines

Oxidation of LDL particles within the subintima is widely accepted to be a cardinal event in the development of the atherosclerotic lesion. The mechanism by which oxidation occurs, however, is unclear. Leukocyte-derived myeloperoxidase may play a particularly important role in the oxidation of subintimal lipid via the production of HOCl. Myeloperoxidase, despite being associated with disease progression, has also been implicated in the development of plaque vulnerability. The recent observation that a single plasma myeloperoxidase measurement in patients presenting with chest discomfort could predict subsequent

adverse cardiac events highlights the potential utility of this biomarker in the risk stratification of patients in the emergency room setting.[70]

Phospholipase A_2 (PLA_2) is a widely distributed membrane-associated enzyme that hydrolyzes phospholipids at the *sn*-2 position to generate free fatty acids and lysophospholipids (specifically lysophosphatidylcholine or lysoPC). LysoPC has been shown *in vivo* to activate endothelial cells, function as a monocyte chemotactic agent, and promote VSMC proliferation, or, under different circumstances, VSMC death.[21]

Elevated levels of lipoprotein-associated phospholipase A_2 (Lp-PLA_2) have been noted in patients with known coronary atherosclerosis, and can predict events.[71] Lp-PLA_2 associates with LDL in the plasma and has been noted in the subintima of both normal and atherosclerotic vessels, suggesting a role in the initiation of disease.[72] Prospective data linking Lp-PLA_2 are inconsistent, however, and there is further evidence suggesting that this molecule may actually serve an antioxidant – and hence an antiatherogenic – function as well.[21]

Secretory PLA_2 type II (sPLA_2-II), a different form of PLA_2, is an acute-phase protein that accumulates in inflammatory fluids, with plasma levels rising in settings of systemic infection or inflammation, analogous to CRP. Induction of sPLA_2 expression can occur following stimulation with proinflammatory cytokines, including TNF-α, IL-1, IL-6, IFN-γ, and ox-LDL. Histologic studies of atherosclerotic lesions have identified sPLA2-II in all cellular components of the lesion, and population studies of patients suggest that sPLA2-II plasma levels predict the development of cardiovascular events.[73,74]

MMP are zinc-containing enzymes with proteolytic activity directed against collagen, elastin, and proteoglycans. Over 20 different MMP isoforms exist, many of which have been identifed in the atherosclerotic plaque and are thought to play an important role in the dissolution of the fibrous cap of the lesion, as well as facilitating monocyte recruitment and VSMC migration.[33] Circulating levels of MMP-9 have been associated with cardiovascular mortality in patients with known cardiovascular atherosclerosis.[75] Further evidence suggests that polymorphisms in the MMP-9 gene may connote an increased risk for atherothrombotic events.[76]

Elevated levels of particular inflammatory cytokines, including TNF-α and IL-6, have been observed to predict initial cardiac events, but are practically difficult to measure, owing in part to their short half-lives.[16] Fibrinogen, also an acute-phase reactant and essential clotting factor, has been evaluated and consistently linked to atherothrombotic events, perhaps underlying the concept that hypercoagulability and inflammation are entwined in the vulnerable patient and not specifically the vulnerable plaque.[77]

Endothelial progenitor cells

Measurement of circulating endothelial progenitor cells (EPC), derived from bone marrow, has yielded tantalizing associations with the development of atherosclerosis. EPC (identified by their uptake of acetylated LDL and binding of *Ulex* lectin) are thought to arise from a monocyte/macrophage lineage and may participate in the maintenance of normally functioning endothelium by localizing and regenerating injured or activated EC.[78] In a small study of 45 patients without known vascular disease, the circulating level of EPCs was inversely related both to Framingham risk score and to normal endothelial function as determined by brachial reactivity.[79] These early findings suggest that depletion of EPC stores may occur in the setting of the chronic endothelial injury observed in atherosclerosis, and may ultimately prove a useful surrogate marker in the assessment of risk.

Pharmacologic interventions

Elucidation of the mechanisms of inflammation that contribute to the development of atherosclerosis has yielded novel targets against which pharmacologic agents have been developed in an effort to retard, halt, or even regress disease. The measurement of clinical biomarkers has already proved efficacious, not only in predicting outcomes, but also in monitoring the overall disease state and the response to these new therapies. Serendipitously, it is commonly observed that agents devised to target one aspect of the inflammatory process beneficially affect other pathways as well, highlighting the complex relationships that ultimately produce the disease phenotype (Table 4.2).

Statin agents were devised to address a risk predisposition present in the majority of patients with atherosclerosis – hypercholesterolemia. Statins inhibit the rate-limiting enzyme in cholesterol synthesis, 3-hydroxy-3-methylglutaryl-coenzyme A reductase, and as such result in the upregulation of LDL receptors in hepatocytes, leading to increased LDL uptake and clearance from the circulation. With statin therapy, serum LDL levels fall considerably and serum HDL levels rise slightly; however, it became evident that the salutory effects of statin therapy transcended their lipid-lowering capabilities. Statins are now widely held to be immunomodulatory drugs with the potential to exert anti-inflammatory effects. Statins have been shown *in vitro* to inhibit IFN-γ-induced major histocompatibility complex II (MHC-II)-mediated T-cell activation, as well as inhibiting peripheral blood monocyte adhesion molecule expression.[80,81] The second-messenger systems Akt and Rho/Rho-kinase are also induced by statins, resulting in a host of potentially beneficial antiatherogenic downstream events, including the potentiation of NO•, in part through eNOS phosphorylation;[82,83] inhibition of EC expression of tissue factor;[84] inhibition of VSMC migration;[85] and mobilization of endothelial progenitor cells.[86] Numerous studies have demonstrated the efficacy of statin treatment in the absence of serum lipid reduction, including a decrease in plaque volume,[87] reduced tissue factor (TF) expression and macrophage accumulation,[88] and reduced VCAM-1 and cytokine expression[89] in experimental animal models. Studies have also observed a reduction in MMP, VCAM-1, and IL-1β expression with statin therapy.[90] Human studies have also suggested a statin benefit, as measured by a reduction in adverse cardiovascular outcomes without significant lipid lowering.[91] Furthermore, the studies of statin therapy and CRP reduction discussed above emphasize an immunomodulatory effect independent of LDL or HDL level.[55]

As atherosclerosis is an inflammatory process, conventional anti-inflammatory agents should be efficacious in slowing disease progression. Despite being clearly beneficial as antithrombotic agents, aspirin and other non-steroidal anti-inflammatory drugs (NSAIDs) have not proved beneficial in retarding atheroma progression. NSAIDs inhibit both cyclooxygenase (COX) isoforms 1 and 2, and thereby slow the generation of prostaglandins from arachidonic acid.

Table 4.2   Immunomodulatory effects of selected pharmacologic agent classes

Drug class	Mechanism of action	Observed benefit
Statin	Inhibition of HMG-CoA reductase	LDL lowering Antioxidant Restoration of endothelial function Antithrombotic Plaque 'stabilizing'
NSAID	COX inhibition	Equivocal effects on endothelial function Both pro- and antithrombotic (varies with specific drug)
Thiazolidinedione	PPAR-α and –γ agonist	May stimulate macrophage uptake of LDL May restore endothelial function

HMG-CoA, 3-hydroxy-3-methylglutaryl coenzyme A ; LDL, low-density lipoprotein; COX, cyclooxygenase; PPAR, peroxisome proliferator-activated receptor

The prostaglandin thromboxane A_2 is a potent platelet activator, and the inhibition of platelet COX-1 slows platelet activation and thrombogenesis. Both COX-1 and COX-2 are expressed in atherosclerotic plaques.[92] The advent of selective COX-2 antagonists prompted evaluation of these new agents as potential immunomodulators that may slow the progression of atherosclerosis. Although there is considerable literature regarding COX-2 inhibition and its propensity for or resistance to thrombosis,[93] studies examining the development of atherosclerosis are inconsistent. COX-2 inhibition has been shown to improve,[94] have a neutral effect on,[95] or exacerbate[96] endothelial cell dysfunction. Moreover, studies of COX-2 inhibition in experimental animals have yielded similarly conflicting results, spanning the spectrum from acceleration to retardation of atherosclerosis.[93] To date, no adequately sized prospective trial of COX-2 antagonists in human atherosclerosis progression has been performed.

The peroxisome proliferator-activated receptor (PPAR) family of nuclear transcriptional regulators are the targets of a unique class of insulin sensitizing agents, the thiazolidinediones (TZD), which serve as PPAR agonists. PPAR-γ is known to be expressed in adipocytes and functions as an important regulator of cellular differentiation and metabolic regulation, controlling the expression of genes such as HMG Co-A reductase, lipoprotein lipase, and apolipoprotein A-I. PPAR-α was known to be more widely expressed (heart, liver, kidney) and to regulate fatty acid β-oxidation and apolipoprotein expression.[97] More recent work has demonstrated both isoforms in the major constituents of the vascular wall (including macrophages, EC, and VSMC), as well as in atherosclerotic lesions.[97] PPAR-γ has been identified as a modulator of inflammation; however, whether it serves a pro- or an anti-inflammatory role remains controversial. Agonists of PPAR-γ have been shown to decrease the inflammatory cytokines TNF-α, IL-1β, IFN-γ, and IL-6, as well as the collagenase MMP-9.[98–101] Conversely, PPAR-γ stimulation by ox-LDL upregulates CD36 expression and potentiates macrophage foam-cell formation.[102] This effect may be balanced by concurrent PPAR-γ induction of cholesterol efflux via the ATP-binding cassette receptor-1 (ABCA1).[26] PPAR-γ may also be involved in the induction of EC apoptosis.[103] There are similar conflicting results concerning the role of PPAR-α as both an anti-inflammatory (through the inhibition of endothelial-cell NFκB activation[104]) and a proinflammatory effector.[105] Early clinical studies evaluating the efficacy of TZD as anti-inflammatory agents have yielded some encouraging results, including the demonstration of a reduction in plasma inflammatory markers, including CRP and fibrinogen in patients with coronary atherosclerosis.[106] Further, PPAR-γ agonism by TZD may help restore the redox balance of the EC in hypercholesterolemia through the suppression of NAD(P)H oxidase expression and subsequent reduction of super-oxide production while potentiating bioavailable NO[107] Although the findings are rather inconsistent, the potential utility of the TZD class as antiatherosclerotic agents remains promising and is the subject of ongoing investigation.

Conclusion

Previously dismissed as an aging process that medical science was powerless to alter, atherosclerosis is now widely viewed as a chronic inflammatory disease that may some day respond to targeted therapy. Advancements in our basic understanding of the molecular mechanisms of vascular wall inflammation are now yielding novel targets for pharmacotherapy and gene therapy that may affect the course of disease. Measurable indices of inflammation predict risk for atherothrombotic events, even in individuals with previously unrecognized atherosclerosis, and may be used to follow response to therapy. Through the prism of inflammation, lines of previously independent investigation now appear to converge, revealing an ever more complex interdependency.

References

1. Ezzati M, Lopez AD, Rodgers A et al. Selected major risk factors and global and regional burden of disease. Lancet 2002; 360:1347–1360.
2. Ross R, Harker L. Hyperlipidemia and atherosclerosis. Science 1976; 193:1094–1100.
3. Poole J, Florey H. Changes in the endothelium of the aorta and the behavior of macrophages in experimental atheroma of rabbits. J Pathol Bacteriol 1958; 75:245–253.
4. Luscinskas PD, Francis W, Gimbrone MA. Endothelial-dependent mechanisms in chronic inflammation leukocyte recruitment. Annu Rev Med 1996; 47:413–421.
5. Rainer de Martin, Hoeth M, Hofer-Warbinek R et al. Transcription factor NF-(kappa)B and the regulation of vascular cell function. Arterioscler Thromb Vasc Biol 2000; 20:83–88.
6. Ruberg F, Leopold J, Loscalzo J. Atherothrombosis: plaque instability and thrombogenesis. Prog Cardiovasc Dis 2002; 44:381–394.
7. Cines DB, Pollak ES, Buck CA et al. Endothelial cells in physiology and in the pathophysiology of vascular disorders. Blood 1998; 91:3527–3561.
8. Libby P. Inflammation in atherosclerosis. Nature 2002; 420:868–874.
9. Loscalzo J. Nitric oxide insufficiency, platelet activation, and arterial thrombosis. Circ Res 2001; 88:756–762.
10. Widlansky M, Gokce N, Keaney JF Jr et al. The clinical implications of endothelial dysfunction. J Am Coll Cardiol 2003; 42:1149–1160.
11. Restrepo C, Tracy R. Variations in human aortic fatty streaks among geographic locations. Atherosclerosis 1975; 21:179–193.
12. Cybulsky M, Gimbrone M. Endothelial expression of a mononuclear leukocyte adhesion molecule during atherogenesis. Science 1991; 251:788–791.
13. Gimbrone M, Bevilacqua M, Cybulsky M. Endothelial-dependent mechanisms of leukocyte adhesion in inflammation and atherosclerosis. Ann NY Acad Sci 1990; 598:77–85.
14. Ruberg F, Loscalzo J. Prothrombotic determinants of coronary atherothrombosis. Vasc Med 2002; 7:289–299.
15. Keaney JF Jr, John F. Atherosclerosis: from lesion formation to plaque activation and endothelial dysfunction. Molec Aspects Med 2000; 21:99–166.
16. Libby P, Ridker P, Maseri A. Inflammation and atherosclerosis. Circulation 2002; 105:1135–1143.
17. Collins T, Cybulsky MI. NF-kappaB: pivotal mediator or innocent bystander in atherogenesis? J Clin Invest 2001; 107:255–264.
18. Walford G, Loscalzo J. Nitric oxide in vascular biology. J Thromb Haemost 2003; 1:2112–2118.
19. Marshall H, Merchant K, Stamler J. Nitrosation and oxidation in the regulation of gene expression. FASEB J 2000; 14:1889–1900.
20. Gimbrone M. Endothelial dysfunction, hemodynamic forces, and atherosclerosis. Thomb Haemost 1999; 82:722–726.
21. Szmitko PE, Wang C-H, Weisel RD et al. Biomarkers of vascular disease linking inflammation to endothelial activation: Part II. Circulation 2003; 108:2041–2048.
22. Boring L, Gosling J, Cleary M et al. Decreased lesion formation in CCR2-/- mice reveals a role for chemokines in the initiation of atherosclerosis. Nature 1998; 394:894–897.
23. Mach F, Sauty A, Iarossi AS et al. Differential expression of three T lymphocyte-activating CXC chemokines by human atheroma-associated cells. J Clin Invest 1999; 104:1041–1050.
24. Haley KJ, Lilly CM, Yang J-H et al. Overexpression of eotaxin and the CCR3 receptor in human atherosclerosis: using genomic technology to identify a potential novel pathway of vascular inflammation. Circulation 2000; 102:2185–2189.
25. Vosper H, Patel L, Graham TL et al. The peroxisome proliferator-activated receptor delta promotes lipid accumulation in human macrophages. J Biol Chem 2001; 276:44258–44265.
26. Chinetti G, Lestavel S, Bocher V et al. PPAR-alpha and PPAR-gamma activators induce cholesterol removal from

human macrophage foam cells through stimulation of the ABCA1 pathway. Nature Med 2001; 7:53–58.

27. Clinton S, Underwood R, Hayes L et al. Macrophage colony-stimulating factor gene expression in vascular cells and in experimental and human atherosclerosis. Am J Pathol 1992; 140:301–316.

28. Mertens A, Holvoet P. Oxidized LDL and HDL: antagonists in atherothrombosis. FASEB J 2001; 15:2073–2084.

29. Durrington PN, Mackness B, Mackness MI. Paraoxonase and atherosclerosis. Arterioscler Thromb Vasc Biol 2001; 21:473–480.

30. Kontush A, Chantepie S, Chapman MJ. Small, dense HDL particles exert potent protection of atherogenic LDL against oxidative stress. Arterioscler Thromb Vasc Biol 2003; 23:1881–1888.

31. Naghavi M, Libby P, Falk E et al. From vulnerable plaque to vulnerable patient: a call for new definitions and risk assessment strategies: Part I. Circulation 2003; 108:1664–1672.

32. Naghavi M, Libby P, Falk E et al. From vulnerable plaque to vulnerable patient: a call for new definitions and risk assessment strategies: Part II. Circulation 2003; 108:1772–1778.

33. Galis ZS, Khatri JJ. Matrix metalloproteinases in vascular remodeling and atherogenesis: the good, the bad, and the ugly. Circ Res 2002; 90:251–262.

34. Visse R, Nagase H. Matrix metalloproteinases and tissue inhibitors of metalloproteinases: structure, function, and biochemistry. Circ Res 2003; 92:827–839.

35. Dollery CM, Owen CA, Sukhova GK et al. Neutrophil elastase in human atherosclerotic plaques: production by macrophages. Circulation 2003; 107:2829–2836.

36. Sukhova GK, Zhang Y, Pan J-H et al. Deficiency of cathepsin S reduces atherosclerosis in LDL receptor-deficient mice. J Clin Invest 2003; 111:897–906.

37. Schonbeck U, Libby P. CD40 signaling and plaque instability. Circ Res 2001; 89:1092–1103.

38. Mach F, Schonbeck U, Sukhova G et al. Reduction of atherosclerosis in mice by inhibition of CD40 signalling. Nature 1998; 394:200–203.

39. Schonbeck U, Gerdes N, Varo N et al. Oxidized low-density lipoprotein augments and 3-hydroxy-3-methylglutaryl coenzyme A reductase inhibitors limit CD40 and CD40L expression in human vascular cells. Circulation 2002; 106:2888–2893.

40. Urbich C, Dernbach E, Aicher A et al. CD40 Ligand inhibits endothelial cell migration by increasing production of endothelial reactive oxygen species. Circulation 2002; 106:981–986.

41. Moulton KS, Vakili K, Zurakowski D et al. Inhibition of plaque neovascularization reduces macrophage accumulation and progression of advanced atherosclerosis. Proc Natl Acad Sci USA 2003; 100:4736–4741.

42. Kolodgie FD, Gold HK, Burke AP et al. Intraplaque hemorrhage and progression of coronary atheroma. N Engl J Med 2003; 349:2316–2325.

43. Klezovitch O, Edelstein C, Scanu AM. Stimulation of interleukin-8 production in human THP-1 macrophages by apolipoprotein(a). Evidence for a critical involvement of elements in its C-terminal domain. J Biol Chem 2001; 276:46864–46869.

44. Ariyo AA, Thach C, Tracy R for the Cardiovascular Health Study Investigators. Lp(a) lipoprotein, vascular disease, and mortality in the elderly. N Engl J Med 2003; 349:2108–2115.

45. Lassegue B, Clempus RE. Vascular NAD(P)H oxidases: specific features, expression, and regulation. Am J Physiol Regul Integr Comp Physiol 2003; 285:R277–297.

46. Brasier AR, Recinos A III, Eledrisi MS. Vascular inflammation and the renin–angiotensin system. Arterioscler Thromb Vasc Biol 2002; 22:1257–1266.

47. Basta G, Lazzerini G, Massaro M et al. Advanced glycation end products activate endothelium through signal-transduction receptor RAGE: a mechanism for amplification of inflammatory responses. Circulation 2002; 105:816–822.

48. Stuhlinger M, Abbasi F, Chu J et al. Relationship between insulin resistance and an endogenous nitric oxide synthase inhibitor. J Am Med Assoc 2002; 287:1420–1426.

49. White MF. Insulin signaling in health and disease. Science 2003; 302:1710–1711.

50. Zhu J, Katz RJ, Quyyumi AA et al. Association of serum antibodies to heat-shock protein 65 with coronary calcification levels. Suggestion of pathogen-triggered autoimmunity in early atherosclerosis. Circulation 2004; 109:36–41.

51. de Kleijn D, Pasterkamp G. Toll-like receptors in cardiovascular diseases. Cardiovasc Res 2003; 60:58–67.

52. Cercek B, Shah PK, Noc M et al. Effect of short-term treatment with azithromycin on recurrent ischaemic events in patients with acute coronary syndrome in the Azithromycin in Acute Coronary Syndrome (AZACS) trial: a randomised controlled trial. Lancet 2003; 361:809–813.

53. O'Connor C, Dunne M, Pfeffer M et al. Azithromycin for the secondary prevention of coronary heart disease events: the WIZARD study: a randomized controlled trial. J Am Med Assoc 2003; 290:1459–1466.

54. Pepys MB, Hirschfield GM. C-reactive protein: a critical update. J Clin Invest 2003; 111:1805–1812.

55. Ridker PM. High-sensitivity C-reactive protein and cardiovascular risk: rationale for screening and primary prevention. Am J Cardiol 2003; 92:17–22.

56. Sesso H, Buring J, Rifai N et al. C-reactive protein and the risk of developing hypertension. J Am Med Assoc 2003; 290:2945–2951.

57. Verma S, Wang C-H, Li S-H et al. A self-fulfilling prophecy: C-reactive protein attenuates nitric oxide production and inhibits angiogenesis. Circulation 2002; 106:913–919.

58. Verma S, Li S-H, Badiwala MV et al. Endothelin antagonism and interleukin-6 inhibition attenuate the proatherogenic effects of C-reactive protein. Circulation 2002; 105:1890–1896.

59. Verma S, Chao-Hung Wang, Weisel RD et al. Hyperglycemia potentiates the proatherogenic effects of C-reactive protein: reversal with rosiglitazone. J Mol Cell Cardiol 2003; 35:417–419.

60. Wang C-H, Li S-H, Weisel RD et al. C-reactive protein upregulates angiotensin type 1 receptors in vascular smooth muscle. Circulation 2003; 107:1783–1790.

61. Ridker PM, Rifai N, Rose L et al. Comparison of C-reactive protein and low-density lipoprotein cholesterol levels in the prediction of first cardiovascular events. N Engl J Med 2002; 347:1557–1565.

62. Ridker PM, Rifai N, Pfeffer MA et al. Inflammation, pravastatin, and the risk of coronary events after myocardial infarction in patients with average cholesterol levels. Circulation 1998; 98:839–844.

63. Kinlay S, Schwartz GG, Olsson AG et al. for the Myocardial Ischemia Reduction with Aggressive Cholesterol Lowering (MIRACL) Study Investigators. High-dose atorvastatin enhances the decline in inflammatory markers in patients with acute coronary syndromes in the MIRACL Study. Circulation 2003; 108:1560–1566.

64. Szmitko PE, Wang C-H, Weisel RD et al. New markers of inflammation and endothelial cell activation: Part I. Circulation 2003; 108:1917–1923.

65. Varo N, de Lemos JA, Libby P et al. Soluble CD40L: risk prediction after acute coronary syndromes. Circulation 2003; 108:1049–1052.

66. Heeschen C, Dimmeler S, Hamm CW et al. for the CAP-TURE Study Investigators. Soluble CD40 ligand in acute coronary syndromes. N Engl J Med 2003; 348:1104–1111.

67. Varo N, Vicent D, Libby P et al. Elevated plasma levels of the atherogenic mediator soluble CD40 ligand in diabetic patients: a novel target of thiazolidinediones. Circulation 2003; 107:2664–2669.

68. Hwang S-J, Ballantyne CM, Sharrett AR et al. Circulating adhesion molecules VCAM-1, ICAM-1, and E-selectin in carotid atherosclerosis and incident coronary heart disease cases: the Atherosclerosis Risk In Communities (ARIC) Study. Circulation 1997; 96:4219–4225.

69. Pradhan AD, Rifai N, Ridker PM. Soluble intercellular adhesion molecule-1, soluble vascular adhesion molecule-1, and the development of symptomatic peripheral arterial disease in men. Circulation 2002; 106:820–825.

70. Brennan M-L, Penn MS, Van Lente F et al. Prognostic value of myeloperoxidase in patients with chest pain. N Engl J Med 2003; 349:1595–1604.

71. Packard CJ, O'Reilly DS, Caslake MJ et al. for the West of Scotland Coronary Prevention Study Group. Lipoprotein-associated phospholipase A2 as an independent predictor of coronary heart disease. N Engl J Med 2000; 343: 1148–1155.

72. Elinder LS, Dumitrescu A, Larsson P et al. Expression of phospholipase A2 isoforms in human normal and atherosclerotic arterial wall. Arterioscler Thromb Vasc Biol 1997; 17:2257–2263.

73. Niessen HW, Krijnen PAJ, Visser CA et al. Type II secretory phospholipase A2 in cardiovascular disease: a mediator in atherosclerosis and ischemic damage to cardiomyocytes? Cardiovasc Res 2003; 60:68–77.

74. Kugiyama K, Ota Y, Takazoe K et al. Circulating levels of secretory type II phospholipase A2 predict coronary events in patients with coronary artery disease. Circulation 1999; 100:1280–1284.

75. Blankenberg S, Rupprecht HJ, Poirier O et al. for the AtheroGene Investigators. Plasma concentrations and genetic variation of matrix metalloproteinase 9 and prognosis of patients with cardiovascular disease. Circulation 2003; 107:1579–1585.

76. Pollanen PJ, Karhunen PJ, Mikkelsson J et al. Coronary artery complicated lesion area is related to functional polymorphism of matrix metalloproteinase 9 gene: an autopsy study. Arterioscler Thromb Vasc Biol 2001; 21:1446–1450.

77. Koenig W. Fibrin(ogen) in cardiovascular disease: an update. Thromb Haemost 2003; 89:601–609.

78. Rehman J, Li J, Orschell CM et al. Peripheral blood 'endothelial progenitor cells' are derived from monocyte/macrophages and secrete angiogenic growth factors. Circulation 2003; 107:1164–1169.

79. Hill JM, Zalos G, Halcox JP et al. Circulating endothelial progenitor cells, vascular function, and cardiovascular risk. N Engl J Med 2003; 348:593–600.

80. Kwak B, Mulhaupt F, Myit S et al. Statins as a newly recognized type of immunomodulator. Nature Med 2000; 6:1399–402.

81. Rezaie-Majd A, Prager GW, Bucek RA et al. Simvastatin reduces the expression of adhesion molecules in circulating monocytes from hypercholesterolemic patients. Arterioscler Thromb Vasc Biol 2003; 23:397–403.

82. Laufs U, La Fata V, Plutzky J et al. Upregulation of endothelial nitric oxide synthase by HMG CoA reductase inhibitors. Circulation 1998; 97:1129–1135.

83. Shishehbor MH, Brennan M-L, Aviles RJ et al. Statins promote potent systemic antioxidant effects through specific inflammatory pathways. Circulation 2003; 108:426–431.

84. Eto M, Kozai T, Cosentino F et al. Statin prevents tissue factor expression in human endothelial cells: role of Rho/Rho-kinase and Akt pathways. Circulation 2002; 105:1756–1759.

85. Laufs U, Marra D, Node K et al. 3-Hydroxy-3-methylglutaryl-CoA reductase inhibitors attenuate vascular smooth muscle proliferation by preventing Rho GTPase-induced down-regulation of p27Kip1. J Biol Chem 1999; 274:21926–21931.

86. Llevadot J, Murasawa S, Kureishi Y et al. HMG-CoA reductase inhibitor mobilizes bone marrow-derived endothelial progenitor cells. J Clin Invest 2001; 108:399–405.

87. Kleemann R, Princen HM, Emeis JJ et al. Rosuvastatin reduces atherosclerosis development beyond and independent of its plasma cholesterol-lowering effect in APOE*3-Leiden transgenic mice: evidence for antiinflammatory effects of rosuvastatin. Circulation 2003; 108:1368–1374.

88. Baetta R, Camera M, Comparato C et al. Fluvastatin reduces tissue factor expression and macrophage accumulation in carotid lesions of cholesterol-fed rabbits in the

absence of lipid lowering. Arterioscler Thromb Vasc Biol 2002; 22:692–698.

89. Sukhova GK, Williams JK, Libby P. Statins reduce inflammation in atheroma of nonhuman primates independent of effects on serum cholesterol. Arterioscler Thromb Vasc Biol 2002; 22:1452–1458.

90. Schieffer B, Drexler H. Role of 3-hydroxy-3-methylglutaryl coenzyme a reductase inhibitors, angiotensin-converting enzyme inhibitors, cyclooxygenase-2 inhibitors, and aspirin in anti-inflammatory and immunomodulatory treatment of cardiovascular diseases. Am J Cardiol 2003; 91:12H–18H.

91. Heart Protection Study Collabrotive Group. MRC/BHF Heart Protection Study of cholesterol lowering with simvastatin in 20536 high-risk individuals: a randomised placebo-controlled trial. Lancet 2002; 360:7–22.

92. Belton O, Byrne D, Kearney D et al. Cyclooxygenase-1 and -2-dependent prostacyclin formation in patients with atherosclerosis. Circulation 2000; 102:840–845.

93. FitzGerald G. COX-2 and beyond: approaches to prostaglandin inhibition in human disease. Nature Rev Drug Discov 2003; 2:879–890.

94. Widlansky ME, Price DT, Gokce N et al. Short- and long-term COX-2 inhibition reverses endothelial dysfunction in patients with hypertension. Hypertension 2003; 42:310–315.

95. Title LM, Giddens K, McInerney MM et al. Effect of cyclooxygenase-2 inhibition with rofecoxib on endothelial dysfunction and inflammatory markers in patients with coronary artery disease. J Am Coll Cardiol 2003; 42:1747–1753.

96. Bulut D LS, Hanefeld C, Koll R et al. Selective cyclo-oxygenase-2 inhibition with parecoxib acutely impairs endothelium-dependent vasodilatation in patients with essential hypertension. J Hypertens 2003; 21:1663–1667.

97. Plutzky J. The potential role of peroxisome proliferator-activated receptors on inflammation in type 2 diabetes mellitus and atherosclerosis. Am J Cardiol 2003; 92:34–41.

98. Jiang C, Ting A, Seed B. PPAR- agonists inhibit production of monocyte inflammatory cytokines. Nature 1998; 391:82–86.

99. Ricote M, Huang J, Fajas L et al. Expression of the peroxisome proliferator-activated receptor gamma (PPARgamma) in human atherosclerosis and regulation in macrophages by colony stimulating factors and oxidized low density lipoprotein. Proc Natl Acad Sci USA 1998; 95:7614–7619.

100. Marx N, Kehrle B, Kohlhammer K et al. PPAR Activators as antiinflammatory mediators in human T lymphocytes: implications for atherosclerosis and transplantation-associated arteriosclerosis. Circ Res 2002; 90:703–710.

101. Marx N, Froehlich J, Siam L et al. Antidiabetic PPAR(gamma)-activator rosiglitazone reduces MMP-9 serum levels in type 2 diabetic patients with coronary artery disease. Arterioscler Thromb Vasc Biol 2003; 23:283–288.

102. Chawla A, Barak Y, Nagy L et al. PPAR-gamma dependent and independent effects on macrophage-gene expression in lipid metabolism and inflammation. Nature Med 2001; 7:48–52.

103. Bishop-Bailey D, Hla T. Endothelial cell apoptosis induced by the peroxisome proliferator-activated receptor (PPAR) ligand 15-deoxy-delta 12,14-prostaglandin J2. J Biol Chem 1999; 274:17042–17048.

104. Marx N, Sukhova GK, Collins T et al. PPAR(alpha) activators inhibit cytokine-induced vascular cell adhesion molecule-1 expression in human endothelial cells. Circulation 1999; 99:3125–3131.

105. Ricote M, Valledor AF, Glass CK. Decoding transcriptional programs regulated by PPARs and LXRs in the macrophage: effects on lipid homeostasis, inflammation, and atherosclerosis. Arterioscler Thromb Vasc Biol 2003: Oct. 30 [Epub ahead of print].

106. Sidhu JS, Cowan D, Kaski J-C. The effects of rosiglitazone, a peroxisome proliferator-activated receptor-gamma agonist, on markers of endothelial cell activation, C-reactive protein, and fibrinogen levels in non-diabetic coronary artery disease patients. J Am Coll Cardiol 2003; 42:1757–1763.

107. Tao L, Liu H-R, Gao E et al. Antioxidative, antinitrative, and vasculoprotective effects of a peroxisome proliferator-activated receptor-(gamma) agonist in hypercholesterolemia. Circulation 2003; 108:2805–2811.

5

Oxidative stress and atherosclerosis

Roland Stocker, John F. Keaney Jr

INTRODUCTION

Over the last 25 years, one aspect of atherosclerosis that has attracted significant interest is the notion that oxidative stress contributes to the pathogenesis of this disease and, perhaps, its clinical sequelae. The sections that follow will provide a historical perspective on the relationship between oxidative stress and atherosclerosis and outline how these concepts have evolved over time, with a particular emphasis on the molecular mechanisms involved.

Oxidative modification hypothesis of atherosclerosis

There is an undeniable association between low-density lipoprotein (LDL) cholesterol and atherosclerosis, based, in part, on data from the general population linking LDL cholesterol to atherosclerotic complications[1] and data showing that LDL cholesterol lowering limits the sequelae of atherosclerosis.[2] Despite this association, early atherosclerosis research was hampered by observations that LDL particles did not appear to be atherogenic *in vitro*. Indeed, macrophages incubated with LDL failed to internalize excess lipoprotein–cholesterol owing to downregulation of the LDL receptor.[3] Thus, foam cell formation was not mediated by the LDL receptor, a fact consistent with the occurrence of atherosclerosis in familial hypercholesterolemia patients without functional LDL receptors. In a search for alternative receptors, Brown and Goldstein observed that acetylation of LDL leads to extensive macrophage cholesterol uptake and foam cell formation. This phenomenon was mediated by a

saturable, specific receptor later termed the 'acetyl-LDL receptor'.[4] Many of these so-called 'scavenger receptors' are known to be present on macrophages and other cell types.[5]

The original description of the acetyl-LDL receptor did acknowledge that there was no plausible means of LDL acetylation *in vivo*;[4] however, Brown and Goldstein did speculate that other LDL modifications might later be found *in vivo* that could facilitate its recognition by this acetyl-LDL receptor. Approximately 2 years later, Henriksen and colleagues[6] observed that LDL incubated with endothelial cells was able to serve as a ligand for macrophage foam cell formation. Since that time, it has been established that several receptors on macrophages and other cells function as 'scavenger' receptors.[7] The molecular identity of the original acetyl-LDL receptor reveals it to exist in two forms, known as scavenger receptors A1 and A2.[8] Other receptors, such as CD68, CD36, SR-B1, and LOX-1, are also known to possess properties similar to those of the classic scavenger receptors.[7]

The notion that oxidative stress could contribute to atherosclerosis was brought to bear in 1989, when Daniel Steinberg and associates proposed the original oxidative modification theory of atherosclerosis (Figure 5.1).[9] This hypothesis proposed that oxidation represents a biologic modification analogous to the chemical modifications discovered by Brown and Goldstein,[4] which give rise to an LDL particle that supports foam cell formation.[9] Accordingly to this hypothesis, oxidized LDL contributed to atherogenesis by (i) aiding the recruitment of circulating monocytes into the intimal space; (ii) inhibiting the ability of resident macrophages to leave the intima; (iii) enhancing the rate of uptake of the lipoprotein, leading to foam cell

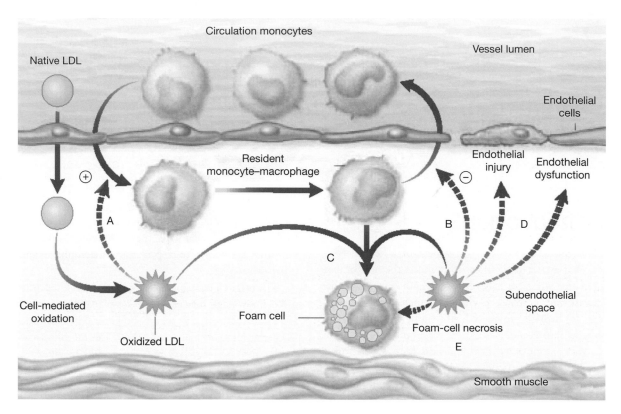

Figure 5.1 The oxidative modification hypothesis of atherosclerosis. Low-density lipoprotein (LDL) becomes entrapped in the subendothelial space, where it may undergo oxidative modification via resident vascular cells, including smooth muscle cells, endothelial cells, and macrophages. Once formed, oxidized LDL stimulates monocyte chemotaxis, which facilitates foam cell formation. Local oxidized LDL also causes endothelial dysfunction and injury. Foam cells necrose as a consequence of oxidized LDL accumulation and release lysosomal enzymes and necrotic debris, further promoting lesion development. (Reproduced with permission from N Engl J Med 1997; 337:408–416)

formation; and (iv) being cytotoxic, leading to loss of endothelial integrity.[10] The latter property provided an important mechanism for fatty streak formation and provided a substrate for progression of the fatty streak to advanced lesions – a process previously outlined in the 'response-to-injury' hypothesis by Ross and colleagues.[11] An attractive feature of the oxidative modification hypothesis was that it did not require endothelial cell injury to initiate atherogenesis, as this part of the pre-existing response to injury was considered a weakness.

The notion that LDL oxidative modification occurs *in vivo* has been addressed. Detailed examination of LDL oxidation reveals that polyunsaturated fatty acids in LDL are the initial targets of oxidation (Figure 5.2a) which subsequently break down into aldehyde species (for review, see reference 12). The aldehydes readily combine with lysine groups on apolipoprotein B-100 to form a Schiff base, altering the surface charge of LDL) (Figure 5.2b). Antibodies have been raised against oxidized epitopes of LDL apolipoprotein B-100 and they avidly stain atherosclerotic lesions in LDL receptor-deficient rabbits,[13,14] apolipoprotein E-deficient mice,[15] and humans,[16,17] with demonstrable colocalization in macrophages[13] and no discernible staining in normal arteries. If one isolates LDL from atherosclerotic lesions, this LDL preparation has physical and chemical properties that are identical to those of LDL oxidized *ex vivo*.[17] Thus, there is considerable evidence that LDL oxidation occurs *in vivo*.

The oxidative modification hypothesis also proposes a proatherogenic activity of oxidized LDL, and experimental data support this contention. For example, the early stages of LDL oxidation are characterized

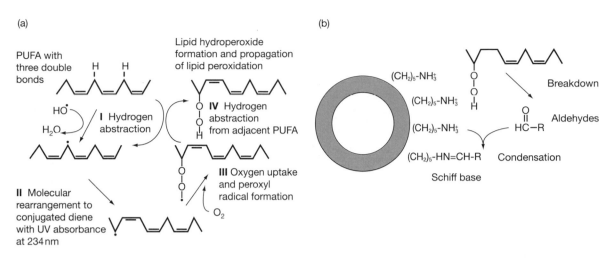

Figure 5.2 Molecular events involved in low-density lipoprotein (LDL) oxidation. (a) In this scheme, hydroxyl radical initiates lipid peroxidation through the abstraction of hydrogen (I) from a bis-allylic methylene group in a polyunsaturated fatty acid (PUFA). The carbon-centered radical thus formed undergoes molecular rearrangement to form a conjugated diene compound exhibiting UV absorbance at 234 nm (II). The carbon-centered radical then reacts readily with molecular oxygen to form a lipid peroxyl radical (III), which may then propagate lipid peroxidation through the abstraction of hydrogen from an adjacent PUFA, forming both a lipid hydroperoxide and another carbon-centered radical (IV). The lipid hydroperoxide species is then subject to breakdown into aldehyde species. The aldehydes readily combine with lysine groups within apolipoprotein B-100 on the LDL surface to form Schiff bases and increase the net negative charge of the LDL particle

by modifications in the genetic program of the vascular wall. Mildly oxidized forms of LDL induce the synthesis of macrophage chemotactic protein-1 (MCP-1) in both smooth muscle and endothelial cells,[18,19] resulting in the recruitment of inflammatory cells.[20] This process occurs *in vivo*,[21] and it appears critical, as mice lacking the MCP-1 receptor are resistant to atherosclerosis.[22,23] Fully oxidized forms of LDL are chemotactic for monocytes[24] and T lymphocytes,[25] and oxidized LDL elicits the production of autoantibodies.[26,27] These data are in keeping with an accumulating body of evidence linking inflammation to atherosclerosis and its clinical sequelae.[28]

There are considerable data to support LDL modification in atherosclerosis, although confirmation that oxidation is the requisite LDL modification for atherosclerosis is not complete. For example, mice lacking the classic type A scavenger receptor are protected from atherosclerosis,[29] as are animals lacking CD36,[30] suggesting that unregulated cholesterol uptake is needed for atherosclerosis; however, not all antioxidants that inhibit LDL oxidation limit atherosclerosis in animals.[31,32] In placebo-controlled large intervention trials, vitamin E and other antioxidants have no benefit

on the incidence of coronary artery disease.[33,34] Consistent with these data, LDL receptor-deficient rabbits develop lipid oxidation in the vessel wall that is abolished by bisphenol, an antioxidant, without any effect on the extent of atherosclerosis.[35] Taken together, the available clinical and animal data indicate that LDL lipid peroxidation does not represent the only manifestation of oxidative stress that is important in atherosclerosis. Emerging data indicate that other oxidative events are present in atherosclerosis and could play a role in modulation of the disease process.

Other manifestations of oxidative stress in atherosclerosis

What is oxidative stress?

The notion of 'oxidative stress' has its origins in early research concerning oxygen activation with X-irradiation[36] and hydroperoxide metabolism in mammalian organs.[37] The actual term 'oxidative stress', owes its origins to Sies,[38] with synonymous terms such as 'oxidant stress' and 'pro-oxidant stress' receiving comparatively less emphasis. The term was described originally[38] as a 'disturbance in the pro-oxidant/antioxidant balance in favor of the former,' and has since been modified to an 'imbalance between oxidants and antioxidants in favor of the oxidants, potentially leading to damage'.[39] Consequently, oxidative stress can be caused by a number of conditions or oxidants that tip the balance toward oxidative damage. Consistent with this notion, and the appreciation of reactive nitrogen species in biology, the term 'nitrosative stress' has also been introduced.[40]

Biological oxidants relevant to atherosclerosis

Free radicals or 1e-oxidants

A free radical is defined as a independently existing species with one or more unpaired electrons.[41] Selected radicals that have relevance to the vasculature are listed in Table 5.1. If two radicals meet, they can combine unpaired electrons to form a covalent bond in reactions that are typically very fast and lead to non-radical products. One such reaction relevant to the vessel wall involves the combination of superoxide ($O_2^{\bullet-}$) with nitric oxide ($^\bullet NO$) to form peroxynitrite ($ONOO^-$) (Reaction 1):

$$O_2^{\bullet-} + {}^\bullet NO \rightarrow ONOO^- \tag{1}$$

More commonly, radicals react with non-radical molecules or abstract hydrogen from a C–H, O–H or S–H bond of non-radical species, as most molecules in biological systems are non-radical species. Typically affected molecules include low molecular weight compounds such as antioxidants, cofactors of enzymes, lipids, proteins, nucleic acids, and carbohydrates. Radical reactions with non-radical species generate a new radical that can set up a chain reaction.

A typical example of such a reaction is the process of lipid peroxidation depicted in Figure 5.2a. The process begins with a radical species ($^\bullet OH$) abstracting from a fatty acid side chain (LH) containing carbon atoms with bis-allelic hydrogens (Reaction 2):

The resulting carbon-centered radical (L$^\bullet$) adds rapidly to O_2 to generate a lipid peroxyl radical (LOO$^\bullet$)

Table 5.1	Examples of free radicals in biological systems (adapted from reference 41)	

Name	Formula	Comments
Carbon-centered radical	$\rangle C^\bullet$	These radicals with the unpaired electron residing on carbon usually react rapidly with O_2 to make peroxyl radicals
Superoxide anion and hydroperoxyl radicals	$O_2^{\bullet-}$, $HO_2^\bullet$	The 'primary' oxygen-centered radical in its anionic and protonated forms
Peroxyl, alkoxyl radicals	$RO_2^\bullet$, $RO^\bullet$	Oxygen-centered radicals that can be formed from reaction of carbon-centered radicals with O_2 ($RO_2^\bullet$), or from the breakdown of organic peroxides, such as lipid hydroperoxides ($RO_2^\bullet$, $RO^\bullet$)
Hydroxyl radical	$^\bullet OH$	Highly reactive, oxygen-centered radical that reacts with all biomolecules
Nitric oxide (nitrogen monoxide) and nitrogen dioxide	$^\bullet NO$, $^\bullet NO_2$	Nitric oxide is formed from L-arginine, and nitrogen dioxide from reaction of $^\bullet NO$ with O_2
Thyl and perthyl radicals	$RS^\bullet$, $RSS^\bullet$	A group of radicals with the unpaired electrons residing on sulfur
Transition-metal ions	Fe, Cu, etc.	Ability to change oxidation numbers by 1, allowing them to accept/donate single electrons; hence they can be catalysts of free-radical reactions

(Reaction 3), which itself can propagate the chain by reacting with a neighboring lipid molecule to generate another L$^{\bullet}$ and lipid hydroperoxide (LOOH) (Reaction 4). In this fashion, many molecules of LOOH may be generated for each initiating radical.

$$LH + {}^{\bullet}OH \rightarrow L^{\bullet} + H_2O \qquad (2)$$

$$L^{\bullet} + O_2 \rightarrow LOO^{\bullet} \qquad (3)$$

$$LOO^{\bullet} + LH \rightarrow L^{\bullet} + LOOH \qquad (4)$$

Highly reactive radicals ($^{\bullet}OH$) abstract H atoms almost without discrimination; less reactive radicals, such as LOO$^{\bullet}$, preferentially abstract H atoms from species with weaker bonds, such as the chromanol O–H bond contained in α-tocopherol (α-TOH). In the latter case, the α-tocopheroxyl radical (α-TO$^{\bullet}$) is produced and, for LOO$^{\bullet}$, a molecule of LOOH (Reaction 5):

$$LOO^{\bullet} + \alpha\text{-TOH} \rightarrow LOOH + \alpha\text{-TO}^{\bullet} \qquad (5)$$

It is important to realize, however, that not all radicals are oxidants and not all oxidants are radicals. Depending upon the situation, a radical may be an oxidizing agent, accepting a single electron from a non-radical, or a reducing agent, donating a single electron to a non-radical. Free radical reactions are governed by thermodynamic and kinetic principles, and among the former the reduction potential is a parameter commonly applied in free radical chemistry to determine the feasibility of a compound X to chemically reduce compound Y. For reference, Buettner[42] has compiled a very useful list of relevant standard reduction potentials that help predict the direction of reactions.

Non-radical reactive species or 2e-oxidants

Several non-radical oxidants are germane to oxidative events in the arterial wall (Table 5.2). The most abundant of these species is hydrogen peroxide (H_2O_2), derived primarily from the action of oxidases on O_2 or from the dismutation of $O_2^{\bullet-}$ (Reaction 6):

$$2\,O_2^{\bullet-} + 2\,H^+ \rightarrow H_2O_2 + O_2 \qquad (6)$$

The reactivity of different non-radical species varies as a function of environment. Hydrogen peroxide is a weak oxidant that is most active toward protein thiol (–SH) groups. Hydrogen peroxide also reacts with certain heme proteins (e.g. myoglobin and cytochrome c) to release iron and/or form ferryl heme and amino acid

Table 5.2 Examples of non-radical oxidants relevant to oxidative stress in the vasculature

Name	Formula	Comments
Hydrogen peroxide	H_2O_2	A diffusible oxidant that is only a weak oxidizing agent and is generally poorly reactive. It may participate in cellular signaling and, in the presence of available transition metals, can give rise to $^{\bullet}OH$
Hypochlorite, hypochlorous acid	^-OCl, HOCl	Weak acid (pK_a ~7.5) but strong oxidant. Reacts with Fe$^{\bullet}$S clusters, metal ions held in proteins by thiolate ligands, heme, amino acid residues (Met, Cys) of proteins and reduced glutathione. Can give rise to secondary reactive species, including chloramines and amino acid-derived aldehydes
Oxoperoxonitrate (1$^-$) or peroxynitrite, peroxynitrous acid	$ONOO^-$, ONOOH	Can be formed via reaction of $O_2^{\bullet-}$ with $^{\bullet}NO$, with k ~10^{10} M^{-1} s^{-1},[220] comparable to the rate at which $O_2^{\bullet-}$ reacts with superoxide dismutase. The protonated form is highly reactive
Alkylperoxynitrites, dinitrogen trioxide, nitryl chloride and nitronium (nitryl) ion	ROONO, N_2O_3, NO_2Cl and NO_2^+	Additional, reactive nitrogen species
Nitrosothiols	RSNO	Formed via reaction of RS$^{\bullet}$ with $^{\bullet}NO$, or thiols with higher oxides of nitrogen. Nitrosothiols are weak oxidants
Singlet oxygen and ozone	$^1O_2^{\bullet}$ O_3	Non-radical oxidants produced from H_2O_2 in the presence of antibodies

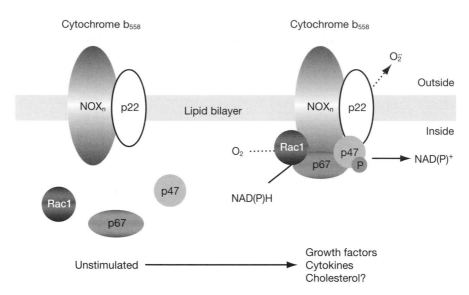

Figure 5.3 The neutrophil oxidase as a paradigm for vascular NADPH oxidases. The oxidase consists of the membrane-bound cytochrome b_{558} that contains two subunits. The first, p22[phox] is ubiquitous, whereas the catalytic subunit varies depending on cell type. There are now five isoforms of catalytic subunits, termed Nox 1–5. Upon stimulation, phosphorylation of p47[phox] affords assembly of the cytosolic components and molecular oxygen is reduced. The precise direction of superoxide production is not yet resolved for all the isoforms. The classic neutrophil oxidase contains Nox2 and generates extracellular superoxide through the reduction of extracellular oxygen

radicals that propagate oxidation reactions via radical chemistry. The classic Haber–Weiss reaction with the formation of $^\bullet$OH is among the more typical mechanisms of oxidative damage resulting from H_2O_2[43] Like H_2O_2, $ONOO^-$ is another weak oxidant; however, when protonated it forms peroxynitrous acid (ONOOH), which is extremely reactive. Since the pK_a of ONOOH is ≈ 7.5,[44] one would expect the formation of $ONOO^-$ in biologic systems to yield a powerful oxidizing environment.

An important feature of non-radical oxidants such as ONOOH[45] and HOCl[46–48] is their predilection for proteins rather than lipids.[49] In particular, these oxidants react qualitatively with cysteine and methionine residues, followed by tyrosine, tryptophan, and phenylalanine, whereas quantitatively lysine residues may be more significant.[50,51] This preference for proteins rather than lipids differentiates non-radical from radical oxidants.

The likelihood of a two-electron oxidant-mediated reaction with amino acid residues in proteins is highly dependent on the local environment. Vicinal thiol and methionine residues are prone to oxidation,[52] and a local environment favoring cysteine residue(s) as thiolate anions (typically via neighboring amino acids low-

ering the cysteine pK_a) greatly accelerates H_2O_2-mediated oxidation. Two examples of this concept are OONOH-mediated oxidation of the zinc thiolate cluster (ZnS_4) of endothelial nitric oxide synthase,[53,54] and HOCl-mediated oxidation of the cysteine-switch domain of pro-metalloproteinases.[55,56]

Sources of oxidants in the vasculature

NAD(P)H oxidases (Nox)

It has long been known that phagocytes, including neutrophils, monocytes, and macrophages, contain a plasma membrane-bound multicomponent oxidase that utilizes NADPH-derived electrons to produce $O_2^{\bullet-}$ from molecular oxygen. The phagocyte NADPH oxidase (Figure 5.3) consists of two membrane-associated units, gp91[phox] and p22[phox], which together form cytochrome $b_{558,}$ and two cytosolic components, p47[phox] and p67[phox].[57] Other proteins, such as Rac1, associate with the oxidase and may participate in its activation. The activation of the phagocyte NADPH oxidase begins with phosphorylation of p47[phox], leading to its association with cytochrome b_{558}.[57] The

---

Table 5.3 Expression of NADPH oxidases in vascular cells

Cell type	Nox expression	mRNA phox expression	Refs
Endothelial cells	Nox4>>Nox2>Nox1	p22, p47, p67	67, 221
Smooth muscle cells	Nox4>Nox1>>Nox2	p22, p47	69, 73
Fibroblasts	Nox4>Nox2=Nox1	p22, p47, p67	61, 71
Monocytes	Nox2>>Nox1	p22, p47, p67	67

Two proteins, p41^{nox} and p51^{nox}, which are homologs of p47^{phox} and p67^{phox}, respectively, have recently been reported,[222] but the vascular cell content of these proteins is unknown.

---

small G-protein Rac also associates with cytochrome b$_{558}$,[58] but independently of both p47^{phox} and p67^{phox} translocation.[59] Activation of the oxidase in phagocytic cells results in large amounts of $O_2^{\bullet-}$ over short periods that appear to be involved in host defense.

There is now convincing evidence that adventitial fibroblasts, vascular smooth muscle and endothelial cells also contain membrane-associated NAD(P)H oxidases that utilize NADH or NADPH to generate $O_2^{\bullet-}$ via 1e-reduction of molecular oxygen (Reaction 8, reviewed in refs[60,61]).

$$NAD(P)H + 2\,O_2 \rightarrow NAD(P)^+ + H^+ + 2\,O_2^{\bullet-} \quad (8)$$

Early evidence indicated that NAD(P)H oxidase activity was a major source of reactive oxygen species in the vasculature.[62–64] In phagocytes, electrons are transferred across the membrane to extracellular oxygen; in vascular smooth muscle cells, $O_2^{\bullet-}$ and H_2O_2 appear to be produced intracellularly and the addition of NAD(P)H to the cells augments $O_2^{\bullet-}$ generation.[60,63] In contrast, data from endothelial cells is consistent with extracellular release of $O_2^{\bullet-}$ based on studies using cell-impermeable spin trapping agents.[65]

There appear to be differences in the component distribution of NAD(P)H oxidases in specific vascular cells (Table 5.3). Fibroblasts and endothelial cells resemble phagocytes in that they contain mRNA for gp91^{phox}, p22^{phox}, p47^{phox}, and p67^{phox}, whereas vascular smooth muscle cells appear to lack gp91^{phox} and p67^{phox}.[60,61] Instead, these cells contain homologs of gp91^{phox} (Nox2), the expression of which can increase cellular $O_2^{\bullet-}$ production.[66] Specific homologs, including Nox1, 3, 4, and 5, have been identified in vascular

cells,[67,68] with endothelial cells expressing very low levels of Nox1, intermediate levels of Nox2, and abundant levels of Nox4 mRNA.[67] In contrast, vascular smooth muscle cells express predominantly Nox4, some Nox1 (which can be induced with angiotensin II),[69] and negligible amounts of Nox2.[67] Continued investigation is likely to define Nox expression further, based on blood vessel type, as Nox2 is more abundant in resistance vessel smooth muscle cells than in conductance artery smooth muscle cells.[70]

The expression of Nox isoforms in endothelial cells, vascular smooth muscle cells, and fibroblasts is associated with constitutive modest $O_2^{\bullet-}$ generation.[60,71] These findings are consistent with observations that Nox2 in endothelial cells appears to be present in a preassembled intracellular complex that includes the p22^{phox}, p47^{phox}, and p67^{phox} subunits.[72] As in phagocytes, NAD(P)H oxidases in vascular cells are subject to activation by specific agonists that include angiotensin II,[69] thrombin,[73] platelet-derived growth factor,[69] tumor necrosis factor-α,[74] interleukin-1[75] and, for endothelial cells, mechanical forces (including shear stress)[76] and vascular endothelial growth factor.[65,74] Activation appears to involve the association of additional proteins with the oxidase components.[65] The upstream signals involved in NADPH oxidase activation in vascular smooth muscle cells treated with angiotensin II indicate a protein kinase C-dependent early phase (30 s), and a prolonged phase (30 min) dependent upon Rac, Src, and phosphatidylinositol 3-kinase.[77] Compared to phagocytes, the amount of $O_2^{\bullet-}$ produced by vascular cells is quite modest and generally thought to modulate key regulatory proteins and cellular responses, rather than precipitating oxidative damage.

With regard to atherosclerosis, there are data indicating that this family of enzymes has a role in the disease process. Early atherosclerosis in Watanabe rabbits (lacking an LDL receptor) demonstrates excess vascular $O_2^{\cdot-}$ production that appears to be due to NAD(P)H oxidase activity.[78] Diet-induced atherosclerosis in primates also exhibits excess vascular $O_2^{\cdot-}$ and upregulation of the NADPH oxidase components p22[phox] and p47[phox], and both phenomena decrease with dietary cholesterol reduction and atherosclerosis regression.[79] Demonstrating a causal role for NAD(P)H oxidase in atherosclerosis has been more problematic. Mice devoid of Nox2 (gp91[phox]) have no change in aortic sinus atherosclerosis using either the apolipoprotein E-null or diet-induced models of atherosclerosis.[80] Two studies have examined the effect of p47[phox] on atherosclerosis in the apolipoprotein E–/– model.[81,82] Neither observed a difference in aortic sinus atherosclerosis as a function of p47[phox]; however, the one study that examined descending aorta atherosclerosis in p47[phox]-null animals found considerably less atherosclerosis than in their counterparts with normal p47[phox].[81]

There are a limited number of studies with human tissue, although in general they support a role for NADPH oxidase in vascular disease. Saphenous vein production of $O_2^{\cdot-}$ increases as a function of cardiovascular risk factors,[83] consistent with NAD(P)H oxidase contributing to atherosclerosis. Sorescu and colleagues[67] found that atherosclerotic lesions in coronary artery segments contained abundant p22[phox] and gp91[phox] near macrophages that correlated with atherosclerosis severity. In contrast, Nox4 was in nonphagocytic cells and varied mostly with cellularity. Vascular tissue in bypass surgery patients with diabetes revealed increased expression of p22[phox], p47[phox], and p67[phox] compared with non-diabetics.[84] The precise contribution of specific Nox isoforms to atherosclerosis and clinical events, however, remains to be determined.

Xanthine oxidase

Xanthine oxidase is an iron–sulfur molybdenum flavoprotein with multiple functions that exists in two forms, xanthine dehydrogenase and xanthine oxidase, the former being predominant.[85] The oxidation of xanthine or hypoxanthine to uric acid is associated with NADH production by the dehydrogenase, whereas the oxidase generates $O_2^{\cdot-}$.[85] The dehydrogenase is readily converted into the oxidase by proteolysis or by reversible oxidation of thiol groups. The role of this enzyme in cellular $O_2^{\cdot-}$ production has been extensively studied in the setting of ischemia–reperfusion.[86] The enzyme has also been implicated in endothelial cell $O_2^{\cdot-}$ production with regard to vascular disease. Cholesterol-fed rabbits demonstrate enhanced endothelial $O_2^{\cdot-}$ production that is inhibited by the xanthine oxidase inhibitor oxypurinol.[87] This increased $O_2^{\cdot-}$ flux from xanthine oxidase contributes to impaired $\cdot$NO bioactivity observed with hypercholesterolemia,[87,88] heavy smoking,[89] and coronary disease.[90] The precise regulation of xanthine oxidase is not yet clear; however, there is evidence that endothelial xanthine oxidase activity is increased by interferon-γ[91] or neutrophil binding to the endothelial surface.[92] Alternatively, there is evidence that endothelial xanthine oxidase is an extracellular enzyme derived from a circulating pool.[93]

Nitric oxide synthases

The nitric oxide synthases catalyse the oxidation of L-arginine to L-citrulline and $\cdot$NO. In the context of atherosclerosis, the endothelial and inducible isoforms have proved most relevant. Reviewing the structure and function of nitric oxide synthases is beyond the scope of this chapter; however, interested readers are referred to several excellent recent reviews.[94–98]

Under specific circumstances endothelial nitric oxide synthase may become 'uncoupled' and thereby an important source of reactive oxygen species. This notion originated with observations that a relative cofactor deficiency for enzyme catalysis allows the enzyme to reduce molecular oxygen rather than transfer electrons to L-arginine, thereby generating $O_2^{\cdot-}$.[99,100] The $O_2^{\cdot-}$ is generated by the oxygenase domain of the enzyme through dissociation of a ferrous–dioxygen complex that is normally stabilized by tetrahydrobiopterin.[101,102]

A number of pathological conditions have been associated with eNOS uncoupling, such as hypercholesterolemia,[103] atherosclerosis,[104,105] and diabetes mellitus.[106] The molecular mechanisms responsible for this phenomenon are not completely understood. In atherosclerosis[104] and diabetes,[107] there is evidence that vascular tetrahydrobiopterin levels may be depressed.

Consistent with this notion, mice that overexpress GTP cyclohydrolase I, the rate-limiting enzyme for tetrahydrobiopterin synthesis, have preserved endothelial NO bioactivity in the setting of diabetes.[108] Other proposed mechanisms for eNOS uncoupling include oxidation of the Zn-thiolate cluster[54] and dephosphorylation of eNOS at residue 497,[109] the latter being a feature of endothelial cells exposed to H_2O_2.[110] Thus, eNOS has the potential to form reactive oxygen species under pathologically relevant conditions.

The function of nitric oxide synthases has important implications for vascular disease. Nitric oxide may react with metal ions, metalloproteins, and $O_2^{\bullet-}$ to form reactive nitrogen species. Perhaps the best characterized of these reactions is the combination of NO and $O_2^{\bullet-}$ to generate $ONOO^-$. Among the most abundant biological targets for $ONOO^-$ is carbon dioxide (CO_2) (reviewed in [111]). The reaction of $ONOO^-$ with CO_2 is complex and initially produces nitrosoperoxycarbonate ($ONOOCO_2^-$), which homolyzes to form a pair of caged radicals $[CO_3^{\bullet-}\ {}^{\bullet}NO_2]$ that may then diffuse apart to become free radicals, or recombine to form nitrocarbonate (O_2NOCO_2), which decomposes to nitrite (NO_3^-) and CO_2. The formation of free nitrogen dioxide (${}^{\bullet}NO_2$) readily leads to protein tyrosine nitration[112] and lipid peroxidation.[113] Thus, uncoupled nitric oxide synthase and the simultaneous generation of ${}^{\bullet}NO$ and $O_2^{\bullet-}$ have important implications for oxidative stress in the vasculature.

Myeloperoxidase

Myeloperoxidase is a heme-containing enzyme that catalyzes the conversion of chloride ion (Cl^-) to the $2e$-oxidant HOCl as the major reaction at physiologic concentrations of chloride (Reaction 9):

$$H_2O_2 + Cl^- + H^+ \rightarrow HOCl + H_2O \qquad (9)$$

Because myeloperoxidase is the only human enzyme that generates HOCl, chlorinated biomolecules are considered specific markers of MPO-mediated oxidation reactions.[114] Myeloperoxidase can yield a number of products, including 3-chlorotyrosine,[115] chlorohydrins from cholesterol and fatty acids,[116] and tyrosyl radicals, with the latter species able to participate in single electron oxidation reactions, including the oxidation of LDL.[117] Another activity of myeloperoxidase and HOCl is to convert L-tyrosine into *p*-hydroxyphenylacetaldehyde[118] which can react with

aminophospholipids[119] and the ε-amino groups of protein lysine residues.[120] The product of these reactions may be subsequently modified by myeloperoxidase to generate a variety of reactive aldehyde residues.[121] Furthermore, L-serine is readily converted by myeloperoxidase to N_e-(carboxymethyl)lysine, a well-characterized advanced glycation end-product.[122] Thus, myeloperoxidase and HOCl can generate a series of secondary oxidation products that may oxidize biomolecules, including LDL, rendering them capable of converting macrophages into foam cells.[123]

Another substrate for myeloperoxidase is nitrite, which can be oxidized to radical species such as nitryl chloride (NO_2Cl) and nitrogen dioxide ($NO_2^{\bullet}$), potent nitrating agents.[124–126] This appears to be an important mechanism for the generation of nitrating species *in vivo* as mice lacking myeloperoxidase do not increase nitrotyrosine levels with inflammation, unlike wildtype mice.[127] Myeloperoxidase also generates high-uptake LDL in the presence of nitrite,[128] lending plausibility to the notion that its activity contributes to atherosclerosis.

The role of myeloperoxidase in atherosclerosis has recently been investigated. Atherosclerotic lesions contain myeloperoxidase that is functionally active.[129] Isolation of LDL from atherosclerotic lesions also reveals the presence of chlorination products,[130] indicative of myeloperoxidase-mediated oxidation reactions. Atherosclerotic tissue also contains high levels of 3-nitrotyrosine,[131] also consistent with myeloperoxidase-mediated oxidation in lesions. These data are also supported by recent clinical trials showing that circulating levels of myeloperoxidase correlate with coronary heart disease[132] and predict clinical events in patients with chest pain.[133] One study testing atherosclerosis in mice found a paradoxical increase in atherosclerosis in animals lacking the myeloperoxidase gene,[134] although most animal models of atherosclerosis are not characterized by myeloperoxidase-mediated oxidation, which calls into question the adequacy of a mouse model in this instance.

Lipoxygenases

Lipoxygenases are iron-containing dioxygenases that catalyze stereospecific insertion of oxygen in polyunsaturated fatty acids, yielding a family of biologically active lipids that includes prostaglandins, thromboxanes, and leukotrienes. The prostaglandins and thromboxanes are often referred to as prostanoids, and are metabolites from arachidonate and similar fatty acids; they are derived from the action of cyclooxygenase I (also prostaglandin G/H synthase I) and contain a cyclopentane ring. The mechanism of catalysis has been studied extensively and was recently reviewed in detail.[135] Enzyme activation requires ambient peroxide as a 'seed' to oxidize a heme-Fe(III) in the active site to generate an oxo-heme species and a protein-tyrosyl radical (compound I). The tyrosyl radical mediates hydrogen atom abstraction from arachidonate to initiate the formation of prostaglandin G_2, followed by reduction to prostaglandin H_2 by the peroxidase component of cyclooxygenase. Both prostaglandin G_2 and H_2 are rapidly transformed into other prostaglandins, such as thromboxane A_2 and prostacyclin, which participate in the regulation of vascular tone and homeostasis.

The non-heme iron-containing lipoxygenases oxidize specific fatty acids at defined positions of their carbon backbone to the corresponding hydroperoxides that serve as the precursors of leukotrienes. Leukotrienes are a family of bioactive lipids that differ from prostanoids in their characteristic conjugated triene structure and in the absence of a cyclopentane ring. These compounds often contribute to inflammatory reactions and increases in vascular permeability. Like cyclooxygenase, lipoxygenases require low levels of 'seeding peroxides' to oxidize inactive Fe^{2+} to the active Fe^{3+} enzyme, and are probably affected by the 'peroxide tone' of cells. *In vitro*, 15-lipoxygenase may oxidize LDL,[136] through both direct and indirect mechanisms.[137,138] The indirect mechanisms refer to the non-enzymatic generation of one-electron oxidants in addition to the specifically oxidized fatty acids – similar to what has been observed with oxidation of other substrates.[139] Similarly, lipid peroxyl radicals are released during the catalytic action of lipoxygenases[140] and may participate in subsequent non-enzymatic lipid peroxidation.[141] Thus, lipoxygenases and cyclooxygenase can generate both oxidized lipids and reactive species that may propagate oxidation reactions.

There is evidence that lipoxygenases participate in the process of atherosclerosis. The 15-lipoxygenase and 5-lipoxygenase are expressed in human lesions[142] and lesions in apolipoprotein E–/– mice, respectively.[143] Consistent with a role for lipoxygenases in atherosclerosis, mice lacking the 12/15-lipoxygenase gene or with decreased 5-lipoxygenase are relatively protected from lesion development in the apolipoprotein E–/– and

LDL receptor–/– models.[143–145] Clinical data also indicate that variant genotypes of the 5-lipoxygenase promoter identify individuals with a greater burden of atherosclerosis and inflammation, further supporting a link between lipoxygenase and this disease.[146] Whether lipoxygenases modulate atherosclerosis through lipid peroxidation or immune modulation, however, is not clear and will require further study.

Mitochondrial respiration

Conventional wisdom dictates that up to 1–2% of electron flow through the respiratory chain may be diverted to molecular oxygen, leading to $O_2^{\bullet-}$ formation.[37] Thus, one must consider the mitochondrion as a potential major intracellular source of reactive oxygen species. Mitochondrial oxidant production is controlled, in part, by the expression of a mitochondrial Mn-containing superoxide dismutase located in the mitochondrial matrix.[147] There is also monoamine oxidase in the outer mitochondrial membrane, which has been proposed as another source of H_2O_2.[148] Within the mitochondria, $O_2^{\bullet-}$ production is thought to occur via complex I (NADH dehydrogenase) or complex III (ubiquinone-cytochrome bc1).[148]

The mitochondrion has become an intense topic of investigation of late, largely owing to the discovery that it plays a critical role in mediating apoptosis.[149] We now know that many cellular responses involve the generation of mitochondrial reactive oxygen species, including growth arrest, apoptosis, and necrosis.[150,151] The most pressing case for vascular disease and the mitochondria relates to diabetes. For example, overproduction of $O_2^{\bullet-}$ has been associated with changes in glycosylation[152] and protein kinase C activation[153] in vascular cells. Overexpression of Mn-superoxide dismutase seems to counteract these deleterious consequences of hyperglycemia.[152,153] A recent study has also linked mitochondrial dysfunction and, presumably, oxidant production to atherosclerotic lesion development,[154,155] and emerging evidence points to a role for mitochondrial dysfunction in a variety of cardiac syndromes, although a truly causal role has yet to be established *in vivo* (for review, see reference 156).

Transition metals and other oxidants

Transition metals such as iron and copper have been studied extensively *in vitro* with regard to radical reactions and damage to biomolecules, as they are strong catalysts for oxidation reactions in the presence of aqueous (H_2O_2) or lipid (LOOH) peroxides.[43,157] With regard to the latter, they catalyze homolytic cleavage of LOOH to lipid alkoxyl radicals that can initiate lipid peroxidation and other oxidation reactions.[157,158] In general, however, the concentration of free transition metals *in vivo* is considered negligible (e.g. [159]), and there is little convincing evidence that they are related to atherosclerosis. In fact, most data imply the opposite, as autopsy examination of patients with hemochromatosis (a disorder of elevated plasma and tissue levels of iron) demonstrates less coronary artery disease than in age- and sex-matched controls;[160] and iron overload of rabbits[161] and mice[162] actually decreases atherosclerosis.

Another prominent risk factor for atherosclerosis is an elevation in serum levels of homocysteine.[163] Although patients having highly elevated homocysteine levels are rare (cystathionine-β-synthase deficient homocysteinuria), epidemiological data indicate that an increased risk of cardiovascular disease exists with even mildly elevated ($> 15\,\mu M$) plasma homocysteine concentrations.[164–166] The mechanism by which homocysteine promotes atherothrombosis remains unclear; however, oxidative stress has been proposed as an important contributing factor.[167] High levels of homocysteine ($> 1\,\mu M$) are cytotoxic to cultured endothelial cells in an H_2O_2-dependent manner,[168,169] lower levels induce endothelial dysfunction via superoxide.[170,171] Homocysteine also promotes oxidative stress by inhibiting cellular glutathione peroxidase (GPx-1) expression in endothelial cells. A recent study demonstrating that both homocysteine and its oxidized form (homocystine) induce lipid peroxidation in endothelial cells[172] would tend to support the notion that oxidative stress is linked to the injurious effect of homocysteine on the endothelium.

Among the more intriguing recent findings is the notion that ozone may be a feature of atherosclerosis. Wentworth and colleagues[173] examined human atherosclerosis specimens taken at the time of surgery and found evidence for ozone-mediated oxidation. The products of ozonolysis include steroid oxidation products that have biologic activity consistent with atherosclerosis, such as cytotoxicity and modification of apolipoprotein B-100. These data are in keeping with previous work demonstrating that antibodies can catalyze ozone formation from singlet oxygen formed during neutrophil action, and that ozone may provide a source of hydroxyl radical-like activity in the absence of transition metal ions.[174]

Reconciling available data on oxidative events and atherosclerosis

There is a wealth of data linking atherosclerosis with a number of oxidative events, ranging from LDL oxidation to the production of intracellular reactive oxygen and nitrogen species. Despite this, it is fundamentally difficult to implicate oxidative stress as a causal feature of atherosclerosis, based on the poor results of antioxidant strategies designed to limit either atherosclerosis or cardiovascular events in human subjects. There are no compelling data that antioxidant supplementation has any effect on the process of atherosclerosis, which calls into question the premise that oxidative stress is required for atherosclerosis.

Several potential explanations come to mind to explain the results of antioxidant trials and, perhaps, reconcile the available data. First and foremost, the most unattractive consideration is that oxidative stress is not causally related to the process of atherosclerosis and its clinical expression. In light of the considerable effort that has been directed toward linking atherosclerosis to oxidative stress, this explanation has been met with limited enthusiasm. A second consideration is that we may not completely understand the relevant oxidants, nor their primary site of action for atherosclerosis, and thus have not really tested the right antioxidants. Indeed, the distinction between one- and two-electron oxidants is germane here, as antioxidant trials to date involved species only active against one-electron oxidants. Finally, oxidative stress may only represent an injury *response* to atherosclerosis. If this latter point proved true, any strategy aimed at oxidation reactions would simply be like treating the symptoms rather than the cause of a disease.

Oxidative events and atherosclerosis are not causally linked

Despite the wealth of data that LDL oxidation is a clear feature of atherosclerosis, the notion that it is both necessary and sufficient is not complete. Although lesions in human[175] and animal[35,176] atherosclerotic tissue contain oxidized lipids, putatively as a consequence of LDL oxidation, lesion formation can be dissociated from lipid peroxidation in the arterial wall.[35] One interpretation for this finding is that LDL oxidation is not necessary for atherosclerosis. One issue supporting the LDL oxidation hypothesis, however, is that scavenger receptors are involved in atherosclerosis, mice lacking type A scavenger receptors[29] or CD36[30] develop fewer lesion than do wildtype mice. There are, however, oxidation-independent mechanisms of foam cell formation to consider.

For example, there is evidence that arterial wall retention of lipoproteins is a determinant of lesion formation. The LDL entry rate into normal arterial segments exceeds its rate of accumulation,[177] consistent with LDL egress as a 'rate-limiting step' for atherosclerosis. Indeed, excess atherogenic lipoproteins are found in lesion-prone arterial sites despite an LDL entry rate comparable to that of normal areas.[178,179] These and other studies tend to suggest that lesion-prone areas exhibit enhanced *retention* of apoB-containing lipoproteins as the inciting event for atherosclerosis.[180–182]

This concept is known as the 'response-to-retention' hypothesis, and it has considerable support in the literature (Figure 5.4). In rabbits injected LDL is followed by arterial LDL retention and microaggregate formation within 2 hours.[183] One mechanism for this process involves extracellular matrix components.[184,185] LDL proteoglycan association is promoted by lipoprotein lipase (LpL)[186] in vessels that have been enriched with LpL,[187] independent of LpL enzymatic activity.[188] Most importantly, LDL retention promotes LDL aggregation, a process stimulated by secretory sphingomyelinase[189] present in the arterial wall.[189]

Entrapment of LDL in the arterial wall sets the stage for foam cell formation, largely independent of oxidation. The interaction of retained LDL with sphingomyelinase[189] can generate ceramides that promote apoptosis and mitogenesis.[190,191] Most importantly, aggregated LDL is readily internalized by macrophages and smooth muscle cells,[192] leading to foam cell formation independent of LDL oxidation.[193] This means of foam cell formation appears quite relevant, as Boren and colleagues[194] constructed a transgenic mouse overexpressing human apoB-100 that develops significant atherosclerosis with dietary hypercholesterolemia. In a

very clever study, they constructed an analogous strain with a human apoB mutant defective in proteoglycan binding (but with intact LDL receptor binding) that did not develop atherosclerotic lesions.[195] Thus, LDL proteoglycan binding is critical for atherosclerotic lesion formation, consistent with the response-to-retention hypothesis. In light of these data, one can propose that LDL aggregation is sufficient for foam cell formation and atherosclerosis. If this were the case, it is possible that LDL oxidation would also occur, but as an epiphenomenon rather than as a cause of atherosclerotic lesion formation. Only further investigation will delineate the relative roles of LDL retention and oxidation in atherosclerosis.

Our knowledge of oxidants in atherosclerosis is incomplete

Among the more compelling early data linking LDL oxidation and atherosclerosis were observations that many structurally distinct antioxidants, such as probucol, vitamin E, and butylated hydroxytoluene, inhibited atherosclerosis in animal models.[196] The rationale for choosing these antioxidant species was their ability to inhibit LDL oxidation by one-electron oxidants such as copper ions or radical generating systems. Almost all human trials (that were based on animal data) utilized these 'traditional' antioxidants. If the oxidative stress of atherosclerosis proves to be due to two-electron oxidants, the aforementioned antioxidant species would actually be expected to fail,[47] consistent with most clinical antioxidant trials to date.

The scenario outlined above is indeed plausible. For example, two-electron oxidants, such as HOCl, oxidize LDL apolipoprotein B-100 preferentially over lipids.[46] The principal source of HOCl, myeloperoxidase, is found in human atherosclerotic lesions and is enzymatically active[129,197] More recently, leukocyte MPO levels have been positively associated with coronary artery disease[132] and the development of acute myocardial infarction in patients presenting to the emergency room.[133] There is also evidence for HOCl-mediated oxidation in atherosclerosis. Lesion-derived LDL and atherosclerotic lesions in humans and Watanabe rabbits immunostain for HOCl-modified epitopes.[47,197–199] Human lesion LDL also contains chlorotyrosine,[130,200] a marker for active MPO and HOCl. Thus, abundant data implicate the two-electron oxidant HOCl in the pathobiology of

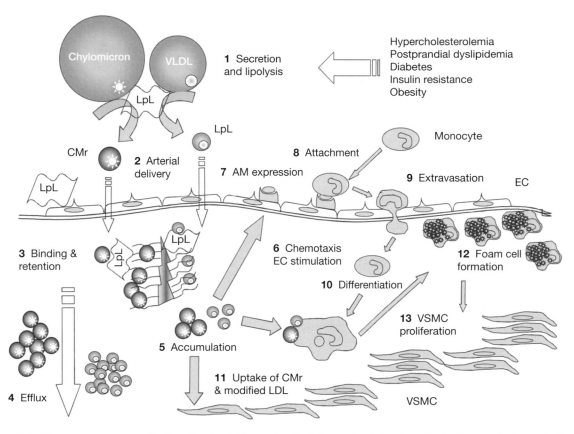

Figure 5.4 The response-to-retention hypothesis of atherosclerosis. Atherosclerosis begins with the lipoprotein lipase (LpL)-mediated delivery (2) and retention (3) of atherogenic lipoproteins on proteoglycans in the arterial wall; non-retained lipoproteins are secreted (4). The accumulation (5) of lipoproteins facilitates (6) chemotaxis and adhesion molecule (AM) expression (7), with attachment of monocytes (8). The accumulated low-density lipoprotein (LDL) also facilitates cellular uptake (11), perhaps through aggregation, leading to foam cell formation (12) and vascular smooth muscle cell (VSMC) proliferation (13). VLDL, very low-density lipoprotein; CMr, chylomicron remnant; EC, endothelial cells. (Adapted from reference 224)

atherogenesis. To the extent that HOCl may contribute causally to atherosclerosis, one must be cognisant that clinical trials with vitamin E would not be expected to alter HOCl-mediated oxidation.

Another two-electron oxidant, H_2O_2, has attracted considerable interest in vascular disease. Specifically, H_2O_2 is known as an intracellular messenger that mediates many maladaptive responses in the vasculature. Mitogenic growth factors promoting cell proliferation have been implicated in atherosclerosis,[201] and growth factor-mediated cell proliferation is, in large part, dependent on intracellular H_2O_2 generation[202-204]. As one might expect, H_2O_2-mediated oxidation is not inhibited by free radical scavengers such as α-tocopherol and ascorbic acid. Thus, to the extent that some features of atherosclerosis are due to unchecked

H_2O_2 production, these responses would not be inhibited by any clinically evaluated antioxidant strategies.

This latter point touches upon a weak link in using antioxidant strategies to limit oxidative stress and ameliorate oxidant-mediated pathology. Successful use of an antioxidant strategy is dependent on a detailed understanding of all relevant oxidants that may promote a disease process. This problem is illustrated in Figure 5.5. The production of superoxide has a number of important consequences that may contribute to vascular disease. Specific antioxidants may scavenge or metabolize some of the relevant oxidizing species, but others escape inactivation. For example, lipid-soluble antioxidants will inhibit lipid peroxidation without any effect on two-electron oxidants that mediate protein modification (OONO or HOCl) or cell signaling by H_2O_2.

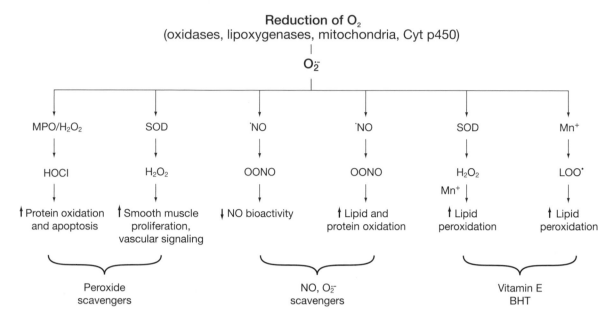

Figure 5.5 Scheme outlining strategies of oxidant scavenging. As stated in the text, many sources of superoxide can beget a number of secondary reactions. Any one 'scavenger' strategy is unlikely to have a material effect on other potentially harmful reactions. Thus, identifying the signals and sources that lead to abnormal ROS/RNS production could prove the preferred strategy for limiting oxidative damage. (Adapted from reference 223)

Alternatively, H_2O_2 scavenging may profoundly limit HOCl-mediated oxidation but have the undesired effect of limiting H_2O_2-mediated signaling that could be necessary. A recent analogy with NO production and the clinical syndrome of sepsis serves as a case in point. Excess NO production underlies vascular leakage and hypotension in sepsis (for review, see reference 205); yet non-specific nitric oxide synthase inhibition failed to improve outcome in this disease.[206] One might anticipate such a problem when physiologic processes go unchecked in disease states (i.e. ROS signaling), as simple scavenging strategies could also interrupt physiologic responses and worsen the clinical situation.

How to resolve the situation? Perhaps one starting point would include a more complete understanding of relevant oxidant sources and the control of their production. Theoretically, this information could be used to devise specific strategies that ameliorate pathologic processes while preserving physiologic ROS signaling. This approach worked well with chronic myelogenous leukemia (CML), a disease previously treated with palliative chemotherapeutic agents although the disease remained incurable. Intense research found that CML involved a chromosomal rearrangement (the so-called

Philadelphia chromosome) that produced a unique fusion gene known as BCR-ABL, encoding a dysregulated tyrosine kinase.[207] This information led to the discovery of a specific tyrosine kinase inhibitor that proved an extremely effective treatment.[208] Thus, understanding the nature of dysregulation can lead to specific therapeutic approaches. Only by a complete understanding of the mechanism(s) of dysregulated oxidant production will a similar result with atherosclerosis be achieved.

Oxidative events are only an injurious response to atherosclerosis

In the light of data linking LDL oxidation to atherosclerosis, considerable effort has been directed at establishing atherosclerosis risk factors as related to LDL oxidation and oxidative stress in vivo. Many studies have linked oxidative stress to atherosclerosis risk factors such as diabetes,[209] hypertension,[60] and smoking.[210] Some have found the link between oxidative stress and atherosclerosis so compelling as to propose that all atherosclerosis risk factors act through excess oxidative stress (Figure 5.6a)[211]. This link between atherosclerosis risk factors and lipid peroxidation was recently tested in the

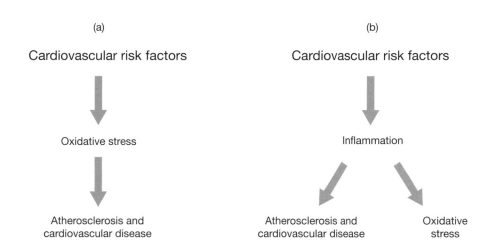

(a)

Cardiovascular risk factors

Oxidative stress

Atherosclerosis and
cardiovascular disease

(b)

Cardiovascular risk factors

Inflammation

Atherosclerosis and
cardiovascular disease

Oxidative
stress

Figure 5.6   Conceptual views of oxidative stress as a cause (a) or a consequence (b) of atherogenesis. In (b), scavenging oxidants and limiting markers of oxidative stress will yield material differences in the process of atherosclerosis

Framingham Study.[212] In that population, lipid peroxidation was linked only to diabetes as an established risk factor for atherosclerosis,[212] and statistical modeling could only explain ~15% of the observed evidence for lipid peroxidation based on cardiovascular risk factors. Thus, lipid peroxidation is only weakly linked to atherosclerosis risk factors.

Inflammation is involved in atherosclerosis (for review, see [213]) and this concept dates back some 25 years, to when Ross[201] observed that adhesion of inflammatory cells to the arterial wall occurred within days of an atherogenic diet. This process is dependent on cellular adhesion molecules such as leukocyte β_1- and β_2-integrins and endothelial vascular cell adhesion molecule-1 and intracellular adhesion molecule-1 (ICAM-1), respectively.[214] Many investigators have demonstrated that circulating markers of inflammation predict atherosclerosis and its clinical sequelae,[215–218] and these data are reviewed in reference 28. One important consequence of inflammation is the generation of oxidants and markers of oxidative damage.[219] Could it be that antioxidant strategies in atherosclerosis have proved disappointing because oxidative events are a consequence, rather than a cause, of the disease (Figure 5.6b)? In this scenario, oxidant scavenging would limit markers of oxidative stress but have little impact on the disease process. Is there evidence to support such a contention? Indeed, the relationship between atherosclerosis risk factors and inflammation is rather tight, in that

all established CVD risk factors are predictive of circulating inflammation markers.[215–218] These findings would suggest that inflammation is a primary process and oxidative stress only secondary.

Conclusions

Atherosclerosis is a disease characterized by arterial lipid deposition and inflammation that, over time, progresses and may precipitate the clinical events of heart attack and stroke. Compelling evidence indicates that oxidative stress is a pervasive aspect of atherosclerosis that contributes to many features of the disease, such as adhesion molecule expression, endothelial dysfunction, and a propensity towards thrombosis. However, direct evidence that oxidative stress, and LDL oxidation in particular, is both necessary and sufficient for atherosclerosis has been difficult to find. There are many potential reasons for this difficulty, not the least of which is our lack of knowledge about the precise molecular events that beget vascular oxidative stress, and the precise mediators involved. Only further investigation will elucidate these events and provide us with the tools to limit oxidative stress at its source and ameliorate all of its secondary phenomena. Only then will we know what components of atherosclerosis are directly due to oxidative stress.

References

1. Wilson PW, Garrison RJ, Castelli WP et al. Prevalence of coronary heart disease in the Framingham Offspring Study: role of lipoprotein cholesterols. Am J Cardiol 1980; 46:649–654.
2. Gotto AM Jr. Treating hypercholesterolemia: looking forward. Clin Cardiol 2003; 26:I21–I28.
3. Goldstein JL, Brown MS. The low-density lipoprotein pathway and its relation to atherosclerosis. Annu Rev Biochem 1977; 46:897–930.
4. Goldstein JL, Ho YK, Basu SK et al. Binding site on macrophages that mediates uptake and degradation of acetylated low density lipoprotein, producing massive cholesterol deposition. Proc Natl Acad Sci USA 1979; 76:333–337.
5. Krieger M, Acton S, Ashkenas J et al. Molecular flypaper, host defense, and atherosclerosis. Structure, binding properties, and functions of macrophage scavenger receptors. J Biol Chem 1993; 268:4569–4572.
6. Henriksen T, Mahoney EM, Steinberg D. Enhanced macrophage degradation of low density lipoprotein previously incubated with cultured endothelial cells: recognition by receptor for acetylated low density lipoproteins. Proc Natl Acad Sci USA 1981; 78:6499–6503.
7. Krieger M. The other side of scavenger receptors: pattern recognition for host defense. Curr Opin Lipidol 1997; 8:275–280.
8. Kodama T, Freeman M, Rohrer L et al. Type I macrophage scavenger receptor contains alpha-helical and collagen-like coiled coils. Nature 1990; 343:531–535.
9. Steinberg D, Parthasarathy S, Carew TE et al. Beyond cholesterol. Modifications of low-density lipoprotein that increase its atherogenicity. N Engl J Med 1989; 320:915–924.
10. Quinn MT, Parthasarathy S, Steinberg D. Endothelial cell-derived chemotactic activity for mouse peritoneal macrophages and the effects of modified forms of low density lipoprotein. Proc Natl Acad Sci USA 1985; 82:5949–5953.
11. Ross R, Glomset J, Harker L. Response to injury and atherogenesis. Am J Pathol 1977; 86:675–684.
12. Esterbauer H, Gebicki J, Puhl H et al. The role of lipid peroxidation and antioxidants in oxidative modification of LDL. Free Radical Biol Med 1992; 13:341–390.
13. Haberland ME, Fong D, Cheng L. Malondialdehyde-altered protein occurs in atheroma of Watanabe heritable hyperlipidemic rabbits. Science 1988; 241:215–218.
14. Boyd HC, Gown AM, Wolfbauer G et al. Direct evidence for a protein recognized by a monoclonal antibody against oxidatively modified LDL in atherosclerotic lesions from a Watanabe heritable hyperlipidemic rabbit. Am J Pathol 1989; 135:815–825.
15. Palinski W, Ord VA, Plump AS et al. ApoE-deficient mice are a model of lipoprotein oxidation in atherogenesis. Demonstration of oxidation-specific epitopes in lesions and high titers of autoantibodies to malondialdehyde-lysine in serum. Arterioscler Thromb 1994; 14:605–616.
16. Palinski W, Rosenfeld ME, Ylä-Herttuala S et al. Low density lipoprotein undergoes oxidative modification in vivo. Proc Natl Acad Sci USA 1989; 86:1372–1376.
17. Ylä-Herttuala S, Palinski W, Rosenfeld ME et al. Evidence for the presence of oxidatively modified low density lipoprotein in atherosclerotic lesions of rabbit and man. J Clin Invest 1989; 84:1086–1095.
18. Cushing SD, Berliner JA, Valente AJ et al. Minimally modified low density lipoprotein induces monocyte chemotactic protein 1 in human endothelial cells and smooth muscle cells. Proc Natl Acad Sci USA 1990; 87:5134–5139.
19. Rajavashisth TB, Andalibi A, Territo MC et al. Induction of endothelial cell expression of granulocyte and macrophage colony-stimulating factors by modified low density lipoproteins. Nature 1990; 344:254–257.
20. Navab M, Imes SS, Hama SY et al. Monocyte transmigration induced by modification of low density lipoprotein in cocultures of human aortic wall cells is due to induction of monocyte chemotactic protein 1 synthesis and is abolished by high density lipoprotein. J Clin Invest 1991; 88:2039–2046.
21. Liao F, Andalibi A, deBeer FC et al. Genetic control of inflammatory gene induction and NF-kappa B-like transcription factor activation in response to an atherogenic diet in mice. J Clin Invest 1993; 91:2572–2579.
22. Boring L, Gosling J, Cleary M et al. Decreased lesion formation in CCR2–/– mice reveals a role for chemokines in the initiation of atherosclerosis. Nature 1998; 394:894–897.
23. Gosling J, Slaymaker S, Gu L et al. MCP-1 deficiency reduces susceptibility to atherosclerosis in mice that overexpress human apolipoprotein B. J Clin Invest 1999; 103:773–778.
24. Quinn MT, Parthasarathy S, Fong LG et al. Oxidatively modified low density lipoproteins: a potential role in recruitment and retention of monocyte/macrophages during atherogenesis. Proc Natl Acad Sci USA 1987; 84:2995–2998.
25. McMurray HF, Parthasarathy S, Steinberg D. Oxidatively modified low density lipoprotein is a chemoattractant for human T lymphocytes. J Clin Invest 1993; 92:1004–1008.
26. Parums DV, Brown DL, Mitchinson MJ. Serum antibodies to oxidized low-density lipoprotein and ceroid in chronic periaortitis. Arch Pathol Lab Med 1990; 114:383–387.
27. Salonen JT, Ylä-Herttuala S, Yamamoto R et al. Autoantibody against oxidised LDL and progression of carotid atherosclerosis. Lancet 1992; 339:883–887.
28. Libby P, Ridker PM, Maseri A. Inflammation and atherosclerosis. Circulation 2002; 105:1135–1143.
29. Suzuki H, Kurihara Y, Takeya M et al. A role for macrophage scavenger receptors in atherosclerosis and susceptibility to infection. Nature 1997; 386:292–296.
30. Febbraio M, Podrez EA, Smith JD et al. Targeted disruption of the class B scavenger receptor CD36 protects against atherosclerotic lesion development in mice. J Clin Invest 2000; 105:1049–1056.
31. Upston JM, Terentis AC, Stocker R. Tocopherol-mediated peroxidation of lipoproteins: implications for vitamin E as a

potential antiatherogenic supplement. FASEB J 1999; 13:977–994.

32. Keaney JF Jr. Antioxidants and atherosclerosis: animal studies. In: Keaney JF Jr, ed. Oxidative stress and vascular disease. Boston: Kluwer, 2000: 195–212.

33. Yusuf S, Dagenais G, Pogue J et al. Vitamin E supplementation and cardiovascular events in high-risk patients. The Heart Outcomes Prevention Evaluation Study Investigators. N Engl J Med 2000; 342:154–160.

34. MRC/BHF Heart Protection Study of antioxidant vitamin supplementation in 20,536 high-risk individuals: a randomised placebo-controlled trial. Lancet 2002; 360:23–33.

35. Witting P, Pettersson K, Ostlund-Lindqvist AM et al. Dissociation of atherogenesis from aortic accumulation of lipid hydro(pero)xides in Watanabe heritable hyperlipidemic rabbits. J Clin Invest 1999; 104:213–220.

36. Gerschman R, Gilbert DL, Nye SW et al. Oxygen poisoning and x-irradiation: a mechanism in common. Science 1954; 119:623–626.

37. Chance B, Sies H, Boveris A. Hydroperoxide metabolism in mammalian organs. Physiol Rev 1979; 59:527–605.

38. Sies H. Introductory remarks. In: Sies H, ed. Oxidative stress. London: Academic Press, 1985: 1.

39. Sies H. Oxidative stress: from basic research to clinical application. Am J Med 1991; 91:31S–38S.

40. Hausladen A, Keng T, Stamler JS. Nitrosative stress: activation of the transcription factor OxyR by S-nitrosothiols. Cell 1996; 86:719–729.

41. Halliwell B, Gutteridge JMC. Free radicals in biology and medicine. Oxford: Clarendon Press, 1999.

42. Buettner GR. The pecking order of free radicals and antioxidants: lipid peroxidation, alpha-tocopherol, and ascorbate. Arch Biochem Biophys 1993; 300:535–543.

43. Haber F, Weiss J. The catalytic decomposition of hydrogen peroxide by iron salts. Proc R Soc London 1934; 147:332–351.

44. Kissner R, Koppenol WH. Product distribution of peroxynitrite decay as a function of pH, temperature, and concentration. J Am Chem Soc 2002; 124:234–239.

45. Thomas SR, Davies MJ, Stocker R. Oxidation and antioxidation of human low-density lipoprotein and plasma exposed to 3-morpholinosydnonimine and reagent peroxynitrite. Chem Res Toxicol 1998; 11:484–494.

46. Hazell LJ, Stocker R. Oxidation of low-density lipoprotein with hypochlorite causes transformation of the lipoprotein into a high-uptake form for macrophages. Biochem J 1993; 290:165–172.

47. Hazell LJ, Stocker R. Alpha-tocopherol does not inhibit hypochlorite-induced oxidation of apolipoprotein B-100 of low-density lipoprotein. FEBS Lett 1997; 414:541–544.

48. Hazell LJ, van den Berg JJ, Stocker R. Oxidation of low-density lipoprotein by hypochlorite causes aggregation that is mediated by modification of lysine residues rather than lipid oxidation. Biochem J 1994; 302 (Pt 1):297–304.

49. Vissers MC, Stern A, Kuypers F et al. Membrane changes associated with lysis of red blood cells by hypochlorous acid. Free Radical Biol Med 1994; 16:703–712.

50. Winterbourn CC. Comparative reactivities of various biological compounds with myeloperoxidase-hydrogen peroxide-chloride, and similarity of the oxidant to hypochlorite. Biochim Biophys Acta 1985; 840:204–210.

51. Pattison DI, Hawkins CL, Davies MJ. Hypochlorous acid-mediated oxidation of lipid components and antioxidants present in low-density lipoproteins: absolute rate constants, product analysis, and computational modeling. Chem Res Toxicol 2003; 16:439–449.

52. Yao Y, Yin D, Jas GS et al. Oxidative modification of a carboxyl-terminal vicinal methionine in calmodulin by hydrogen peroxide inhibits calmodulin-dependent activation of the plasma membrane Ca-ATPase. Biochemistry 1996; 35:2767–2787.

53. Raman CS, Li H, Martasek P et al. Crystal structure of constitutive endothelial nitric oxide synthase: a paradigm for pterin function involving a novel metal center. Cell 1998; 95:939–950.

54. Zou MH, Shi C, Cohen RA. Oxidation of the zinc–thiolate complex and uncoupling of endothelial nitric oxide synthase by peroxynitrite. J Clin Invest 2002; 109:817–826.

55. Van Wart HE, Birkedal-Hansen H. The cysteine switch: a principle of regulation of metalloproteinase activity with potential applicability to the entire matrix metalloproteinase gene family. Proc Natl Acad Sci USA 1990; 87:5578–5582.

56. Fu X, Kassim SY, Parks WC, Heinecke JW. Hypochlorous acid oxygenates the cysteine switch domain of pro-matrilysin (MMP-7). A mechanism for matrix metalloproteinase activation and atherosclerotic plaque rupture by myeloperoxidase. J Biol Chem 2001; 276:41279–41287.

57. Babior BM, Lambeth JD, Nauseef W. The neutrophil NADPH oxidase. Arch Biochem Biophys 2002; 397:342–344.

58. Parkos CA, Allen RA, Cochrane CG et al. Purified cytochrome b from human granulocyte plasma membrane is comprised of two polypeptides with relative molecular weights of 91,000 and 22,000. J Clin Invest 1987; 80:732–742.

59. Heyworth PG, Bohl BP, Bokoch GM et al. Rac translocates independently of the neutrophil NADPH oxidase components p47phox and p67phox. Evidence for its interaction with flavocytochrome b558. J Biol Chem 1994; 269:30749–30752.

60. Griendling KK, Sorescu D, Ushio-Fukai M. NAD(P)H oxidase: role in cardiovascular biology and disease. Circ Res 2000; 86:494–501.

61. Rey FE, Pagano PJ. The reactive adventitia: fibroblast oxidase in vascular function. Arterioscler Thromb Vasc Biol 2002; 22:1962–1971.

62. Mohazzab-H K, Wolin MS. Properties of a superoxide anion-generating microsomal NADH oxidoreductase, a potential pulmonary artery P_{O_2} sensor. Am J Physiol 1994; 267:L823–L831.

63. Pagano PJ, Ito Y, Tornheim K et al. An NADPH oxidase superoxide generating system in rabbit aorta. Am J Physiol 1995; 268:H2274–H2280.

64. Rajagopalan S, Kurz S, Münzel T et al. Angiotensin II-mediated hypertension in the rat increases vascular superoxide production via membrane NADH/HADPH oxidase activation. Contribution to alterations of vasomotor tone. J Clin Invest 1996; 97:1916–1923.

65. Ushio-Fukai M, Tang Y, Fukai T et al. Novel role of gp91(phox)-containing NAD(P)H oxidase in vascular endothelial growth factor-induced signaling and angiogenesis. Circ Res 2002; 91:1160–1167.

66. Suh YA, Arnold RS, Lassegue B et al. Cell transformation by the superoxide-generating oxidase Mox1. Nature 1999; 401:79–82.

67. Sorescu D, Weiss D, Lassegue B et al. Superoxide production and expression of nox family proteins in human atherosclerosis. Circulation 2002; 105:1429–1435.

68. Cheng G, Cao Z, Xu X et al. Homologs of gp91phox: cloning and tissue expression of Nox3, Nox4, and Nox5. Gene 2001; 269:131–140.

69. Lassegue B, Sorescu D, Szocs K et al. Novel gp91(phox) homologues in vascular smooth muscle cells : nox1 mediates angiotensin II-induced superoxide formation and redox-sensitive signaling pathways. Circ Res 2001; 88:888–894.

70. Touyz RM, Chen X, Tabet F et al. Expression of a functionally active gp91phox-containing neutrophil-type NAD(P)H oxidase in smooth muscle cells from human resistance arteries: regulation by angiotensin II. Circ Res 2002; 90:1205–1213.

71. Pagano PJ, Clark J, Cifuentes-Pagano ME et al. Localization of a constitutively active, phagocyte-like NADPH oxidase in rabbit aortic adventitia: enhancement by angiotensin II. Proc Natl Acad Sci USA 1997; 94:14483–14488.

72. Li JM, Shah AM. Intracellular localization and preassembly of the NADPH oxidase complex in cultured endothelial cells. J Biol Chem 2002; 277:19952–19960.

73. Patterson C, Ruef J, Madamanchi NR et al. Stimulation of a vascular smooth muscle cell NAD(P)H oxidase by thrombin. Evidence that p47(phox) may participate in forming this oxidase in vitro and in vivo. J Biol Chem 1999; 274:19814–19822.

74. Li JM, Mullen AM, Yun S et al. Essential role of the NADPH oxidase subunit p47(phox) in endothelial cell superoxide production in response to phorbol ester and tumor necrosis factor-alpha. Circ Res 2002; 90:143–150.

75. Gu Y, Xu YC, Wu RF et al. p47phox participates in activation of RelA in endothelial cells. J Biol Chem 2003; 278:17210–17217.

76. Hwang J, Saha A, Boo YC et al. Oscillatory shear stress stimulates endothelial production of O2- from p47phox-dependent NAD(P)H oxidases, leading to monocyte adhesion. J Biol Chem 2003; 278:47291–47298.

77. Seshiah PN, Weber DS, Rocic P et al. Angiotensin II stimulation of NAD(P)H oxidase activity: upstream mediators. Circ Res 2002; 91:406–413.

78. Warnholtz A, Nickenig G, Schulz E et al. Increased NADH-oxidase-mediated superoxide production in the early stages of atherosclerosis: evidence for involvement of the renin–angiotensin system. Circulation 1999; 99:2027–2033.

79. Hathaway CA, Heistad DD, Piegors DJ et al. Regression of atherosclerosis in monkeys reduces vascular superoxide levels. Circ Res 2002; 90:277–283.

80. Kirk EA, Dinauer MC, Rosen H et al. Impaired superoxide production due to a deficiency in phagocyte NADPH oxidase fails to inhibit atherosclerosis in mice. Arterioscler Thromb Vasc Biol 2000; 20:1529–1535.

81. Barry-Lane PA, Patterson C, van der Merwe et al. p47phox is required for atherosclerotic lesion progression in ApoE(–/–) mice. J Clin Invest 2001; 108:1513–1522.

82. Hsich E, Segal BH, Pagano PJ et al. Vascular effects following homozygous disruption of p47(phox): an essential component of NADPH oxidase. Circulation 2000; 101:1234–1236.

83. Guzik TJ, West NE, Black E et al. Vascular superoxide production by NAD(P)H oxidase: association with endothelial dysfunction and clinical risk factors. Circ Res 2000; 86:E85–E90.

84. Guzik TJ, Mussa S, Gastaldi D et al. Mechanisms of increased vascular superoxide production in human diabetes mellitus: role of NAD(P)H oxidase and endothelial nitric oxide synthase. Circulation 2002; 105:1656–1662.

85. Harrison R. Structure and function of xanthine oxidoreductase: where are we now? Free Radical Biol Med 2002; 33:774–797.

86. McCord JM. Oxygen-derived free radicals in postischemic tissue injury. N Engl J Med 1985; 312:159–163.

87. Ohara Y, Peterson TE, Harrison DG. Hypercholesterolemia increases endothelial superoxide anion production. J Clin Invest 1993; 91:2546–2551.

88. Cardillo C, Kilcoyne CM, Cannon RO III et al. Xanthine oxidase inhibition with oxypurinol improves endothelial vasodilator function in hypercholesterolemic but not in hypertensive patients. Hypertension 1997; 30:57–63.

89. Guthikonda S, Sinkey C, Barenz T et al. Xanthine oxidase inhibition reverses endothelial dysfunction in heavy smokers. Circulation 2003; 107:416–421.

90. Spiekermann S, Landmesser U, Dikalov S et al. Electron spin resonance characterization of vascular xanthine and NAD(P)H oxidase activity in patients with coronary artery disease: relation to endothelium-dependent vasodilation. Circulation 2003; 107:1383–1389.

91. Dupont GP, Huecksteadt TP, Marshall BC et al. Regulation of xanthine dehydrogenase and xanthine oxidase activity and gene expression in cultured rat pulmonary endothelial cells. J Clin Invest 1992; 89:197–202.

92. Wakabayashi Y, Fujita H, Morita I et al. Conversion of xanthine dehydrogenase to xanthine oxidase in bovine carotid artery endothelial cells induced by activated neutrophils: involvement of adhesion molecules. Biochim Biophys Acta 1995; 1265:103–109.

93. White CR, Darley-Usmar V, Berrington WR et al. Circulating plasma xanthine oxidase contributes to vascular dysfunction in hypercholesterolemic rabbits. Proc Natl Acad Sci USA 1996; 93:8745–8749.

94. Alderton WK, Cooper CE, Knowles RG. Nitric oxide synthases: structure, function and inhibition. Biochem J 2001; 357:593–615.

95. Shaul PW. Regulation of endothelial nitric oxide synthase: location, location, location. Ann Rev Physiol 2002; 64:749–774.

96. Roman LJ, Martasek P, Masters BS. Intrinsic and extrinsic modulation of nitric oxide synthase activity. Chem Rev 2002; 102:1179–1190.

97. Fleming I. Brain in the brawn: the neuronal nitric oxide synthase as a regulator of myogenic tone. Circ Res 2003; 93:586–588.

98. Cirino G, Fiorucci S, Sessa WC. Endothelial nitric oxide synthase: the Cinderella of inflammation? Trends Pharmacol Sci 2003; 24:91–95.

99. Vasquez-Vivar J, Kalyanaraman B, Martasek P et al. Superoxide generation by endothelial nitric oxide synthase: the influence of cofactors. Proc Natl Acad Sci USA 1998; 95:9220–9225.

100. Xia Y, Tsai AL, Berka V et al. Superoxide generation from endothelial nitric-oxide synthase. A Ca2+/calmodulin-dependent and tetrahydrobiopterin regulatory process. J Biol Chem 1998; 273:25804–25808.

101. Bec N, Gorren AC, Voelker C et al. Reaction of neuronal nitric-oxide synthase with oxygen at low temperature. Evidence for reductive activation of the oxy-ferrous complex by tetrahydrobiopterin. J Biol Chem 1998; 273:13502–13508.

102. Gorren AC, Bec N, Schrammel A et al. Low-temperature optical absorption spectra suggest a redox role for tetrahydrobiopterin in both steps of nitric oxide synthase catalysis. Biochemistry 2000; 39:11763–11770.

103. Pritchard KA Jr, Groszek L, Smalley DM et al. Native low-density lipoprotein increases endothelial cell nitric oxide synthase generation of superoxide anion. Circ Res 1995; 77:510–518.

104. Vasquez-Vivar J, Duquaine D, Whitsett J et al. Altered tetrahydrobiopterin metabolism in atherosclerosis: implications for use of oxidized tetrahydrobiopterin analogues and thiol antioxidants. Arterioscler Thromb Vasc Biol 2002; 22:1655–1661.

105. Laursen JB, Somers M, Kurz S et al. Endothelial regulation of vasomotion in apoE-deficient mice: implications for interactions between peroxynitrite and tetrahydrobiopterin. Circulation 2001; 103:1282–1288.

106. Hink U, Li H, Mollnau H et al. Mechanisms underlying endothelial dysfunction in diabetes mellitus. Circ Res 2001; 88:E14–E22.

107. Shinozaki K, Kashiwagi A, Nishio Y et al. Abnormal biopterin metabolism is a major cause of impaired endothelium-dependent relaxation through nitric oxide/O$_2^-$ imbalance in insulin-resistant rat aorta. Diabetes 1999; 48:2437–2445.

108. Alp NJ, Mussa S, Khoo J et al. Tetrahydrobiopterin-dependent preservation of nitric oxide-mediated endothelial function in diabetes by targeted transgenic GTP-cyclohydrolase I overexpression. J Clin Invest 2003; 112:725–735.

109. Lin MI, Fulton D, Babbitt R et al. Phosphorylation of threonine 497 in endothelial nitric-oxide synthase coordinates the coupling of L-arginine metabolism to efficient nitric oxide production. J Biol Chem 2003; 278:44719–44726.

110. Thomas SR, Chen K, Keaney JF Jr. Hydrogen peroxide activates endothelial nitric oxide synthase through coordinated phosphorylation and dephosphorylation via a phosphoinositide 3-kinase-dependent signaling pathway. J Biol Chem 2002; 277:6017–6024.

111. Squadrito GL, Pryor WA. Oxidative chemistry of nitric oxide: the roles of superoxide, peroxynitrite, and carbon dioxide. Free Radical Biol Med 1998; 25:392–403.

112. Gow AJ, Duran D, Malcolm S et al. Effects of peroxynitrite-induced protein modifications on tyrosine phosphorylation and degradation. FEBS Lett 1996; 385:63–66.

113. Byun J, Mueller DM, Fabjan JS et al. Nitrogen dioxide radical generated by the myeloperoxidase-hydrogen peroxide-nitrite system promotes lipid peroxidation of low density lipoprotein. FEBS Lett 1999; 455:243–246.

114. Heinecke JW, Hsu FF, Crowley JR et al. Detecting oxidative modification of biomolecules with isotope dilution mass spectrometry: sensitive and quantitative assays for oxidized amino acids in proteins and tissues. Methods Enzymol 1999; 300:124–144.

115. Hazen SL, Crowley JR, Mueller DM et al. Mass spectrometric quantification of 3-chlorotyrosine in human tissues with attomole sensitivity: a sensitive and specific marker for myeloperoxidase-catalyzed chlorination at sites of inflammation. Free Radical Biol Med 1997; 23:909–916.

116. Heinecke JW, Li W, Mueller DM et al. Cholesterol chlorohydrin synthesis by the myeloperoxidase-hydrogen peroxide-chloride system: potential markers for lipoproteins oxidatively damaged by phagocytes. Biochemistry 1994; 33:10127–10136.

117. Savenkova MI, Mueller DM, Heinecke JW. Tyrosyl radical generated by myeloperoxidase is a physiological catalyst for the initiation of lipid peroxidation in low density lipoprotein. J Biol Chem 1994; 269:20394–20400.

118. Hazen SL, Hsu F, Heinecke JW. p-Hydroxyphenylacetaldehyde is the major product of L-tyrosine oxidation by activated human phagocytes. J Biol Chem 1996; 271:1861–1867.

119. Hazen SL, Heller J, Hsu FF et al. Synthesis, isolation, and characterization of the adduct formed in the reaction of p-hydroxyphenylacetaldehyde with the amino headgroup of phosphatidylethanolamine and phosphatidylserine. Chem Res Toxicol 1999; 12:19–27.

120. Hazen SL, Gaut JP, Hsu FF et al. p-Hydroxyphenylacetaldehyde, the major product of L-tyrosine oxidation by the myeloperoxidase–H$_2$O$_2$–chloride system of phagocytes, covalently modifies epsilon-amino groups of protein lysine residues. J Biol Chem 1997; 272:16990–16998.

121. Anderson MM, Hazen SL, Hsu FF et al. Human neutrophils employ the myeloperoxidase–hydrogen peroxide–chloride system to convert hydroxy-amino acids into glycolaldehyde, 2-hydroxypropanol, and acrolein. A mechanism for the generation of highly reactive alpha-hydroxy and alpha,beta-unsaturated aldehydes by phagocytes at sites of inflammation. J Clin Invest 1997; 99:424–432.

122. Anderson MM, Requena JR, Crowley JR et al. The myeloperoxidase system of human phagocytes generates *N*-epsilon-(carboxymethyl)lysine on proteins: a mechanism for producing advanced glycation end products at sites of inflammation. J Clin Invest 1999; 104:103–113.

123. Kawamura M, Heinecke JW, Chait A. Increased uptake of alpha-hydroxy aldehyde-modified low density lipoprotein by macrophage scavenger receptors. J Lipid Res 2000; 41:1054–1059.

124. Eiserich JP, Cross CE, Jones AD et al. Formation of nitrating and chlorinating species by reaction of nitrite with hypocholorous acid. J Biol Chem 1996; 271:19199–19208.

125. van der Vliet A, Eiserich JP, Halliwell B et al. Formation of reactive nitrogen species during peroxidase-catalyzed oxidation of nitrite. J Biol Chem 1997; 272:7617–7625.

126. Eiserich JP, Hristova M, Cross CE et al. V. Formation of nitric oxide-derived inflammatory oxidants by myeloperoxidase in neutrophils. Nature 1998; 391:393–397.

127. Gaut JP, Byun J, Tran HD et al. Myeloperoxidase produces nitrating oxidants in vivo. J Clin Invest 2002; 109:1311–1319.

128. Podrez EA, Schmitt D, Hoff HF et al. Myeloperoxidase-generated reactive nitrogen species convert LDL into an atherogenic form in vitro. J Clin Invest 1999; 103:1547–1560.

129. Daugherty A, Dunn JL, Rateri DL et al. Myeloperoxidase, a catalyst for lipoprotein oxidation, is expressed in human atherosclerotic lesions. J Clin Invest 1994; 94:437–444.

130. Hazen SL, Heinecke JW. 3-Chlorotyrosine, a specific marker of myeloperoxidase-catalyzed oxidation, is markedly elevated in low density lipoprotein isolated from human atherosclerotic intima. J Clin Invest 1997; 99:2075–2081.

131. Leeuwenburgh C, Hardy MM, Hazen SL et al. Reactive nitrogen intermediates promote low density lipoprotein oxidation in human atherosclerotic intima. J Biol Chem 1997; 272:1433–1436.

132. Zhang R, Brennan ML, Fu X et al. Association between myeloperoxidase levels and risk of coronary artery disease. J Am Med Assoc 2001; 286:2136–2142.

133. Brennan ML, Penn MS, Van Lente F et al. Prognostic value of myeloperoxidase in patients with chest pain. N Engl J Med 2003; 349:1595–1604.

134. Brennan ML, Anderson MM, Shih DM et al. Increased atherosclerosis in myeloperoxidase-deficient mice. J Clin Invest 2001; 107:419–430.

135. Rouzer CA, Marnett LJ. Mechanism of free radical oxygenation of polyunsaturated fatty acids by cyclooxygenases. Chem Rev 2003; 103:2239–2304.

136. Belkner J, Wiesner R, Rathman J et al. Oxygenation of lipoproteins by mammalian lipoxygenases. Eur J Biochem 1993; 213:251–261.

137. Upston JM, Neuzil J, Witting PK et al. Oxidation of free fatty acids in low density lipoprotein by 15-lipoxygenase stimulates nonenzymic, alpha-tocopherol-mediated peroxidation of cholesteryl esters. J Biol Chem 1997; 272:30067–30074.

138. Kuhn N, Heydeck D, Hugou I et al. In vivo action of 15-lipoxygenase in early stages of human atherosclerosis. J Clin Invest 1997; 99:888.

139. Samokyszyn VM, Marnett LJ. Hydroperoxide-dependent cooxidation of 13-*cis*-retinoic acid by prostaglandin H synthase. J Biol Chem 1987; 262:14119–14133.

140. Chamulitrat W, Mason RP. Lipid peroxyl radical intermediates in the peroxidation of polyunsaturated fatty acids by lipoxygenase. Direct electron spin resonance investigations. J Biol Chem 1989; 264:20968–20973.

141. Upston JM, Neuzil J, Stocker R. Oxidation of LDL by recombinant human 15-lipoxygenase: evidence for alpha-tocopherol-dependent oxidation of esterified core and surface lipids. J Lipid Res 1996; 37:2650–2661.

142. Ylä-Herttuala S, Rosenfeld ME, Parthasarathy S et al. Colocalization of 15-lipoxygenase mRNA and protein with epitopes of oxidized low density lipoprotein in macrophage-rich areas of atherosclerotic lesions. Proc Natl Acad Sci USA 1990; 87:6959–6963.

143. Mehrabian M, Allayee H, Wong J et al. Identification of 5-lipoxygenase as a major gene contributing to atherosclerosis susceptibility in mice. Circ Res 2002; 91:120–126.

144. Cyrus T, Witztum JL, Rader D et al. Disruption of the 12/15-lipoxygenase gene diminishes atherosclerosis in apo E-deficient mice. J Clin Invest 1999; 103:1597–1604.

145. George J, Afek A, Shaish A et al. 12/15-Lipoxygenase gene disruption attenuates atherogenesis in LDL receptor-deficient mice. Circulation 2001; 104:1646–1650.

146. Dwyer JH, Allayee H, Dwyer KM et al. Arachidonate 5-lipoxygenase promoter genotype, dietary arachidonic acid, and atherosclerosis. N Engl J Med 2004; 350:29–37.

147. Kinnula VL, Crapo JD. Superoxide dismutases in the lung and human lung diseases. Am J Respir Crit Care Med 2003; 167:1600–1619.

148. Cadenas E, Davies KJ. Mitochondrial free radical generation, oxidative stress, and aging. Free Radical Biol Med 2000; 29:222–230.

149. Liu X, Kim CN, Yang J et al. Induction of apoptotic program in cell-free extracts: requirement for dATP and cytochrome c. Cell 1996; 86:147–157.

150. Quillet-Mary A, Jaffrezou JP, Mansat V et al. Implication of mitochondrial hydrogen peroxide generation in ceramide-induced apoptosis. J Biol Chem 1997; 272:21388–21395.

151. Li AE, Ito H, Rovira II et al. A role for reactive oxygen species in endothelial cell anoikis. Circ Res 1999; 85:304–310.

152. Du XL, Edelstein D, Rossetti L et al. Hyperglycemia-induced mitochondrial superoxide overproduction activates the hexosamine pathway and induces plasminogen activator inhibitor-1 expression by increasing Sp1 glycosylation. Proc Natl Acad Sci USA 2000; 97:12222–12226.

153. Nishikawa T, Edelstein D, Du XL et al. Normalizing mitochondrial superoxide production blocks three pathways of hyperglycaemic damage. Nature 2000; 404:787–790.

154. Knight-Lozano CA, Young CG, Burow DL et al. Cigarette smoke exposure and hypercholesterolemia increase

mitochondrial damage in cardiovascular tissues. Circulation 2002; 105:849–854.

155. Ballinger SW, Patterson C, Knight-Lozano CA et al. Mitochondrial integrity and function in atherogenesis. Circulation 2002; 106:544–549.

156. Ramachandran A, Levonen AL, Brookes PS et al. Mitochondria, nitric oxide, and cardiovascular dysfunction. Free Radical Biol Med 2002; 33:1465–1474.

157. Keaney JF Jr, Frei B. Antioxidant protection of low-density lipoprotein and its role in the prevention of atherosclerotic vascular disease. In: Frei B, ed. Natural antioxidants in human health and disease. San Diego: Academic Press, 1994: 303–352.

158. Minotti G, Aust SD. The role of iron in the initiation of lipid peroxidation. Chem Phys Lipids 1987; 44:191–208.

159. Rae TD, Schmidt PJ, Pufahl RA et al. Undetectable intracellular free copper: the requirement of a copper chaperone for superoxide dismutase. Science 1999; 284:805–808.

160. Miller M, Hutchins GM. Hemochromatosis, multiorgan hemosiderosis, and coronary artery disease. J Am Med Assoc 1994; 272:231–233.

161. Dabbagh AJ, Shwaery GT, Keaney JF Jr et al. Effect of iron overload and iron deficiency on atherosclerosis in the hypercholesterolemic rabbit. Arterioscler Thromb Vasc Biol 1997; 17:2638–2645.

162. Kirk EA, Heinecke JW, LeBoeuf RC. Iron overload diminishes atherosclerosis in apoE-deficient mice. J Clin Invest 2001; 107:1545–1553.

163. McCully KS. Vascular pathology of homocysteinemia: implications for the pathogenesis of atherosclerosis. Am J Pathol 1969; 56:111–128.

164. Clarke RL, Daly L, Robinson K et al. Hperhomocysteinemia: an independent risk factor for vascular disease. N Engl J Med 1991; 324:1145–1155.

165. Stampfer MJ, Malinow MR, Willett WC et al. A prospective study of plasma homocyst(e)ine and risk of myocardial infarction in US physicians. J Am Med Assoc 1992; 268:877–881.

166. Selhub J, Jaques PF, Bostom AG et al. Association between plasma homocyst(e)ine concentrations and extracranial carotid artery stenosis. N Engl J Med 1995; 332:328–329.

167. Welch GN, Loscalzo J. Homocyst(e)ine and atherothrombosis. N Engl J Med 1998; 338:1042–1050.

168. Starkbaum G, Harlan JM. Endothelial cell injury due to copper-catalyzed hydrogen peroxide generation from homocysteine. J Clin Invest 1986; 77:1370–1376.

169. Wall RT, Harlan JM, Harker LA et al. Homocysteine-induced endothelial cell injury in vitro: a model for the study of vascular injury. Thromb Res 1980; 18:113–121.

170. Lang D, Kredan MB, Moat SJ et al. Homocysteine-induced inhibition of endothelium-dependent relaxation in rabbit aorta: role for superoxide anions. Arterioscler Thromb Vasc Biol 2000; 20:422–427.

171. Zhang X, Li H, Jin H et al. Effects of homocysteine on endothelial nitric oxide production. Am J Physiol Renal Physiol 2000; 279:F671–F678.

172. Heydrick SJ, Weiss N, Thomas SR et al. L-homocysteine and L-homocystine steriospecifically induce eNOS-dependent lipid peroxidation in endothelial cells. Free Radical Biol Med 2004; 36:632–640.

173. Wentworth P Jr, Nieva J, Takeuchi C et al. Evidence for ozone formation in human atherosclerotic arteries. Science 2003; 302:1053–1056.

174. Wentworth P Jr, Wentworth AD, Zhu X et al. Evidence for the production of trioxygen species during antibody-catalyzed chemical modification of antigens. Proc Natl Acad Sci USA 2003; 100:1490–1493.

175. Suarna C, Dean RT, May J et al. Human atherosclerotic plaque contains both oxidized lipids and relatively large amounts of α-tocopherol and ascorbate. Arterioscler Thromb Vasc Biol 1995; 15:1616–1624.

176. Witting PK, Pettersson K, Letters JM et al. Site-specific anti-atherogenic effect of probucol in apolipoprotein E-deficient mice. Arterioscler Thromb Vasc Biol 2000; 20:E26–E30.

177. Carew TE, Pittman RC, Marchand ER et al. Measurement in vivo of irreversible degradation of low density lipoprotein in the rabbit aorta. Predominance of intimal degradation. Arteriosclerosis 1984; 4:214–224.

178. Schwenke DC, Zilversmit DB. The arterial barrier to lipoprotein influx in the hypercholesterolemic rabbit. 1. Studies during the first two days after mild aortic injury. Atherosclerosis 1989; 77:91–103.

179. Schwenke DC, Zilversmit DB. The arterial barrier to lipoprotein influx in the hypercholesterolemic rabbit. 2. Long-term studies in deendothelialized and reendothelialized aortas. Atherosclerosis 1989; 77:105–115.

180. Schwenke DC, Carew TE. Initiation of atherosclerotic lesions in cholesterol-fed rabbits. I. Focal increases in arterial LDL concentration precede development of fatty streak lesions. Arteriosclerosis 1989; 9:895–907.

181. Schwenke DC, Carew TE. Initiation of atherosclerotic lesions in cholesterol-fed rabbits. II. Selective retention of LDL vs. selective increases in LDL permeability in susceptible sites of arteries. Arteriosclerosis 1989; 9:908–918.

182. Falcone D, Hajjar D, Minick C. Lipoprotein and albumin accumulation in reendothelialized and deendothelialized aorta. Am J Pathol 1984; 114:112–120.

183. Nievelstein PF, Fogelman AM, Mottino G et al. Lipid accumulation in rabbit aortic intima 2 hours after bolus infusion of low density lipoprotein. A deep-etch and immunolocalization study of ultrarapidly frozen tissue. Arterioscler Thromb 1991; 11:1795–1805.

184. Ylä-Herttuala S, Solakivi T, Hirvonen MR et al. Glycosaminoglycans and apolipoproteins B and A-1 in human aortas: chemical and immunological analysis of lesion-free aortas from children and adults. Arteriosclerosis 1987; 7:333–340.

185. Camejo G, Hurt-Camejo E, Olsson U et al. Proteoglycans and lipoproteins in atherosclerosis. Curr Opin Lipidol 1993; 4:385–391.

186. Williams KJ, Fless GM, Petrie K et al. Mechanisms by which lipoprotein lipase alters cellular metabolism of lipoprotein(a), low-density lipoprotein, and nascent lipoproteins. Roles for low-density lipoprotein receptors and heparan sulfate proteoglycans. J Biol Chem 1992; 267:13284–13292.

187. Rutledge JC, Goldberg IJ. Lipoprotein lipase (LpL) affects low density lipoprotein (LDL) flux through vascular tissue: evidence that LpL increases LDL accumulation in vascular tissue. J Lipid Res 1994; 35:1152–1160.

188. Williams KJ, Fless GM, Petrie K et al. Mechanisms by which lipoprotein lipase alters cellular metabolism of lipoprotein(a), low density lipoprotein, and nascent lipoproteins: roles for low density lipoprotein receptors and heparan sulfate proteoglycans. J Biol Chem 1992; 267:13284–13292.

189. Xu X, Tabas I. Sphingomyelinase enhances low density lipoprotein uptake and ability to induce cholesteryl ester accumulation in macrophages. J Biol Chem 1991; 266:24849–24858.

190. Hannun YA. The sphingomyelin cycle and the second messenger function of ceramide. J Biol Chem 1994; 269:3125–3128.

191. Joseph C, Wright SD, Bornmann W et al. Bacterial lipopolysaccharide has structural similarity to ceramide and stimulates ceramide-activated protein kinase in myeloid cells. J Biol Chem 1994; 269:17606–17610.

192. Ismail N, Alavi M, Moore S. Lipoprotein-proteoglycan complexes from injured rabbit aortas accelerate lipoprotein uptake by arterial smooth muscle cells. Arteriosclerosis 1994; 105:79–87.

193. Vijayagopal P, Srinivasan SR, Radhakrishnamurthy B et al. Lipoprotein–proteoglycan complexes from atherosclerotic lesions promote cholesteryl ester accumulation in human monocytes/macrophages. Arterioscler Thromb 1992; 12:237–249.

194. Boren J, Olin K, Lee I et al. Identification of the principal proteoglycan-binding site in LDL. A single-point mutation in apo-B100 severely affects proteoglycan interaction without affecting LDL receptor binding. J Clin Invest 1998; 101:2658–2664.

195. Skalen K, Gustafsson M, Rydberg EK et al. Subendothelial retention of atherogenic lipoproteins in early atherosclerosis. Nature 2002; 417:750–754.

196. Keaney JF Jr. Antioxidants and vascular disease: animal studies. In: Tardif JC, Bourassa MG, eds. Antioxidants and cardiovascular disease. Rotterdam: Kluwer, 2000: 101–116.

197. Malle E, Waeg G, Schreiber R et al. Immunohistochemical evidence for the myeloperoxidase/H2O2/halide system in human atherosclerotic lesions: colocalization of myeloperoxidase and hypochlorite-modified proteins. Eur J Biochem 2000; 267:4495–4503.

198. Malle E, Wag G, Thiery J et al. Hypochlorite-modified (lipo)proteins are present in rabbit lesions in response to dietary cholesterol. Biochem Biophys Res Commun 2001; 289:894–900.

199. Malle E, Hazell L, Stocker R et al. Immunologic detection and measurement of hypochlorite-modified LDL with specific monoclonal antibodies. Arterioscler Thromb Vasc Biol 1995; 15:982–989.

200. Fu S, Wang H, Davies M et al. Reactions of hypochlorous acid with tyrosine and peptidyl-tyrosyl residues give dichlorinated and aldehydic products in addition to 3-chlorotyrosine. J Biol Chem 2000; 275:10851–10858.

201. Ross R. Atherosclerosis – an inflammatory disease. N Engl J Med 1999; 340:115–126.

202. Heeneman S, Haendeler J, Saito Y et al. Angiotensin II induces transactivation of two different populations of the platelet-derived growth factor beta receptor. Key role for the p66 adaptor protein Shc. J Biol Chem 2000; 275:15926–15932.

203. Sundaresan M, Yu ZX, Ferrans VJ et al. Requirement for generation of H2O2 for platelet-derived growth factor signal transduction. Science 1995; 270:296–299.

204. Chen K, Thomas SR, Keaney JF Jr. Beyond LDL oxidation: ROS in vascular signal transduction. Free Radical Biol Med 2003; 35:117–132.

205. Shah NS, Billiar TR. Role of nitric oxide in inflammation and tissue injury during endotoxemia and hemorrhagic shock. Environ Health Perspect 1998; 106(Suppl 5):1139–1143.

206. Cobb JP. Use of nitric oxide synthase inhibitors to treat septic shock: the light has changed from yellow to red. Crit Care Med 1999; 27:855–856.

207. Shtivelman E, Lifshitz B, Gale RP et al. Fused transcript of abl and bcr genes in chronic myelogenous leukaemia. Nature 1985; 315:550–554.

208. Druker BJ, Sawyers CL, Kantarjian H et al. Activity of a specific inhibitor of the BCR-ABL tyrosine kinase in the blast crisis of chronic myeloid leukemia and acute lymphoblastic leukemia with the Philadelphia chromosome. N Engl J Med 2001; 344:1038–1042.

209. Gopaul NK, Änggård EE, Mallet AI et al. Plasma 8-epi-PGF2alpha levels are elevated in individuals with non-insulin dependent diabetes mellitus. FEBS Lett 1995; 368:225–229.

210. Morrow JD, Frei B, Longmire AW et al. Increase in circulating products of lipid peroxidation (F2-isoprostanes) in smokers. Smoking as a cause of oxidative damage. N Engl J Med 1995; 332:1198–1203.

211. Alexander RW. Theodore Cooper Memorial Lecture. Hypertension and the pathogenesis of atherosclerosis. Oxidative stress and the mediation of arterial inflammatory response: a new perspective. Hypertension 1995; 25:155–161.

212. Keaney JF Jr, Larson MG, Vasan RS et al. Obesity and systemic oxidative stress: clinical correlates of oxidative stress in the Framingham study. Arterioscler Thromb Vasc Biol 2003; 23:434–439.

213. Pearson TA, Mensah GA, Alexander RW et al. Markers of inflammation and cardiovascular disease: application to clinical and public health practice: a statement for healthcare professionals from the Centers for Disease Control and Prevention and the American Heart Association. Circulation 2003; 107:499–511.

214. Zimmerman GA, Prescott SM, McIntyre TM. Endothelial cell interactions with granulocytes: tethering and signaling molecules. Immunol Today 1992; 13:93–100.

215. Hwang SJ, Ballantyne CM, Sharrett AR et al. Circulating adhesion molecules VCAM-1, ICAM-1, and E-selectin in carotid atherosclerosis and incident coronary heart disease cases: the Atherosclerosis Risk in Communities (ARIC) study. Circulation 1997; 96:4219–4225.

216. Ridker PM, Hennekens CH, Roitman-Johnson B et al. Plasma concentration of soluble intercellular adhesion molecule 1 and risks of future myocardial infarction in apparently healthy men. Lancet 1998; 351:88–92.

217. Malik I, Danesh J, Whincup P et al. Soluble adhesion molecules and prediction of coronary heart disease: a prospective study and meta-analysis. Lancet 2001; 358:971–976.

218. Pradhan AD, Rifai N, Ridker PM. Soluble intercellular adhesion molecule-1, soluble vascular adhesion molecule-1, and the development of symptomatic peripheral arterial disease in men. Circulation 2002; 106:820–825.

219. Nathan C. Points of control in inflammation. Nature 2002; 420:846–852.

220. Kissner R, Nauser T, Bugnon P et al. Formation and properties of peroxynitrite as studied by laser flash photolysis, high-pressure stopped-flow technique, and pulse radiolysis. Chemical Res Toxicol 1997; 10:1285–1292.

221. Jones SA, O'Donnell VB, Wood JD et al. Expression of phagocyte NADPH oxidase components in human endothelial cells. Am J Physiol 1996; 271:H1626–H1634.

222. Takeya R, Ueno N, Kami K et al. Novel human homologues of p47phox and p67phox participate in activation of superoxide-producing NADPH oxidases. J Biol Chem 2003; 278:25234–25246.

223. Munzel T, Keaney JF Jr. Are ace inhibitors a 'magic bullet' against oxidative stress? Circulation 2001; 104:1571–1574.

224. Proctor SD, Vine DF, Mamo JC. Arterial retention of apolipoprotein B48- and B100-containing lipoproteins in atherogenesis. Curr Opin Lipid 2002; 13:461–470.

6

Thrombosis and atherosclerosis

Jane E. Freedman, Joseph Loscalzo

Introduction

The majority of acute coronary events are related to disruption of a 'vulnerable' atherosclerotic plaque, leading to the exposure of subintimal contents and the formation of a platelet-rich thrombus. The importance of platelet activation in the events leading to vessel occlusion in acute coronary syndromes is supported by the clear clinical benefit of treatment with aspirin for both primary and secondary prevention strategies.[1] This process, however, is complex and influenced by a wide variety of cellular and plasma-derived mediators that determine the balance between occlusive and non-occlusive thrombosis. In this chapter, the events that contribute to the process of thrombosis in the setting of the atherosclerotic plaque will be reviewed.

Mechanisms of plaque rupture

In advanced fibrolipid lesions the atheromatous contents are separated from the vascular lumen by a fibrous cap. The thinnest portion of this cap occurs in the region adjoining the normal intima. Rupture occurs when strain within this fibrous cap exceeds the deformability of its components. The process of rupture is thought to occur from the shear stress or pressure changes transpiring in an artery. Ruptured plaques are associated with decreased collagen as well as larger numbers of macrophages, T cells, and smooth muscle cells than those found in unruptured plaques.[2] These findings have suggested that the process of plaque rupture may be one of localized inflammatory process. The action of enzymes within the macrophages may lead to a weakening of the fibrous cap and can also predispose it to rupture.

The mechanical stability of the plaque is a pivotal determinant of this process. A plaque predisposed to rupture is normally lipid rich with a thin fibrous cap that lacks the normal support from collagen and smooth muscle cells.[3] Treatment with lipid-lowering agents over time stabilizes plaques, probably by depletion of plaque lipid and through a reduction in inflammatory cell activity.[4] These changes, in turn, appear to lead to a reduction in thrombosis by decreasing platelet activity and tissue factor expression.[4] This paradigm is consistent with the significant reduction in clinical events observed in large randomized trials of lipid-lowering therapies in the setting of little or no plaque regression.[5]

Thrombosis and the ruptured plaque

Thrombus formation within a coronary vessel is the precipitating event in myocardial infarction and unstable angina, as shown in angiographic[6] and pathologic[7] studies. The angiographic severity of coronary stenoses does not adequately predict sites of subsequent acute coronary syndromes. For this reason, rupture of atheromatous plaque in relatively mildly stenosed vessels and subsequent thrombus formation is believed to underlie the majority of acute coronary syndromes.[8,9] Either superficial intimal injury caused by endothelial denudation or deep intimal injury caused by plaque rupture exposes collagen and von Willebrand factor to circulating platelets (Figure 6.1).[9] Platelets can then adhere directly to collagen or indirectly via the binding of von Willebrand factor to glycoprotein Ib/IX. Local platelet activation (by tissue factor-mediated thrombin generation or by collagen) stimulates further thrombus

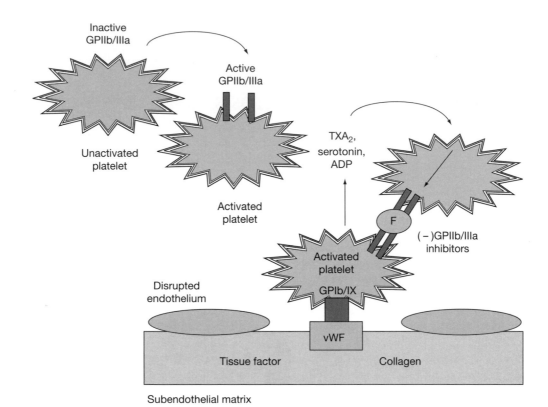

Figure 6.1 Vascular injury exposes subendothelial von Willebrand factor (vWF) to the circulating blood. Platelets adhere to the site of injury when glycoprotein (GP)Ib/IX expressed on the platelet surface binds to the subendothelial vWF. This triggers signaling events causing the synthesis and release of ADP, thromboxane (TX)A$_2$, and serotonin, leading to platelet activation. These events cause a conformational change in GPIIb/IIIa, enabling the high-affinity binding of fibrinogen (F). As local platelet activation and recruitment occurs, fibrinogen bivalently bonds to the activated platelet GPIIb/IIIa receptors, resulting in platelet thrombus formation

formation, which leads to additional platelet recruitment caused by cell-surface thrombin formation and the release of serotonin, ADP, and thromboxane A$_2$. After activation, thrombus forms as platelets aggregate via the binding of bivalent fibrinogen to glycoprotein IIb/IIIa (Figure 6.1).

The clinical relevance of these pathways is supported by the increased platelet-derived thromboxane and prostaglandin metabolites detected in patients with acute coronary syndromes.[10] Thrombi contained within a ruptured plaque are often composed of multiple layers of different age, suggesting repetitive recurrences of rupture. Interestingly, some patients with unstable coronary syndromes have been shown to have multiple thrombi by intracoronary angioscopy.[11,12] Some of the thrombi may lead to complete occlusion, whereas others do not obstruct the lumen. These findings suggest that in specific high-risk patients a systemic process is at play, leading to vulnerability of several plaque locations.[11,12] Consistent with these observations is the increasing understanding of the contribution of inflammation to atherosclerosis (see below).

The interaction between thrombosis and inflammation

The importance of platelet-dependent thrombosis has made the platelet aggregate a common therapeutic target in acute coronary syndromes. Recently, such therapies have included the use of aspirin, thienopyridines, and direct glycoprotein IIb/IIIa inhibitors. Although

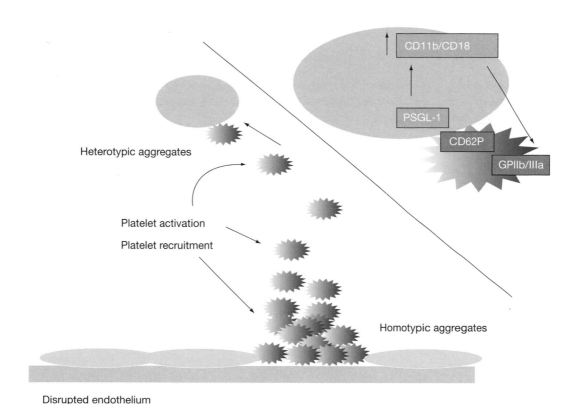

Figure 6.2 Patients with acute coronary syndromes have not only increased interactions between platelets (homotypic aggregates), but also increased interactions between platelets and leukocytes (heterotypic aggregates). Heterotypic aggregates form when platelets are activated and undergo degranulation, after which they adhere to circulating leukocytes. Platelets bind via P-selectin (CD62P) expressed on the surface of activated platelets to the leukocyte receptor, P-selectin glycoprotein ligand-1 (PSGL-1). This leads to increased expression of CD11b/CD18 (Mac-1) on leukocytes, which may support interactions with platelets via bivalent fibrinogen linking this integrin with its platelet surface counterpart glycoprotein IIb/IIIa

the mechanisms of action of these various agents differ, they all inhibit fibrinogen-dependent platelet–platelet association. As highlighted by the disappointing clinical results of trials using oral glycoprotein IIb/IIIa inhibitors,[13] however, merely preventing the process of platelet aggregation may not always translate into clinical efficacy. Platelets are also known to be involved in the inflammatory response and produce mediators, including platelet-derived growth factor, platelet factor-4, and transforming growth factor-β. Patients with acute coronary syndromes have not only increased interactions between platelets (homotypic aggregates), but also increased interactions between platelets and leukocytes (heterotypic aggregates) detectable in circulating blood (Figure 6.2). These latter aggregates form

when platelets are activated and undergo degranulation, after which they adhere to circulating leukocytes.

Heterotypic aggregates commonly form in inflammatory states (Figure 6.2).[14] Platelets bind via P-selectin (CD62P) expressed on the surface of activated platelets to the leukocyte receptor P-selectin glycoprotein ligand-1 (PSGL-1).[15] This association leads to increased expression of CD11b/CD18 (Mac-1) on leukocytes,[16] which itself supports interactions with platelets, perhaps via bivalent fibrinogen linking this integrin with its platelet surface counterpart glycoprotein IIb/IIIa.[17,18] The relevance of platelet–leukocyte aggregates in vascular disease is supported by a study demonstrating that the infusion of recombinant human PSGL-1 in an animal model of vascular injury reduced myocardial reperfusion injury and preserved vascular endothelial function.[19]

In unstable coronary syndromes, markers of cardiac necrosis may not provide adequate information about plaque disruption. As platelet–leukocyte aggregates potentially reflect plaque instability, including ongoing vascular thrombosis and inflammation, their measurement may be a useful index of the propensity for acute atherothrombotic vascular syndromes. In addition, platelet–leukocyte aggregates may also be a more sensitive marker of platelet activation than surface P-selectin expression, as degranulated platelets rapidly lose surface P-selectin *in vivo* but continue to be detected in the circulation.[20] Supportive of this view is a recent study demonstrating that after acute myocardial infarction, circulating monocyte–platelet aggregates are a more sensitive marker of *in vivo* platelet activation than platelet surface P-selectin.[21] Neutrophil activation and neutrophil–platelet adhesion measurements in patients with unstable angina have also been shown to be significantly increased compared to those patients with stable angina.[22]

The interaction between platelets and leukocytes in acute coronary syndromes highlights the relation between inflammation and thrombosis in cardiovascular disease. In addition to triggering thrombosis directly, plaque rupture promotes activation of the inflammatory response. The expression of tissue factor on both endothelial cells and monocytes is partially regulated by proinflammatory cytokines, including tumor necrosis factor and interleukin-1.[23] Tissue factor also interacts with P-selectin, accelerating fibrin formation and deposition.[23] In addition, platelet surface P-selectin induces the expression of tissue factor on monocytes[24] and enhances monocyte cytokine expression,[25] as well as promoting CD11b/CD18 expression.[16]

Also bridging the thrombotic, atherosclerotic, and inflammatory processes are interactions between CD40 and CD40 ligand (CD40L or CD154).[26] Ligation of CD40 on various vascular cells contributes to the pathogenesis of atherosclerosis and thrombosis.[26,27] On endothelial cells or monocytes the engagement of CD40 leads to the synthesis of adhesion molecules, chemokines, and tissue factor, and causes the activation of matrix metalloproteinases.

CD40L has also been detected in platelets[26] where, after stimulation, it is translocated to the platelet surface (Figure 6.3). CD40L is upregulated on platelets in a fresh thrombus.[26] The surface-expressed CD40L is cleaved from the platelet over a period of minutes to hours, generating a soluble fragment (soluble CD40L, or sCD40L).[28] It is estimated that more than 95% of the circulating sCD40L is derived from platelets.[28] Found to be increased on platelets in arterial thrombus,[26] sCD40L has been shown to be elevated in cardiovascular disease[29,30] and associated with increased cardiovascular risk in apparently healthy women.[31] Although sCD40L has been characterized as a marker of thrombotic disease, much less is known about its direct role in platelet function. It has been suggested that CD40L is an $\alpha_{IIb}\beta_3$ ligand, a platelet agonist, and contributes to the stability of arterial thrombi.

Thrombosis: the role of reactive oxygen species and antioxidants

Even in the setting of a ruptured atherosclerotic plaque, activation and recruitment of platelets is tightly regulated. Adhesion of platelets to the endothelium is prevented by several mechanisms, including endothelial cell production of prostacyclin and nitric oxide (NO).[32,33] The presence or absence of NO from the vascular endothelium is important in vascular occlusion and has been extensively characterized. Endothelium-dependent dilation is impaired in animal models of atherosclerosis and in isolated atherosclerotic human coronary arteries.[34] In addition, it is well established that cardiovascular disease and coronary risk factors, including cholesterol level, male gender, family history, and age, are associated with impaired endothelium-dependent vasodilation in coronary arteries.[35]

Nitric oxide inhibits platelet activation[36,37] and prevents thrombosis.[38] It is also directly released from platelets, and appears to regulate the recruitment of additional platelets and the process of thrombosis.[39] Importantly, platelets from patients with acute myocardial infarction and unstable angina despite aspirin treatment are still partially activated, as measured by platelet surface expression of P-selectin and active glycoprotein IIb/IIIa,[40] supporting the importance of activation processes independent of the eicosanoid pathway.

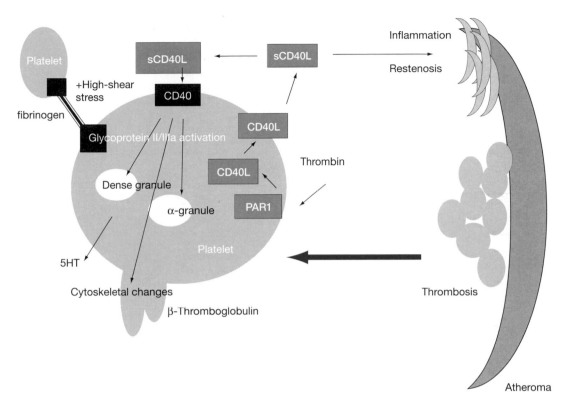

Figure 6.3 After platelet stimulation via the thrombin receptor (PAR1), CD40 ligand (CD40L) is translocated to the platelet surface. Surface-expressed CD40L is then cleaved from the platelet over a period of minutes to hours, subsequently generating a soluble fragment, sCD40L. Soluble CD40L can then bind to CD40 and promote inflammatory or thrombotic responses by causing further platelet activation and the release of substances from both dense (5HT) and α-granules, as well as the expression of active glycoprotein IIb/IIIa. Release of sCD40L can also lead to smooth muscle cell proliferation or, in high-shear settings, enhance the formation of homotypic aggregates via fibrinogen

A prominent feature of both abnormal platelet function and dysfunctional endothelium-dependent vasodilation in the setting of cardiovascular disease is oxidative stress (Figure 6.4). Superoxide anion is an important source of oxidative stress and limits the biological activity of NO. Excessive vascular superoxide production has been demonstrated in hypercholesterolemia as well as other disease states associated with endothelial dysfunction.[41,42]

Evidence also suggests that oxidative stress is important for normal platelet function. Platelet aggregation is associated with a burst of oxygen consumption[43] and a marked rise in glutathione disulfide.[44] Whereas dramatic changes in platelet NO redox status occur during normal aggregation, conditions that provoke oxidative stress without inducing a florid aggregation response have also been shown to be prothrombotic. Reactive oxygen species contribute causally to many pathophysiologic conditions, including atherosclerosis, and have been detected in both resting and activated platelets (Figure 6.4). Superoxide is produced by platelets,[45] as are hydroperoxy derivatives of long-chain fatty acids (12-HpETE). Superoxide in particular is known to augment platelet aggregation responses.[46] The reactive oxygen species produced by platelets can evoke an oxidative stress that supports lipid peroxidation, induces cellular activation, and promotes endothelial dysfunction. Superoxide (in the presence of transition metals) promotes lipid peroxidation, leading to the generation of lipid alkoxyl and peroxyl radicals and causing lipid radical chain propagation reactions.[47,48] This process can be terminated by NO. By reacting with superoxide or lipid peroxyl radicals, NO can form peroxynitrite and lipid peroxynitrites, respectively, with a resultant loss of NO bioactivity.[48]

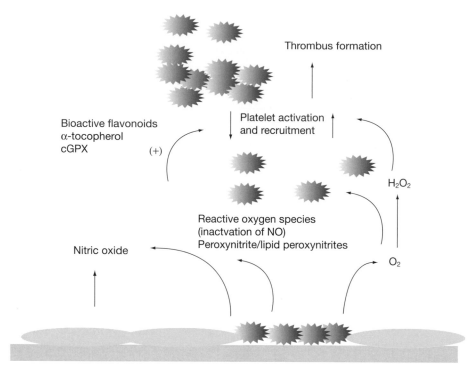

Figure 6.4 Oxidative stress is important for normal platelet function. Platelet aggregation is associated with a burst of oxygen consumption and rise in glutathione disulfide. Reactive oxygen species have been detected in both resting and activated platelets. Superoxide, NO, and hydroperoxy derivatives of long-chain fatty acids (12-HpETE) are produced by platelets. The reactive oxygen species produced by platelets can evoke an oxidative stress that supports lipid peroxidation, induces cellular activation, and promotes endothelial dysfunction. Antioxidants or bioactive flavonoids may indirectly inhibit platelets through metabolism of reactive oxygen species, many of which alter platelet function

Antioxidants may indirectly inhibit platelets through the metabolism of reactive oxygen species, many of which alter platelet function. Hydroperoxides produced by the platelet (PGG$_2$, 12-HpETE, and PLOOH) are metabolized by the selenium-dependent enzyme glutathione peroxidase (cGPx). Glutathione peroxidase potentiates the inhibition of platelet function by NO by reducing LOOH,[49] and impairment of this process can lead to a clinical thrombotic disorder.[50] This important antioxidant role of plasma glutathione peroxidase may be of broader relevance than this rare thrombotic disorder first described in children. Glutathione peroxidase is a selenium-containing enzyme, and selenium deficiency has been reported in patients with acute myocardial infarction and coronary atherothrombotic disease.[51]

There is also ample clinical evidence to suggest that antioxidant status is important in normal platelet function. In patients with coronary artery disease, decreased plasma and platelet antioxidant activity is associated with increased platelet aggregability.[52,53] Clinical studies have shown that vitamin E supplementation is associated with increased hemorrhagic stroke, emphasizing the platelet inhibitory properties of α-tocopherol.[54] Although epidemiological studies initially suggested that dietary antioxidant consumption is inversely associated with the development of coronary artery disease,[55] recent prospective studies of vitamin supplementation have presented less favorable results.[56,57]

Related to vitamin supplementation, dietary intake of specific nutrients has been suggested as a means of modifying the progression of cardiovascular disease and thrombosis. In particular, epidemiological studies have reported an inverse relationship between the total dietary intake of plant flavonoids and the incidence of cardiovascular disease,[54,58] and it has been suggested that red wine consumption may reduce coronary disease.[59,60] The source of this beneficial effect is believed to be flavonoids, polyphenol derivatives of diphenylpyrans that are found in plant but not animal food products; large, prospective trials evaluating diets rich in flavonoids are currently lacking.

A proposed mechanism for the beneficial cardiovascular effects of both flavonoids and vitamins is enhanced bioactivity of NO, and it has been suggested that select flavonoids may inhibit thrombosis and enhance vasodilation by a NO-dependent process.[61,62] Reported mechanisms for the flavonoid- or vitamin-dependent increase in NO include metabolism of reactive oxygen species, as well as regulation of endothelial NO synthase transcriptional or signaling pathways.[52]

The role of genetics in atherothrombotic disease

Approximately half of the thrombotic events in cardiovascular disease occur in patients without traditional risk factors. This has led to more recent studies focusing on the molecular genetics of atherothrombosis, seeking to identify novel determinants. Although many specific genetic abnormalities have been found to contribute to the risk of venous thrombosis, the search for relevant genetic variants in arterial thrombosis has been less successful. This may be because atherothrombosis is a complex and highly prevalent polygenic disease in the population, and the phenotype is rarely due to an isolated genetic abnormality or variant.[63] Importantly, a recent report from the Framingham Heart Study demonstrated that heritable factors play a major role in determining platelet aggregation, and measured covariates play a lesser role.[64] In this study, the best-characterized prothrombotic polymorphisms (glycoprotein IIIa PI(A2) and fibrinogen Hind III β-148) contributed less than 1% to the overall variance. The authors conclude that 'future studies are warranted to identify the key genetic variants that regulate platelet function'.[64]

Recently, an association between atherosclerotic disease and spontaneous venous thrombosis was reported, suggesting that these two conditions may share common risk factors.[65] This observation suggests that the traditional genetic risk factors associated with venous thrombosis may contribute to atherothrombotic disease. Abnormalities in the factor V Leiden gene have been clearly associated with increased risk of venous thrombosis, and this abnormality may also increase the risk of myocardial infarction.[66] Elevated fibrinogen levels have also been associated with arterial thrombotic disease,[67] and it is believed that increased fibrinogen levels may lead to enhanced blood viscosity, greater clot formation, or increased platelet aggregation. Fibrinogen levels in the plasma have been related to various polymorphisms in the gene coding for its three polypeptide chains.[68] Polymorphisms of the factor VII gene have also been associated with variable plasma levels, and there is a suggestion that elevated levels contribute to the risk of coronary artery disease.[69] These associations are, however, not entirely established, as there are also many studies reporting a lack of association for variants contributing to the coagulation cascade.[70,71]

Another possible candidate gene responsible for the regulation of thrombosis is eNOS, a polymorphic variation in the genotype of which may account for differences in NO production. eNOS is located on chromsome 7q35–36, and estimates suggest that genetic variations contribute to at least 30% of the variance in plasma NO levels in the population.[72,73] Multiple polymorphic variants of the eNOS gene have been described, and the most extensively characterized is the 894-G/T polymorphism in exon 7 of the gene, resulting in a glutamate or aspartate at position 298. Healthy individuals with the 894T allele have higher plasma levels of nitrogen oxides,[74] and epidemiologic studies have shown an increased risk of hypertension, myocardial infarction, and stroke in patients homozygous for the Glu298Asp variant[75–78]. Another eNOS polymorphism, designated ecNOS4a, has been identified on intron 4. This variant has four tandem 27 bp repeats, compared to the wildtype allele which has five tandem repeats (ecNOS4b). The ecNOS4a allele has been associated with premature coronary artery disease,[79] and with a history of myocardial infarction.[79]

Variants of eNOS have been shown to influence platelet function and NO release to a variable degree. The polymorphisms in the promoter region ($p = 0.002$)

and in exon 7 ($p = 0.007$), but not in intron 4 ($p > 0.05$), are associated with lower levels of platelet-derived NO.[49] The eNOS gene polymorphisms do not affect ADP-induced platelet aggregation, but the exon 7 variant does alter collagen-induced aggregation. Taken together, these data suggest that select eNOS variants may influence thrombotic propensity.

Summary

Arterial thrombosis causing unstable cardiovascular disease is due to disruption of the vulnerable atherosclerotic plaque, leading to exposure of the subintimal contents to flowing blood and the formation of a platelet-rich thrombus. The importance of platelet activation in the events leading to vessel occlusion in acute coronary syndromes has been clearly shown, and the factors that contribute to thrombosis in this setting continue to be explored. This complex process is influenced by a wide variety of cellular and plasma-derived mediators that are influenced by diverse, yet related, processes, including redox state, genetic status, inflammation, as well as traditional cardiovascular risk factors. In concert, these processes determine the balance between occlusive and non-occlusive thrombosis in the setting of the ruptured atherosclerotic plaque, and to the clinical syndromes that accompany these processes.

References

1. Antiplatelet Trialists Collaboration. Collaborative overview of randomised trials of antiplatelet therapy: I: prevention of death, myocardial infarction, and stroke by prolonged antiplatelet therapy in various categories of patients. Br Med J 1994; 308:81–106.
2. Pasterkamp G, Schoneveld AH, van der Wal AC et al. Inflammation of the atherosclerotic cap and shoulder of the plaque is a common and locally observed feature in unruptured plaques of femoral and coronary arteries. Arterioscler Thromb Vasc Biol 1999; 19:54–58.
3. Ambrose JA, Martinez EE. A new paradigm for plaque stabilization. Circulation 2002; 105:2000–2004.
4. Maron DJ, Fazio S, Linton MF. Current perspectives on statins. Circulation 2000; 101:207–213.
5. Brown BG, Zhao XQ, Chait A et al. Simvastatin and niacin, antioxidant vitamins, or the combination for the prevention of coronary disease. N Engl J Med 2001; 345:1583–1592.
6. DeWood MA, Spores J, Notske R et al. Prevalence of total coronary occlusion during the early hours of transmural myocardial infarction. N Engl J Med 1980; 303:897–902.
7. Falk E. Unstable angina with fatal outcome: dynamic coronary thrombosis leading to infarction and/or sudden death. Autopsy evidence of recurrent mural thrombosis with peripheral embolization culminating in total vascular occlusion. Circulation 1985; 71:699–708.
8. Falk E. Plaque rupture with severe pre-existing stenosis precipitating coronary thrombosis. Characteristics of coronary atherosclerotic plaques underlying fatal occlusive thrombi. Br Heart J 1983; 50:127–134.
9. Davies MJ, Thomas AC. Thrombosis and acute coronary-artery lesions in sudden cardiac ischemic death. N Engl J Med 1984; 310:1137–1140.
10. Fitzgerald DJ, Roy L, Catella F, FitzGerald A. Platelet activation in unstable coronary disease. N Engl J Med 1986; 315:983–989.
11. Ueda Y, Asakura M, Yamaguchi O et al. The healing process of infarct-related plaques. Insights from 18 months of serial angioscopic follow-up. J Am Coll Cardiol 2001; 38:1916–1922.
12. Asakura M, Ueda Y, Yamaguchi O et al. Extensive development of vulnerable plaques as a pan-coronary process in patients with myocardial infarction: an angioscopic study. J Am Coll Cardiol 2001; 37:1284–1288.
13. Chew DP, Bhatt DL, Sapp S et al. Increased mortality with oral platelet glycoprotein IIb/IIIa antagonists: a meta-analysis of phase III multicenter randomized trials. Circulation 2001; 103:201–206.
14. Arber N, Berliner S, Pras E et al. Heterotypic leukocyte aggregation in the peripheral blood of patients with leukemia, inflammation and stress. Nouv Rev Fr Hematol 1991; 33:251–255.
15. Rinder HM, Bonan JL, Rinder CS et al. Dynamics of leukocyte-platelet adhesion in whole blood. Blood 1991; 78:1730–1737.
16. Neumann FJ, Zohlnhofer D, Fakhoury L et al. Effect of glycoprotein IIb/IIIa receptor blockade on platelet-leukocyte interaction and surface expression of the leukocyte integrin Mac-1 in acute myocardial infarction. J Am Coll Cardiol 1999; 34:1420–1426.
17. Gawaz MP, Loftus JC, Bajt ML et al. Ligand bridging mediates integrin alpha IIb beta 3 (platelet GPIIB-IIIA) dependent homotypic and heterotypic cell–cell interactions. J Clin Invest 1991; 88:1128–1134.
18. Simon DI, Ezratty AM, Francis SA et al. Fibrin(ogen) is internalized and degraded by activated human monocytoid cells via Mac-1 (CD11b/CD18): a nonplasmin fibrinolytic pathway. Blood 1993; 82:2414–2422.
19. Hayward R, Campbell B, Shin YK et al. Recombinant soluble P-selectin glycoprotein ligand-1 protects against myocardial ischemic reperfusion injury in cats. Cardiovasc Res 1999; 41:65–76.
20. Michelson AD, Barnard MR, Hechtman HB et al. In vivo tracking of platelets: circulating degranulated platelets rapidly lose surface P-selectin but continue to circulate and function. Proc Natl Acad Sci USA 1996; 93:11877–11882.
21. Michelson AD, Barnard MR, Krueger LA et al. Circulating monocyte–platelet aggregates are a more sensitive marker of

in vivo platelet activation than platelet surface P-selectin: studies in baboons, human coronary intervention, and human acute myocardial infarction. Circulation 2001; 104:1533–1537.

22. Ott I, Neumann FJ, Gawaz M et al. Increased neutrophil–platelet adhesion in patients with unstable angina. Circulation 1996; 94:1239–1246.

23. Shebuski RJ, Kilgore KS. Role of inflammatory mediators in thrombogenesis. J Pharmacol Exp Ther 2002; 300:729–735.

24. Celi A, Pellegrini G, Lorenzet R et al. P-selectin induces the expression of tissue factor on monocytes. Proc Natl Acad Sci USA 1994; 91:8767–8771.

25. Neumann FJ, Marx N, Gawaz M et al. Induction of cytokine expression in leukocytes by binding of thrombin-stimulated platelets. Circulation 1997; 95:2387–2394.

26. Henn V, Slupsky JR, Grafe M et al. CD40 ligand on activated platelets triggers an inflammatory reaction of endothelial cells. Nature 1998; 391:591–594.

27. Mach F, Schonbeck U, Sukhova GK et al. Reduction of atherosclerosis in mice by inhibition of CD40 signalling. Nature 1998; 394:200–203.

28. Andre P, Prasad KS, Denis CV et al. CD40L stabilizes arterial thrombi by a beta3 integrin-dependent mechanism. Nature Med 2002; 8:247–252.

29. Freedman JE. CD40 ligand – assessing risk instead of damage? N Engl J Med 2003; 348:1163–1165.

30. Heeschen C, Dimmeler S, Hamm CW et al. Soluble CD40 ligand in acute coronary syndromes. N Engl J Med 2003; 348:1104–1111.

31. Schonbeck U, Varo N, Libby P et al. Soluble CD40L and cardiovascular risk in women. Circulation 2001; 104:2266–2268.

32. de Graaf JC, Banga JD, Moncada S et al. Nitric oxide functions as an inhibitor of platelet adhesion under flow conditions. Circulation 1992; 85:2284–2290.

33. Radomski MW, Palmer MJ, Moncada S. The role of nitric oxide and cGMP in platelet adhesion to vascular endothelium. Biochem Biophys Res Commun 1987; 148:1482–1489.

34. Bossaller C, Habib GB, Yamamoto H et al. Impaired muscarinic endothelium-dependent relaxation and cyclic guanosine 5'-monophosphate formation in atherosclerotic human coronary artery and rabbit aorta. J Clin Invest 1986; 79:170–174.

35. Vita JA, Treasure CB, Nabel EG et al. Coronary vasomotor response to acetylcholine relates to risk factors for coronary artery disease. Circulation 1990; 81:491–497.

36. Stamler J, Mendelsohn ME, Amarante P et al. *N*-acetylcysteine potentiates platelet inhibition by endothelium-derived relaxing factor. Circ Res 1989; 65:789–795.

37. Cooke JP, Stamler J, Andon N et al. Flow stimulates endothelial cells to release a nitrovasodilator that is potentiated by reduced thiol. Am J Physiol 1990; 259:H804–H812.

38. Shultz PJ, Raij L. Endogenously synthesized nitric oxide prevents endotoxin-induced glomerular thrombosis. J Clin Invest 1992; 90:1718–1725.

39. Freedman JE, Loscalzo J, Barnard MR et al. Nitric oxide released from activated platelets inhibits platelet recruitment. J Clin Invest 1997; 100:350–356.

40. Langford E, Wainwright R, Martin J. Platelet activation in acute myocardial infarction and angina is inhibited by nitric oxide donors. Arterioscler Thromb Vasc Biol 1996; 16:51–55.

41. Lynch S, Frei B, Morrow J et al. Vascular superoxide dismutase deficiency impairs endothelial vasodilator function through direct inactivation of nitric oxide and increased lipid peroxidation. Arterioscler Thromb Vasc Biol 1997; 17:2975–2981.

42. Vita JA, Keaney JF Jr. Endothelial function: a barometer for cardiovascular risk? Circulation 2002; 106:640–642.

43. Bressler N, Broekman M, Marcus A. Concurrent studies of oxygen consumption and aggregation in stimulated human platelets. Blood 1979; 53:167–178.

44. Burch J, Burch P. Glutathione disulfide production during arachidonic acid oxygenation in human platelets. Prostaglandins 1990; 39:123–124.

45. Freedman J, Keaney JF Jr. NO and superoxide in human platelets. In: Packer L, ed. Nitric oxide, Part C: Biological and antioxidant activities. San Diego, CA: Academic Press, 1999: 61–67.

46. Handin R, Karabin R, Boxer G. Enhancement of platelet aggregation by superoxide anion. J Clin Invest 1987; 59:959–965.

47. O'Donnell VB, Freeman BA. Interactions between nitric oxide and lipid oxidation pathways: implications for vascular disease. Circ Res 2001; 88:12–21.

48. Beckman J, Beckman T, Chen J et al. Apparent hydroxyl radical production by peroxynitrite: implications for endothelial injury from nitric oxide and superoxide. Proc Natl Acad Sci USA 1990; 87:1620–1624.

49. Freedman JE, Frei B, Welch GN et al. Glutathione peroxidase potentiates the inhibition of platelet function by S-nitrosothiols. J Clin Invest 1995; 96:394–400.

50. Freedman JE, Loscalzo J, Benoit SE et al. Decreased platelet inhibition by nitric oxide in two brothers with a history of arterial thrombosis. J Clin Invest 1996; 97:979–987.

51. Keaney J, Stamler J, Folts J et al. NO forms a stable adduct with serum albumin that has potent antiplatelet properties in vivo. Clin Res 1992; 40:194A.

52. Freedman JE, Keaney JF Jr. Vitamin E inhibition of platelet aggregation is independent of antioxidant activity. J Nutr 2001; 131:374S–377S.

53. Steiner M. Effect of alpha-tocopherol administration on platelet function in man. Thromb Haemost 1983; 49:73–77.

54. Keli SO, Hertog MG, Feskens EJ et al. Dietary flavonoids, antioxidant vitamins, and incidence of stroke: the Zutphen study. Arch Intern Med 1996; 156:637–642.

55. D'Odorico A, Martines D, Kiechl S et al. High plasma levels of alpha- and beta-carotene are associated with a lower risk of atherosclerosis: results from the Bruneck study. Atherosclerosis 2000; 153:231–239.

56. Yusuf S, Dagenais G, Pogue J et al. Vitamin E supplementation and cardiovascular events in high-risk patients. The Heart Outcomes Prevention Evaluation Study Investigators. N Engl J Med 2000; 342:154–160.

57. Collaborative Group of the Primary Prevention Project. Low-dose aspirin and vitamin E in people at cardiovascular risk: a randomised trial in general practice. Lancet 2001; 357:89–95.

58. Hertog MG, Feskens EJ, Hollman PC et al. Dietary antioxidant flavonoids and risk of coronary heart disease: the Zutphen Elderly Study. Lancet 1993; 342:1007–1011.

59. Renaud S, DeLorgeril M. Wine, alcohol, platelets and the French paradox for coronary artery heart disease. Lancet 1992; 296:320–331.

60. St. Leger A, Cochrane A, Moore F. Factors associated with cardiac mortality in developed countries with particular reference to the consumption of wine. Lancet 1979; 124:1017–1720.

61. Freedman JE, Parker C 3rd, Li L et al. Select flavonoids and whole juice from purple grapes inhibit platelet function and enhance nitric oxide release. Circulation 2001; 103:2792–2798.

62. Stein J, Keevil J, Wiebe D et al. Purple grape juice improves endothelial function and reduces the susceptibility of LDL cholesterol to oxidation in patients with coronary artery disease. Circulation 1999; 100:1050–1055.

63. Voetsch B, Loscalzo J. Genetic determinants of arterial thrombosis. Arterioscler Thromb Vasc Biol 2004; 24:216–229.

64. O'Donnell CJ, Larson MG, Feng D et al. Genetic and environmental contributions to platelet aggregation: the Framingham heart study. Circulation 2001; 103:3051–3056.

65. Prandoni P, Bilora F, Marchiori A et al. An association between atherosclerosis and venous thrombosis. N Engl J Med 2003; 348:1435–1441.

66. Doggen CJ, Cats VM, Bertina RM et al. Interaction of coagulation defects and cardiovascular risk factors: increased risk of myocardial infarction associated with factor V Leiden or prothrombin 20210A. Circulation 1998; 97:1037–1041.

67. Meade TW, Mellows S, Brozovic M et al. Haemostatic function and ischaemic heart disease: principal results of the Northwick Park Heart Study. Lancet 1986; 2:533–537.

68. van 't Hooft FM, von Bahr SJ, Silveira A et al. Two common, functional polymorphisms in the promoter region of the beta-fibrinogen gene contribute to regulation of plasma fibrinogen concentration. Arterioscler Thromb Vasc Biol 1999; 19:3063–3070.

69. van 't Hooft FM, Silveira A, Tornvall P et al. Two common functional polymorphisms in the promoter region of the coagulation factor VII gene determining plasma factor VII activity and mass concentration. Blood 1999; 93:3432–3441.

70. Doggen CJ, Bertina RM, Cats VM et al. Fibrinogen polymorphisms are not associated with the risk of myocardial infarction. Br J Haematol 2000; 110:935–938.

71. Doggen CJ, Cats VM, Bertina RM et al. A genetic propensity to high factor VII is not associated with the risk of myocardial infarction in men. Thromb Haemost 1998; 80:281–285.

72. Marsden PA, Heng HH, Scherer SW et al. Structure and chromosomal localization of the human constitutive endothelial nitric oxide synthase gene. J Biol Chem 1993; 268:17478–17488.

73. Wang XL, Mahaney MC, Sim AS et al. Genetic contribution of the endothelial constitutive nitric oxide synthase gene to plasma nitric oxide levels. Arterioscler Thromb Vasc Biol 1997; 17:3147–3153.

74. Yoon Y, Song J, Hong SH et al. Plasma nitric oxide concentrations and nitric oxide synthase gene polymorphisms in coronary artery disease. Clin Chem 2000; 46:1626–1630.

75. Lacolley P, Gautier S, Poirier O et al. Nitric oxide synthase gene polymorphisms, blood pressure and aortic stiffness in normotensive and hypertensive subjects. J Hypertens 1998; 16:31–35.

76. Shimasaki Y, Yasue H, Yoshimura M et al. Association of the missense Glu298Asp variant of the endothelial nitric oxide synthase gene with myocardial infarction. J Am Coll Cardiol 1998; 31:1506–1510.

77. Elbaz A, Poirier O, Moulin T et al. Association between the Glu298Asp polymorphism in the endothelial constitutive nitric oxide synthase gene and brain infarction. The GENIC Investigators. Stroke 2000; 31:1634–1639.

78. Hingorani AD, Liang CF, Fatibene J et al. A common variant of the endothelial nitric oxide synthase (Glu298→Asp) is a major risk factor for coronary artery disease in the UK. Circulation 1999; 100:1515–1520.

79. Wang XL, Sim AS, Badenhop RF et al. A smoking-dependent risk of coronary artery disease associated with a polymorphism of the endothelial nitric oxide synthase gene. Nature Med 1996; 2:41–45.

7

Endothelial dysfunction in atherosclerosis: mechanisms of impaired nitric oxide bioactivity

Naomi M. Hamburg, Joseph A. Vita

Introduction

Located at the juncture between flowing blood and the vessel wall, the vascular endothelium participates in the maintenance of vascular health, and according to the current paradigm, loss of endothelial function is a central mediator of atherogenesis.[1] In the normal state the endothelium produces a variety of factors that regulate vasomotor tone, inflammation, coagulation, and the composition of the vascular wall (Table 7.1). The term 'endothelial dysfunction' refers to the phenotypic transformation that endothelial cells undergo when exposed to an atherogenic environment.[2] The dysfunctional endothelium promotes vasoconstriction, inflammation, thrombosis, and abnormal cellular proliferation; thus, it facilitates the development of atherosclerosis (Figure 7.1). Growing evidence connecting endothelial abnormalities to cardiovascular events has strengthened our appreciation of the clinical significance of this systemic pathophysiologic state.[3]

Whereas risk factors induce broad-based changes in endothelial phenotype, a defining element – although not the only determinant – of endothelial dysfunction is insufficiency of nitric oxide (NO). In 1980, Furchgott and Zawadzki[4] described the endothelium-dependent release of a vasodilator substance termed endothelium-derived relaxing factor that was subsequently identified as NO.[5] Over the last 23 years, subsequent work has

---

Table 7.1 Factors released by the endothelium to maintain vascular homeostasis

Maintenance of vascular tone

Vasodilator factors	*Vasoconstrictor factors*
Nitric oxide	Endothelin-1
Endothelium-derived	Angiotensin II
hyperpolarizing factor	Thromboxane A_2
Prostacyclin	

Control of local thrombosis

Anti-thrombotic factors	*Prothrombotic factors*
Nitric oxide	Tissue factor
Tissue plasminogen activator	Von Willebrand's factor
Heparans	

Control of vascular inflammation

Anti-inflammatory factors	*Proinflammatory factors*
Nitric oxide	Monocyte chemotactic factor-1
	Vascular cell adhesion molecule-1
	Intercellular adhesion molecule-1
	Selectins
	Interleukins 1, 6, and 18

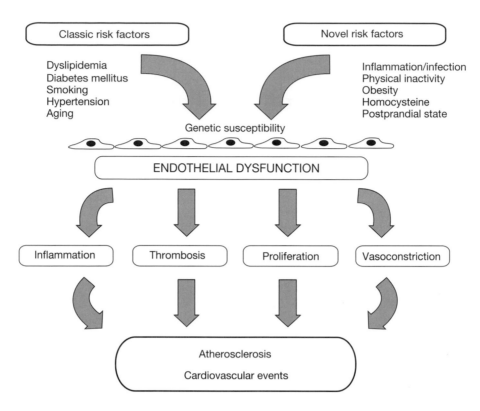

Figure 7.1 The role of endothelial dysfunction in atherogenesis. Cardiovascular risk factors combined with intrinsic susceptibility impair endothelial homeostatic functions. The dysfunctional endothelium promotes multiple deleterious processes and contributes to the development of atherosclerotic lesions and clinical cardiac events

identified NO as a principal mediator of the vasoprotective actions of the endothelium (for a detailed review, the reader is referred to Loscalzo and Vita[6]). NO suppresses the endothelial release of inflammatory cytokines and the expression of adhesion molecules, and thus blocks vascular infiltration of leukocytes. NO also limits vascular smooth muscle proliferation, intimal fibrosis, and platelet aggregation. Thus the synthesis of appropriate amounts of NO sustains vascular health, and its loss characterizes the atherothrombotic milieu.

The vasodilator properties of NO facilitate assessment of its bioactivity in humans. Arterial dilation in response to various endothelium-dependent agonists, including acetylcholine and shear stress, reflects the local bioactivity of NO, and these responses have therefore evolved into useful measures of endothelial health.[3] Studies using this approach have provided compelling evidence for reduced NO bioactivity in human atherosclerosis. For example, intracoronary acetylcholine

infusion produces paradoxical vasoconstriction in individuals with coronary atherosclerosis, reflecting loss of acetylcholine-stimulated NO production and the unopposed constrictor effects of acetylcholine on vascular smooth muscle.[7] Investigations of individuals with both classic and novel cardiac risk factors have shown an early loss of endothelium-dependent vasodilation.[8] Numerous prospective studies have reported an increase in cardiovascular events associated with abnormal endothelial responses.[3] Taken together, these findings strongly support a role for NO insufficiency in the generation of atherosclerosis and its later clinical expression.

Recent work has enriched our understanding of the precise molecular pathways that modulate NO synthesis and bioavailability in health and disease. This chapter will focus on the perturbations in these molecular pathways that contribute to endothelial dysfunction in atherosclerosis. Decreased NO bioactivity can be accounted for by three fundamental mechanisms:

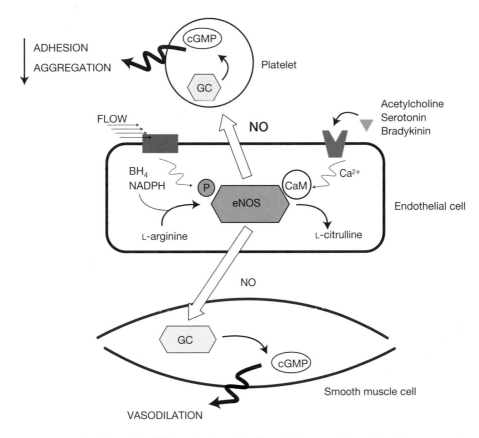

Figure 7.2 Mechanisms of nitric oxide (NO) synthesis and action in the vasculature. Agonists augment endothelial NO synthase (eNOS) activity via receptor-mediated increases in calcium levels that enhance binding to calmodulin (CaM). Stimulating factors such as flow also activate eNOS by increasing phosphorylation at certain residues. eNOS synthesizes NO by converting L-arginine to L-citrulline in a reaction that requires tetrahydrobiopterin (BH_4) and NADPH as cofactors. NO diffuses from the endothelium into target cells, where it activates guanylyl cyclase (GC) conversion of guanosine triphosphate (GTP) to cyclic guanosine monophosphate (cGMP). cGMP stimulates smooth muscle cell relaxation and inhibits platelet adhesion and aggregation

impaired endothelial NO production, accelerated NO degradation and inactivation, and decreased responsiveness to NO in target cells. First, a very brief overview of endothelial NO production and signaling in the normal state will be given, followed by a review of some of the pathological mechanisms responsible for suppressing NO synthesis and/or accelerating its destruction under atherogenic conditions.

Mechanisms of NO production by the endothelium

The production and local actions of endothelium-derived NO are shown in Figure 7.2. As shown,

endothelial cells synthesize NO through the conversion of L-arginine to L-citrulline by the action of endothelial NO synthase (eNOS), and regulation of this enzyme in endothelial cells has been extensively reviewed.[9–15] The enzyme eNOS is constitutively expressed by the gene *NOS3* and requires homodimerization for activity. Post-translational modifications target eNOS to the plasma membrane, particularly to caveolae, where association with repressor proteins such as caveolin-1 limits basal activity. The enzyme is rapidly activated by a number of agonists, including acetylcholine and bradykinin, that increase intracellular calcium levels and promote an interaction with calmodulin. Other factors, including vascular endothelial growth factor (VEGF), shear stress, and estrogen, can also activate the enzyme without a sustained increase in intracellular calcium via phosphorylation of specific amino acid residues. There are a number of additional cofactors necessary for the generation of NO by eNOS, including tetrahydrobiopterin, NADPH, and flavins. Once produced, NO diffuses into the vessel lumen and underlying vascular smooth muscle cell layer. Platelet activity is reduced and vascular smooth muscle cell relaxation occurs as NO activates guanylyl cyclase and raises cyclic guanosine monophosphate (cGMP) levels in these cells. NO also relaxes vascular smooth muscle by non-guanylyl cyclase-dependent mechanisms, including activation of calcium-dependent potassium channels in the cell membrane.[16]

Mechanisms of impaired endothelial NO production

Consistent with the complex regulation of NO production, there are many potential sites for dysregulation under pathologic conditions (Figure 7.3). For example, the rate of NO synthesis may depend on the amount, activity, and cellular location of the eNOS enzyme, as well as on the availability of substrate and cofactors. This section will review specific mechanisms in atherosclerosis and related conditions that may adversely affect NO synthesis. An improved understanding of these mechanisms may provide new targets for therapeutic interventions for the disease.

eNOS expression

Depressed expression of eNOS may play an important role in atherogenesis.[12] Consistent with this theory, endothelial cells obtained from human arteries with advanced atherosclerotic plaques have diminished eNOS transcript and protein content compared to cells from normal arteries.[17] Factors associated with atherogenesis, including oxidized low-density lipoprotein (oxLDL)[18] and tumor necrosis factor-α (TNF-α),[19] lower eNOS levels and reduce NO production in cultured endothelial cells. Further support for altered eNOS expression in atherosclerosis derives from experiments showing that antiatherogenic interventions, such as statins,[20] and increased shear stress,[21] elevate eNOS protein levels in endothelial cells.

Deficiency of eNOS protein reflects lower eNOS transcript concentrations and may imply disturbances at both transcriptional and post-transcriptional levels. Recent findings have highlighted destabilization of the mRNA transcript as the primary mechanism for impaired eNOS expression in the setting of certain agents. In cells exposed to inflammatory cytokines and oxLDL, eNOS mRNA is more rapidly degraded.[18,19] The shortened mRNA half-life is accompanied by loss of protein binding to elements in the stabilizing 3' untranslated region.[22]

The direct contribution of diminished eNOS protein levels to the development of endothelial dysfunction in humans remains to be determined. One recent clinical investigation, however, raised the intriguing possibility that abnormal eNOS expression and endothelial dysfunction are reversible by a therapeutic intervention. Arterial specimens taken from patients with coronary artery disease who participated in an intensive exercise program contained higher amounts of eNOS and displayed improved flow-mediated dilation than did those from sedentary controls.[23] Thus, risk factor modification may have the potential to improve endothelial vasomotor function by restoring eNOS expression levels.

Protein interactions

Multiple cellular proteins have been identified that interact directly with eNOS and affect its activity, as depicted in Figure 7.4. Although the ability of calmodulin to activate eNOS has long been recognized, recent work highlights the role of additional proteins critical for proper eNOS regulation. In the normal state, these molecular interactions allow the tight control of NO synthesis. Evidence is accumulating that an imbalance between inhibitory and stimulatory proteins contributes to NO insufficiency in atherosclerosis.

In the absence of stimulatory inputs, endothelial cells release NO only at a low level, owing to tonic suppression by proteins bound to eNOS. Caveolin-1 plays a key structural role in the formation of caveolae, which are cholesterol-rich invaginations of the plasma membrane that organize components of a number of signal transduction complexes, including eNOS.[11] In addition, many *in vitro* experiments have demonstrated that caveolin-1 binds to eNOS and inhibits its

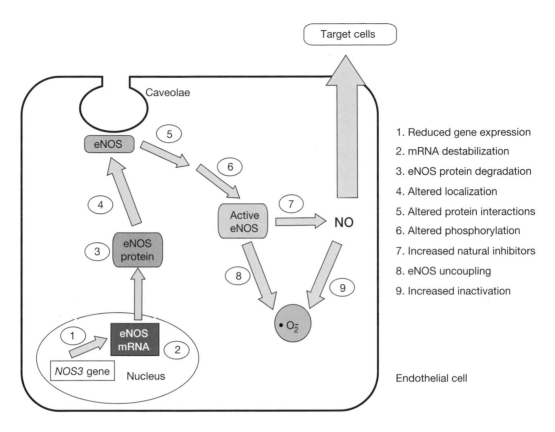

Figure 7.3 Potential mechanisms of decreased nitric oxide (NO) bioactivity in atherosclerosis. Reduced *NOS3* gene transcription, shortened endothelial NO synthase (eNOS) transcript half-life, and accelerated eNOS enzyme degradation decrease eNOS protein levels. Abnormal intracellular localization, imbalanced stimulatory and inhibitory protein interactions, and specific alterations in protein phosphorylation favor eNOS inactivity and reduce NO synthesis. Endogenous inhibitors of eNOS accumulate and suppress NO production. Suboptimal concentrations of substrate and cofactors disrupt eNOS-catalytic function, resulting in the production of superoxide instead of NO. Superoxide and other reactive oxygen species react with NO, leading to its inactivation and degradation

activity.[24] After exposure to agonists such as acetylcholine that elevate intracellular calcium levels, calmodulin competitively disrupts the binding of caveolin-1 to eNOS and converts eNOS into the active state.[25] In intact vessels, strategies that increase caveolin-1 levels are associated with reduced NO synthesis.[26] Conversely, genetically modified animals with reduced caveolin-1 expression display enhanced endothelium-dependent arterial dilation.[27] These results strongly suggest that caveolin-1 inhibits NO generation by eNOS, and that this modulation plays a role in determining endothelial function.

Proatherosclerotic conditions may strengthen the interaction between caveolin-1 and eNOS, resulting in decreased NO production and endothelial dysfunc-

tion. For example, human hypercholesterolemic serum or LDL cholesterol increase the formation of caveolin–eNOS complexes in cultured endothelial cells and decrease NO release.[28] Conversely, statin therapy is associated with decreased affinity of caveolin for eNOS and enhanced NO production in endothelial cells.[29] Pigs consuming a high-fat diet have increased coronary artery caveolin content and an associated decrease in endothelium-dependent vasorelaxation.[30] An anti-atherogenic effect of lowering caveolin levels is also supported by a study of apo E-deficient mice with an additional disruption of the caveolin gene. The mice without caveolin showed markedly reduced aortic atheroma formation.[31] Together, these findings suggest that increased caveolin blockade of eNOS activity disturbs endothelial function and participates in the development of atherosclerosis.

Coupling with cellular proteins can also increase eNOS activity, and these interactions may be suppressed during atherogenesis. Though mainly associated with the chaperone system responsible for correct protein folding, heat-shock protein 90 (hsp90) is now recognized as a participant in eNOS regulation.[32] By partnering with eNOS to form hsp90–eNOS complexes, hsp90 promotes the activation of NO synthesis following stimulation with a number of agonists, including VEGF, histamine, and shear stress.[32] In intact vessels, inhibition of hsp90 reduces endothelium-dependent vasodilation in response to both acetylcholine and flow,[32,33] although these results must be interpreted with some caution as the hsp90 inhibitor, geldanamycin, itself augments superoxide production.[34] Whether or not reduced interaction between hsp90 and eNOS accounts for pathologic endothelial function in the atherosclerotic vessel is not known. Similarly, the relevance of other eNOS-associated regulatory proteins, such as dynamin 2, eNOS-interacting protein (NOSIP), and eNOS traffic inducer (NOSTRIN), to endothelial dysfunction in atherosclerosis remains to be determined.

Intracellular location

The location of eNOS within endothelial cells may influence its enzymatic activity.[11] In post-translational processing, eNOS is both myristoylated and palmitoylated and, thereby, targeted to plasma membranes.[35,36] The majority of eNOS activity is found in the membrane portion containing caveolae.[37] In endothelial cells, disruption of normal eNOS localization reduces agonist-stimulated NO release.[38] The relevance of this mechanism to atherosclerosis is supported by the observation that incubation of endothelial cells with oxidized LDL depletes caveolar cholesterol, displaces eNOS from caveolae, and decreases agonist-induced NO synthesis.[39] Further work is required to elucidate the precise interactions between localization, eNOS activation, and vascular function in human atherosclerosis.

Phosphorylation state

Recently, there has been considerable interest in the modulation of eNOS activity by dynamic changes in its phosphorylation state. A number of phosphorylation sites have been identified at serine, threonine, and tyrosine residues that increase or decrease NO synthesis (Figure 7.4).[40] Although recent experimental reports emphasize the complexity of eNOS regulation by phosphorylation, we here focus on two locations that have the clearest pathophysiologic role: the stimulatory site, serine 1177 (corresponding to the bovine serine 1179), and the inhibitory site, threonine 495 (corresponding to bovine threonine 497).

It is well established that phosphorylation of eNOS at serine 1177 activates the enzyme. Multiple factors that stimulate endothelial NO release, such as shear stress,[41] VEGF,[41] and bradykinin,[42] have been shown to increase phosphorylation at serine 1177. Maximal endothelium-dependent dilation to acetylcholine also appears to depend on serine 1177 phosphorylation.[43] Agonist-induced serine 1177 phosphorylation may be mediated by several different kinases, including Akt,[41] AMP-activated kinase,[44] and protein kinase A.[40] Thus, this site appears to integrate input from an array of signaling pathways relevant to atherosclerosis.

Several additional lines of evidence support the clinical relevance of serine 1177 phosphorylation. For example, statin treatment[45] increases serine 1177 phosphorylation in cultured endothelial cells. A similar effect was observed following exposure to high-density lipoprotein (HDL),[46] possibly contributing to the known association between high levels of HDL and reduced atherosclerotic risk. In patients with atherosclerosis, exercise-induced improvements in the endothelial function of the internal mammary artery are associated with activation of Akt and increased phosphorylation of serine 1177.[23] Thus, a number of interventions known to improve endothelial function and reduce cardiovascular risk have favorable effects on eNOS phosphorylation and consequent NO production.

In contrast to the effects of serine 1177 phosphorylation, phosphorylation at threonine 495 has an inhibitory effect on eNOS activity,[47] and a number of stimuli exert their effects by phosphorylating one site and dephosphorylating the other.[10] Phosphorylation at threonine 495 appears to reduce eNOS activity by blocking the binding of calmodulin.[42] Protein kinase C (PKC) plays a role in maintaining threonine 495 phosphorylation in the resting state,[48] and non-specific PKC inhibition results in dephosphorylation of this

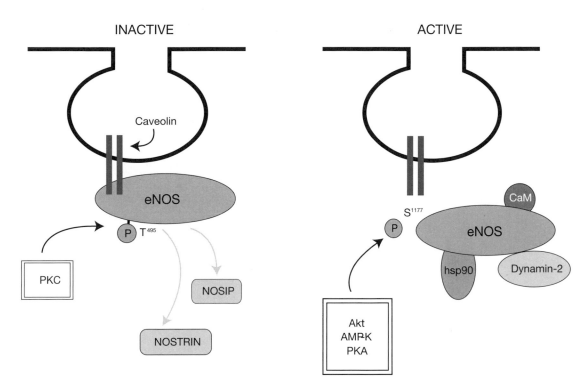

Figure 7.4 Mechanisms of post-translational eNOS regulation. Complex protein networks determine eNOS activity. Binding to caveolin and threonine 495 (T^{495}) phosphorylation by protein kinase C (PKC) decreases eNOS activity. eNOS interacting protein (NOSIP) and eNOS traffic inducer (NOSTRIN) induce translocation to the cytoplasm and attenuate NO synthesis. In contrast, interactions with calmodulin, hsp90, and dynamin-2 activate eNOS. Phosphorylation at serine 1177 (S^{1177}) by Akt, AMP-activated protein kinase (AMPK), and protein kinase A (PKA) stimulates NO production. In atherogenesis, multiple abnormalities favor inhibitory over stimulatory signals and thus limit NO synthesis

residue and increased eNOS activity.[49] Oral administration of a PKC-ß inhibitor has also been shown to protect against hyperglycemia-induced endothelial dysfunction in the human forearm;[50] whether or not this vasoprotective effect is due to changes in eNOS phosphorylation remains to be determined.

Endogenous eNOS inhibitors

Endogenous antagonists of eNOS have generated great interest for their potential role in reducing NO production in vascular disease. Asymmetric dimethyl arginine (ADMA) is a metabolite of the eNOS substrate that is generated by protein catabolism and competitively inhibits eNOS at physiologic concentrations.[51] Several factors associated with atherogenesis, including hyperhomocysteinemia,[52] LDL,[53] and TNF-α,[54] all increase endothelial cell production of ADMA. In

humans, circulating ADMA concentrations are higher in individuals with atherosclerosis and with risk factors, such as hypercholesterolemia, hypertension, and diabetes mellitus.[55] Furthermore, ADMA levels correlate with endothelial dysfunction in hypercholesterolemic individuals,[56] and in hyperhomocysteinemia induced by methionine.[57] Studies suggest that ADMA accumulation may be explained, in large part, by impaired activity of dimethylarginine dimethylaminohydrolase (DDAH), the enzyme responsible for ADMA breakdown.[58] DDAH function can be reduced by hyperlipidemia,[54] homocysteine,[52] hyperglycemia,[59] and other forms of increased oxidative stress.[54] These data are consistent with a model in which a proatherogenic environment leads to impaired ADMA metabolism, excess concentrations of this inhibitor compared to L-arginine, and hence impaired endothelial NO release.

The relevance of ADMA has been extended to the clinical setting as investigations have shown that higher plasma levels of ADMA are associated with increased risk for cardiovascular events.[60,61] The contribution of ADMA to endothelial dysfunction is also supported by the observation that L-arginine supplementation has beneficial effects in patients with cardiovascular disease.[62] Normal plasma levels of L-arginine far exceed the eNOS K_m (Michaelis–Menton constant), and thus arginine supplementation would not be expected to increase NO synthesis. In the presence of a competitive inhibitor such as ADMA, however, substrate supplementation has the potential to increase eNOS activity and improve endothelial function. Collectively, the available evidence supports an important role for ADMA in the pathogenesis of endothelial dysfunction in atherosclerosis.

Genetic polymorphisms of eNOS

The interest in genomic medicine has prompted several studies examining the relation of *NOS3* variants to endothelial function. Such polymorphisms have the potential to alter the expression or activity of the enzyme, and thus could predispose affected individuals to vascular disease.[63] To date, however, the findings linking eNOS gene polymorphisms, endothelial dysfunction, and atherosclerosis have been contradictory.

Multiple polymorphisms have been identified within the promoter, coding, and intronic regions of the *NOS3* gene.[64] Two polymorphisms have the best-characterized pathophysiologic role: the T786C promoter polymorphism, which may decrease eNOS expression,[65] and the G894T polymorphism in exon 7 that may accelerate eNOS protein degradation.[66] Some investigators have reported an increased risk of coronary artery disease and myocardial infarction associated with these polymorphisms;[67–70] however, other groups have found no predisposition to atherosclerosis or cardiac events in the presence of these alleles.[67,71,72]

Erbs and colleagues[73] addressed the impact of these two eNOS polymorphisms on endothelial function in a group of patients with established coronary disease. Subjects with the T786C promoter polymorphism alone, the G894T exon 7 polymorphism alone, or both mutations displayed blunted endothelium-dependent dilation of microvessels compared to unaffected individuals. Neither polymorphism was associated with an abnormality of conduit artery endothelial

function; however, the explanation for or relevance of such a differential effect on endothelial function according to arterial size is not immediately apparent.

Two studies have indicated an interaction between genetic and environmental factors in the development of endothelial dysfunction. Rossi and colleagues[74] observed that the T786C polymorphism is associated with endothelial dysfunction in patients with hypertension, but not in normotensive subjects. Similarly, Leeson and colleagues[75] found diminished brachial artery flow-mediated dilation in smokers who carried the G894T polymorphism, but no effect of the polymorphism in non-smokers. Together, these results suggest that variations in eNOS genotype may confer a predisposition to the development of an abnormal endothelial phenotype in the setting of other risk factors for vascular dysfunction, and suggest an inability to compensate under pathologic conditions. Further studies involving much larger numbers of patients will be required to define fully the clinical relevance of eNOS polymorphisms for endothelial dysfunction in various forms of cardiovascular disease.

Mechanisms of NO inactivation

Whereas inefficient production contributes to NO deficiency in atherosclerosis, studies also substantiate the role of increased NO 'inactivation' during the development of vascular diseases. In aerobic conditions, normal vascular cell metabolism generates many reactive oxygen species (ROS),[76] including superoxide anion, hydrogen peroxide, lipid hydroperoxides, hypochlorous acid, and, as most recently described, ozone.[77] A number of these have been shown to be present in atherosclerotic lesions and have the potential to interact with NO and limit its bioactivity, or to induce other changes that reduce its availability. Many studies have focused particularly on superoxide anion, which rapidly combines with NO to generate peroxynitrite and effectively eliminates the biological activity of NO.[78] In the healthy vasculature, multiple antioxidant defense systems limit oxidative NO inactivation. Proatherosclerotic conditions increase ROS flux, overwhelm depleted antioxidant systems, and disrupt NO signaling by a number of mechanisms, including inactivation of NO.

Oxidative stress and endothelial dysfunction

Many lines of evidence support a critical role for increased oxidative stress in atherosclerosis-associated endothelial dysfunction. In animal models of atherosclerosis, blood vessels release greater quantities of superoxide anion.[79] This increase is associated with impairment of endothelium-dependent vasorelaxation that is reversible with specific superoxide scavengers.[79,80] Further support for the role of oxidant stress in endothelial dysfunction comes from studies of antioxidant interventions in animal models and in humans, and this subject has been extensively reviewed.[79,81–83]

In human subjects, the strongest direct evidence for the importance of NO inactivation by ROS is provided by studies demonstrating rapid improvement of endothelial function following short-term intra-arterial infusion of antioxidants, particularly ascorbic acid. Ascorbic acid infusion reverses endothelial dysfunction in patients with diabetes mellitus,[84] hypercholesterolemia,[85] hypertension,[86] a history of cigarette smoking,[87] and coronary artery disease.[88] Importantly, superphysiologic concentrations of ascorbic acid are required (1–10 mM),[86] a finding that is consistent with the kinetics of the interactions between superoxide, NO, and ascorbic acid.[89]

The clinical relevance of oxidative stress-induced endothelial dysfunction was recently demonstrated in a prospective study of patients with coronary artery disease. An increase in endothelium-dependent vasodilation after ascorbic acid infusion was associated with an elevated risk of future cardiovascular events.[88] Thus, oxidative mechanisms play a central role in altered endothelial function and may facilitate the occurrence of adverse clinical outcomes.

It is important to point out, however, that endothelial dysfunction in atherosclerosis is not always rapidly reversible with short-term antioxidant infusion. Widlansky and colleagues[90] recently observed no effect of high-concentration ascorbic acid on endothelial function in atherosclerotic coronary arteries. This finding is consistent with the developing understanding that ROS have complex effects on endothelial cell phenotype beyond the direct inactivation of NO and oxidation of LDL (for a recent review see Chen and colleagues[91]). These observations may explain the failure of simple antioxidant strategies to reduce cardiovascular disease risk,[92] and have focused attention on strategies that act to reduce oxidative stress by inhibiting cellular sources of ROS.

Vascular sources of reactive oxygen species

Diverse cellular systems, including mitochondrial enzymes, cytochrome P450-related enzymes, cyclooxygenases, and lipoxygenases, are all potential contributors to increased oxidative stress (Figure 7.5). Nonenzymatic sources of ROS have also been identified. Recent work highlights dysregulation of oxidase enzymes as a major determinant of ROS production and reduced NO bioactivity in vascular disease. In particular, evidence links endothelial dysfunction to elevated output of ROS by NAD(P)H oxidases, xanthine oxidase, mycloperoxidase, and eNOS.

NAD(P)H oxidases

NAD(P)H oxidases contribute significantly to leukocyte antimicrobial function, but isoforms of these enzymes also are expressed in vascular cells and contribute to superoxide anion production in the vascular wall.[82] Diverse stimuli implicated in atherogenesis, including hypercholesterolemia, angiotensin, disturbed flow, stretch, and inflammatory cytokines, upregulate NAD(P)H oxidase expression and activity, suggesting a mechanism for higher superoxide production in these states.[82] In human atherosclerotic lesions, NAD(P)H subunit expression correlates with disease severity and superoxide level.[93] Moreover, NAD(P)H oxidase-mediated superoxide release is increased in coronary arteries from patients with atherosclerosis.[94]

There is extensive evidence suggesting that NAD(P)H-derived oxidants contribute to endothelial dysfunction.[82] For example, mice lacking the gp91[phox] subunit of an endothelial NAD(P)H oxidase have decreased endothelium-derived ROS production and an associated increase in NO bioactivity as demonstrated by augmented aortic relaxation to acetylcholine.[95] In humans, superoxide production by saphenous veins harvested from patients with atherosclerosis was NAD(P)H dependent and correlated with endothelium-dependent vasodilation as well as coronary risk factor burden.[96] These findings suggest that a specific inhibitor of NAD(P)H oxidase might

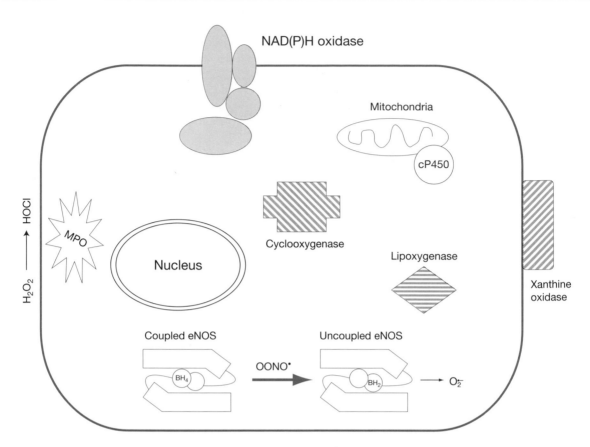

Figure 7.5   Vascular sources of reactive oxygen species. Multiple enzymatic sources of reactive oxygen species are present in the vasculature during atherogenesis, including NAD(P)H oxidase, myeloperoxidase, mitochondrial enzymes, cytochrome P450 (cP450), lipoxygenase, cyclooxygenase, and uncoupled eNOS

have therapeutic promise. Although such inhibitors are not currently available, it is notable that one effect of statin therapy is to inhibit the proper assembly of NAD(P)H oxidase,[97] and that statin therapy reduces oxidative stress[98] and improves endothelial function in humans.[2]

Xanthine oxidase

Superoxide production in the vasculature is also dependent on the action of xanthine oxidase, a molybdoenzyme involved in purine metabolism. Treatment with xanthine oxidase inhibitors restored normal vascular superoxide production levels and improved NO-dependent vasorelaxation in hypercholesterolemic rabbits.[99] Likewise, the xanthine oxidase inhibitor oxypurinol enhanced endothelium-dependent vasodilation in patients with hypercholesterolemia.[100] Using

electron spin resonance spectroscopy, Spiekermann and colleagues[94] showed elevated *in vivo* superoxide production by xanthine oxidase in subjects with coronary artery disease.[94] Furthermore, increased xanthine oxidase activity was associated with both impaired flow-mediated dilation and enhanced vascular response to ascorbic acid in these patients. These findings suggest a pathophysiologic connection between superoxide elaborated by xanthine oxidase and reduced NO bioactivity during human atherogenesis.

Myeloperoxidase

The significance of inflammatory cell-mediated oxidative processes to vascular dysfunction is becoming clear. Activated macrophages release the enzyme myeloperoxidase (MPO) into the extracellular space, where it generates hypochlorous acid, a potent oxidant species. Numerous investigations have shown MPO within atherosclerotic lesions, as well as evidence for its activity, including MPO-modified LDL and proteins.[101,102] Hypochlorous acid lowers agonist-stimulated NO release from endothelial cells and vascular tissue.[103,104] It is notable that, as a two-electron oxidant, hypochlorous acid is not scavenged by antioxidant vitamins, such as vitamin E or ascorbic acid, providing a further potential explanation for the failure of large-scale clinical trials to show a benefit of these antioxidants.

Although the MPO product hypochlorous acid may reduce NO bioactivity by a variety of mechanisms, MPO also has the unique ability to consume NO directly in a catalytic fashion and induce endothelial dysfunction.[105] Consistent with such an effect, myeloperoxidase impairs NO-dependent vasodilation in isolated arterial rings and decreases NO bioavailability in cultured cells.[104,106] Importantly, myeloperoxidase is rapidly taken up by endothelial cells via a transcytotic process that involves caveolae, and the enzyme accumulates in the subendothelial space, positioning it anatomically to interfere with the effects of NO in the vessel wall.[106,107] The relevance of MPO to endothelial dysfunction in humans is the subject of ongoing investigation.

eNOS

Finally, evidence is accumulating that implicates eNOS itself as a significant site of vascular superoxide production. A number of factors linked to atherosclerosis, including LDL, oxLDL, and glucose, induce eNOS-dependent superoxide production in endothelial cells. In the healthy endothelium, eNOS synthesizes NO in a reaction that transfers electrons from NADPH to L-arginine. Multiple *in vitro* studies have shown that pathologic conditions can interrupt proper electron flow within eNOS, resulting in the conversion of oxygen to superoxide. This 'uncoupling' of eNOS occurs particularly when cellular reserves of L-arginine or cofactors are insufficient.

Recent work has focused on the role of tetrahydrobiopterin (BH_4) in modulating superoxide production by eNOS. BH_4 is an essential cofactor for eNOS activity; its deficiency is associated with eNOS uncoupling in purified protein systems and endothelial dysfunction in animal models of atherosclerosis,[108] diabetes,[109] and hypertension.[110] Selective endothelial overexpression of GTP cyclohydrolase I, the rate-limiting enzyme in endogenous BH_4 synthesis, restored NO-dependent vasodilation in diabetic mice.[111] Pharmacologic supplementation with BH_4 improves endothelial vasomotor function in humans with atherosclerosis[112] and coronary risk factors,[113,114] implying underlying BH_4 depletion and potential eNOS uncoupling during atherogenesis.

One mechanism leading to relative BH_4 deficiency is cellular oxidant stress. In the presence of oxidant species BH_4 is oxidized to BH_2, which is unable to participate in eNOS enzymatic activity. Peroxynitrite has been shown to induce this conversion and to increase eNOS-dependent superoxide production in murine arteries. In cultured endothelial cells, treatment with the antioxidant ascorbic acid augments NO release, in part by preserving optimal BH_4 concentration.[115] A similar effect was observed after chronic administration of ascorbic acid to hypercholesterolemic mice; treated animals had lower vascular levels of BH_2 in association with improved endothelial function.[116] Thus, eNOS uncoupling may represent a self-activating process as increased oxidant stress degrades BH_4 and, in turn, augments eNOS superoxide production.

Alterations in endogenous antioxidant mechanisms

The healthy vasculature possesses antioxidant defense mechanisms that protect it from normal ROS production. Alterations in these defensive systems may contribute to oxidant stress and endothelial pathology in atherogenesis. For example, extracellular superoxide dismutase contributes significantly to the metabolism of superoxide anion, and animals deficient in this enzyme display hypertension and impaired endothelium-dependent vasodilation.[117] Similarly, the enzyme glutathione peroxidase contributes to the metabolism of hydrogen peroxide and lipid hydroperoxides, and animal studies demonstrate that deficiency of this antioxidant enzyme is associated with endothelial dysfunction under conditions of increased oxidative stress.[118,119] The relevance of these mechanisms for endothelial function has not been substantiated in clinical studies; however, it is notable that individuals with low levels of glutathione peroxidase have a higher risk of cardiovascular events.[120]

With regard to low molecular weight antioxidants, there is evidence that cellular levels of glutathione influence NO bioactivity. A polymorphism in the glutamate–cysteine ligase modifier gene, a rate-limiting enzyme for glutathione synthesis, is associated with endothelial dysfunction[121] and increased risk for myocardial infarction.[122] Further support for the relevance of glutathione status for endothelial function is provided by the observations that treatment with a glutathione precursor, or with glutathione itself, restores endothelium-dependent vasodilation in patients with coronary artery disease[123] and with risk factors.[124]

Reduced levels of cofactors for antioxidant enzymes may also be important for the pathogenesis of endothelial dysfunction. For example, NADPH is an important cofactor for the activity of glutathione reductase, catalase, and, indirectly, glutathione peroxidase.[125,126] The primary source of NADPH in cells is the enzyme glucose-6-phosphate dehydrogenase (G6PD). Recent studies suggest that reduced G6PD activity is associated with increased oxidative stress and a loss of biologic activity in endothelial cells,[126] whereas overexpression of G6PD has the opposite effect.[125] Preliminary studies support the clinical relevance of these mechanisms in humans with G6PD deficiency, which is particularly common in African-Americans.[127,128]

Conclusions

It is now clear that diverse mechanisms interfere with the ability of the endothelium to maintain adequate NO availability. Collectively, these findings strongly support a model in which cardiovascular risk factors reduce vascular NO, disrupt the functional integrity of the endothelium, and in this way produce clinical disease. The importance of NO deficiency in atherogenesis affords a treatment possibility. By augmenting NO production and minimizing oxidative stress, therapies may restore endothelial function. Many established[2,129] and novel therapeutics[130,131] have been shown to reverse endothelial dysfunction in subjects with coronary artery disease. Future studies are needed to establish whether improving endothelial function retards the development of atherosclerosis and prevents cardiac events.

Acknowledgments

Dr Hamburg is supported by National Institutes of Health Training Grant T32 HL 07224. Dr Vita is supported by grants from the National Institutes of Health (HL55993 and PO1HL60886).

References

1. Vita JA, Keaney JF Jr. Endothelial function: a barometer for cardiovascular risk? Circulation 2002; 106:640–642.
2. Levine GN, Keaney JF Jr, Vita JA. Cholesterol reduction in cardiovascular disease: clinical benefits and possible mechanisms. N Engl J Med 1995; 332:512–521.
3. Widlansky ME, Gokce N, Keaney JF Jr et al. The clinical implications of endothelial dysfunction. J Am Coll Cardiol 2003; 42:1149–1160.
4. Furchgott RF, Zawadzki JV. The obligatory role of endothelial cells in the relaxation of arterial smooth muscle by acetylcholine. Nature 1980; 288:373–376.
5. Ignarro LJ, Buga GM, Wood KS et al. Endothelium-derived relaxing factor produced and released from artery and vein is nitric oxide. Proc Natl Acad Sci USA 1987; 84:9265–9269.
6. Loscalzo J, Vita JA. Nitric oxide and the cardiovascular system. Totowa, NJ: Humana Press, 2000.
7. Ludmer PL, Selwyn AP, Shook TL et al. Paradoxical vasoconstriction induced by acetylcholine in atherosclerotic coronary arteries. N Engl J Med 1986; 315:1046–1051.
8. Gokce N, Vita JA. Clinical manifestations of endothelial dysfunction. In: Loscalzo J, Schafer AI, eds. Thrombosis and hemorrhage. Philadelphia: Lippincott Williams & Wilkins, 2002: 685–706.
9. Michel T, Feron O. Nitric oxide synthases: which, where, how, and why? J Clin Invest 1997; 100:2146–2152.
10. Fleming I, Busse R. Molecular mechanisms involved in the regulation of the endothelial nitric oxide synthase. Am J Physiol Regul Integr Comp Physiol 2003; 284:R1–12.
11. Shaul PW. Regulation of endothelial nitric oxide synthase: location, location, location. Annu Rev Physiol 2002; 64:749–774.
12. Tai SC, Robb GB, Marsden PA. Endothelial nitric oxide synthase: a new paradigm for gene regulation in the injured blood vessel. Arterioscler Thromb Vasc Biol 2004; 24:1–8.
13. Boo YC, Jo H. Flow-dependent regulation of endothelial nitric oxide synthase: role of protein kinases. Am J Physiol Cell Physiol 2003; 285:C499–C508.
14. Fulton D, Gratton JP, Sessa WC. Post-translational control of endothelial nitric oxide synthase: why isn't calcium/calmodulin enough? J Pharmacol Exp Ther 2001; 299:818–824.
15. Govers R, Rabelink TJ. Cellular regulation of endothelial nitric oxide synthase. Am J Physiol Renal Physiol 2001; 280:F193–F206.
16. Bolotina VM, Najibi S, Palacino JJ et al. Nitric oxide directly activates calcium-dependent potassium channels in vascular smooth muscle. Nature 1994; 368:850–853.

17. Wilcox JN, Subramanian RR, Sundell CL et al. Expression of multiple isoforms of nitric oxide synthase in normal and atherosclerotic vessels. Arterioscler Thromb Vasc Biol 1997; 17:2479–2488.

18. Liao JK, Shin WS, Lee WY et al. Oxidized low-density lipoprotein decreases the expression of endothelial nitric oxide synthase. J Biol Chem 1995; 270:319–324.

19. Yoshizumi M, Perrella MA, Burnett JC Jr et al. Tumor necrosis factor downregulates an endothelial nitric oxide synthase mRNA by shortening its half-life. Circ Res 1993; 73:205–209.

20. Laufs U, La Fata V, Plutzky J et al. Upregulation of endothelial nitric oxide synthase by HMG CoA reductase inhibitors. Circulation 1998; 97:1129–1135.

21. Uematsu M, Ohara Y, Navas JP. Regulation of endothelial cell nitric oxide synthase mRNA expression by shear stress. Am J Physiol 1995; 269:C1371–C1378.

22. Lai PF, Mohamed F, Monge JC et al. Downregulation of eNOS mRNA expression by TNFalpha: identification and functional characterization of RNA-protein interactions in the 3'UTR. Cardiovasc Res 2003; 59:160–168.

23. Hambrecht R, Adams V, Erbs S et al. Regular physical activity improves endothelial function in patients with coronary artery disease by increasing phosphorylation of endothelial nitric oxide synthase. Circulation 2003; 107:3152–3158.

24. Minshall RD, Sessa WC, Stan RV et al. Caveolin regulation of endothelial function. Am J Physiol Lung Cell Mol Physiol 2003; 285:L1179–L1183.

25. Michel JB, Feron O, Sacks D et al. Reciprocal regulation of endothelial nitric-oxide synthase by Ca^{2+}-calmodulin and caveolin. J Biol Chem 1997; 272:15583–15586.

26. Bucci M, Gratton JP, Rudic RD et al. In vivo delivery of the caveolin-1 scaffolding domain inhibits nitric oxide synthesis and reduces inflammation. Nature Med 2000; 6:1362–1367.

27. Drab M, Verkade P, Elger M et al. Loss of caveolae, vascular dysfunction, and pulmonary defects in caveolin-1 gene-disrupted mice. Science 2001; 293:2449–2452.

28. Feron O, Dessy C, Moniotte S et al. Hypercholesterolemia decreases nitric oxide production by promoting the interaction of caveolin and endothelial nitric oxide synthase. J Clin Invest 1999; 103:897–905.

29. Feron O, Dessy C, Desager JP et al. Hydroxy-methylglutaryl-coenzyme A reductase inhibition promotes endothelial nitric oxide synthase activation through a decrease in caveolin abundance. Circulation 2001; 103:113–118.

30. Thompson MA, Henderson KK, Woodman CR et al. Exercise preserves endothelium-dependent relaxation in coronary arteries of hypercholesterolemic male pigs. J Appl Physiol 2003; 96:1114–1126.

31. Frank PG, Lee H, Park DS et al. Genetic ablation of caveolin-1 confers protection against atherosclerosis. Arterioscler Thromb Vasc Biol 2003; 24:98–105.

32. Garcia-Cardena G, Fan R, Shah V et al. Dynamic activation of endothelial nitric oxide synthase by Hsp90. Nature 1998; 392:821–824.

33. Viswanathan M, Rivera O, Short BL. Heat shock protein 90 is involved in pulsatile flow-induced dilation of rat middle cerebral artery. J Vasc Res 1999; 36:524–527.

34. Dikalov S, Landmesser U, Harrison DG. Geldanamycin leads to superoxide formation by enzymatic and non-enzymatic redox cycling. Implications for studies of Hsp90 and endothelial cell nitric-oxide synthase. J Biol Chem 2002; 277:25480–25485.

35. Busconi L, Michel T. Endothelial nitric oxide synthase. N-terminal myristoylation determines subcellular localization. J Biol Chem 1993; 268:8410–8413.

36. Garcia-Cardena G, Oh P, Liu J et al. Targeting of nitric oxide synthase to endothelial cell caveolae via palmitoylation: implications for nitric oxide signaling. Proc Natl Acad Sci USA 1996; 93:6448–6453.

37. Shaul PW, Smart EJ, Robinson LJ et al. Acylation targets emdothelial nitric-oxide synthase to plasmalemmal caveolae. J Biol Chem 1996; 271:6518–6522.

38. Sessa WC, Garcia-Cardena G, Liu J et al. The Golgi association of endothelial nitric oxide synthase is necessary for the efficient synthesis of nitric oxide. J Biol Chem 1995; 270:17641–17644.

39. Blair A, Shaul PW, Yuhanna IS et al. Oxidized low density lipoprotein displaces endothelial nitric-oxide synthase (eNOS) from plasmalemmal caveolae and impairs eNOS activation. J Biol Chem 1999; 274:32512–32519.

40. Boo YC, Jo H. Flow-dependent regulation of endothelial nitric oxide synthase: role of protein kinases. Am J Physiol Cell Physiol 2003; 285:C499–C508.

41. Dimmeler S, Fleming I, Fisslthaler B et al. Activation of nitric oxide synthase in endothelial cells by Akt-dependent phosphorylation. Nature 1999; 399:601–605.

42. Fleming I, Fisslthaler B, Dimmeler S et al. Phosphorylation of Thr(495) regulates Ca(2+)/calmodulin-dependent endothelial nitric oxide synthase activity. Circ Res 2001; 88:E68–E75.

43. Scotland RS, Morales-Ruiz M, Chen Y et al. Functional reconstitution of endothelial nitric oxide synthase reveals the importance of serine 1179 in endothelium-dependent vasomotion. Circ Res 2002; 90:904–910.

44. Chen ZP, Mitchelhill KI, Michell BJ et al. AMP-activated protein kinase phosphorylation of endothelial NO synthase. FEBS Lett 1999; 443:285–289.

45. Kureishi Y, Luo Z, Shiojima I et al. The HMG-CoA reductase inhibitor simvastatin activates the protein kinase Akt and promotes angiogenesis in normocholesterolemic animals. Nature Med 2000; 6:1004–1010.

46. Mineo C, Yuhanna IS, Quon MJ et al. High density lipoprotein-induced endothelial nitric-oxide synthase activation is mediated by Akt and MAP kinases. J Biol Chem 2003; 278:9142–9149.

47. Harris MB, Ju H, Venema VJ et al. Reciprocal phosphorylation and regulation of endothelial nitric-oxide synthase in response to bradykinin stimulation. J Biol Chem 2001; 276:16587–16591.

48. Michell BJ, Chen ZZ, Tiganis T et al. Coordinated control of endothelial nitric-oxide synthase phosphorylation by

protein kinase C and the cAMP-dependent protein kinase. J Biol Chem 2001; 276:17625–17628.

49. Hirata K, Kuroda R, Sakoda T et al. Inhibition of endothelial nitric oxide synthase activity by protein kinase C. Hypertension 1995; 25:180–185.

50. Beckman JA, Goldfine AB, Gordon MB et al. Inhibition of protein kinase C beta prevents impaired endothelium-dependent vasodilation caused by hyperglycemia in humans. Circ Res 2002; 90:107–111.

51. Vallance P, Leone A, Calver A et al. Accumulation of an endogenous inhibitor of nitric oxide synthesis in chronic renal failure. Lancet 1992; 339:572–575.

52. Stuhlinger MC, Tsao PS, Her JH et al. Homocysteine impairs the nitric oxide synthase pathway: role of asymmetric dimethylarginine. Circulation 2001; 104:2569–2575.

53. Boger RH, Sydow K, Borlak J et al. LDL cholesterol upregulates synthesis of asymmetrical dimethylarginine in human endothelial cells: involvement of S-adenosylmethionine-dependent methyltransferases. Circ Res 2000; 87:99–105.

54. Ito A, Tsao PS, Adimoolam S et al. Novel mechanism for endothelial dysfunction: dysregulation of dimethylarginine dimethylaminohydrolase. Circulation 1999; 99:3092–3095.

55. Boger RH. The emerging role of asymmetric dimethylarginine as a novel cardiovascular risk factor. Cardiovasc Res 2003; 59:824–833.

56. Boger RH, Bode-Boger SM, Szuba A et al. Asymmetric dimethylarginine (ADMA): a novel risk factor for endothelial dysfunction: its role in hypercholesterolemia. Circulation 1998; 98:1842–1847.

57. Stuhlinger MC, Oka RK, Graf EE et al. Endothelial dysfunction induced by hyperhomocyst(e)inemia: role of asymmetric dimethylarginine. Circulation 2003; 108:933–938.

58. Dayoub H, Achan V, Adimoolam S et al. Dimethylarginine dimethylaminohydrolase regulates nitric oxide synthesis: genetic and physiological evidence. Circulation 2003; 108:3042–3047.

59. Lin KY, Ito A, Asagami T et al. Impaired nitric oxide synthase pathway in diabetes mellitus: role of asymmetric dimethylarginine and dimethylarginine dimethylaminohydrolase. Circulation 2002; 106:987–992.

60. Valkonen VP, Paiva H, Salonen JT et al. Risk of acute coronary events and serum concentration of asymmetrical dimethylarginine. Lancet 2001; 358:2127–2128.

61. Zoccali C, Bode-Boger S, Mallamaci F et al. Plasma concentration of asymmetrical dimethylarginine and mortality in patients with end-stage renal disease: a prospective study. Lancet 2001; 358:2113–2117.

62. Maxwell AJ, Cooke JP. L-arginine. In: Loscalzo J, Vita JA, eds. Nitric oxide and the cardiovascular system. Totowa, NJ: Humana Press, 2000: 547–585.

63. Loscalzo J. Functional polymorphisms in a candidate gene for atherothrombosis: unraveling the complex fabric of a polygenic phenotype. J Am Coll Cardiol 2003; 41:946–948.

64. Wattanapitayakul SK, Mihm MJ, Young AP et al. Therapeutic implications of human endothelial nitric oxide synthase gene polymorphism. Trends Pharmacol Sci 2001; 22:361–368.

65. Nakayama M, Yasue H, Yoshimura M et al. T-786ÆC mutation in the 5'-flanking region of the endothelial nitric oxide synthase gene is associated with coronary spasm. Circulation 1999; 99:2864–2870.

66. Tesauro M, Thompson WC, Rogliani P et al. Intracellular processing of endothelial nitric oxide synthase isoforms associated with differences in severity of cardiopulmonary diseases: cleavage of proteins with aspartate vs. glutamate at position 298. Proc Natl Acad Sci USA 2000; 97:2832–2835.

67. Rossi GP, Cesari M, Zanchetta M et al. The T-786C endothelial nitric oxide synthase genotype is a novel risk factor for coronary artery disease in Caucasian patients of the GENICA study. J Am Coll Cardiol 2003; 41:930–937.

68. Nakayama M, Yasue H, Yoshimura M et al. T(-786)→ C mutation in the 5'-flanking region of the endothelial nitric oxide synthase gene is associated with myocardial infarction, especially without coronary organic stenosis. Am J Cardiol 2000; 86:628–634.

69. Shimasaki Y, Yasue H, Yoshimura M et al. Association of the missense Glu298Asp variant of the endothelial nitric oxide synthase gene with myocardial infarction. J Am Coll Cardiol 1998; 31:1506–1510.

70. Hingorani AD, Liang CF, Fatibene J et al. A common variant of the endothelial nitric oxide synthase (Glu298→Asp) is a major risk factor for coronary artery disease in the UK. Circulation 1999; 100:1515–1520.

71. Cai H, Wilcken DE, Wang XL. The Glu-298→Asp (894G→T) mutation at exon 7 of the endothelial nitric oxide synthase gene and coronary artery disease. J Mol Med 1999; 77:511–514.

72. Poirier O, Mao C, Mallet C et al. Polymorphisms of the endothelial nitric oxide synthase gene – no consistent association with myocardial infarction in the ECTIM study. Eur J Clin Invest 1999; 29:284–290.

73. Erbs S, Baither Y, Linke A et al. Promoter but not exon 7 polymorphism of endothelial nitric oxide synthase affects training-induced correction of endothelial dysfunction. Arterioscler Thromb Vasc Biol 2003; 23:1814–1819.

74. Rossi GP, Taddei S, Virdis A et al. The T-786C and Glu298Asp polymorphisms of the endothelial nitric oxide gene affect the forearm blood flow responses of Caucasian hypertensive patients. J Am Coll Cardiol 2003; 41:938–945.

75. Leeson CPM, Hingorani AD, Mullen MJ et al. Glu298Asp endothelial nitric oxide synthase gene polymorphism interacts with environmental and dietary factors to influence endothelial function. Circ Res 2002; 90:1153–1158.

76. Heinecke JW. Sources of vascular oxidative stress. In: Keaney JF Jr, ed. Oxidative stress and vascular disease. Boston: Kluwer Academic, 2000: 9–25.

77. Wentworth P Jr, Nieva J, Takeuchi C et al. Evidence for ozone formation in human atherosclerotic arteries. Science 2003; 302:1053–1056.

78. Beckman JS, Koppenol WH. Nitric oxide, superoxide, and peroxynitrite: the good, the bad, and the ugly. Am J Physiol.1996; 271:C1424–C1437.

79. Keaney JF Jr. Atherosclerosis, oxidative stress, and endothelial function. In: Keaney JF Jr, ed. Oxidative stress and vascular disease. Boston: Kluwer Academic, 2000: 155–181.

80. Gryglewski RJ, Palmer RM, Moncada S. Superoxide anion is involved in the breakdown of endothelium-derived vascular relaxing factor. Nature 1986; 320:454–456.

81. Cai H, Harrison DG. Endothelial dysfunction in cardiovascular diseases: the role of oxidant stress. Circ Res 2000; 87:840–844.

82. Griendling KK, Fitzgerald GA. Oxidative stress and cardiovascular injury: Part I: basic mechanisms and in vivo monitoring of ROS. Circulation 2003; 108:1912–1916.

83. Tomasian D, Keaney JF Jr, Vita JA. Antioxidants and the bioactivity of endothelium-derived nitric oxide. Cardiovasc Res 2000; 47:426–435.

84. Ting HH, Timimi FK, Boles KS et al. Vitamin C improves endothelium-dependent vasodilation in patients with non-insulin-dependent diabetes mellitus. J Clin Invest 1996; 97:22–28.

85. Ting HH, Timimi FK, Haley EA et al. Vitamin C improves endothelium-dependent vasodilation in forearm resistance vessels of humans with hypercholesterolemia. Circulation 1997; 95:2617–2622.

86. Sherman DL, Keaney JF Jr, Biegelsen ES et al. Pharmacological concentrations of ascorbic acid are required for the beneficial effects on endothelial vasomotor function in hypertension. Hypertension 2000; 35:936–941.

87. Motoyama T, Kawano H, Kugiyama K et al. Endothelium-dependent vasodilation in the brachial artery is impaired in smokers: effect of vitamin C. Am J Physiol 1997; 273:H1644–H1650.

88. Heitzer T, Schlinzig T, Krohn K et al. Endothelial dysfunction, oxidative stress, and risk of cardiovascular events in patients with coronary artery disease. Circulation 2001; 104:2673–2678.

89. Jackson TS, Xu A, Vita JA et al. Ascorbate prevents the interaction of superoxide and nitric oxide only at very high physiological concentrations. Circ Res 1998; 83:916–922.

90. Widlansky ME, Biegelsen ES, Hamburg NM et al. Coronary endothelial dysfunction is not rapidly reversible with ascorbic acid. Free Radical Biol Med 2004; 36:123–130.

91. Chen K, Thomas SR, Keaney JF Jr. Beyond LDL oxidation: ROS in vascular signal transduction. Free Radical Biol Med 2003; 35:117–132.

92. Yusuf S, Dagenais G, Pogue J et al. Vitamin E supplementation and cardiovascular events in high-risk patients. The Heart Outcomes Prevention Evaluation Study Investigators. N Engl J Med 2000; 342:154–160.

93. Sorescu D, Weiss D, Lassegue B et al. Superoxide production and expression of nox family proteins in human atherosclerosis. Circulation 2002; 105:1429–1435.

94. Spiekermann S, Landmesser U, Dikalov S et al. Electron spin resonance characterization of vascular xanthine and NAD(P)H oxidase activity in patients with coronary artery disease: relation to endothelium-dependent vasodilation. Circulation 2003; 107:1383–1389.

95. Gorlach A, Brandes RP, Nguyen K et al. A gp91phox containing NADPH oxidase selectively expressed in endothelial cells is a major source of oxygen radical generation in the arterial wall. Circ Res 2000; 87:26–32.

96. Guzik TJ, West NE, Black E et al. Vascular superoxide production by NAD(P)H oxidase: association with endothelial dysfunction and clinical risk factors. Circ Res 2000; 86:E85–E90.

97. Wagner AH, Kohler T, Ruckschloss U et al. Improvement of nitric oxide-dependent vasodilatation by HMG-CoA reductase inhibitors through attenuation of endothelial superoxide anion formation. Arterioscler Thromb Vasc Biol 2000; 20:61–69.

98. Shishehbor MH, Aviles RJ, Brennan ML et al. Association of nitrotyrosine levels with cardiovascular disease and modulation by statin therapy. J Am Med Assoc 2003; 289:1675–1680.

99. Ohara Y, Peterson TE, Harrison DG. Hypercholesterolemia increases endothelial superoxide anion production. J Clin Invest 1993; 91:2546–2551.

100. Cardillo C, Kilcoyne CM, Cannon RO et al. Xanthine oxidase inhibition with oxypurinol improves endothelial vasodilator function in hypercholesterolemic but not in hypertensive patients. Hypertension 1997; 30:57–63.

101. Daugherty A, Dunn JL, Rateri DL et al. Myeloperoxidase, a catalyst for lipoprotein oxidation, is expressed in human atherosclerotic lesions. J Clin Invest 1994; 94:437–444.

102. Hazell LJ, Arnold L, Flowers D et al. Presence of hypochlorite-modified proteins in human atherosclerotic lesions. J Clin Invest 1996; 97:1535–1544.

103. Jaimes EA, Sweeney C, Raij L. Effects of the reactive oxygen species hydrogen peroxide and hypochlorite on endothelial nitric oxide production. Hypertension 2001; 38:877–883.

104. Zhang C, Patel R, Eiserich JP et al. Endothelial dysfunction is induced by proinflammatory oxidant hypochlorous acid. Am J Physiol Heart Circ Physiol 2001; 281:H1469–H1475.

105. Abu-Soud HM, Hazen SL. Nitric oxide is a physiological substrate for mammalian peroxidases. J Biol Chem 2000; 275:37524–37532.

106. Eiserich JP, Baldus S, Brennan ML et al. Myeloperoxidase, a leukocyte-derived vascular NO oxidase. Science 2002; 296:2391–2394.

107. Baldus S, Eiserich JP, Mani A et al. Endothelial transcytosis of myeloperoxidase confers specificity to vascular ECM proteins as targets of tyrosine nitration. J Clin Invest 2001; 108:1759–1770.

108. Laursen JB, Somers M, Kurz S et al. Endothelial regulation of vasomotion in apoE-deficient mice: implications for interactions between peroxynitrite and tetrahydrobiopterin. Circulation 2001; 103:1282–1288.

109. Hink U, Li H, Mollnau H et al. Mechanisms underlying endothelial dysfunction in diabetes mellitus. Circ Res 2001; 88:E14–E22.

110. Landmesser U, Dikalov S, Price SR et al. Oxidation of tetrahydrobiopterin leads to uncoupling of endothelial cell nitric oxide synthase in hypertension. J Clin Invest 2003; 111:1201–1209.

111. Alp NJ, Mussa S, Khoo J et al. Tetrahydrobiopterin-dependent preservation of nitric oxide-mediated endothelial function in diabetes by targeted transgenic GTP-cyclohydrolase I overexpression. J Clin Invest 2003; 112:725–735.

112. Tiefenbacher CP, Bleeke T, Vahl C et al. Endothelial dysfunction of coronary resistance arteries is improved by tetrahydrobiopterin in atherosclerosis. Circulation 2000; 102:2172–2179.

113. Heitzer T, Brockhoff C, Mayer B et al. Tetrahydrobiopterin improves endothelium-dependent vasodilation in chronic smokers: evidence for a dysfunctional nitric oxide synthase. Circ Res 2000; 86:E36–E41.

114. Stroes E, Kastelein J, Cosentino F et al. Tetrahydrobiopterin restores endothelial function in hypercholesterolemia. J Clin Invest 1997; 99:41–46.

115. Huang A, Vita JA, Venema RC et al. Ascorbic acid enhances endothelial nitric oxide synthase activity by increasing intracellular tetrahydrobiopterin. J Biol Chem 2000; 275:17399–17406.

116. d'Uscio LV, Milstien S, Richardson D et al. Long-term vitamin C treatment increases vascular tetrahydrobiopterin levels and nitric oxide synthase activity. Circ Res 2003; 92:88–95.

117. Jung O, Marklund SL, Geiger H et al. Extracellular superoxide dismutase is a major determinant of nitric oxide bioavailability: in vivo and ex vivo evidence from ecSOD-deficient mice. Circ Res 2003; 93:622–629.

118. Forgione MA, Weiss N, Heydrick S et al. Cellular glutathione peroxidase deficiency and endothelial dysfunction. Am J Physiol Heart Circ Physiol 2002; 282:H1255–H1261.

119. Forgione MA, Cap A, Liao R et al. Heterozygous cellular glutathione peroxidase deficiency in the mouse: abnormalities in vascular and cardiac function and structure. Circulation 2002; 106:1154–1158.

120. Blankenberg S, Rupprecht HJ, Bickel C et al. Glutathione peroxidase 1 activity and cardiovascular events in patients with coronary artery disease. N Engl J Med 2003; 349:1605–1613.

121. Nakamura SI, Sugiyama S, Fujioka D et al. Polymorphism in glutamate-cysteine ligase modifier subunit gene is associated with impairment of nitric oxide-mediated coronary vasomotor function. Circulation 2003; 108:1425–1427.

122. Nakamura S, Kugiyama K, Sugiyama S et al. Polymorphism in the 5'-flanking region of human glutamate-cysteine ligase modifier subunit gene is associated with myocardial infarction. Circulation 2002; 105:2968–2973.

123. Vita JA, Frei B, Holbrook M et al. L-2-oxothiazolidine-4-carboxylic acid reverses endothelial dysfunction in patients with coronary artery disease. J Clin Invest 1998; 101:1408–1414.

124. Kugiyama K, Ohgushi M, Motoyama T et al. Intracoronary infusion of reduced glutathione improves endothelial vasomotor response to acetylcholine in human coronary circulation. Circulation 1998; 97:2299–2301.

125. Leopold JA, Zhang YY, Scribner AW et al. Glucose-6-phosphate dehydrogenase overexpression decreases endothelial cell oxidant stress and increases bioavailable nitric oxide. Arterioscler Thromb Vasc Biol 2003; 23:411–417.

126. Leopold JA, Cap A, Scribner AW et al. Glucose-6-phosphate dehydrogenase deficiency promotes endothelial oxidant stress and decreases endothelial nitric oxide bioavailability. FASEB J 2001; 15:1771–1773.

127. Forgione MA, Loscalzo J, Holbrook M, et al. Glucose-6-phosphate dehydrogenase deficiency, lipid peroxidation, and vascular oxidant stress in African Americans. Circulation 2001; 104:II-295.

128. Forgione MA, Loscalzo J, Holbrook M et al. The A326G (A+) variant of the glucose-6-phosphate dehydrogenase gene is associated with endothelial dysfunction in African Americans. J Am Coll Cardiol 2003; 41:249A.

129. Mancini GB, Henry GC, Macaya C et al. Angiotensin-converting enzyme inhibition with quinapril improves endothelial vasomotor dysfunction in patients with coronary artery disease. The TREND (Trial on Reversing ENdothelial Dysfunction) Study. Circulation 1996; 94:258–265.

130. Duffy SJ, Keaney JF Jr, Holbrook M et al. Short- and long-term black tea consumption reverses endothelial dysfunction in patients with coronary artery disease. Circulation 2001; 104:151–156.

131. Hambrecht R, Wolf A, Gielen S et al. Effect of physical exercise on coronary endothelial function in coronary artery disease. N Engl J Med 2000; 342:454–460.

8

Lipoproteins and atherogenesis

Vassilis I. Zannis, Kyriakos E. Kypreos, Angeliki Chroni, Dimitris Kardassis, Eleni E. Zanni

General overview of the lipoprotein pathways and their contribution to lipid homeostasis and to atherosclerosis

The lipoprotein pathways

The transport of free cholesterol, cholesteryl esters, triglycerides, phospholipids and other lipids in the circulation is achieved by the packing of the lipid moieties into water-soluble lipoproteins. The plasma lipoproteins are either spherical particles or discoidal particles. The spherical particle has a core of non-polar neutral lipid consisting of cholesteryl esters (CE) and triglycerides (TG), and coats of relatively polar materials such as phospholipids, cholesterol, and proteins (Figure 8.1a, Table 8.1).[1] The discoidal particle consists of mostly polar lipids and proteins, and is in a bilayer conformation (Figure 8.1a).[1,2]

Plasma lipoproteins have traditionally been grouped into five major classes and various subclasses, based on their buoyant density (Figure 8.1a): chylomicrons, very low-density lipoproteins (VLDL), intermediate-density lipoproteins (IDL), low-density lipoproteins (LDL), and high-density lipoproteins (HDL). Lipoprotein (a) (Lp(a)), which will be discussed later, floats in the LDL region.[2,3]

Lipoproteins are synthesized and catabolized in three distinct pathways: the chylomicron pathway, the VLDL/IDL/LDL pathway, and the HDL pathway, all of which are metabolically interrelated (Figure 8.1b–d). Several different proteins, including apolipo-proteins, plasma enzymes, lipid transfer proteins, lipoprotein receptors, and lipid transporters, participate in these pathways and contribute to lipid homeostasis. The properties of the apolipoproteins, plasma enzymes and lipid transfer proteins, lipoprotein receptors, and receptors for modified lipoproteins (scavenger receptors) are shown in Tables 8.2, 8.3, 8.4, and 8.5, respectively.

The assembly of chylomicrons and VLDL occurs intracellularly, whereas that of HDL occurs extracellularly.[4,5] In the chylomicron pathway, synthesis of chylomicrons occurs in the intestine. Following food uptake, dietary lipids assemble with apoB-48 in intestinal epithelial cells to form chylomicrons. The assembly and subsequent secretion of chylomicrons in the lymph requires microsomal triglyceride transfer protein (MTP). In the absence of apoB-48 or MTP, chylomicrons are not formed. Following secretion, the TG of chylomicrons are hydrolyzed in plasma by lipoprotein lipase, which is anchored on the surface of microvascular endothelial cells and is activated by apolipoprotein CII (apoCII). Triglyceride hydrolysis converts chylomicrons to chylomicron remnants rich in CE. These remnants contain apoE on their surface and are cleared rapidly by the liver mainly through the LDL receptor and possibly other members of the LDL receptor family. This family includes the LDL receptor-related protein (LRP), the megalin/gp330, the apoE receptor-2 (apoER2), and the VLDL receptor (VLDLr), which are discussed later.

Known genetic alterations in the different steps of the chylomicron pathway, associated with human diseases, are shown schematically in Figure 8.1b. Diseases associated with lipoprotein abnormalities have been extensively reviewed:[5–7]

Table 8.1 Properties and composition of major human plasma lipoproteins (modified from references 1 and 388`)

Properties and compositions	Chylomicrons	VLDL	LDL	HDL	Lp(a)
Source	Intestine	Liver	VLDL	Liver and intestine	Liver
Size (Å)	750–12 000	300–800	180–300	50–120	250–300
Density (g/ml)	< 0.94	0.94–1.006	1.019–1.063	1.063–1.21	1.040–1.090
Molecular mass (kDa)	~400 000	10–80 000	2300	175–360	3000–8000
Triglycerides (%wt)	80–95	45–65	4–8	2–7	~1
Phospholipids (%wt)	3–6	15–20	18–24	26–32	~22
Free cholesterol (%wt)	1–3	4–8	6–8	3–5	~8
Esterified cholesterol (%wt)	2–4	16–22	45–50	15–20	~37
Protein (%wt)	1–2	6–10	18–22	45–55	~32
Major apolipoproteins	apoA-I, apoA-IV, apoB-48, apoCI, apoCIII, apoE	apoB-100, apoE, apoCI, apoCII, apoCIII	apoB-100	apoA-I, apoA-II	apoB-100, apo(a)
Minor apolipoproteins	apoA-II, apoCII	apoA-I, apoA-II, apoA-IV, apoCIV, apoAV	apoCI, apoCII, apoCIII, apoE	apoCI, apoCII, apoCIII, apoD, apoE, apoJ, apoAV	–

VLDL, very low-density lipoproteins; LDL, low-density lipoprotein; HDL, high-density lipoproteins;Lp(a), lipoprotein (a); apo, apolipoprotein

(a)

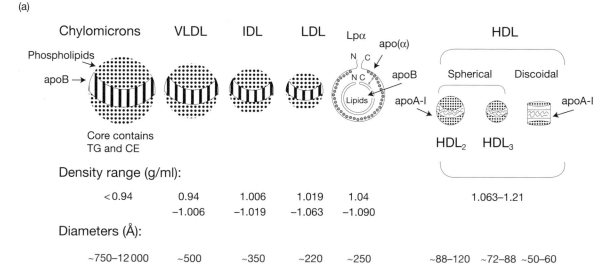

Figure 8.1 (a) Schematic representation of plasma lipoproteins and their metabolic pathways. The major apolipoproteins of low- and high-density lipoproteins (LDL and HDL) are depicted to shield the fatty acyl chains of the phospholipids. The schematic representation of lipoprotein(a) (LP(a)) is designed to depict the position of apolipoprotein B (apoB) and apo(a). TG, triglycerides; CE, cholesteryl esters

(b)

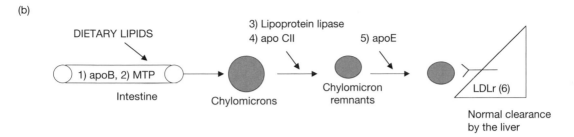

(1) Homozygous hypobetalipoproteinemia due to generation of truncated apoB
    forms (i.e. apoB-30 etc.)
(2) Abetalipoproteinemia due to mutations in MTP
(3) Familial type I hyperlipoproteinemia (hypertriglyceridemia) due to lack of lipoprotein lipase
(4) Familial type I hyperlipoproteinemia (hypertriglyceridemia) due to lack of apoCII
(5) Familial type III hyperlipoproteinemia due to mutations in apoE

Figure 8.1 (b) Schematic representation of the pathway of the biosynthesis and catabolism of chylomicrons. Numbers 1–6 indicate the proteins of the pathway and their association with diseases. These are: (1) apoB, (2) microsomal triglyceride transfer protein (MTP), (3) lipoprotein lipase (LPL), (4) apoCII, (5) apoE, (6) LDL receptor (LDLr)

(c)

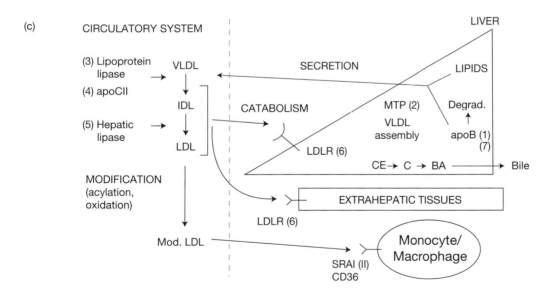

(1) Homozygous hypobetalipoproteinemia due to the generation of truncated apoB forms
(2) Abetalipoproteinemia due to mutations in MTP
(3) Familial type I hyperlipoproteinemia (hypertriglyceridemia) due to mutations in lipoprotein lipase
(4) Familial type I hyperlipoproteinemia (hypertriglyceridemia) due to mutations in apoCII
(5) Hepatic lipase deficiency due to mutations in hepatic lipase
(6) Familial hypercholesterolemia due to mutations in the LDL receptor
(7) Familial defective apoB-100 and other apoB mutations that affect the affinity of LDL for
    the LDL receptor

Figure 8.1 (c) Schematic representation of the pathway of the biosynthesis and catabolism of very low-density lipoprotein (VLDL). Numbers 1–6 indicate the proteins of the pathway and their association with diseases. These are: (1) apoB, (2) MTP, (3) LPL, (4) apoCII, (5) apoE, (6) LDLr

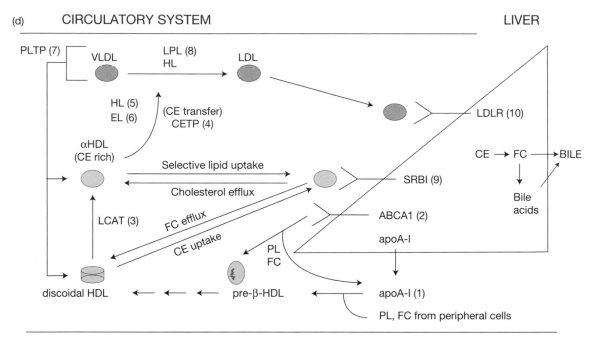

(1) ApoA-I deficiency due to chain termination mutations or deletions of the apoA-I gene
(2) Tangier disease due to mutations in the ABCA1 transporter
(3) LCAT deficiency (inability to esterify cholesterol on HDL and LDL) and fish eye disease (inability to esterify cholesterol on HDL only) due to mutations in LCAT
(4) CETP deficiency due to mutations in CETP
(5) Hepatic lipase deficiency due to mutations in hepatic lipase
(6) Endothelial lipase
(7) Phospholipid transfer protein
(8) Lipoprotein lipase
(9) Scavenger receptor type BI
(10) LDL receptor

Figure 8.1 (d) Schematic representation of the pathway of biogenesis and catabolism of HDL by liver. Numbers 1–10 indicate key cell membrane or plasma proteins shown to influence HDL levels or composition and their association with diseases. These are: (1) apoA-I; (2) ATP-binding cassette A1 (ABCA1); (3) lecithin : cholesterol acyltransferase (LCAT); (4) cholesteryl ester transfer protein (CETP); (5) hepatic lipase (HL); (6) endothelial lipase (EL); (7) phospholipids transfer protein (PLTP); (8) LPL; (9) scavenger receptor type BI (SRBI); (10) LDLr

The diseases associated with the chylomicron pathway are:

- *Homozygous hypobetalipoproteinemia* is characterized by lack of synthesis and secretion of chylomicrons, and is the result of chain termination mutations that generate truncated apoB forms.

- *Abetalipoproteinemia* is characterized by a lack of chylomicron synthesis and secretion, and is the result of mutations in MTP.

- *Familial type I hyperlipoproteinemia (hypertriglyceridemia)* is characterized by high plasma triglyceride levels, and is the result of mutations in lipoprotein lipase or an inhibitor of lipoprotein lipase.

- *Familial type I hyperlipoproteinemia (hypertriglyceridemia)* is characterized by high plasma triglyceride levels, and is the result of mutations in apoCII.

- *Familial type III hyperlipoproteinemia* is characterized by high plasma cholesterol and usually high triglyceride levels which accumulate in the VLDL and IDL regions, and is the result of mutations in apoE.

Two additional conditions of unknown or uncertain molecular etiology are:

- *Type V hyperlipoproteinemia* is characterized by the presence of chylomicrons in fasting plasma, and moderate to severe hypertriglyceridemia.[6] This syndrome was described by Fredrickson and Lees,[8] and encompasses a diverse group of patients with primary and secondary causes of hypertriglyceridemia.[8,9]

- *Chylomicron retention disease* is characterized by defective secretion of chylomicrons and fat malabsorption.

Biogenesis of LDL occurs in the liver. In this pathway, apoB assembles intracellularly with lipids in the hepatocytes by the action of MTP to form VLDL, which is then secreted into the plasma. Lack of MTP or unavailability of lipids leads to apoB degradation and inhibits VLDL assembly and secretion. More details on the assembly and secretion of VLDL, chylomicrons, and Lp(a) are provided in later chapters. Following secretion, the TG of VLDL are hydrolyzed by the action of lipoprotein lipase (which is activated by apoCII) to produce IDL, which is further converted to LDL by the action of hepatic lipase. IDL and LDL are recognized and catabolized by the LDL receptor (Figure 8.1c). An increase in the plasma LDL levels or the formation of small dense LDL particles is associated with an increased risk for atherosclerosis.[10] Mutations in the LDL pathway underlying human diseases are shown in Figure 8.1c and have been extensively reviewed:[5,6,11]

These diseases are:

- *Homozygous hypobetalipoproteinemia* (see above).

- *Abetalipoproteinemia* (see above).

- *Familial hypertriglyceridemia* is characterized by the accumulation of chylomicrons, high plasma triglyceride levels and is the result of mutations in the LPL or in apoCII, or an inhibitor of LPL.

These three diseases have been described in the chylomicron pathway

- *Hepatic lipase deficiency* is characterized by the accumulation of large-size HDL and LDL, and is the result of mutations in the hepatic lipase (HL).

- *Familial hypercholesterolemia* is characterized by high plasma cholesterol and xanthomatosis, and is the result of mutations in the LDL receptor.

- *Familial defective apoB-100 and other apoB mutations* that affect the affinity of LDL for the LDL receptor. They are characterized by moderate increases in the LDL levels.

One additional disease of unknown molecular etiology is:

- *Familial combined hyperlipidemia* is characterized by increased plasma cholesterol and in some cases increased triglyceride levels, and is the result of overproduction of apoB.

The LDL pathway is discussed in more detail in a later chapter.

Biogenesis of HDL occurs mainly in the liver through a complex pathway. In the early steps of this pathway, apolipoprotein A-I (apoA-I) is secreted mostly lipid free by the liver, and acquires phospholipid and cholesterol via its interactions with the ATP-binding cassette A1 (ABCA1) lipid transporter and other processes. Through a series of intermediate steps that are poorly understood, apoA-I is gradually lipidated and proceeds to form discoidal particles that are converted to spherical particles by the action of lecithin: cholesterol acyl transferase (LCAT). Both the discoidal and the spherical HDL particles interact functionally with the HDL receptor/scavenger receptor class B type I (SRBI) as will be discussed later. The interactions of apoA-I with SRBI are important for the atheroprotective functions of HDL. The late steps of the HDL pathway involve the transfer of cholesteryl esters to VLDL/LDL for eventual catabolism by the LDL receptor, the hydrolysis of phospholipids and residual triglycerides by the various lipases (LPL, HL, and endothelial lipase (EL)), and the transfer of phospholipids from VLDL/LDL to HDL by the action of phospholipid transfer protein (PLTP) (Figure 8.1d and Table 8.3).

Known mutations in the HDL pathway that may affect this pathway are shown in Figure 8.1d and have been reviewed extensively.[4,6,12,13] The diseases are:

- *ApoA-I deficiency* is characterized by the absence of HDL, and is the result of chain determination mutations or deletions of the apoA-I gene.

- *Tangier disease* is characterized by the absence of HDL, and is the result of mutations in the ABCA1 transporter.

- *LCAT deficiency.* Mutations in the enzyme LCAT are associated with two phenotypes. The classical LCAT

Table 8.2 Summary of apolipoprotein structure and functions[388]

Apolipo-protein	Amino acids*	Lipoprotein	Function	Association with disease
ApoA-I	243	HDL	Activates LCAT, interacts with SRBI and promotes selective lipid uptake and cholesterol efflux, interacts with ABCA1 and promotes lipid efflux and HDL biogenesis, has atheroprotective functions in the arterial wall	Deletion of apoA-I, apoCIII, apoA-IV loci and inversion of the apoA-I, CIII, loci are associated with atherosclerosis
ApoA-II	77	HDL	Inhibits the activity of hepatic lipase Atherogenic in some mice models	ApoA-II deficiency in humans does not affect HDL levels or susceptibility to coronary heart disease
ApoA-IV	376	d < 1.21 g/ml	Activates LCAT moderately Is antiatherogenic in transgenic mice Has functional similarities with apoA-I Promotes cholesterol efflux, protects from atherosclerosis	Deletion of apoA-I, apoCIII, apoA-IV loci and inversion of the apoA-I, CIII, loci are associated with atherosclerosis
ApoB	4536	LDL, VLDL, Lp(a)	Ligand for the LDL receptor promotes the formation of nascent VLDL	Abetalipoproteinemia, hypobetalipoproteinemia, LDL receptor binding defects familial apoB-100 deficiency
ApoCI	57	VLDL, LDL, HDL	Activates LCAT moderately	
ApoCII	79	VLDL, LDL, HDL	Activates lipoprotein lipase	Familial type I hyperlipoproteinemia (hypertriglyceridemia)
ApoCIII	79	VLDL, LDL, HDL	Inhibits the catabolism of triglyceride-rich lipoproteins	Deletion of apoA-I, CIII, A-IV loci and inversion of apoA-I, CIII loci is associated with atherosclerosis
Apo CIV[389,390]	102	VLDL	Increased VLDL, is expressed at very low levels in human liver, nearly undetectable in plasma. May contribute to plasma triglyceride levels	None Overexpression increases plasma triglycerides
ApoAV[391]	345	VLDL, HDL	May contribute to plasma triglyceride homeostasis	Overexpression reduces plasma triglyceride levels
ApoE	299	VLDL, LDL, HDL	Ligand for the LDL receptor. Binds *in vitro* to other apoE-recognizing receptors. Activates LCAT moderately Interacts functionally with SR-B1 Essential for the clearance of lipoprotein remnants. Atheroprotective	Familial type III hyperlipoproteinemia Late-onset of Alzheimer's disease
Apo(a)	4529	Lp(a)	Co-localizes with lipid deposition in the arterial wall. Has protease activity different from that of plasmin. Interferes with fibrinolysis, induces proinflammatory and proliferative conditions in the vascular wall and induces atherosclerosis in transgenic mice	Increased Lp(a) levels are associated with cardiovascular disease Lp(a) may contribute to thrombosis

* Refers to the sequence of the mature protein without the signal peptide and in the case of apoA-I without the 6-amino acid-long amino terminal prosegment.

HDL, high-density lipoprotein; apo, apolipoprotein; LCAT, lecithin : cholesterol acyltransferase; SRBI, scavenger receptor class B type I; ABCA1, ATP-binding cassette A1; LDL, low-density lipoprotein; VLDL, very low-density lipoprotein; Lp(a), lipoprotein (a)

Table 8.3 Plasma enzymes and lipid transfer proteins

Enzyme/ protein	Amino acids*	Site of synthesis	Function	Association with disease
Lipoprotein lipase (LPL)	448	High level in adipose tissue, heart, muscle, brain; low level in most other tissues Undetectable liver, spleen and white blood cells	Hydrolysis of 1 and 3 ester bonds of chylomicron and VLDL triglycerides	Type I hyperlipoproteinemia, (hypertriglyceridemia)
Hepatic lipase (HL)	476	Liver	Hydrolysis of mono- and diacylglycerol and phospholipids of HDL2 and IDL	Hepatic lipase deficiency causes increased plasma cholesterol and triglycerides, abnormal lipoprotein profiles, premature atherosclerosis in some cases
Lecithin cholesterol acyltrans-ferase (LCAT)	416	Liver, brain, testis	Esterification of free cholesterol on HDL and LDL using the C2 acyl group of lecithin	Familial LCAT deficiency, fish eye disease In LCAT deficiency there is accumulation of discoidal HDL particles Kidney disease and atherosclerosis in some cases
Cholesteryl ester transfer protein (CETP)	476	Liver, small intestine, spleen, adipose tissue, muscle and adrenal, kidney (lesser extent)	Exchange or transfer of cholesteryl ester, triglycerides and phospholipids between lipoproteins. CETP transfers cholesteryl esters primarily from VLDL and LDL to HDL	Familial CETP deficiency. It is characterized by hyperalphalipoproteinemia CHD is observed only in some populations with CETP mutations
Phospholipid transfer protein (PLTP)	476	Ubiquitously expressed; liver, ovary, thymus, placenta, and adipose tissue	Transfers phospholipid from chylomicrons and VLDL to HDL. Converts HDL3 into populations of larger and smaller HDL particles	PLTP activity is inversely correlated with the serum triglyceride levels
Endothelial lipase (EL)	482	Liver, lung, kidney, placenta (endothelial cells)	Phospholipase activity and limited triglyceride lipase activity HDL is the primary substrate	Overexpression decreases HDL EL deficiency increases HDL
Microsomal triglyceride transfer protein dimer of 55 kDa and 97 kDa subunits	876 aa (97 kDa subunit)	55 kDa disulfide isomerase subunit ubiquitous expression, 97kDa subunit liver intestine	Assembly of VLDL and chylomicrons	Mutations in MTP are associated with abetalipoproteinemia

* Refers to the sequence of the mature protein without the signal pepide
VLDL, very low-density lipoprotein; HDL, high-density lipoprotein; IDL, intermediate-density lipoprotein

Table 8.4 Summary of low-density lipoprotein (LDL) receptor family members[137]

Name	Amino acids*	Tissue-specific	Ligand	Recognition	Function
LDL receptor	839	Ubiquitous	LDL, remnants	ApoB, apoE	Binds and internalizes lipoproteins that contain apoB and apoE on their surface (LDL, β-VLDL, IDL, HDL with apoE); is subjected to feedback regulation by extracellular cholesterol levels Is essential for the clearance of LDL and apoE-containing lipoprotein remnants
ApoER2	922	Brain, testis, ovary, placenta	β-VLDL apoE-containing lipoproteins	ApoE	Binds *in vitro* apoE-containing lipoproteins such as β-VLDL and other apoE-containing lipoproteins; does not bind LDL; may play a role in cholesterol homeostasis in the brain
VLDL receptor	819	Heart, muscle, adipose tissue	VLDL, β-VLDL, IDL	ApoE	Binds *in vitro* VLDL, β-VLDL, and IDL (does not bind LDL)
LRP	4525	Liver, brain, lung	Multiligand receptor binds apoE-enriched β-VLDL, other ligands	ApoE	Physiological function unknown, inactivation of the LRP gene leads to embryonic lethality Binds *in vitro* and internalizes lipoproteins enriched with apoE such as β-VLDL. Also binds α2-macroglobulin–protease complex plasminogen activator. Inhibitor complex lactopherin lipoprotein lipase. Role in lipoprotein metabolism *in vivo* is unclear

* Refers to the mature sequence without the signal peptide.
Apo, apolipoprotein; VLDL, very low-density lipoprotein; IDL, intermediate-density lipoprotein; HDL, high-density lipoprotein; LRP, LDL receptor-related protein

deficiency is characterized by the inability of the mutant LCAT to esterify cholesterol on HDL and LDL, and the accumulation of discoidal HDL in plasma. The fish eye disease is characterized by the inability of the mutant LCAT to esterify cholesterol on HDL only. Both diseases are characterized by low HDL levels.

- *Cholesteryl ester transfer protein (CETP) deficiency* is characterized by an increase in HDL, and is the result of mutations in CETP.
- *Hepatic lipase.*

Based on studies in animal models that are discussed later, HDL structure and function can also be affected by defects in:

- *Endothelial lipase*
- *Phospholipid transfer protein*
- *Lipoprotein lipase*
- *Scavenger receptor BI.*

Finally, low levels of HDL and apoA-I predispose to atherosclerosis.[10]

Apolipoproteins

The protein components of lipoproteins are called apolipoproteins and have been named apoA-I, apoA-II, apoA-IV, apoB, apoCI, apoCII, apoCIII, apoCIV, apoD, apoE, apo(a), and apoJ, etc.[1,14] A hallmark of most of the apolipoproteins, such as apoA-I, apoA-IV, and apoE, is the presence of amphipathic α-helices consisting of either 22 or 11 residues in their secondary structure.[15] These amphipathic helices contribute to the lipid-binding properties and possibly some other functions of the apolipoproteins. ApoB is characterized by the presence of extensive regions of amphipathic β sheet(s), which contribute to lipid binding.[16] Examples of how the apolipoproteins apoB and apoA-I assemble with lipids and form LDL and HDL are discussed later.

In addition to their lipid-binding functions, the apolipoproteins have several other specific functions. Lipid-bound apoA-I is a ligand for SRBI.[17] Lipid-free apoA-I is a ligand for ABCA1.[18] Both lipid-bound and lipid-free apoA-I are ligands for cubilin, which is

Table 8.5 Summary of scavenger receptors (SR)[392]

Name	Amino acids*	Character	Tissue-specific	Ligands known	Function
Class A					
SRAI	453	–	Macrophages	AcLDL, oxLDL, modified BSA, mal-BSA, fucoidan, dextran sulfate, poly G/poly I polyribonucleotides, Gram-negative bacteria, apoptotic cells, silica, LPS, LTA, Aβ-peptide, AGE-modified proteins	Plays a role in phagocytosis
SRAII	349	Lacks the 106 C-terminal residues	Macrophages	AcLDL, oxLDL, modified BSA, fucoidan, dextran sulfate, poly G/poly I polyribonucleotides, Gram-negative bacteria, apoptotic cells, silica, LPS, Aβ-peptide, AGE-modified proteins	Mediates macrophage adhesion *in vitro*
Class B					
SRBI	509	–	Liver and steroidogenic tissues	AcLDL, oxLDL, LDL, HDL, malBSA, phosphatidylserine, apoptotic cells	Recognize HDL particles via apoA-I and promotes selective lipid uptake and cholesterol efflux The affinity of the ligand is apoA-I~ pre-β1-HDL <<HDL<rHDL[apoA-I]
SRBII[393]	506	Differs from SRBI in the C-terminal cytoplasmic tail Generated by alternative splicing	Liver and steroidogenic tissues	HDL, LDL and modified LDL	Has 25% of selective lipid uptake and cholesterol efflux capacity of SRBI
CD36	471	–	Platelets, microvascular endothelial cells, erythroid precursors, adipocytes, striated muscle, breast, retina, monocyte/macrophages	Thrombospordin, modified LDL, oxidized lipids Apoptotic cells *Plasmodium*-infected erythrocytes	Mediates macrophage scavenging of modified lipoproteins of senescent polymorphonuclear cells Long-chain fatty acid transporter Primary receptor for platelet adhesion in muscle and heart CD36 deficiency in humans is associated with reduced uptake of oxLDL

*Refers to the mature sequence without the signal peptide

Ac, acetylated; ox, oxidized; LDL, low-density lipoprotein; BSA, bovine serum albumin; mal, maleylated; LPS, lipopolysaccharides; LTA, lipoteichoic acid; AGE, advanced glycation end products; HDL, high-density lipoprotein an HDL receptor.[19] ApoA-I, and to a lesser extent apoA-IV, apoCII, and apoE, are activators of LCAT,[20,21] and apoCII is an activator of LPL.[22] ApoB-100 and apoE are ligands for the LDL receptor (LDLr).[7,23] ApoE *in vitro* is also a ligand for apoE receptor 2 (apoER2), LDLr-related protein (LRP), gp 330/megalin, VLDL receptor (VLDLr), and other lipoprotein receptors.[1,23] Apolipoprotein functions and their associations with human disease are summarized in Table 8.2.

Enzymes and lipid transfer proteins

Following biosynthesis, lipoproteins are modified in plasma by the action of plasma enzymes and lipid transfer proteins, and are subsequently recognized by different types of cell receptor. These modifications are very important for the function and catabolism of lipoproteins. The enzymes and lipid transfer proteins involved in these modifications are LPL, HL, LCAT, CETP, and PLTP.[4,6,12] Their properties, sites of expression, and associations with human disease are summarized in Table 8.3.

LPL

LPL is a glycoprotein synthesized mainly by adipose tissue, cardiac and skeletal muscle, and monocyte-derived macrophages. It hydrolyzes preferentially the 1- and 3-ester bonds of the triglycerides of chylomicron and VLDL, generating free fatty acids and mainly 2-monoglycerides. LPL is secreted and binds to endothelial cells via its heparin-binding sites. The enzyme is activated by apoCII[6] and inhibited by 1 M NaCl. Deficiency in LPL is associated with severe hypertriglyceridemia.[6]

HL

HL is a glycoprotein synthesized by the liver. It is secreted and binds to the surfaces of sinusoidal endothelial cells.[6] HL hydrolyzes mono- and diacylglycerols and phospholipids of IDL and HDL, resulting in the generation of more dense lipoprotein particles.[24] *In vivo* and *in vitro* studies have shown that HL hydrolyzes large, apoE-enriched HDL particles.[6] Deficiency of HL in human and experimental animals is associated with increased levels of triglycerides and phospholipids in HDL and IDL. Variation in the activity of HL is due to genetic or environmental factors. Increase in HL activity is associated with small

dense LDL and decrease in HDL2.[6] Cholesterol-lowering drugs and other treatments may affect the size of LDL and HDL.[25]

EL

EL is structurally and functionally related to the other members of the lipase gene family. Similar to HL, EL has primarily phospholipase activity and limited triglyceride lipase activity.[26–28] EL is expressed by endothelial cells, macrophages, liver, and other tissues, including lung, kidney, testis, and placenta.[26–28] Overexpression of EL dramatically reduces the HDL and apoA-I levels and causes only a small decrease in non-HDL cholesterol levels.[26,27,29,30] In contrast, inactivation of EL in mice decreased clearance of HDL and increased plasma HDL and apoA-I levels.[29,30] The findings indicate that EL affects the structure, concentration, and metabolism of HDL. The role of this novel lipase in atherogenesis has yet to be determined.

LCAT

LCAT is a glycoprotein synthesized by the liver. Following secretion, it associates with HDL and LDL. It is responsible for the esterification of free cholesterol of HDL and LDL, using the fatty acyl group on the position C-2 of lecithin as the acyl donor.[13] Mutations in LCAT are associated with either the classical LCAT deficiency, characterized by the inability of the enzyme to esterify the cholesterol of HDL and LDL,[13] or with fish eye disease, characterized by the inability of the enzyme to esterify cholesterol on HDL, but not on LDL.[31]

CETP

CETP is a highly hydrophobic glycoprotein synthesized by the liver, the small intestine, and several other tissues.[32] It catalyzes an exchange of neutral lipids, particularly triglyceride and cholesteryl esters, between all the major lipoprotein classes. Net transport of CE by the action of CETP depends mainly on the availability of suitable triglyceride-rich acceptor particles.[1] Cholesteryl ester transport to VLDL and LDL is associated with reciprocal but not equimolar transport of triglycerides.[33] CETP deficiency in humans is characterized by increased HDL levels and a low prevalence of coronary heart disease (CHD), whereas heterozygotes for another CETP mutation have increased risk for CHD.[4]

PLTP

PLTP is a glycoprotein synthesized principally by the liver and the adipose tissue. PLTP facilitates the exchange and net transfer of phospholipids from VLDL to HDL, and does not have cholesteryl ester or triglyceride transfer activity. PLTP can also remodel the HDL.[34,35] PLTP activity is increased in diabetes mellitus, in obesity, and in insulin resistance.[34] The role of the lipases and lipid transfer proteins in atherogenesis is discussed later, as they appear in the different lipoprotein pathways.

Under normal conditions, existing homeostatic mechanisms in the body help to maintain physiological concentrations of the various classes of lipoproteins and their derivatives in plasma. When the function or regulation of synthesis of one or more proteins of the lipoprotein system is altered, the concentration or the function(s) of one of the lipoproteins may be altered. These changes may affect the levels of cholesterol and/or triglycerides in plasma and, in some instances, promote atherosclerosis and other complications.

Lipoproteins and atherogenesis

Factors contributing to atherogenesis

Our ability to understand better the role of apolipoproteins, plasma enzymes, lipid transfer proteins, lipoprotein receptors and lipid transporters in the homeostasis of cholesterol and other lipids and their contribution to atherogenesis was assessed first in human studies. This knowledge has been greatly enhanced during the last 15 years by the generation of animal models in which one or more protein(s) have been altered by the addition or subtraction of the corresponding gene(s). Following alterations of one or more gene(s) of the pathway of interest, the parameters analyzed in the experimental animals are the lipid and lipoprotein profile, the pathogenesis of atherosclerosis, or other physiological changes. The combined knowledge from the study of human subjects and animal models is summarized in Tables 8.6, 8.7, 8.8, and 8.9, and is discussed in further detail in later sections.

Atherosclerosis is a focal disease of the arterial wall that appears usually in areas of disturbed blood flow where gene expression is altered,[36] and affects large- and medium-sized arteries. In response to proatherogenic conditions, such as those created by hypercholesterolemia, monocytes bind to adhesion molecules on the endothelial cell surface and migrate to the subendothelial space, where they differentiate to macrophages. Induction of adhesion molecules is promoted by proinflammatory stimuli.[37] Recruitment and migration of monocytes into the subendothelial space is promoted by oxidized LDL, as well as by monocyte chemattractant factor (MCP-1), which binds to the MCP-1 receptor CCR2.[38] These proteins are expressed by endothelial cells, smooth muscle cells, and monocyte/macrophages, and are induced in hypercholesterolemia.[39] These cells, through the scavenger receptors (SRAI, SRAII, and CD36)[40,41] and possibly other processes, are loaded with cholesteryl ester, which is later deposited in the site of the lesion and contributes to the evolution of the atherosclerotic plaque.[42]

The initial lesion created by macrophages is called the fatty streak, and is reversible.[43–46] The lesions may progress with the recruitment of additional monocytes and T cells and migration into the intima (Figure 8.2).[47] Signals secreted by the blood-borne cells, as well as by the activated endothelial cells,[48] promote migration of smooth muscle cells from the media into the intima, which subsequently proliferate and synthesize matrix components such as collagen and proteoglycans.[42] As the development of lesions progresses, cholesteryl ester-laden monocytes/macrophages and smooth muscle cells in the plaque die. This leads to the creation of the necrotic core with extracellular cholesterol clefts, which characterize the advanced lesions.[49] The luminal face of the lesion often forms a fibrous cap consisting of smooth muscle cells, matrix components, and calcium deposits. This cap is produced by the smooth muscle cells and stabilizes the plaque. In humans, a clinical event, such as myocardial infarction or stroke, may occur as a result of rupture of unstable plaques that are enriched with lipid-filled macrophages and have weak fibrous caps, or from intraplaque hemorrhage that leads to the generation of a thrombogenic event that will occlude the plaque.[50,51] It was shown recently that in late stages of necrosis or with thin caps, the region containing cholesterol clefts is enriched in glycophorin A and iron deposits. The findings suggest that erythrocytes contribute to cholesterol deposition, macrophage infiltration, enlargement of the necrotic core, and destabilization of the plaque.[52]

The involvement of lipoproteins and other factors in the cascade of events that leads to the initiation of

Table 8.6   Role of the chylomicron pathway in lipid homeostasis and in atherogenesis: lessons from animal models and human studies

Protein affected	Susceptibility to atherosclerosis	Lipoprotein profile	Other pathologies
ApoCI transgenic[394,395]	–	Moderate to severe hypertriglyceridemia	
ApoCII deficiency in humans[4]	None	Severe hypertriglyceridemia	Recurrent pancreatitis
ApoCII transgenic[396]	–	Severe hypertriglyceridemia	–
ApoCIII transgenic[88,397]	Increased atherosclerosis compared to control	Severe hypertriglyceridemia	–
ApoCIII–/–[398]		Reduced TG	
ApoCIII × apoA-I transgenic ApoCIII × CETP transgenic ApoCIII × apoA-I × CETP transgenic[4,399,400]	Reduced atherosclerosis compared to apoCIII transgenic	Severe hypertriglyceridemia Low HDL	–
ApoCIV transgenic[390]	–	Two-fold increase in TG	–
ApoE transgenic[84]	Low levels of expression are protective	Mice overexpressing apoE developed severe hypertriglyceridemia[86]	–
ApoE knockout (ApoE–/–)[87,286]	Very susceptible mice develop spontaneous atherosclerosis at 8–10 weeks of age and have been used as models to study early and advanced atherosclerotic lesions	8–25-fold increase in plasma cholesterol Accumulation of lipoprotein remnants	–
Lipoprotein lipase deficiency in humans[6]	None	Severe hypertriglyceridemia	Recurrent pancreatitis
MTP knockout mice[401]	–	In heterozygotes MTP+/– LDL↓ Lipoprotein secretion impaired	MTP–/– embryonic lethal Accumulation of cytosolic fat in the visceral endoderm of the yolk sac in MTP+/– and MTP–/–
ApoE2, apoE3, apoE4 knockin[287]	Susceptibility follows the order mouse E<h apoE3<h apoE4<h apoE2	Increase in VLDL and triglyceride follows the order apoE3<apoE4<apoE2	

Continued...

Table 8.6 Continued

Protein affected	Susceptibility to atherosclerosis	Lipoprotein profile	Other pathologies
Transplantation of apoE–/– mice with normal bone marrow[275] or bone marrow of apoE–/– mice transduced with an apoE-expressing retrovirus[294]	Reduced atherosclerosis in young animals No change in the extent of atherosclerotic lesions in older animals	No change in plasma lipids and lipoproteins	–
Transplantation of normal mice with apoE–/– bone marrow[293]	Induction of atherosclerosis	No change in lipid levels	–
Adenovirus-mediated gene transfer of apoE3/apoE4 in apoE–/– normal or nude mice[288,289]	ApoE3 limited progression of early lesions and advanced regression of advanced lesions. ApoE4 was less effective	Reduction of plasma cholesterol, VLDL and remnant lipoproteins Increase of HDL cholesterol	–
Adenovirus-mediated gene transfer of apoE in LDLr–/– mice[290]	Reduction of advanced lesions	No change in lipid levels	–
Adenovirus-mediated gene transfer of C-terminal truncated apoE forms to apoE–/– mice[86]	–	Normalized plasma lipid and lipoprotein levels The truncated apoE had a dominant effect when coexpressed with full-length apoE	–
Gene transfer of apoE by a helper-dependent adenovirus[297]	Low levels of apoE expression Prevented atherosclerosis	Low levels of apoE expression Normalization of plasma lipid levels	–

Apo, apolipoprotein; TG, triglyceride; HDL, high-density lipoprotein; CETP, cholesteryl ester transfer protein; LDL, low-density lipoprotein; VLDL, very low-density lipoprotein; LDLr, LDL receptor

the atherosclerotic lesion is shown in Figure 8.2[53,54] and discussed in detail in other chapters. It is believed that atherogenic lipoproteins, such as LDL and lipoprotein remnants that float in the VLDL/IDL region, promote atherosclerosis, and antiatherogenic lipoproteins, such as HDL, protect from atherosclerosis. It has been proposed that when the concentration of LDL and other atherogenic lipoprotein particles is high, they enter the subendothelium. In atherosclerosis-prone mice, lipid and lipoprotein aggregates are found in the subendothelial space of the arteries.[55] The retention of LDL in the vessel wall depends on their interaction with extracellular proteoglycans. Transgenic mice expressing a mutant apoB-100 form which has defective binding to glycosaminoglycans have substantially less initial atheroma.[56]

The tendency of LDL to adhere to proteoglycans increases with treatment of LDL using phospholipase A$_2$. This generates small, dense LDL which is atherogenic.[57] Phospholipase A$_2$ transgenic mice on a high- or a low-fat diet have decreased HDL and paraoxonase levels, and slightly increased LDL levels, and develop more aortic lesions than do control mice.[58,59]

Table 8.7 Role of the low-density lipoprotein (LDL) pathway in lipid homeostasis and in atherogenesis: lessons from animal models and human studies

Protein affected	Susceptibility to atherosclerosis	Lipoprotein profile	Other pathologies
ApoB transgenic[80]	Increased atherosclerosis in response to atherogenic diet	LDL↑	–
ApoB-100 transgenics with mutations in the proteoglycan-binding domain of apoB[56]	Less atherosclerosis than normal apoB-100 transgenics	Similar lipoprotein profile and cholesterol levels with apoB transgenics	–
LDLr–/– × apoB transgenic defective in apoB editing[71]	Increased atherosclerosis on chow diet	LDL ↑	–
LDLr knockout[402]	Increased atherosclerosis in response to atherogenic diet	LDL↑, VLDL↑, HDL↓	–
ApoB transgenic × LDL receptor knockout[72]	Increased atherosclerosis in response to chow diet; used as models to study development of early and advanced atherosclerosis	LDL↑, VLDL↑, HDL↓	–
Hepatic lipase deficiency in humans[6] *See HL transgenic and deficient animal models in Table 8.8*	Susceptible, starts at the age of 40–50	VLDL remnants↑ TG-enriched LDL and HDL	–
Human apo(a) transgenic[223,224]	Increased atherosclerosis in response to atherogenic diets	Apo(a) is found in d > 1.21 g/ml Lp(a) is formed after infusion of LDL	–
ApoA-I × apo(a) transgenic[246]	Decreased atherosclerosis; fewer lesions compared to apo(a) transgenics	Two-fold increase in HDL	–
ApoB x apo(a) transgenics[248]	Modest increase in atherosclerosis compared to either apoB or apo(a) transgenics	Four-fold increase in LDL Lipoprotein profile resembles that of humans	–
ApoB transgenic × LDLr–/– × apo(a) transgenic[72]	Severe atherosclerosis on chow or atherogenic diet, but quantitatively similar to the levels observed in apoB transgenic × LDLr–/– mice	Increased LDL Decreased HDL	–

Unless otherwise stated, 'transgenic' indicates transgenic mice expressing the human transgene.
Apo, apolipoprotein; LDLr, LDL receptor; VLDL, very low-density lipoprotein; TG, triglyceride; HDL, high-density lipoprotein; Lp(a), lipoprotein (a)

Table 8.8   Role of the high-density lipoprotein (HDL) pathway in lipid homeostasis and in atherogenesis: lessons from animal models and human studies

Protein affected	Susceptibility to atherosclerosis	Lipoprotein profile	Other pathologies
ApoA-I transgenic (Tg)[79]	Similar to WT	HDL↑	–
ApoA-I Tg rabbits[403]	Reduced atherosclerosis by 50% in response to atherogenic diet	Two-fold increase in HDL. ApoB lipoproteins did not change	–
ApoA-I Tg × apoE–/– mice[319]	Reduced atherosclerosis compared to apoE–/–	–	–
Adenovirus-mediated gene transfer of apoA-I to LDLr–/– mice [325]	Reduced atherosclerosis compared to LDLr–/–	HDL↑	–
ApoA-I Tg × LDLr–/– rabbits[419]	Reduced atherosclerosis compared to LDLr–/–	HDL↑	–
ApoA-I–/– × apoB Tg [321,322]	Increased atherosclerosis as compared to apoB transgenic	HDL↓	–
ApoA-I-deficient in humans[4]	CHD at age 11–52 in different probands	Absence of HDL	–
ApoA-I knockout mice[323]	No phenotype	HDL↓	–
ApoA-II transgenic[82,83]	Increased atherosclerosis	Abnormal composition, HDL↑	–
ApoA-II deficiency in humans[4]	None	Normal lipids	–
ApoA-II–/– mice[404]	–	50% reduction in HDL due to increased catabolism	Decreased FFA insulin and glucose levels
ApoA-I × apoA-II Tg[405]	15-fold increase in atherosclerosis as compared to apoA-I transgenics in response to atherogenic diet	Cholesterol and HDL were similar in apoA-I and apoA-I × apoA-II transgenics	–
Gene transfer of apoA-I to LDLr–/– or apoE–/–[324,325,327]	Reduced atherosclerosis of LDLr–/– or apoE–/–	Increased HDL	–
ApoA+/+ × apoE–/– transplanted with normal bone marrow[326]	Reduced atherosclerosis. Reduced cholesterol content of atherosclerotic aorta compared to apoA–/– × apoE–/– transplanted with normal bone marrow	Cholesterol levels of apoA–/– × apoE–/– reduced compared to apoA-I+/+ × apoE–/– mice	–
Human apoA-IV Tg × apoE–/– mice[89]	Reduced atherosclerosis compared to apoE–/–	Cholesterol ↑ HDL not affected	–
Mouse apoA-IV Tg[90]	Reduced atherosclerosis	Increased HDL	–
ApoA-V–/–[391]	–	Four-fold increase in plasma TG	
ApoA-V Tg [391]	–	Decreased plasma TG No change in HDL	–

Continued…

Table 8.8 Continued

Protein affected	Susceptibility to atherosclerosis	Lipoprotein profile	Other pathologies
ABCA1 mutations (Tangier disease in humans)[13]	Partially susceptible	Lack of HDL, reduced LDL	–
ABCA1–/– mice[340]	None	Low cholesterol. Absence of HDL, deficiency in fat-soluble vitamins A, E, K	Impaired growth and neuronal development. Hemolysis, platelet abnormalities
ABCA1 Tg[339]	Protected from diet-induced atherosclerosis	Two- to three-fold increase in HDL, apoE and apoA-I Decreased apoB and LDL	–
ABCA1 Tg × apoE–/–[339]	Increased atherosclerosis compared to apoE–/– mice	Lipids and lipoproteins same as in apoE–/– mice	–
Transplantation of ABCA1–/– bone marrow in LDLr–/– mice[342]	Increased atherosclerosis	Lipid levels same as in LDLr–/– mice	–
Transplantation of ABCA1–/– bone marrow in apoE–/– mice[406]	Increased atherosclerosis	Lipid levels same as in LDLr–/– and apoE–/– mice	–
Transplantation of normal marrow in ABCA1–/– mice[341]	–	Minimal effect on HDL levels	
SRBI Tg [353,360–362]	–	HDL↓ apoA-I↓ VLDL↓ LDL↓ Accelerated clearance of HDL Decreased cholesterol content of steroidogenic tissues and increased bile excretion	–
SRBI–/– mice[407]	–	HDL↑ Abnormal composition	Impaired oocyte development and red blood cell maturation
SRBI+/– × LDLr–/– [363]	Increased atherosclerosis	Increased LDL cholesterol	
SRBI–/– × apoE–/– [355,356,364]	Occlusive coronary atherosclerosis	HDL↑	Cardiac dysfunction Die at 8 weeks of age
SRBI Tg × LDLr+/–[360]	Reduced atherosclerosis compared to LDLr+/– mice	VLDL↓ LDL↓ HDL↓	
SRBI Tg × apoB transgenics[361]	Reduced atherosclerosis at low levels of SRBI expression, not at high levels	HDL↓	–
LCAT deficiency in humans[12]	Susceptible	Total C↓ TG↑ HDL↓ Discoidal HDL Small, spherical HDL	Corneal opacity Renal failure

Continued...

Table 8.8 Continued

Protein affected	Susceptibility to atherosclerosis	Lipoprotein profile	Other pathologies
Fish eye disease[12]	Susceptible	Total C↓ TG↑ HDL↓ Increased HDL catabolism	Corneal opacity
LCAT−/− mice[408,409]	None	HDL apoA-I↓ Total C↓ TG↑. Discoidal HDL	Renal lesions
LCAT Tg rabbits[410]	Reduced diet-induced atherosclerosis	HDL↑ and apoA-I↑	Decrease in HDL catabolism
LCAT Tg × LDLr−/− rabbits[411,412]	Similar diet-induced atherosclerosis as the LDLr−/− rabbits	HDL↑ and apoA-I↑ Decrease in apoA-I catabolism Increase in apoA-I synthesis	–
LCAT Tg mice or LCAT Tg × apoA-I Tg or LCAT Tg × apoA-II Tg[371,372]	Increased atherosclerosis	HDL apoA-I↑ LDL normal HDL dysfunctional	–
LCAT Tg × CETP Tg mice[373]	Atherogenic profile of LCAT Transgenic reversed	HDL normal function	–
LCAT Tg × HL−/− mice[413]	Atherogenic profile of LCAT Transgenic reversed	No change in HDL cholesterol and apoA-I levels	–
LCAT × CETP Tg mice[373]	Reduced atherosclerosis compared to LCAT Tg	Increase in plasma cholesterol	–
Gene transfer of human LCAT to non-human primates[414]	–	HDL and apoA-I↑ LDL and apoB↓	–
HL Tg mice[385]	Reduction of atherosclerosis	HDL↓ apoA-I↑	–
HL Tg rabbits[386,387]	Same as WT rabbits	HDL↓ apoA-I↑	–
HL−/− × apoE−/− mice[384]	Reduced atherosclerosis relative to apoE−/−		–
HL−/− mice[383]	Reduced atherosclerosis in arteries	Large HDL enriched in phospholipids↑	–
Endothelial lipase (EL) transgenic mice[29,30]	–	HDL↓	–
EL knockout mice[30]	–	HDL↑	–
Mouse CETP Tg[415]	Severe atherosclerosis	VLDL↑ LDL↑	–
CETP × apoE−/− or CETP × LDLr−/− [369]	Increased atherosclerosis compared to apoE−/− or LDLr−/− mice	Same profile as apoE−/− and LDLr−/− mice HDL↓	–
CETP deficiency in humans[4]	Variable susceptibility Some mutations, increased CHD, others do not	HDL↑ Abnormal composition	–
CETP × apoA-I Tg mice[368]	–	HDL↑ apoA-I↑. Compared to CETP transgenics	–

Continued...

Table 8.8   Continued

Protein affected	Susceptibility to atherosclerosis	Lipoprotein profile	Other pathologies
CETP Tg mice[367]	–	HDL↓ and apoA-I↓ Increased HDL clearance	–
CETP × apoCIII Tg mice[399]	–	HDL↓ TG↑	–
PLTP Tg[375]	–	Small or no changes in HDL	–
PLTP gene transfer[416]	–	HDL↓. Formation of preβ HDL	–
PLTP–/–[376,377]	–	Decreased HDL and apoA-I due to hypercatabolism of HDL. Increased VLDL and LDL on high-fat diet Increase in apoA-IV	–
PLTP–/– × apoB Tg or PLTP–/– × apoE–/–[378]	Reduced atherosclerosis comparedto apoB transgenic or apoE–/– mice	VLDL↓ LDL↓	–
Paraoxanase–/– × apoE–/–[337]	Increased atherosclerosis	No changes in lipid and lipoproteins Increased lipoprotein oxidation	–
LPL–/–[379]	–	Severe hypertriglyceridemia Neonatal death	–
Cardial muscle-specific LPL Tg[381]	–	Increased HDL	–

Apo, apolipoprotein; WT, wild-type; LDLr, low-density lipoprotein receptor; CHD, coronary heart disease; FFA, free fatty acid; VLDL, very low-density lipoprotein; SRBI, scavenger receptor type BI; LCAT, lecithin : cholesterol acyl transferase; CETP, cholesteryl ester transfer protein

Modification of LDL is mediated by products of lipid peroxidation in plasma and in the subendothelial space. Oxidized LDL is taken up by the scavenger receptors SRAI, SRAII, and CD36, leading to the accumulation of cholesteryl esters in these cells.[40,60] The atheroprotective function of HDL may involve inhibition of oxidation of LDL by HDL,[61] SRBI- and ABCA1-mediated efflux of cholesterol to HDL and apoA-I, respectively,[62] HDL-mediated increase in the activity of endothelial nitric oxide synthase (eNOS),[63,64] and possibly through other mechanisms. Mice are generally resistant to the development of atherosclerosis, and the genetic background of the mouse strain influences their susceptibility.[65–68] Mice can, however, become susceptible to atherosclerosis on normal diets or atherogenic western-type diets by mutations in the apoE or the LDL receptor genes, by overexpression of apoB-100, or by crosses within atherogenic mouse lines[69–72]. In addition, atherosclerosis-susceptible strains can become resistant by transfer into susceptible strains of an atherosclerosis resistance gene locus derived from a resistant strain.[68] Analysis of atherosclerotic lesions of normocholesterolemic children aged 1–13 who died of trauma or other causes indicated that maternal hypercholesterolemia during pregnancy may influence the susceptibility to atherosclerosis of the offspring.[73] Similar observations were made in normocholesterolemic offspring of New

Table 8.9 Other genes affecting atherogenesis

Protein affected	Susceptibility to atherosclerosis	Lipoprotein profile
P-selectin–/–× apoE–/– mice[92]	Less susceptible to atherosclerosis than apoE–/–	No significant change in plasma lipids and lipoproteins
P-selectin–/–× E selectin–/–× LDLr–/– mice[93]	Less atherosclerosis than the LDLr–/– mice	No significant change in plasma lipids and lipoproteins
Inducible NO synthase–/–× apoE–/–[111]	Modest reduction in atherosclerosis but little change in lesion composition	No significant change in plasma lipids and lipoproteins
12/15 lipoxygenase–/– × apoE–/–[105]	Reduced atherosclerosis. Reduced levels of autoantibodies to oxLDL	No significant change in plasma lipids and lipoproteins
15 lipoxygenase Tg × LDLr–/–[106]	Increased atherosclerosis	No significant change in plasma lipids and lipoproteins
LPL–/– fetal liver cells or bone marrow transplantation in C57BL/6 mice[295,382]	Reduced susceptibility to atherosclerosis	No significant change in plasma lipids and lipoproteins
Transplantation of ACAT–/– bone marrow in apoE–/– or LDLr–/– mice[417]	Similar susceptibility to atherosclerosis as apoE–/– or LDLr–/– Reduced levels of macrophages and lipids in advanced lesions	Significant reduction in VLDL levels
Transplantation of myeloperoxidase–/– bone marow in LDLr–/– mice[110,418]	Increased atherosclerosis	No change in plasma lipid levels
MCP–/–× apoE–/– MCP-1–/–× apoB transgenic[98–100]	Reduced atherosclerosis	No significant change in plasma lipidsand lipoproteins
Transplantation of LDLr–/– mice with CXCR2-deficient bone marrow[101]	Reduced atherosclerosis	No significant change in plasma lipids and lipoproteins
M-CSF–/–× apoE–/– mice[102,103]	Resistant to atherosclerosis	No significant change in plasma lipids and lipoproteins
ICAM–/–× apoE–/– mice[94]	Reduced atherosclerosis. Reduced monocyte recruitment to lesions	No significant change in plasma lipids and lipoproteins
SRAI–/– × LDLr–/– or SRAI–/–× apoE–/–[200,201]	Reduced lesion size	
Transplantation of apoE–/– or LDLr–/– mice with SRAI overexpressing bone marrow[218]	No effect on atherosclerosis	Reduced VLDL remnants compared to apoE–/– mice
CD36–/–× apoE–/–[218]	80% reduction in aortic lesion than apoE–/– on western-type diet and reduced atherosclerosis with low-fat diet as compared with apoE–/– mice	Modest decreases in HDL and VLDL
CD36–/–[217]	–	Increased HDL cholesterol and VLDL triglycerides
CD36 muscle-specific Tg[211]	–	Decreased VLDL triglycerides, increased fatty acid oxidation in the muscle

Apo, apolipoprotein; LDL, low-density lipoprotein; LDLr, LDL receptor; ox, oxidized; VLDL, very low-density lipoprotein; LPL, lipoprotein lipase; MCP, monocyte chemoattractant protein; SR, scavenger receptor; ICAM, intercellular adhesive molecule

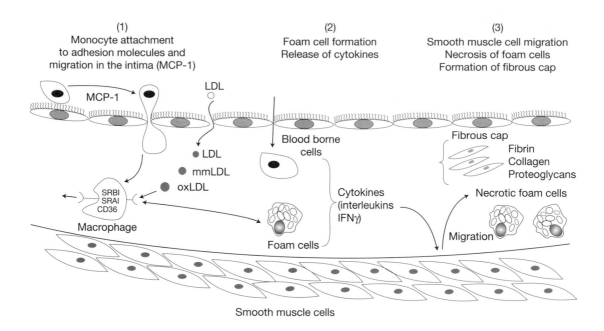

Figure 8.2 Schematic representation of the cascade of events which promote the initiation of atherosclerotic lesions and the formation of fatty streak and complex lesions. MCP, monocyte chemoattractant protein; LDL, low-density lipoprotein; mm, minimally modified; ox, oxidized; SR, scavenger receptor; IFN, interferon

Zealand White rabbits[74] and LDLr–/– mice.[75] Offspring of LDLr–/– mice showed that maternal hypercholesterolemia altered patterns of gene expression in the non-atherosclerotic descending aorta of the offspring. Although not rigorously proven, it is possible that hypercholesterolemia reprograms the expression of proatherogenic genes in the offspring, and that these changes may persist after birth and predispose to atherogenesis. In various mouse models the extent of atherosclerosis is assessed by measuring the area of aortic root lesions at the fatty streak stage or in the stage of advanced lesions.[43,76]

The role of apolipoproteins in lipid homeostasis and in atherogenesis

Existing biochemical and genetic data suggest that increased plasma apoA-I and decreased plasma apoB levels can decrease the LDL/HDL ratio and thus protect humans against atherosclerosis.[10] Consistent with the human data, studies of transgenic mice showed that the plasma levels of apoB and apoA-I are correlated directly with plasma LDL and HDL levels[77,78] and,

as predicted, apoA-I transgenics are protected from atherosclerosis, whereas the apoB transgenic mice develop atherosclerosis.[79,80] Overexpression of apoA-II leads to high triglyceride levels and abnormal composition of HDL and predisposes to atherosclerosis, particularly when plasma triglycerides are elevated.[81–83] ApoE expression may positively or negatively affect the catabolism of chylomicrons, depending on the plasma apoE levels,[84–86] whereas, as will be discussed in detail later, lack of apoE predisposes to atherosclerosis.[87] Overexpression of apoCIII, as well as apoCI, apoE, apoCII, and apoA-II, or diminished expression of apoCII, is associated with hypertriglyceridemia owing to inhibition of the hydrolysis of triglycerides of chylomicrons and VLDL.[81,88] Finally, overexpression of apoA-IV in mice increases HDL levels and protects from atherosclerosis, most probably by assuming some of the beneficial functions of apoA-I and HDL.[89,90] LDL levels may be increased by mutations in the LDL receptor, and these changes are associated with increased atherosclerosis.[71] HDL levels may be affected by a variation in all the genes involved in the HDL pathway.[86] The involvement of apoE, the LDL receptor, proteins of the HDL pathway, some inflammatory mediators, scavenger receptors, and enzymes bound to HDL in atherogenesis are discussed in subsequent sections.

The role of oxidized lipoproteins, adhesion and immunoregulatory proteins, cytokines, chemokines and NO in atherogenesis

As discussed above, adhesion molecules, chemokines and their receptors, and inflammatory mediators have been implicated in the pathogenesis of atherosclerosis (Figure 8.2).[91] The contribution of these molecules to atherogenesis has been studied in atherosclerosis-prone apoE–/– or LDLr–/– mice (Table 8.9). Studies in P-selectin–/– × apoE–/– mice showed that at 4 months of age aortic root lesions were small, consisting primarily of fatty streaks, and had fewer smooth muscle cells than in apoE–/– mice. By 15 months of age the animals had developed fibrous plaques throughout the aorta, although the progression in lesion development was delayed compared to apoE–/– mice.[92] The P-selectin–/– and E-selectin–/– × LDLr–/– mice[93] reduced monocyte adhesion to endothelial cells, and had reduced atherosclerosis as compared to LDLr–/– mice. Similarly, ICAM–/– × apoE–/– mice had small but significant reductions in monocyte recruitment to atherosclerotic lesions compared to apoE–/– mice.[94] Minimally oxidized LDL in cell culture studies promoted the expression of MCP-1[95] and macrophage colony-stimulating factor (M-CSF),[96] and increased the adhesion of monocytes to endothelial cells.[97] Disruption of the MCP-1 or CCR2 genes markedly reduced the development of atherosclerosis in apoE–/– or apoB-overexpressing mice, respectively, indicating the importance of chemotaxis in atherogenesis.[98–100] Transplantation of LDLr–/– mice with bone marrow cells lacking CXCR2 (high-affinity receptors for IL-8) resulted in significantly less atherosclerosis than in mice reconstituted with wild-type bone marrow cells.[101] Furthermore, deficiency of the gene encoding M-CSF in an apoE–/– background promotes extreme resistance to the development of atherosclerosis, thereby indicating the importance of macrophage differentiation in atherogenesis.[102,103] Although atherosclerosis occurs in LDLr–/– mice, expression of the LDL receptor in macrophages promoted the formation of foam cell-rich lesions under conditions of moderate hypercholesterolemia.[104]

Lipoprotein oxidation is considered a key event in atherogenesis.[53] 12/15 Lipoxygenase, 5 lipoxygenase (5-LO) and myeloperoxidase are three enzymes that contribute to lipoprotein oxidation. Double-deficient mice that were 12/15-lipoxygenase–/– × apoE–/– had decreased aortic atherosclerosis, and reduced levels of autoantibodies to oxidized LDL epitopes compared to apoE–/– mice.[105] In contrast, overexpression of 15-lipoxygenase in LDLr–/– mice resulted in larger aortic lesions.[106] In a study of 470 healthy volunteers of 5-LO promoter genotypes, a variant was statistically associated with increased intima-media thickness.[107] Other studies point to the importance of the 5-LO gene in atherogenesis. Mehrabian et al. identified a major locus for atherosclerosis on mouse chromosome 6 in an atherosclerosis-resistant strain (CAST) which contained the 5-LO gene. A congenital strain containing the atherosclerosis-resistant locus had 20% of the normal 5-LO mRNA and protein levels compared to the control strain.[108] Dietary arachidonic acid, enhanced and *n*-3 fatty acid blunted the atherogenic effect of the variant genotype.[107] In human patients, increased plasma myeloperoxidase level was a risk factor for myocardial infarction and other major cardiac events.[109] On the other hand, transplantation of LDLr–/– mice with myeloperoxidase–/– bone marrow increased by 50% the atherosclerotic lesions as compared to LDLr–/– mice transplanted with normal bone marrow.[110] The involvement of macrophage-derived NO in atherogenesis was studied in double-deficient (inducible (i)) NOS–/– × apoE–/–) mice. In the C57BL/6 background, the double-deficient mice did not differ in early lesion formation as compared to apoE–/– mice,[111] however, iNOS–/– × apoE–/– mice of a mixed genetic background fed a western-type diet had a reduction in lesion area compared with apoE–/– mice, with little change in lesion composition.[111] Inhibition of iNOS also inhibited the progression of coronary atherosclerosis in cholesterol-fed hypercholesterolemic rabbits.[112]

The induction of neonatal tolerance to oxidized lipoproteins reduced atherosclerosis in apoE–/– mice, indicating that attenuation of the immune response has a beneficial effect on the progression of the disease.[113] The involvement of immunoregulatory CD40 signaling was examined by injecting LDLr–/– mice fed an atherogenic diet with antibody to CD40 ligand. This treatment limited the progression of aortic atherosclerosis, increased collagen and smooth muscle, decreased the macrophage cell content, and reduced the number of lesions.[114]

The biogenesis, functions, and catabolism of apoB-containing lipoproteins

Intracellular biogenesis of apoB-containing lipoproteins

Structure and biosynthesis of apoB-100 and apoB-48 forms

Apolipoprotein B is the main protein component of LDL and comprises 23.8% of the weight of the LDL particle.[1,5] The primary sequence of human apoB-100 was originally deduced by four independent research groups from the corresponding sequence of overlapping cDNA clones.[115] The mature apoB-100 protein contains 4536 amino acids.[115] Based on a molecular mass (Mr) of 513 kDa, it can be calculated that there is one apoB-100 molecule per LDL particle.[115]

ApoB is synthesized by the liver and the intestine and has two protein forms designated apoB-100 and apoB-48. These forms are generated by a post-transcriptional modification that converts the CAA triplet of the apoB mRNA, which encodes for Gln-2153, to a chain termination codon UAA.[116] The editing enzyme is a site-specific deaminase, apobec-1, which converts the C residue of the 2153 codon to U.[116]

The receptor and lipid-binding functions of apoB

ApoB-100 and apoB-48 are required for the assembly and secretion of VLDL and chylomicrons, respectively, and this process is prevented in abetalipoproteinemia and some forms of homozygous hypobetalipoproteinemia.[5] ApoB is the ligand that mediates the recognition of LDL by the LDL receptor. As discussed later, the LDL receptor–apoB interaction mediates the clearance of LDL from plasma and regulates cellular cholesterol biosynthesis.[117] Several independent studies showed that the carboxy-terminal domain of apoB-100 between residues 3000 and 3700 is probably involved

in receptor binding. The sequence between residues 3359 and 3367 of apoB has 63% homology to the apoE sequence between residues 142 and 150, which has been implicated in receptor binding.[1,115] A naturally occurring R3500Q apoB point mutation is responsible for decreased receptor binding of the variant LDL. This condition was named familiar defective apoB-100.[118] Reduced receptor binding is also caused by an R3531C point mutation.[5,119] Finally, truncated apoB forms extending to apoB-75 bind LDL efficiently, whereas shorter apoB forms do not, and are associated with hypobetalipoproteinemia syndromes.[1,5]

Analysis of the lipid-binding properties of apoB peptides showed that the carboxy-terminal end (residues 4101–4536) and a domain in the middle of the molecule (residues 1701–3070) and some regions between residues 1001 and 1700, may represent the major lipid-binding domains of apoB.[1]

Based on the analysis of hydrophobicity and hydrophobic moment of the apoB sequence, it has been calculated that apoB consists of three regions enriched in amphipathic α-helices, separated by two regions of enriched amphipathic β-sheets. These domains were designated α, β, α2, β2, α3, and it has been proposed that they contribute to lipid binding. The approximate boundaries of these domains are α1 (aa 58–795), β1 (aa 827–2001), α2 (aa 2045–2587), β2 (aa 2571–4032), α3 (4017–4515).[16]

Intracellular assembly of VLDL and chylomicrons

VLDL assembly in the hepatocytes and chylomicron assembly in enterocytes involve a two-step process.[5,120] In the first step(s) of VLDL (chylomicron) assembly, apoB acquires small amounts of phospholipids cotranslationally in the rough endoplasmic reticulum (ER), along with a small amount of triglycerides. These lipids are interpreted in the lipovitellin-like lipid-binding domain that is found in the amino-terminal region of apoB by the action of MTP.[120] As apoB translation proceeds, more core lipids are added by the action of MTP and, eventually, spherical particles are formed and released from the ribosomes. In a parallel process that is catalyzed by MTP, a VLDL-sized particle free of apoB is formed in the smooth ER and migrates in the junctions between smooth and rough ER. In a second step of VLDL (chylomicron) assembly, the apoB-free/triglyceride-rich particles fuse with the apoB-containing lipoprotein particles. VLDL (chylomicron) particles formed are transferred to the Golgi, where apoB is *N*-glycosylated and some additional phospholipids are added. Secretory vesicles containing VLDL (chylomicrons) migrate and fuse to the basolateral membranes of hepatocytes (enterocytes), and the lipoproteins are exocytosed.

MTP is a dimer consisting of a 55-kDa disulfide isomerase subunit, which is a ubiquitous protein, and a 97-kDa subunit found mainly in the liver and intestine.[5,121] MTP, which acts in the first step of VLDL chylomicron assembly, can transfer both triglycerides, cholesteryl esters, and, to some extent, phospholipids between lipid vesicles. Mutations in the 97-kDa subunit of MTP are associated with abetalipoproteinemia.[5,121] If apoB does not assemble with lipids, it is degraded.[1]

Small, dense LDL

Small, dense LDL represents a subpopulation of LDL particles that can be separated by ultracentrifugation in the range of 1.025–1.034 g/ml.[24] The presence of small, dense LDL in plasma can also be assayed by non-denaturing polyacrylamide gradient gel electrophoresis (GGE) or nuclear magnetic resonance (NMR).[24] The levels of small, dense LDL in plasma are affected by age, sex, pregnancy, diseases (such as insulin resistance, obesity, diabetes mellitus, hypertriglyceridemia, AIDS),[24] and by certain drugs (such as β-adrenergic receptor blockers).[24,122] Small, dense LDL is one of the features of the metabolic syndrome. This condition is also associated with abdominal obesity, dyslipidemia (elevated triglyceride), low HDL cholesterol, increased blood pressure, insulin resistance (with or without glucose intolerance), and prothrombotic and proinflammatory states. In subjects with elevated LDL levels, small, dense LDL may contribute to the risk for atherosclerosis.[24,122] The Physician's Health Study, which included 14 916 men, indicated that small LDL particles, when adjusted for plasma triglyceride levels, were not a good risk indicator for myocardial infarction. In contrast, plasma triglyceride levels were associated with increased relative risk.[123] Genetic studies of small kindreds showed that monogenic factors contributed to the presence of small, dense LDL in between 9 and 21% of the subjects at a young age, whereas at later ages monogenic factors accounted for the presence of small, dense LDL in 47–95% of the subjects in different studies.[124–127]

Small, dense LDL has a lower affinity for the LDL receptors, remains longer in the circulation (and thus has greater susceptibility to oxidation), is better retained by proteoglycans in the subendothelium, and is more cytotoxic than larger LDL.[24] Small, dense LDL may be generated by hydrolysis of triglycerides of IDL/LDL by hepatic lipase.[25] Load score-based linkage analysis of 19 families that included 142 members did not find a linkage of small, dense LDL with Mn superoxide dismutase, apoAII, apoCII, apoCIII, LPL, HL, MTP, insulin receptor, or LDL receptor.[126] However, other studies indicated an increase in small, dense LDL in subjects with LPL gene mutations, the apoE4 phenotype, a CETP promoter polymorphism, increased plasma PA-1 and fibrinogen levels.[124,128–130] Linkage analysis showed association between a HL promoter polymorphism and increased small, dense LDL levels in families with familial combined hyperlipidemia. However, this association was not detected by a genome scan of a subset of these families.[130] It is clear from the numerous linkage studies that several genes contribute to the size and heterogeneity of LDL in humans. It appears that exercise, which increases LPL and reduces HL levels, as well as a reduction in body mass,[131] a low-fat diet,[132] a polyunsaturated fat diet,[133] and lipid-lowering drugs (statins, niacin, fibrates) contribute to the reduction of the small, dense LDL levels.

The LDL receptor pathway, familial hypercholesterolemia and atherogenesis

Our current understanding of the molecular events involved in the receptor-mediated catabolism of lipoproteins has been shaped mainly by the pioneering work of Goldstein, Brown and colleagues, who first demonstrated the presence of a specific receptor on cell surfaces that recognizes, binds, and internalizes LDL.[1,11,117,134] Since then, several other members of the LDL receptor family have been described.[1,11,135–142] Ligands for the LDL receptor are the LDL, which contains apoB, and the apoE-containing lipoproteins, such as IDL, βVLDL, and HDL with apoE,[11,143] as well as apoE-containing proteoliposomes.[144] The affinity of HDL with apoE for the LDL receptor was more than 20 times greater than that for LDL itself. The structures of the LDL receptor family members are shown in Figure 8.3, and their properties are summarized in Table 8.4.

Functional definition of the LDL receptor: its intracellular itinerary and the feedback regulatory mechanisms

Early biochemical and genetic studies established that the cell surface of cultured human fibroblasts and other cell types contains high-affinity receptors for LDL. The presence of these receptors was initially assayed by binding of [^{125}I]-LDL to cell cultures (Figure 8.4a). Based on these assays, it was found that patients with familial hypercholesterolemia (FH) either lack or have defective receptors.[11,117,134]

Binding of LDL to the LDL receptor can be detected at 4°C, but the receptor is not internalized.[11,117,134] When cell cultures are incubated at 37°C, the coated pits containing the LDL receptor complex invaginate into the cell and pinch off to form endocytic vesicles called endosomes, which carry LDL to lysosomes (Figure 8.5a).[11,117,134,145] Following dissociation of the clathrin, several endocytic vesicles fuse to form endosomes.[145] The endosome develops an acidic pH by the action of an ATP-driven protein pump,[146] which mediates the dissociation of the lipoprotein receptor complex.[147] The free receptor in recycling vesicles returns to the cell surface prior to the fusion of endosomes with primary lysosomes.[147] Fusion of endosomes with primary lysosomes results in the hydrolytic degradation of apoB to amino acids, and hydrolysis of cholesteryl esters by the lysosomal enzyme acid lipase.[1,11,117,134] Liberated cholesterol is used by cells for membrane synthesis. The kinetics of receptor internalization hydrolysis of apoB and cholesterol esterification are saturable processes, as indicated in Figure 8.4b.

Regulatory mechanisms that follow the interaction of LDL with the LDL receptor

Hydrolysis of cholesteryl esters by acid lipase triggers three regulatory responses that contribute to cellular cholesterol homeostasis: inhibition of cholesterol synthesis by reduction of the activity of HMG-CoA reductase gene, the rate-limiting enzyme of cholesterol biosynthesis (Figure 8.4b),[148] a decrease in the number of surface LDL receptors, which prevents additional cholesterol influx into the cell (Figure 8.5a),[11,117,134] and activation of acyl-CoA:cholesterol acyltransferase

(ACAT2), which re-esterifies excess cholesterol preferentially with oleic acid, resulting in cytoplasmic storage of cholesteryl ester droplets (Figure 8.5a).[149] As will be discussed later, the decrease of the LDL receptor number is regulated at the level of transcription.[1,11] Furthermore, HMG-CoA reductase, located in the ER, contains a cholesterol-sensing domain, and the increase in the membrane cholesterol content triggers the rapid ubiquitin-dependent proteosomal degradation of the enzyme and, ultimately, inhibition of cholesterol biosynthesis.[11]

Purification of the LDL receptor, cloning of cDNA and the gene encoding for the LDL receptor

Following the initial cell culture-based assays for the LDL receptor activity and the cellular regulatory responses, an assay was developed for LDL receptor activity using cell membrane preparations.[150] This development allowed the purification of the LDL receptor from bovine adrenal cortex.[151] The mature receptor is an acetic glycoprotein of apparent molecular mass of 160 kDa and isoelectric point 4.3.[11,152] Sequencing of peptides obtained from the purified bovine LDL receptor allowed the synthesis of degenerate oligonucleotides, which were used as probes for cloning of cDNA encoding for the bovine LDL receptor,[153] and subsequently for the cDNA and the gene encoding the human LDL receptor.[154] This represents a basic approach that was also used for the isolation of cDNA and genes that encode several proteins of the lipoprotein system (Tables 8.2–8.5).

The LDL receptor mRNA is 5.3 kb long, including a 2.6 kb long 3′ untranslated region. The LDL receptor gene is 45 kb long and contains 17 exons and 18 introns;[154] it maps to the short arm of chromosome 19 (p13.1–p13.3).[11]

The human LDL receptor cDNA and gene encode a protein of 860 amino acids, including a 21-residue long signal peptide.[153,154] Computer analysis of the receptor sequence showed that it consists of five domains as illustrated in Figure 8.3a. It is important to note that the cytoplasmic domain contains a conserved NPVY sequence between residues 804 and 807, which is required for movement of the receptor to the coated pits. Computer analysis of the structure of the LDL receptor showed the presence of seven imperfect amino terminal repeats, designated 1–7 (Figure 8.3a). Two

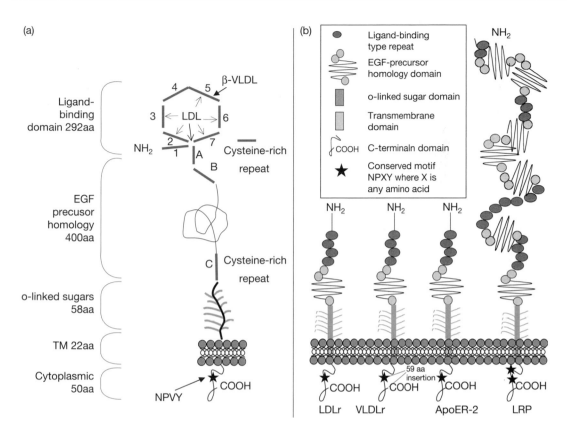

Figure 8.3 (a) Schematic representation depicting the low-density lipoprotein receptor (LDLr) and the five different structural domains of the receptor. (b) Schematic representation of the LDLr and some members of the LDLr family. The symbols used in the diagram are defined in the box. (Adapted from reference 137, 155 with permission). EGF, epidermal growth factor; TM, transmembrane; LPR, LDLr-related protein; apo, apolipoprotein

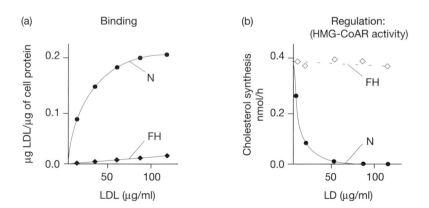

Figure 8.4 A representative experiment of binding of [^{125}I]-LDL (low-density lipoprotein) to cultured skin fibroblasts containing normal and deficient LDL receptors and the regulatory feedback mechanism that ensues following the entry of LDL into the cell. (a) Receptor binding. (b) A representative experiment of cholesterol synthesis (HMG-CoAR activity) following uptake of LDL by the cells. The kinetics of receptor internalization, hydrolysis of apolipoprotein (apoB) and cholesterol esterification (reflecting the ACAT-activity) are similar to that of panel A. (Adapted from reference 134, with permission). N, normal; FH, familial hypercholesterolemia

(a)

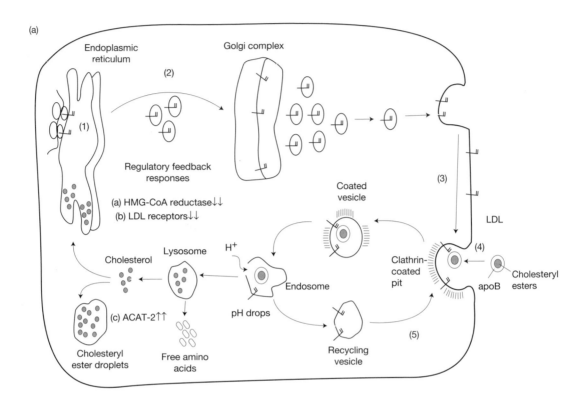

(b)

Class of mutation	Lack of synthesis	Defective transport from ER to Golgi	Defective binding of LDL	Defective clustering in coated pits	Defective recycling	Response to statins and bile acid resins
1	X					−
2	⟶ X					−
3	⟶ X					+
4	⟶ X					−
5	⟶ X					−
Heterozygosity for classes 1–5						+

(c)

Principles of cholesterol lowering

Statins: HMG-CoA reductase↓   Cellular C↓   LDLr↑↑   Plasma C↓↓
Bile acid resins: BA↓   Cellular C→BA   LDLr↑   Plasma C↓
Combinations of statins   HMG-CoA reductase↓ ⎫   Cellular C↓↓   LDLr↑↑↑   Plasma C↓↓↓
and bile acid resins: BA↓ ⎭

(d)

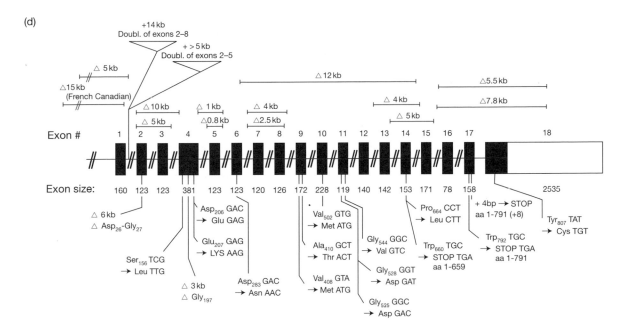

Figure 8.5 (a) Schematic representation of the biosynthesis and the itinerary of the low-density lipoprotein (LDL) receptor and the feedback regulatory mechanisms that follow the entry of cholesterol into the cell. Numbers 1–5 represent different steps of biosynthesis, modifications, positioning into the coated pits, intracellular transfer and recycling of the receptor. (b) Classes of the LDL receptor based on different steps of the receptor itinerary, and pharmacogenetic predictions on how patients with mutations will respond to HMG-CoA reductase inhibitors (statins) and bile acid (BA)-binding resins (adapted from reference 134 with permission). (c) Principles of cholesterol lowering using statins and BA-binding resins. The response to BA-binding resins alone is smaller, owing to feedback cellular response to increase cholesterol biosynthesis. (d) Schematic representation of the human LDL receptor gene and the various mutations associated with familial hypercholesterolemia. The mutations are described in the text.[1,135] ER, endoplasmic reticulum; C, cholesterol

adjacent repeats, designated A and B, are located in the epidermal growth factor precursor homology region.[154] Deletion or oligonucleotide-directed mutagenesis within each of the repeated sequences, and functional analysis of the mutant receptors following expression in COS cells, confirmed the importance of these regions for ligand binding. This analysis also showed that repeats 2, 3, 6, 7, and A are required for maximum binding of LDL (via apoB) but not βVLDL (via apoE), whereas repeat 5 is required for maximum binding of both LDL and βVLDL (Figure 8.3a).[155,156]

Biosynthesis and post-translational modifications and recycling of the LDL receptor

Following synthesis, the LDL receptor protein is modified post-translationally in the ER and Golgi by *N*- and *O*-linked glycosylation.[152,157] The modified receptors reach the cell surface, are initially incorporated in various areas of the plasma membrane, and subsequently cluster in the clathrin-coated pits (Figure 8.5a).

Mutations in the LDL receptor gene are associated with familial hypercholesterolemia

Familial hypercholesterolemia (FH) is an autosomal dominant disease characterized clinically by increased LDL cholesterol, xanthomas in tendons and skin, and premature coronary atherosclerosis. Homozygotes are more severely affected than heterozygotes. The frequency of heterozygotes is approximately 1 in 500 persons, and these individuals have plasma cholesterol 350–550 mg/dl from birth. Tendon xanthomas and coronary atherosclerosis appear after ages 20 and 30, respectively. Homozygotes have a frequency of 1 in 1 000 000 and cholesterol levels 650–1000 mg/dl; they develop cutaneous xanthomas by the fourth year of life, and without treatment die from myocardial infarction by the age of 20.[11]

The functional, biochemical and genetic analysis of the LDL receptor facilitated enormously the delineation of the molecular defects that underlie familial hypercholesterolemia. The LDL receptor deficiency prevents the uptake of IDL and LDL, and increases the conversion of IDL to LDL.[158] Based on the new molecular information, a variety of defects in the LDL receptor identified previously with binding studies could be assigned to one of five classes (Figure 8.5b). The class 1 mutants are characterized by the absence of receptor protein, owing to either gross alterations (insertions, deletions) in the receptor gene or nonsense mutations leading to premature chain termination.[1,11,136] The class 2 mutants are characterized by defective modification of the precursor *N*- and *O*-linked carbohydrates.[159,160] These mutations consist mostly of amino acid deletions or substitutions, and have been localized in exons 2, 4, 6, 11, and 14,[1,11,136] and cause the entrapment of a precursor form of <Mr>=120 kDa in the ER.[160] The Watanabe heritable hyperlipidemic (WHHL) rabbit mutation (discussed later) belongs in this category. The class 3 mutants are characterized by receptors of either normal or aberrant apparent <Mr> that are modified, normally reach the cell surface, but have reduced affinity for LDL. Such mutants result from deletions/insertions or amino acid substitutions in exons 2–8[1,11,136] in the cysteine-rich domain of the receptor. The class 4 mutants are characterized by normal synthesis, modification, and transport to the cell surface, but inability to cluster into the coated pits. As a result, these mutant receptors bind LDL normally but do not internalize the complex.[1,11,136] All these mutants have alterations within the first 21 residues of the cytoplasmic tail. Functional analysis of either naturally occurring mutants or mutants generated by *in vitro* mutagenesis showed that substitutions of Tyr807 by Cys or other non-aromatic amino acids were sufficient to create an internalization defect.[161] The class 5 mutations are characterized by receptors that are synthesized, secreted, and internalized normally, but cannot be released from the endosomes, and hence cannot recycle to the cell surface. These mutations are found in the epidermal growth factor (EGF) precursor homology domain and may involve residues located on or in the vicinity of repeats A, B, and C (Figure 8.3a).[11,155,162] The EGF precursor

homology domain may mediate the dissociation of the receptor–ligand complex in the ER as a result of the lowering of the pH in this organelle.[11,163] Figure 8.5b shows how patients with different types of mutation may respond to cholesterol-lowering therapies. Figure 8.5c shows the principle of cholesterol lowering using 3-hydroxyl-3-methyl-glutaryl-CoA (HMG-CoA) reductase inhibitors (statins) and bile acid-binding resins. The mutations described for the LDL receptor have been reviewed extensively;[136] several known mutations are shown in Figure 8.5d.

A rare form of familiar hypercholesterolemia with an autosomal recessive mode of inheritance has been described.[164,165] Cultured lymphocytes of the patients have normal or increased receptor binding but defective internalization. The disease is caused by mutations in the phosphotyrosine-binding domain of a protein designated autosomal recessive hypercholesterolemia (ARH).[166] ARH binds to the NPVY domain of the LDL receptor (Figure 8.3a), and may function to chaperone the LDL receptor to the coated pits and anchor it to the clathrin and AP-2.[165] Alternatively, ARH may act as an adaptor molecule by binding to the LDL receptor after it reaches the coated pits and anchoring it to the clathrin and AP-2.[165]

HMG-CoA reductase inhibitors (statins) increases the LDL receptor numbers on the cell surface and hence the clearance of plasma cholesterol. As shown in Figure 8.5b, statins can only be used for the treatment of LDL heterozygotes and homozygotes of the third class of mutations, which may bind LDL with reduced affinity. Combination of statins with bile acid-binding resins that bind and remove bile acids from the intestine, or new drugs that affect intestinal sterol absorption, have an even greater cholesterol-lowering effect.[167,168]

How a cell senses fluctuations in cholesterol levels, and the effect of receptor mutations

As shown in Figure 8.5a, when the cell senses excess intracellular cholesterol it inhibits the endogenous cholesterol biosynthesis and decreases the LDL receptor number. The HMG-CoA reductase activity is decreased by proteosome-mediated degradation of this enzyme. The cell also increases the esterification of excess cholesterol in order to store limited amounts of cholesteryl esters in the form of lipid droplets. In the

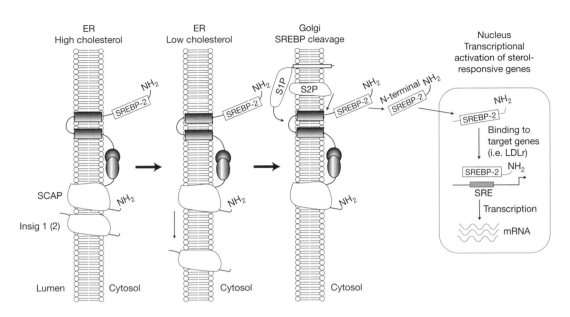

Figure 8.6 Schematic representation of proteolytic activation of sterol regulatory element-binding protein (SREBP) through a cholesterol sensing mechanism which leads to the release of the N-terminal segment of SREBP, which translocates to the nucleus and activates target genes. (Adapted from reference 169, with permission). ER, endoplasmic reticulum; LDLr, low-density lipoprotein receptor; SCAP, SREBP cleavage activating protein

opposite situation, when the cell is deprived of cholesterol it increases the LDL receptor numbers to import more cholesterol via the LDL receptor pathway.

The mechanism through which a cell senses cholesterol levels has recently been clarified and involves a membrane-bound transcription factor named sterol regulatory element-binding protein-2 (SREBP-2) (Figure 8.6).[11,169] This membrane-bound basic helix–loop–helix transcription factor controls genes involved in cellular cholesterol homeostasis.[170] Another major member of the family, SREBP-1, controls genes involved in fatty acid biosynthesis.[171] All members of the family have a highly acidic amino-terminal activation domain that is recognized by the transcriptional coactivator CREB-binding protein (CBP).[172] When cholesterol is in excess, membrane protein SREBP cleavage activating protein (SCAP), present in the ER, interacts with SREBP as well as another cholesterol-sensing protein, insig1(2), and all three proteins remain anchored in the ER membrane. Under conditions of cholesterol depletion, insig1(2) dissociates from the complex and allows SREBP and SCAP to move via vesicular transport to the Gogli, where SREBP are cleaved by two proteases designated site 1 (S1P) and site 2 (S2P); SP1 cleaves the loop connecting

the two transmembrane regions in the Golgi lumen, and SP2 cleaves within the first transmembrane domain.[169,173–175] The cleaved aminoterminal fragment containing ~480 amino acids of SREBP containing the bHLHZip motif that includes the DNA binding, and the activation domain, translocates to the nucleus and induces transcription of several genes involved in cholesterol or fatty acid biosynthesis and transport.[11]

Animal models with LDL receptor deficiency or abundance

Transgenic mice overexpressing the human LDL receptor catabolize LDL effectively, leading to very low levels of plasma LDL,[176] and are protected from atherosclerosis in response to atherogenic diets.[177] In contrast, LDLr–/– mice, which have mild hypercholesterolemia but eightfold elevated IDL and LDL cholesterol, develop atherosclerosis in response to atherogenic diets.[178] Atherosclerosis is exacerbated in LDLr–/– × apoE–/– mice[179] and in LDLr–/– × apoB transgenic mice.[72] The use of LDLr-deficient mouse models to test the atherogenicity of the other genes is discussed in later sections.

Other members of the LDL receptor family that recognize apoE-containing lipoproteins

In mammalian species, the LDL receptor gene family contains four additional structurally and evolutionarily-related members:[11,137–142] the LDL receptor-related protein (LRP), the megalin/gp330, the VLDL receptor (VLDLr), and the apoE receptor-2 (apoER2) (Figure 8.3, Table 8.4).

LRP   In 1988, a protein of 4525 amino acids was cloned from a human lymphocyte cDNA library with homology to the LDL receptor and was named LRP.[138] LRP, which is identical to protease-activated α_2-macroglobulin,[180] is synthesized as a precursor of Mr 600 kDa and is cleaved in the *trans* Golgi to two subunits of Mr 515 and 85 kDa, respectively, which associate non-covalently on the cell surface.[181] LRP has regions which are homologous to the cysteine-rich domain, the EGF precursor domain, and the cytoplasmic tail of the LDL receptor (Figure 8.3b). LRP mRNA and protein are present in various tissues, including liver, brain, and lung.[138] Studies with LDL receptor-negative skin fibroblasts showed that LRP-mediated binding and the uptake of βVLDL by the cells are stimulated by apoE and inhibited by apoCI and, to a lesser extent, by apoCII.[23,182] LRP also binds with high affinity and mediates the uptake of activated α_2-macroglobulin–protease complexes,[180] plasminogen activator–inhibitor complexes,[183,184] lactopherin,[183] and lipoprotein lipase, hormones and carrier proteins for vitamins.[137,139] Inactivation of the LRP gene in mice leads to embryonic lethality at around the implantation stage.[184]

Megalin   Megalin, also known as gp330, is a large protein similar in size and domain structure to LRP.[185] It resides in coated pits on the apical surface of epithelial cells in the renal glomerulus and proximal tubule. Megalin is associated with Heymann-type autoimmune nephritis in rats.[186] The function of megalin/gp330 is unknown. It binds apoE-containing lipoproteins and most of the ligands that are recognized by LRP.[137,183]

VLDLr   VLDLr was initially isolated from rabbit and human cDNA libraries.[140,141] VLDLr is an evolutionarily conserved protein that has a striking homology to the LDL receptor. The domain structures of cysteine repeats, the EGF homology, the serine–threonine-rich domain, the transmembrane spanning, and the cytoplasmic regions are highly preserved between the two

proteins. The intron–exon organization of the human VLDLr and LDLr genes is the same, except for the presence of an additional repeat in the ligand-binding domain of VLDLr.[141] The VLDLr is expressed abundantly in heart, muscle, and adipose tissue, and is barely detectable in the liver.[140] The findings suggest that VLDLr may be involved in the catabolism of triglyceride-rich VLDL by muscle and the adipose tissue. Inactivation of the VLDLr gene in mice did not affect the lifespan or the plasma lipid and lipoprotein levels.[187]

ApoER2   ApoER2 is highly homologous and has a similar domain structure to LDLr and VLDLr, and has three different forms resulting from alternate splicing.[188] ApoER2 binds with high affinity apoE-rich β-migrating VLDL and apoE proteoliposomes, but does not bind to LDL.[142,189] The difference in ligand specificity has been attributed to structural differences between the two receptors in the linker sequence, which connects with cysteine-rich repeats 4 and 5.[155] ApoER2 is expressed abundantly in the brain, and to a lesser extent in the testes and ovaries.[142] The tissue distribution indicates that apoER2 may contribute to lipid homeostasis in the brain.[189] Studies in double-deficient VLDLr–/– × apoER2–/– mice indicated that these receptors may also play an important role in brain development and functions, mediated via its interaction with the brain protein Reelin which is expressed in the cortex and cerebellum and activation of intracellular signaling pathways.[190]

The scavenger receptors SRAI and SRAII, and CD36

Functional definition of the scavenger receptor class A types I and II (SRAI and SRAII)

It has been shown that the protein and lipid moieties of LDL can be modified *in vivo* by malonyldialdehyde (MDA) and other short-chain aldehydes that are released by platelets or produced during lipid peroxidation or by oxidation of LDL in the intima.[191,192] These changes render the modified LDL substrate for a new class of receptors, called scavenger receptors. It has been estimated that in normal humans two-thirds of LDL is catabolized through the LDL receptor pathway and one-third by a receptor-independent pathway that may reside in scavenger cells.[116] It was initially shown that mouse peritoneal macrophages and human monocyte-derived macrophages contain receptors that bind specifically and with high affinity to modified LDL.[193] The bound, modified LDL is internalized, the protein moiety degraded to amino acids, and the cholesteryl esters of the modified LDL hydrolyzed, presumably by a non-lysosomal cholesteryl ester hydrolase.[193,194] When the cells are grown in medium containing serum, half of the free cholesterol is secreted and the remainder is re-esterified by ACAT-1 and stored in the cytoplasm as cholesteryl ester droplets.[193] In the continuous presence of modified LDL in the culture medium the macrophages apparently fail to downregulate their scavenger receptor activity, and this results in a dramatic increase in cellular content and cholesteryl esters.[195] The accumulation of cholesteryl esters in the monocyte–macrophages may lead to the formation of foam cells characteristic of atherosclerotic lesions.[193]

Structure and functions of the scavenger receptors SRAI and SRAII

Kodama, in Krieger's laboratory, purified the receptor for modified lipoprotein to near homogeneity from bovine lung,[196] and cloned the corresponding cDNA.[197,198] cDNA encoding the human receptor has also been obtained from a monocyte-derived cell line (THP1).[199] This analysis showed two forms of the human and the bovine receptor, type I (SRAI) (453 aa) and type II (SRAII) (349 aa) (Table 8.5).[196–198] Computer analysis of the predicted primary protein sequence showed that SRAI contains a 50-amino acid long amino-terminal cytoplasmic domain, a 26-amino acid long membrane-spanning domain, a 32-amino acid long membrane spacer region with two potential N-glycosylation sites, a rod-like structure which contains 163 residues that form an α-helical coiled coil and contains five potential N-glycosylation sites, 72 residues that form a collagen-like domain, and an 110 amino acid cysteine-rich carboxy-terminal domain. The SRAII is identical to the SRAI receptor, except that it contains only a six-residue carboxy-terminal domain. A schematic representation of the different domains of the SRAI and SRAII is shown in Figure 8.7. The rod-like structure is generated in the trimeric receptor by the merger of a triple-stranded left-handed superhelix formed by the α-helical coiled coil and a right-handed collagen-like triple helix.[196] The binding of modified LDL to both types of the receptor is similar,[197] suggesting that the carboxy-terminal cysteine-rich domain is not involved in receptor binding. Functional studies showed that the same receptor recognizes both acetyl LDL and oxidized LDL with different specificities, and that receptor binding is diminished by deletion of residues −320 to −342 of the collagen-like domain.[1]

The contribution of SRAI in atherogenesis has been studied by crossing SRAI-deficient mice with atherosclerosis-prone mice. SRAI−/− × LDLr−/− or SRAI−/− × apoE−/− mice have smaller lesions.[200,201] Transplantation of bone marrow cells overexpressing SRAI in apoE−/− or LDLr−/− mice did not affect atherosclerosis, although it reduced VLDL remnants in the apoE−/− mice.[202,203] SRAI−/− × apoE$_3$ Leiden-transgenic mice develop more complex lesions, with calcification, necrosis, cholesterol clefts, and fibrosis than do apoE3 Leiden-transgenic mice.[204]

CD36

CD36 is a membrane protein with two short cytoplasmic amino- and carboxy-terminal membrane domains and belongs to the scavenger receptor B family (Figure 8.7).[60,205,206] CD36 is expressed in a variety of cells and tissues, including monocyte-derived macrophages, microvascular endothelial cells, adipocytes, platelets, and striated muscle and heart (Table 8.5).[60,206] CD36 is a multiligand receptor that binds modified lipoprotein and apoptotic cells and may contribute to foam cell formation.[207,208] It also binds bacteria parasites and viruses.[208,209] The expression of CD36 in macrophages is induced by oxidized LDL, which is one of its ligands.[206] LDL modified by monocyte-reactive nitrogen species generated by myeloperoxidase is a CD36 ligand.[210] CD36 functions as a long-chain fatty acid translocase that transports fatty acids across the membrane, and contributes to energy metabolism.[211,212] CD36 is also involved in platelet adhesion and angiogenesis,[213] and modulates TGF-β activation[214] and the inflammatory response.[215] Owing to these properties, CD36 is thought to play an important role in atherosclerosis and other complex diseases, such as diabetes and cardiomyopathies.[60,206] Monocyte-derived macrophages from humans with CD36 deficiency have reduced binding and uptake of oxidized LDL compared to normal controls.[210]

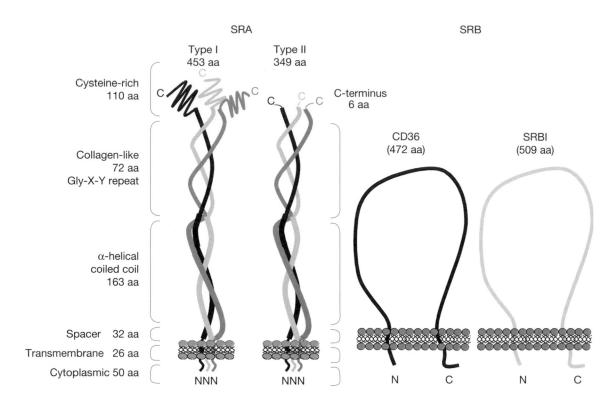

Figure 8.7 Schematic representation of class A and class B members of the scavenger receptor (SR) family. Adapted from references 137 and 315 with permission

Transgenic mice overexpressing CD36 in muscle had decreased circulating TG, fewer TG in VLDL, and increased fatty acid oxidation in muscle.[211] Replacement of the mutant CD36 locus by a wild-type locus ameliorated insulin resistance and lowered serum fatty acids in spontaneous hypertensive rats.[216] CD36–/– mice had reduced fatty acid uptake in heart, skeletal muscle, and adipose tissue, and increased HDL cholesterol and VLDL triglycerides.[217] Compared to apoE–/– mice, CD36–/– × apoE–/– mice had an 80% reduction in aortic lesions on an atherogenic diet, and a significant reduction in lesions on a normal diet (Table 8.9).[218]

Lp(a)

Structure, biosynthesis, and catabolism

Lp(a) represents a distinct class of lipoprotein particles found mostly in the LDL density region but in other lipoprotein classes as well, including triglyceride-rich

fractions.[3,219] The lipid moieties of these particles are similar to that of LDL (Table 8.1).[3,219] Apo(a) is a glycoprotein of 4529 amino acids synthesized by the liver, and contains approximately 30% of carbohydrate moieties.[3,220] The protein moiety of Lp(a) consists of one molecule of apoB-100 and one of apo(a). These proteins are linked by a single intradisulfide bridge between Cys4326 of apoB and Cys4057 (located on kringle IV-9) of apo(a) (Figure 8.1a).[3]

Transgenic mice expressing human apo(a) secrete lipid-free apo(a), which could be converted to Lp(a) by intravenous injection of human LDL. Furthermore, human apo(a) × apoB-100 transgenics secrete Lp(a).[221,222] These findings support the extracellular assembly of LDL with Lp(a) and indicate that Lp(a) assembly does not require any enzymes or other protein *in vivo*.[223,224] The assembly of Lp(a) appears to be a two-step process. The first step is the docking of apo(a) to the LDL; the second is the formation of the disulfide bridge between Cys 4057 of apo(a) and Cys 4326 of apoB.[3]

The concentration of Lp(a) in plasma is determined by the rate of secretion of apo(a)/Lp(a) by liver cells, and is genetically determined.[225] Turnover studies have shown that the catabolism of Lp(a) *in vitro* is lower than that of LDL.[3] The mechanism and sites of Lp(a) catabolism remain unknown; it may involve the kidney, and to a lesser extent the liver and may require members of the LDL receptor family.

Genetics

The structure of apo(a) has been derived from the cDNA sequence of overlapping cDNA clones.[220] Human apo(a) consists of a protease domain which has 94% homology to that of plasminogen, one domain which has homology to kringle V of plasminogen, and a variable number of domains (ranging from 15 to 40) with homology to kringle IV of plasminogen.[220] Lp(a) has proteolytic activity that is different from that of plasmin.[220,226] An extensive polymorphism for apo(a) has been observed in humans. The different apo(a) isoforms differ in molecular mass, ranging from 400 to 800 kDa, and their transmission follows Mendelian inheritance.[3] The difference in Lp(a) size arises from the different number of kringle IV repeats, which ranges from 2 to 40.[3,227] The Lp(a) concentration in subjects with the same phenotype is determined primarily by differences in the production rates.[3] Epidemiological studies have shown that the Lp(a) size is inversely related to the plasma Lp(a) concentration.[227] The plasma Lp(a) levels are controlled by the apo(a) locus as well as by other genetic factors, such as LDL receptor defects, and environmental factors such as drugs and hormones.[3]

Functions

It has been suggested that Lp(a) may contribute to the pathogenesis of atherosclerosis, and possibly thrombosis, by interfering with the metabolism of LDL and plasminogen, respectively. It is believed that Lp(a) modulates the balance between fibrinolysis and clotting by binding to a forming fibrin thrombus. Existing evidence suggests that Lp(a) may inhibit fibrinolysis by interfering with the binding of plasminogen to fibrinogen.[3] Lp(a) also competes for the binding of plasminogen to fibrin.[228,229] Lp(a) inhibits the streptokinase-mediated activation of plasminogen,[230] inhibits the urokinase or tissue plasminogen activator (tPA)-mediated activation of plasminogen,[229,231,232] affects the synthesis of plasminogen activator inhibitor-1 (PAI-1),[233] and inhibits the binding of plasminogen to tetranectin, an interaction that enhances plasminogen activation by tPA.[232] All these functions of Lp(a) can interfere with fibrinolysis.

Lp(a) has been found in atherosclerotic lesions,[234] and there are several *in vitro* and *in vivo* studies indicating that Lp(a)/apo(a) has proatherogenic properties. Lp(a) is a substrate for factor XIIIa,[235] which may crosslink Lp(a) to fibrin, fibrinogen, and fibronectin in atherosclerotic lesions *in vivo*. Lp(a) also binds proteoglycans.[236] Peptide fragments generated by the proteolytic activity of Lp(a) can be taken up by macrophages and might contribute further to atherogenesis.[3] Apo(a)/Lp(a) interacts with the extracellular matrix, including fibrin,[237] fibronectin,[226] tetranectin,[232] proteoglycans (e.g. decorin),[236] and macrophage receptors,[238] and thus may contribute to atherogenesis.

Lp(a) has chemoattractant activity for monocytes,[239] and induces the release of monocyte chemotactic activity (MCA) from endothelial cells.[240] Through its inhibition of the conversion of plasminogen to plasmin, apo(a)/Lp(a) also inhibits the plasmin-catalyzed activation of transforming growth factor-β (TGF-β).[241] Decreased TGF-β levels promote cell proliferation and migration of smooth muscle cells *in vitro*[242] and *in vivo* in apo(a) transgenic mice.[243] In addition, Lp(a) stimulates the expression of ICAM-1, VCAM-1, and E-selectin at the surface of endothelial cells,[244,245] all of which participate in the recruitment of leukocytes to the vessel wall. These properties may explain the atherogenicity of Lp(a).

The role of Lp(a) in atherogenesis is supported by studies in transgenic mice. The apo(a) transgenics developed plaques when fed a high-cholesterol atherogenic diet.[224] Atherosclerotic lesions were shown to be significantly reduced in human apo(a) × apoA-I transgenic mice.[246] Transgenics for a mutant human apo(a) in which the lysine-binding sites of apo(a) were altered failed to develop lesions.[247] An increase in atherosclerosis was observed in human apo(a) × apoB double transgenic mice.[248] Similarly, apo(a) × apoB transgenic × LDLr−/− mice and apoB transgenic × LDLr−/− mice developed severe atherosclerosis which was similar in both of these mouse lines (Table 8.7).[72]

Lp(a) and atherothrombotic vascular disease

In studies in different ethnic groups, in patients with familial hypercholesterolemia,[3,249] or in subjects with high LDL levels, it was shown that high plasma Lp(a) levels are associated with coronary heart disease (CHD) and early myocardial infarction.[3,250] Numerous prospective studies have shown that Lp(a) is an independent risk factor for CHD, and in 14 out of 18 studies high levels of Lp(a) were associated with CHD.[3] High Lp(a) is also associated with peripheral vascular disease and stroke.[3,251] Lp(a) levels were significantly reduced in a group of hypertriglyceridemic patients by treatment with nicotinic acid;[252] however, currently there are no well-established pharmacological treatments for high Lp(a) levels in the general population.[3]

In vivo antifibrinolytic activity of Lp(a) was demonstrated only in the transgenic mice.[253] Most studies did not find an association between fibrinolytic parameters and Lp(a) levels.[3,254] Moreover, several studies failed to find a strong connection between plasma Lp(a) levels and thrombogenicity.[3] There is, however, a strong association between increased Lp(a) levels and the occurrence of thrombotic events in patients with immune-mediated diseases. It is possible that Lp(a) β_2-glycoprotein I interactions may be a link between thrombosis and autoimmune disease.[255] The affinity of Lp(a) for fibrin is increased by homocysteine,[256] and this may explain the atherosclerosis and thromboembolic phenomena associated with hyperhomocysteinemia.

The contribution of lipid and bile acid transporters in whole-body cholesterol homeostasis

Lipid and bile acid transporters in the liver and the intestine

To understand overall lipid homeostasis in humans, we must also consider the absorption of dietary lipids in the intestine, the biosynthesis of bile acids in the liver, the uptake and efflux of sterols, phospholipids, and bile acids by the liver and the intestine, and the excretion of bile in the feces. Liver contains the enzymes that synthesize bile acids from precursor cholesterol molecules.[257–259] Bile acids are exported into the bile by the ABCB11 transporter, also known as bile salt export pump (BSEP) or sister of *p*-glycoprotein (SPGP), and possibly by other transporters.

Phospholipids are also exported from the liver by the initial action of ABCB4 flippase, and cholesterol is exported into the bile by the ABCG5/ABCG8 transporter (Figure 8.8; Table 8.10).[260,261]

The role of ABCB4 and ABCB11 in bile acid metabolism has been supported by studies in human subjects and animal models. Thus, transgenic mice overexpressing murine ABCB11 in the liver have increased hepatobiliary secretion but normal fecal bile acid secretion.[262] ABCB11 deficiency in mice fed a cholic acid-supplemented diet led to the development of severe cholestasis.[263] Mutation of ABCB4 in humans is associated with cholelithiasis.[264]

Exported phospholipid, cholesterol, and bile acids form micelles and, through ducts, concentrate in the gallbladder. In response to dietary fats, bile is released into the lumen of the small intestine to promote their solubilization and catabolism.[257]

Dietary sterols are taken through an unknown carrier in the intestine. Ninety-nine per cent of the plant sterols (PS) and shellfish sterols are resecreted into the intestinal lumen by the ABCG5/ABCG8 transporters and removed in the feces. Mutations in either ABCG5 or ABCG8 cause sitosterolemia in humans.[260] Bile acids are transported into the enterocytes by the ileal bile acid transporter (IBAT), a Na^+-linked symporter. Bile acids are carried in the cytosol by the cytosolic ileal bile acid-binding protein (IBABP), and are released in the bloodstream by the action of an unknown transporter. The bile acids that reach the liver via the enterohepatic circulation are imported into the liver by a Na^+-linked symporter, the sodium taurocholate cotransporting polypeptide (NTCP).[169,257,261]

Normally, 5% of bile acids are excreted into the feces. As will be discussed further, bile acid sequestrants, such as cholestyramine, which bind and remove bile acids via the feces, are used as hypocholesterolemic drugs, usually in combination with statins (Figure 8.5c).[168]

Dietary fats absorbed into the intestine assemble intracellularly into chylomicrons and are secreted into the lymph and reach the circulation. Similarly, fatty acids taken up by the liver (via albumin and other mechanisms) are incorporated into VLDL. ApoA-I secreted by the hepatocytes and enterocytes accepts cellular phospholipids and cholesterol from ABCA1 to form precursor HDL particles, which are converted to mature spherical HDL (Figure 8.8a).

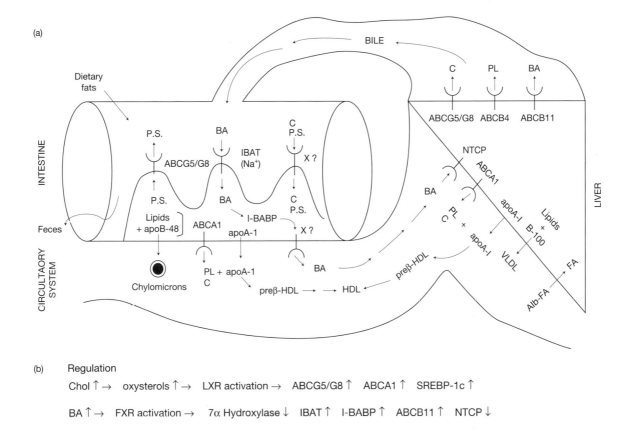

Chol ↑ → oxysterols ↑ → LXR activation → ABCG5/G8 ↑ ABCA1 ↑ SREBP-1c ↑

BA ↑ → FXR activation → 7α Hydroxylase ↓ IBAT ↑ I-BABP ↑ ABCB11 ↑ NTCP ↓

Figure 8.8 (a) Schematic representation of whole-body sterol homeostasis that takes into account the dietary sterol uptake, the biosynthesis and transport of bile acids (BA), cholesterol (C) and phospholipids (PL), and the excretion of bile. (b) Nuclear receptor-mediated regulation of intestinal and hepatic transporters of BA sterols and plant sterols (PS). (Adapted from reference 315). ABC, ATP-binding casette; IBAT, ileal bile acid transporter; IBABP, ileal bile acid binding protein; LDL, low-density lipoprotein; HDL, high-density lipoprotein; apo, apolipoprotein; NTCP, sodium taurocholate co-transporting polypeptide; FA, fatty acid; Alb, albumin; VLDL, very low-density lipoprotein; FXR, farnesol X receptor; LXR, liver X receptor; SREBP, sterol regulatory element-binding protein

Bile acids activate hormone nuclear receptors and affect lipid homeostasis

The liver contains 70% of the body's LDL receptors. Nuclear hormone receptors represent a superfamily of transcriptional factors that are activated by hormones, such as retinoids, steroids, thyroid hormone, prostaglandins, products of lipid metabolism, vitamin D oxysterols, and bile acids, and regulate cell differentiation, development, homeostasis, and reproduction.[265] The nuclear receptor superfamily also includes numerous orphan receptors. Liver X receptors (LXRα and LXRβ) and farnesol X receptors

(FXRα and FXRβ) are nuclear hormone receptors that are activated by heterodimerization with retinoid X receptor (RXR) in the presence of their permissive ligands, as well as by 9-*cis*-retinoic acid.[266] Ligands for LXRα are 22-*R*-hydroxycholesterol and other oxysterols.[266,267] Ligands for FXRα are bile acids such as chenodeoxycholic acid, lithocholic acid and deoxycholic acid.[268–270] When bile acids levels increase, FXR, which is expressed in hepatocytes and intestinal epithelial cells, is activated and represses the transcription of 7α hydroxylase, which is the rate-limiting enzyme in the synthesis of bile acids (Figure 8.8b).

Table 8.10 Phospholipid, sterol, and bile acid transporters

Name/site	Function	Other pathologies
ABCA1 hepatic and intestinal, basolateral, membrane bound	ATP-dependent efflux of cellular cholesterol and phospholipid to apoA-I and other acceptors	Tangier disease
NTCP (sodium taurocholate cotransporting polypeptide) hepatic, basolateral, membrane-bound	Binds and imports into the hepatocyte 1 molecule of bile acid along with 2 molecules of Na^+	–
I-BABP (ileal bile acid binding protein) Cytosolic	Binds intracellularly and promotes the transport of bile acid to the basolateral membrane of the enterocytes. Bile acids are subsequently exported via an unknown membrane bound transporter	–
ABCB4 hepatic, apical, membrane bound	Flips phospholipids from the inner to the outer membrane leaflet which is then transferred to bile	–
ABCB11 hepatic apical membrane bound	ATP dependent, exports phospholipid into bile	-
ABCG5/ABCG8 intestinal, apical and hepatic membrane bound	In the intestine, exports into the intestinal lumen plant sterols (PS), shellfish sterols and cholesterol These sterols have been absorbed from the intestinal lumen by an unknown apical transporter In the liver, promotes the apical transport of cholesterol into the bile	Sitosterolemia characterized by high concentrations of plant and shellfish sterols in the bloodstream
I-BAT (ileal bile acid transporter protein) intestinal apical membrane bound	Binds and imports into the enterocyte 1 molecule of bile acid and 2 molecules of Na^+	–
Unknown transporter(s), intestinal, apical membrane bound	Binds and imports into the enterocyte cholesterol and plant sterols (PS) and shellfish sterols	–
Unknown transporter(s) intestinal, basolateral membrane bound	Binds and exports from the enterocyte bile acid	–

When cellular sterols increase in the liver the level of oxysterols also increases, leading to the activation of LXR and the transcription of target genes such as ABCG5/ABCG8 and ABCA1 that promote efflux of hepatic cholesterol as well as SREBP-1c, which upregulates genes involved in fatty acid biosynthesis. The activation of these genes provides cholesteryl esters and phospholipids to balance the increased levels of free cholesterol.[169] FXR also controls the enterohepatic circulation of bile acids by increasing the transcription of IBAT in the intestine, and increasing the expression of ABCB11 and decreasing the expression of NTCP in the liver (Figure 8.8b).

Role of apoE in cholesterol and triglyceride homeostasis and in atherogenesis:molecular causes of type III hyperlipoproteinemia

Apolipoprotein E

Apolipoprotein E (apoE) is a component of VLDL, IDL, HDL, chylomicrons, and chylomicron remnants, and is required for the clearance of lipoprotein remnants from the circulation (Figure 8.1b). Lipoprotein-bound apoE is the ligand for the LDL receptor, as well as for other receptors.[1,140,142,189,271] *In vitro* and *in vivo* studies have shown that mutations in apoE that prevent binding of apoE-containing lipoproteins to the LDL receptor are associated with high plasma cholesterol levels and cause premature atherosclerosis in humans and experimental animals.[87,272] ApoE is also involved in cholesterol efflux processes, and is atheroprotective.[273–275] ApoE may also modulate the macrophage- and T lymphocyte-mediated immune response in atheroma.[47]

In humans, three common alleles at a single genetic locus exist, which give rise to three homozygous and three heterozygous apoE phenotypes.[276] The phenotype E2/2 is associated with cardiovascular disease,[277] and the phenotype E4/4 is a risk factor for Alzheimer's disease (Figure 8.9 a and b).[278] Similar to apoA-I and apoA-IV, apoE contains mostly 22 amino acid repeats and few 11 amino acid repeats which, based on X-ray crystallography and computer modeling, are organized in amphipathic α-helices.[279,280] These a helices contribute to the ability of apoE to bind to lipids and form lipoproteins. X-ray crystallography of the amino-terminal 22 kDa fragment of apoE showed that this region forms a four-helix bundle that is stabilized by hydrophobic interactions and salt bridges.[280]

It is possible that disturbances in lipid homeostasis,[189] as well as interactions of apoE with other brain proteins, may contribute to the neurodegeneration observed in Alzheimer's disease (Figure 8.10).[281]

ApoE structure and functions

Certain apoE phenotypes and genotypes are associated with type III hyperlipoproteinemia (type III HLP)

Familial type III HLP, also called familial dysbetalipoproteinemia, or broad β, or floating β disease, is characterized by xanthomas, elevated plasma cholesterol and triglyceride levels, cholesterol-enriched βVLDL and IDL particles, increased plasma apoE levels, and premature coronary and peripheral atherosclerosis.[7] The frequency of the disease was estimated to be 0.01–0.1% in the population. The great majority of the patients with type III HLP have the E2/2 phenotype,[277] which results from the substitution of Cys for Arg-158. This mutation, combined with other genetic or

(a)

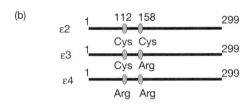

Common apoE alleles
(allele frequency)

α Large and small spheres represent the unmodified and modified apoE forms, respectively. The symbols * and + indicate phenotype associated with type III hyperlipoproteinemia and Alzheimer's disease, respectively

Figure 8.9 (a) Schematic representation of the common and rare apolipoprotein E (apoE) alleles and apoE phenotypes. Large and small spheres represent the unmodified and the O-glycosylated sialylated forms of apoE, respectively. The symbols * and + indicate phenotype associated with type III hyperlipoproteinemia and Alzheimer's disease, respectively. (b) Amino acid differences between the ε2 ε3 and ε4 alleles

environmental factors, affects the catabolism of apoE-containing lipoproteins and causes type III HLP.[7] Another feature of type III HLP is that it results in the accumulation in plasma of remnants of lipoprotein metabolism enriched in cholesteryl esters and apoE.[282]

Dominant and recessive forms of type III hyperlipoproteinemia

The Arg-158→Cys mutation in the homozygote state, depending on other genetic or environmental factors,

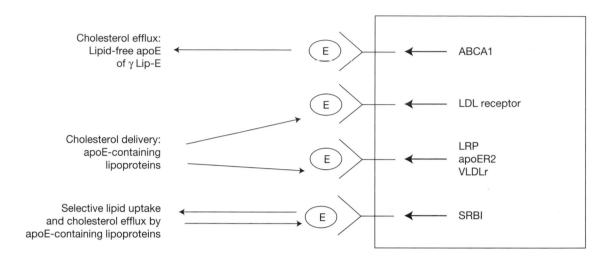

Figure 8.10   Contribution of apolipoprotein E (apoE), apoE-containing lipoproteins, low-density lipoprotein receptor (LDLr) family members, ATP-binding cassette-A1 (ABCA1) and scavenger receptor type BI (SRBI) in cellular cholesterol homeostasis. VLDLr, very low-density lipoprotein; apoER2, apoE receptor 2

may result in type III hyperlipoproteinemia. This form of type III HLP is inherited in an autosomal recessive fashion.[7] A variety of rare apoE mutations have also been described,[7] some of which are associated with a dominant mode of inheritance of type III HLP, which is expressed at an early age. These include substitutions Arg-136→Ser, Arg-142→Cys, Arg-145→Cys, Lys-146→Gln, Lys-146→Glu, Arg-147→Trp and an insertion of seven amino acids (duplication of residues 121–127).[1] These apoE mutations which are associated with dominant forms of type III HLP are between residues 136 and 152. The importance of the 136–152 region of apoE for receptor binding was also assessed by *in vitro* mutagenesis.[1] Mutations within this region reduced the receptor-binding activity to 10–50% of control.[283]

In vitro and in vivo analysis of the molecular basis of a human disease associated with apoE deficiency

A rare form of type III HLP associated with familial apoE deficiency was first described in a family in 1981.[284] Familial apoE deficiency in humans is associated with increased plasma cholesterol, the accumulation of remnants in the VLDL and IDL region, and premature atherosclerosis.[272] The biochemical and clinical features of patients with apoE deficiency were lack of plasma apoE; Chol 529 ± 74 mg/dl, TG 221 ± 62 mg/dl, VLDL Chol 243 ± 9 mg/dl, IDL Chol 230 ± 41 mg/dl; cholesterol-rich VLDL and IDL remnants which could be lowered by diets. The patients had tuboeruptive and palmar xanthomas; and the development of premature atherosclerosis.[272,284]

Initial studies using cultures of peripheral blood human monocyte–macrophages obtained from an apoE-deficient patient and normal controls showed that the apoE-deficient cultures synthesized low amounts of two aberrant forms of apoE mRNA[285] (Figure 8.11a) and did not produce any immunoprecipitable forms of apoE.[285] Both aberrant mRNA contained termination codons within the intronic sequences of the mRNA, and were predicted to encode short peptides that could not be detected in the culture medium (Figure 8.11b).

Generation of animal models of apoE deficiency and type III hyperlipoproteinemia

The importance of apoE for the clearance of lipoprotein remnants has been established by the generation of mice deficient in apoE (Table 8.6). Comparison of the lipid and lipoprotein profiles of the deficient and

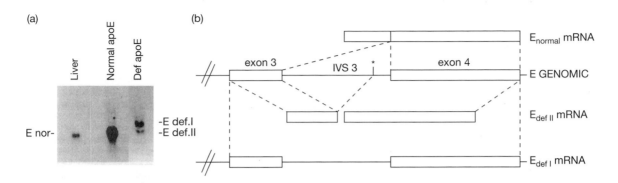

Figure 8.11 (a) Autoradiograph of blotting analysis of RNA isolated from human liver and transformed mouse C127 cells expressing either the normal or apolipoprotein E (apoE)-deficient gene. First lane: mRNA (5 µg) obtained from fetal human liver. Second and third lanes: RNA isolated from one 50 mm diameter Petri dish of clones of C127 cells expressing the normal or deficient apoE gene, respectively. (b) Schematic representation of the mRNA species that are generated by aberrant splicing in the apoE-deficient (E_{def}) gene. The symbol ˙ indicates the position of the activated cryptic splice site, as determined by S1 nuclease mapping and sequence analysis of the deficient apoE gene[198]

control mice on a normal chow diet showed that there was a dramatic increase in total cholesterol in the deficient mice, from approximately 60 mg/dl to 490 mg/dl. All of this increase could be accounted for by increases in the VLDL and LDL cholesterol.[87] More dramatic increases in total VLDL and IDL cholesterol occur when the apoE-deficient mice were fed western-type diets rich in cholesterol and saturated fats (Figure 8.12a). A vitamin A fat tolerance test performed on the apoE-deficient and normal mice showed that the administration of an intragastric bolus of retinol in corn oil impaired the clearance of retinol palmitate esters (which accumulate in the chylomicron remnant fractions) in the deficient but not in the control mice. These observations established that apoE is required for the clearance of the remnants of lipoprotein metabolism which are rich in cholesteryl esters. Patient information as well as genetic mouse studies has established that the formation of these remnants occurs independently of apoE synthesis; however, clearance of these remnants, which float in the VLDL and IDL region, is critically dependent on the presence of apoE. Deficient mice develop coronary and pulmonary atherosclerotic lesions within 10 weeks on a chow diet, which is accelerated further when the animals are placed on western-type diets (Figure 8.12b). Thus, the biochemical and clinical features of apoE deficiency in mice resembles closely the picture observed previously in apoE-deficient humans.

The lesions generated in apoE–/– mice resemble those seen in humans.[286] In mice expressing the human apoE isoforms, aortic root atherosclerosis increased in the following order: murine apoE<apoE3<apoE4<apoE2 (Table 8.6).[287] The extent of atherosclerosis was highly correlated with VLDL clearance.[287] ApoE3- and apoE4 expression in the liver by adenovirus-mediated gene transfer in apoE–/– and apoE–/– nude mice showed that apoE3 limited progression and induced regression of early and advanced lesions, whereas apoE4 had only limited lesion progression but little or no effect on regression. Lesions in apoE3- and apoE4-expressing mice had fewer foam cells, less lipid, and an increased fibrous cap.[288,289]

Adenovirus-mediated gene transfer of apoE in LDLr–/– mice inhibited progression, caused regression of advanced lesions and reduced the content of isoprostanes without a change in lipid or lipoprotein levels, which is a specific marker of lipid peroxidation.[290,291] The lesions had reduced macrophage content and increased extracellular matrix component. In most (but not all cases),[292] low levels of apoE expression by bone marrow transplantation or retroviral gene transfer protected from atherosclerosis.[275,293,294] A reduction in lesions following bone marrow transplantation was found in young animals, but not in older animals with established lesions.[294]

Macrophages derived from apoE3 Leiden and apoE2 transgenics did not protect apoE–/– mice from atherosclerosis, although high levels of expression of

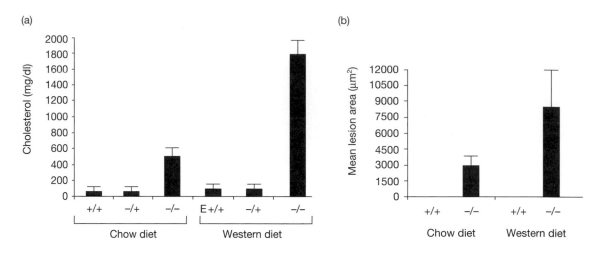

Figure 8.12   (a) Plasma cholesterol levels of apolipoprotein E (apoE)-deficient and control mice maintained on two different diets. Left side, normal chow diet. Right side, western-type diet, consisting of modified chow containing 21% (w/w) fats P/S 0.07, 19.5% (w/w) casein, 0.15% cholesterol, and lacking sodium cholate. (b) Quantitative analysis of atherosclerosis determined in the proximal aorta in apoE-deficient and control mice fed both the mouse chow and western-type diets. Values summarized in the figure represent mean ± standard deviation; +/+, control mice; -/-, homozygous apoE-deficient mice; +/-, heterozygous mice for apoE deficiency. (Adapted from reference 87, with permission)

apoE3 Leiden in apoE–/– × apoE3 Leiden transgenics reduced atherosclerosis.[295] Low expression of apoE in the adrenals protected apoE–/– and LDLr–/– mice from atherosclerosis without a change in plasma lipid levels.[296]

Recently a helper-dependent apoE-expressing adenovirus was used to correct the high-cholesterol profile of apoE–/– mice.[297] It was found that lifelong correction of the high cholesterol profile was achieved in two mice using the appropriate helper virus serotype with one initial injection and reinjection of the virus after 18 months. It is remarkable that, despite the fact that the plasma apoE levels of the cured mice ranged from 1 to 7 mg/dl, the plasma cholesterol was, for most of their lifespan, below 100 mg/dl and the mice were protected from atherosclerosis.[297]

New insights on the in vivo functions of apoE in cholesterol and triglyceride homeostasis using adenovirus-mediated gene transfer

Specific effect of the carboxy-terminal domain of apoE in the induction of hypertriglyceridemia   In humans, apoE levels correlate with plasma triglyceride levels.[282] Similar observations have been reported for experimental animals.[85,298] A series of recent studies used

adenoviruses expressing full-length and truncated genomic apoE sequences to correct the high cholesterol profile of the apoE-deficient (apoE–/–) mice. It was shown that overexpression of full-length apoE (by infection of mice with 1–2 × 10⁹ pfu) did not correct the high cholesterol levels of the apoE–/– mice: in contrast, it induced high triglyceride levels; however, the high cholesterol profile of apoE–/– mice was corrected by infection with truncated apoE forms (Figure 8.13a).[299–302] These studies also showed that infection of C57BL/6 mice with adenoviruses expressing truncated apoE forms that lack the carboxy-terminal region did not change the plasma lipid and lipoprotein profile of the mice, whereas overexpression of full-length apoE induced combined hyperlipidemia, characterized by high cholesterol and high triglyceride levels.[299,302] The greatest concentration of the cholesterol and triglycerides induced by apoE was in the VLDL and IDL region.[299–302] The data suggested either increased production of VLDL or defect(s) in lipolysis and/or remnant clearance.

Other experiments showed that the increase in triglycerides was caused by increased VLDL secretion and decreased lipolysis of the hypertriglyceridemic VLDL. When mice were coinfected with adenoviruses expressing full-length apoE and lipoprotein lipase,

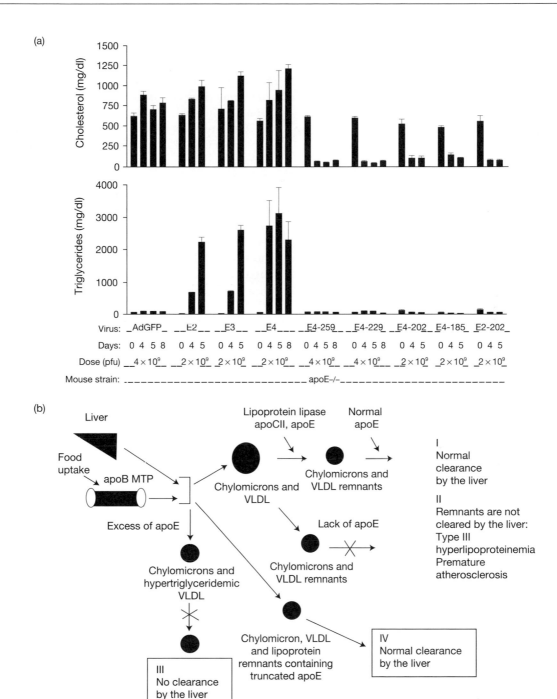

Figure 8.13 (a) Cholesterol and triglyceride levels of apolipoprotein E (apoE) -/- mice infected with the control adenovirus AdGFP, or recombinant adenoviruses expressing apoE2, apoE3, apoE4 or apoE4 carboxy-terminal deletion mutants. (b) Schematic representation of the pathway of biosynthesis and catabolism of chylomicrons. I Normal catabolism. II Defective catabolism of chylomicron remnants due to deficiency in apoE. III Defective catabolism of chylomicrons due to overexpression of apoE. IV Normal clearance of chylomicron, VLDL and lipoprotein remnants by the truncated apoE forms

hypertriglyceridemia was corrected, indicating that under conditions of apoE overexpression the endogenous lipoprotein lipase activity may be rate limiting for the lipolysis and/or clearance of VLDL.

The hypertriglyceridemic effect of the full-length apoE was dose dependent. In transgenic mice expressing human apoE2, dyslipidemia could be corrected by low doses ($2–5 \times 10^8$ pfu) of recombinant adenoviruses expressing full-length apoE, or by high doses of truncated apoE; however, dyslipidemia was aggravated by high doses of full-length apoE.[300,303]

The role of the carboxy-terminal segment of apoE in hypertriglyceridemia is also supported by one additional set of experiments that involved remnant clearance in apoE and LDL receptor double-deficient (apoE–/– × LDLr–/–) mice by truncated apoE forms. This analysis showed that although overexpression of truncated apoE2-202 or apoE4-202 can normalize the high cholesterol and triglyceride profiles of the apoE–/– mice, similar doses of apoE2-202 or apoE4-202 did not correct the high cholesterol profiles of the apoE–/– × LDLr–/– double-deficient mice but did not induce hypertriglyceridemia.[302] On the other hand, infection of the double-deficient mice with the full-length apoE2 or apoE4 induced hypertriglyceridemia in these mice.[302]

Based on *in vivo* and *in vitro* studies, it appears that the truncated apoE forms extending from residue 1 to residues 185 or 202 or 229 or 259 maintain their ability to associate with pre-existing lipoproteins.[299–302] Once apoE is lipoprotein bound, it may be taken up by the LDL receptor and possibly other apoE-recognizing receptors.[299–302] Hypertriglyceridemia may result from a distorted conformation of full-length apoE on the surface of triglyceride-rich lipoprotein particles that mask their receptor-binding domain.

Mechanism of type III hyperlipoproteinemia caused by the E2/E2 phenotype   The E2/E2 phenotype represents an interesting case because it is generally believed that the C for R158 substitution reduces the affinity of apoE for the LDL receptor and results in type III hyperlipoproteinemia.[277,304] Adenovirus-mediated gene transfer of full-length and truncated apoE forms showed that overexpression of apoE2 in apoE–/– mice is associated with high cholesterol and triglyceride levels, whereas overexpression of the truncated apoE2-202 normalizes cholesterol levels of apoE–/– mice and does not trigger hypertriglyceridemia (Figure 8.13a).

Thus, full-length apoE2 behaved *in vivo* like the apoE3 and apoE4 isoforms,[299–302] except that it exacerbated the high cholesterol levels of apoE–/– mice (Figure 8.13a). Unexpectedly, however, the truncated apoE2-202 form behaves *in vivo* like the truncated apoE4-202 form, despite the fact that apoE2-202 retains the C for R158 substitution (Figure 8.13a). Full-length apoE2 induces combined hyperlipidemia in C57BL/6 mice, characterized by high plasma cholesterol and triglyceride levels.

Receptor-binding experiments showed that the removal of the carboxy-terminal 203–299 amino acids of apoE2 increased the affinity of apoE-containing proteoliposomes for the LDLr.[302] A coinfection experiment with full-length apoE2 and lipoprotein lipase suggested that the activity of lipoprotein lipase, rather than apoCII, becomes rate limiting for the clearance of VLDL triglycerides.

Hypertriglyceridemia occurs in a subfraction of individuals who have the apoE2/2 phenotype,[277,305] and it is possible that these dyslipidemic subjects may present the same remnant-clearance defect as the mice overexpressing full-length apoE2, apoE3, and apoE4 isoforms.[277,299–302,305] It is possible that binding of apoE2 to triglyceride-rich VLDL may distort or mask the receptor-binding site of apoE, thus preventing receptor-mediated clearance of triglyceride-rich VLDL.

The LDL receptor may be the predominant receptor for remnant clearance   Experiments using apoE–/– × LDLr–/– double-deficient mice showed that neither the full-length apoE2 or apoE4 nor the truncated apoE2-202 or apoE4-202 corrected the high cholesterol profiles of the apoE–/– × LDLr–/– double-deficient mice.[302] The data indicate that lipoprotein clearance by the truncated apoE forms is mediated mostly by the LDL receptor.

Therapeutic potential of truncated apoE forms   Expression of apoE within a physiological range clears lipoprotein remnants,[303] whereas overexpression of full-length apoE results in hypertriglyceridemia.[299–302] The undesirable side-effect of apoE overexpression significantly diminishes its therapeutic potential. The ability of the truncated apoE forms that lack the carboxy-terminal helices from residues 185 to 299 to clear cholesterol without induction of hypertriglyceridemia[299–302] makes them attractive therapeutic targets in future gene therapy applications to correct remnant removal disorders. Overall, the adenovirus-mediated gene transfer studies reviewed provide the following new information on apoE (Figure 8.13b).

The amino-terminal 1–185 domain of apoE is sufficient to direct receptor-mediated lipoprotein clearance *in vivo*; clearance is mediated mainly by the LDL receptor; the carboxy-terminal 261–299 domain of apoE induces hypertriglyceridemia. Hypertriglyceridemia results partially from increased VLDL secretion, diminished lipolysis, and inefficient VLDL clearance. The dyslipidemia induced by E2 in mice (and possibly in humans) may not be only the result of C for R158 substitution, and can be partially attributed to the carboxy-terminal segment of apoE. Truncated apoE forms have a dominant effect in remnant clearance, and may have future therapeutic applications for the correction of remnant removal disorders (Figure 8.13b).

The HDL pathway: the roles of apoA-I, the ABCA1 lipid transporter and the HDL receptor (SRBI) in the biogenesis and the atheroprotective functions of HDL

Apolipoprotein A-I and HDL

ApoA-I is the major protein component of HDL and plays a key role in the biogenesis and function of HDL. In the absence of apoA-I HDL is not formed.[4,13,18,306–309] ApoA-I has a unique structure that may underlie its functions. ApoA-I contains 22- and 11-amino acid repeats[15] which, based on X-ray crystallography[310] and physicochemical studies,[15] are organized predominantly in amphipathic α-helices (Figure 8.14a). Based on the crystal structure and several structural studies, detailed belt- as well as hairpin-shaped models have been proposed that describe the binding of apoA-I in discoidal and spherical HDL particles (Figure 8.14b).[311,312]

In the belt model, two apolipoprotein A-I molecules are wrapped beltwise around a small discoidal patch of bilayer containing 160 lipid molecules. Each

apoA-I monomer forms a curved, planar, amphipathic α-helical ring (Figure 8.14b). The apoA-I amphipathic helices have an average of approximately 3.67 residues per helical turn (instead of 3.60 residues for the conventional α-helices) and binding to the discoidal HDL with the hydrophobic surface facing inward toward the fatty acyl chains. This apoA-I helix makes three full turns every 11 residues, and provides a physiological meaning to the 11-residue repeats of apoA-I. When the cholesterol of the discoidal particle is esterified, the discs are converted to spheres and apoA-I structure has to readjust on the helical surface. This structure of apoA-I helices contributes to its lipid-binding properties.[312]

Lipid-bound apoA-I activates the enzyme LCAT.[313] Lipid-free apoA-I interacts functionally with ABCA1 to promote lipid efflux from cells.[18] Lipid-bound apoA-I also interacts functionally with SRBI.[17,314,315] On binding to HDL, SRBI mediates selective uptake of cholesteryl esters and other lipids from HDL by cells, and net efflux of excess cholesterol.[315]

Lipid-binding and LCAT activation properties of apoA-I in vitro and in vivo

Analysis of the ability of point mutants in a different region of apoA-I to solubilize multilamellar phospholipid vesicles showed that substitution of a series of charged amino acids between residues 191 and 239 in apoA-I did not substantially affect the ability of the mutant proteins to bind to HDL. In contrast, substitution of the positively charged lysine for specific hydrophobic residues in helix 10 (Leu222, Phe225, Phe229), or substitution of valine residues for the more bulky leucine residues in helix 9 (Leu 211, Leu214, Leu218, Leu219), dramatically altered the ability of the mutant protein to solubilize multilamellar 1,2-dimyristoyl-L-phosphatidylcholine (DMPC) vesicles and to bind to HDL.[315]

Adenovirus-mediated gene transfer in apoA-I-deficient (apoA-I–/–) mice was used to assess the role of the carboxy-terminal amino acids of apoA-I in the biogenesis of HDL.[306] These analyses showed that mutations that prevent binding of apoA-I to phospholipid and HDL *in vitro* result in low apoA-I and HDL levels *in vivo* following gene transfer of mutant apoA-I forms in apoA-I–/– mice. The low apoA-I and HDL levels in these animal models are the result of defective maturation of HDL *in vivo* that traps HDL at the stage of discoidal particles.[306]

Atheroprotective functions of apoA-I and HDL

ApoA-I and HDL have been implicated in the inhibition or regression of atherosclerosis in humans and experimental animals.[316–318] Initial studies showed that overexpression of the apoA-I gene in the atherosclerosis-susceptible C57BL/6 mouse protected the transgenic mice from atherosclerosis in response to a high-fat diet, compared to non-transgenic controls placed on the same diet (Table 8.8).[79] The same effect was observed in atherosclerosis-prone apoE-deficient mice, in which the expression of apoA-I gene significantly reduced lesion formation.[319] Expression of human apoA-I in apoE−/− mice does not influence the expression of VCAM-1 and the early stages of lipid deposition in the subendothelial matrix and monocyte adhesion to the endothelium, indicating that apoA-I exerts its atheroprotective functions through other mechanisms.[320]

ApoB transgenic × apoA-I−/− mice had a 1.8–3.0-fold increase in fatty streak lesions on an atherogenic diet compared to apoB transgenics.[321,322] In addition, when human apoA-I transgenic rabbits were crossed with WHHL rabbits (lacking the LDL receptor), the apoA-I × LDL−/− rabbits had increased HDL cholesterol levels and were protected from atherosclerosis, compared to the control LDL−/− WHHL rabbits.[89] It remains a paradox that apoA-I−/− mice that lack HDL did not develop atherosclerosis on normal or atherogenic diets.[323] It is possible that apoE and apoA-IV associated with HDL may assume some of the antiatherogenic functions of apoA-I and HDL. Human patients with specific defects in apoA-I develop atherosclerosis.[4]

Gene transfer of apoA-I in apoE−/− × apoA-I transgenic or LDLr−/− mice fed a western diet limited the progression of fatty streak lesions and led to lesion regression.[324,325] The expression of apoA-I was necessary to reduce atherosclerosis in apoE−/− mice which express apoE only in macrophages.[326]

Stable expression of apoA-I in LDLr−/− mice using a helper-dependent apoA-I-expressing adenovirus did not alter significantly the plasma lipid profile of the mice.[327] However, the treatment reduced by more than

50% the development of atherosclerosis in response to an atherogenic diet over the 24-month period. It also altered the composition of the atherosclerotic lesions.[327] Most recently, intravenous administration in five doses at weekly intervals of 15 mg/kg of apoA-I Milano/phospholipid complexes in patients with acute coronary syndrome caused a small but statistically significant reduction of coronary atherosclerosis, as determined by intravascular ultrasound.[318] However, the small number of patients studied, and limitations in the methodologies used, necessitates that these suggestive findings be confirmed with larger studies.

HDL and apoA-I have been reported to have antioxidant and anti-inflammatory properties, can alter prostacyclin levels and platelet function, and modulate NO release following interaction of HDL with SRBI.[63,64,328] All these properties may contribute to atheroprotection by HDL.[329]

ApoA-I may directly or indirectly protect against oxidation of LDL. *In vitro*, apoA-I renders LDL resistant to lipoxygenase-mediated oxidation.[61,330,331] An indirect effect rests on the presence on HDL of the antioxidant enzymes paraoxonase and platelet-activating factor-acetyl hydrolase (PAFAH), which prevents the formation of oxidized LDL *in vitro*.[332–334] ApoA-I transgenics both in C57BL/6 and in apoE−/− background or apoA-I gene transfer in apoE−/− mice, resulted in increased levels of both of these antioxidant enzymes.[335] In mice with advanced lesions,[336] the overexpression of human apoA-I or PAFAH reduced macrophage adhesion to the vessel wall. Paraoxonase −/− × apoE−/− mice had increased lipoprotein oxidation and atherosclerosis compared to control mice (Table 8.8).[337]

It has been proposed that oxidized LDL binds to CD36 receptor and disrupts endothelial nitric oxide (eNOS) activation, and that this is reversed by binding of HDL to SRBI.[328] The beneficial effect of HDL on the arterial wall was also demonstrated in subjects with heterozygote deficiency of ABCA1. Low HDL levels in these subjects are associated with impairment in basal and stimulated NO bioactivity, and this defect could be corrected by infusion of discoidal phosphatidylcholine/apoA-I particles.[338]

Functional interactions between apoA-I and ABCA1 in vitro and in vivo

Functional interactions between apoA-I and ABCA1 promote the efflux of cellular cholesterol and

(a) ApoA-I

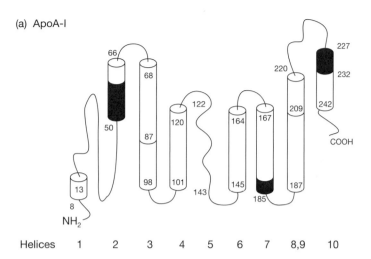

(b) Discoidal HDL

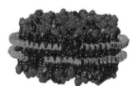

Helices   1   2   3   4   5   6   7   8,9   10

Structure: ApoA-I consists of repeated units that form ten amphipathic α-helices
Functions: ApoA-I is essential for the biogenesis of HDL and has atheroprotective functions
ApoA-I activates LCAT, interacts functionally with ABCA1 and promotes efflux of
cholesterol and phospholipids and interacts functionally with the HDL receptor (SRBI) and
promotes selective lipid uptake and cholesterol efflux

(c) ABCA1

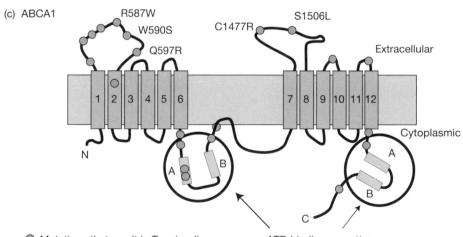

◯ Mutations that result in Tangier disease   ATP-binding cassettes

- ABCA1 is involved in the efflux of cellular cholesterol and phospholipids
- Tangier patients and ABCA1 knockout mice have very low apoA-I and HDL levels
- ABCA1 transgenic mice have decreased plasma cholesterol and apoB levels, have 2–3-fold
  increase in HDL and apoA-I levels and are protected from diet-induced atherosclerosis
- The ABCA1 deficiency in mice did not affect the lipid content and the secretion rates of bile

Figure 8.14   (a) Schematic representation of the boundaries of the α-helical regions of apolipoprotein A (apoA)-I based on computer modeling,[15] X-ray crystallography, and physicochemical studies.[263] Cylinders represent amphipathic α-helices. Predicted amphipathic α-helices are shown in white; additional α-helical regions that were observed by X-ray crystallography are shown in black. (b) Belt model of apolipoprotein (apoA)-I conformation on discoidal high-density lipoprotein (HDL) particles. The figure is adapted from Segrest et al,[312] with permission. (c) Schematic representation of the structure of the ATP-binding cassette A1 (ABCA1) transporter and summary of its functions.[346] Some representative mutations that result in Tangier disease are indicated in the figure. LCAT, lecithin: cholesterol acyltransferase

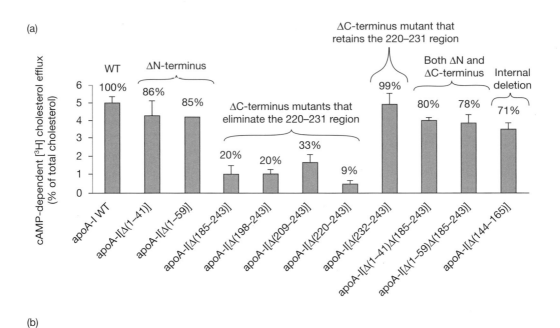

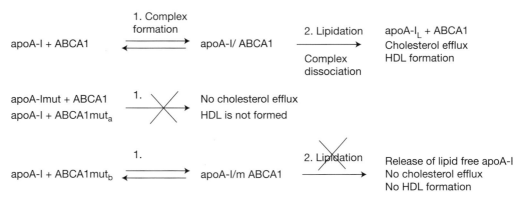

Figure 8.15 (a) cAMP-dependent (ATP-binding cassette-A1 (ABCA1)-mediated) cholesterol efflux in J774 mouse macrophages. Cholesterol efflux studies were performed as described.[18] (b) Two-step model of cholesterol efflux that explains Tangier disease and high-density lipoprotein (HDL) deficiencies. The first step involves complex formation between apolipoprotein (apoA)-I and ABCA1, and the second step involves lipidation of apoA-I and release of the complex. Defects in the two steps may result from either lack of association due to the mutations in apoA-I or ABCA1, or lack of lipidation of the apoA-I acceptor. Both types of defect will inhibit HDL biogenesis

phospholipids and, through a series of intermediate steps, lead to the formation of HDL in the circulation. Human patients or animal models that lack or have defective forms of apoA-I or ABCA1 fail to form HDL. Recent studies established that ABCA1, a member of the ABC family of transporters, is responsible for Tangier disease.[13] ABCA1 is a ubiquitous membrane protein containing 12 membrane-spanning regions and two ATP-binding cassette motifs (Figure 8.14c). ABCA1 is expressed abundantly in the liver, macrophages, lung, adrenal gland, intestine, brain, and other tissues, and at lower levels in the stomach, testis, and other tissues.[13]

Transgenic mice overexpressing human ABCA1 had decreased plasma cholesterol and apoB levels, but a more than two fold increase in HDL-cholesterol and apoA-I levels, and were better protected from atherosclerosis than C57BL/6 mice in response to atherogenic diets (Table 8.8).[339] Unexpectedly, ABCA1 overexpression in apoE−/− mice resulted in a 2–2.6-fold increase in aortic atherosclerosis despite showing little effect on their plasma lipid profile.[339] These findings suggested the potential involvement of ABCA1 in the atheroprotective functions of apoE.

ABCA1−/− mice have lower total serum cholesterol and lipid deposition in various tissues and impaired growth and neuronal development, thus mimicking the phenotype of human Tangier disease patients.[340] ABCA1−/− mice had moderately increased cholesterol absorption in response to a high-cholesterol diet compared to WT mice.[308] Transplantation of normal bone marrow in ABCA1−/− mice indicated that expression of ABCA1 in monocyte/macrophages contributes minimally to HDL formation.[341]

Bone marrow transplantation of ABCA1−/− leukocytes to LDLr−/− did not affect HDL levels, but it increased the amount of macrophages in peripheral blood leukocytes in spleen and liver and also increased atherosclerosis.[342] Similar bone marrow transplantation of ABCA1−/− macrophages in apoE−/− or LDLr−/− mice increased foam cell accumulation and accelerated atherosclerosis in apoE−/− mice.[308]

The role of ABCA1 on the lipid content of bile salts and on bile secretion is not clear. One study found that in ABCA1−/− mice the bile acid content and the secretion rates of biliary cholesterol, bile salts, and phospholipid were not impaired.[343] Another study showed that cholesterol and phospholipid concentrations in the bile of human ABCA1-transgenic mice were increased 1.8-fold, indicating that overexpression of ABCA1 increases biliary lipid secretion.[344]

Domains of apoA-I required for cholesterol efflux, and mode of interaction between apoA-I and ABCA1

Although it is clear that functions of both apoA-I and ABCA1 are critical for the formation of HDL, the question that persisted was, what is the nature of the functional interactions between these two very important proteins.

Systematic *in vitro* studies using a variety of apoA-I mutants showed that:

- The amino-terminal deletions do not affect the ABCA1-mediated lipid efflux.
- The carboxy-terminal deletions that remove the 220–231 region diminished the ABCA1-mediated lipid efflux.
- The carboxy-terminal (232–243) deletion that retains the 220–231 region does not affect the ABCA1-mediated lipid efflux.
- Double amino-terminal and carboxy-terminal deletions which contain only the central helices 3–7 of apoA-I restored the ABCA1-mediated lipid efflux.
- Point mutations and deletions in the central helices 3–7 of apoA-I do not affect ABCA1-mediated lipid efflux (Figure 8.15a).[18,345]

Other studies using direct binding and competition crosslinking experiments showed that apoA-I mutants that fail to promote cholesterol efflux crosslink inefficiently with ABCA1, and those that promote cholesterol efflux crosslink efficiently.[345]

The end-product of the functional interactions between apoA-I and ABCA1 is the biogenesis of HDL. Thus a fundamental question, based on the *in vitro* analysis, is how cholesterol efflux is related to the biogenesis of HDL. This question was addressed by a combination of *in vitro* experiments and adenovirus-mediated gene transfer of apoA-I mutants to apoA-I-deficient mice.[18,306,345–347] These studies showed that:

- ApoA-I mutants that promote cholesterol efflux crosslink efficiently to ABCA1 and vice versa.
- ApoA-I mutants that lack the 220–231 domain are defective in the efflux of cellular cholesterol and phospholipids, and crosslink poorly to ABCA1.
- The carboxy-terminal mutants fail to form discoidal or spherical HDL particles.
- The central region of apoA-I alone, which contains helices 3–7, has the capacity to promote ABCA1-mediated lipid efflux and to form discoidal HDL particles *in vivo*.

Several models have been advanced to explain the ABCA1/apoA-I interactions that lead to lipid efflux. Some proposed that there is no direct association between ABCA1 and apoA-I; rather, they suggested that ABCA1 generates an unstable membrane domain by flipping phosphatidylserine to the outer leaflet of the plasma membrane, which allows docking and subsequent lipidation of the amphipathic helices of apoA-I.[348,349] One of the models, designated hybrid model, proposed that an initial tethering of apoA-I to membranes occurs through the carboxy-terminal apoA-I region, followed by association of apoA-I with ABCA1.[350]

A third intuitive model is the direct association model, which assumes physical interactions between apoA-I and ABCA1,[346] and is supported by *in vitro* and *in vivo* studies by us and others.[345–347] The information obtained from the *in vitro* and *in vivo* studies was used to explain the mode of interaction between apoA-I and ABCA1.

A two-step model in the ABCA1-mediated cholesterol efflux that explains Tangier disease and HDL deficiencies

Previous studies showed that an ABCA1 mutant, ABCA1[W590S], crosslinks more efficiently to apoA-I than wild-type (WT) ABCA1 at 37°C; however, the W590S mutant has defective lipid efflux and is associated with Tangier disease.[346] Analysis of the dissociation of the complexes formed between apoA-I and ABCA1 showed that the rate of dissociation was similar for the WT ABCA1 and the ABCA1[W590S] mutants;[347] however, the apoA-I released from WT ABCA1 was bound to lipids, whereas the apoA-I released from ABCA1[W590S] was lipid free.[347] Taking together all the available *in vitro* and *in vivo* data, we suggest a two-step model of cholesterol efflux that can explain the functional interactions of ABCA1 with apoA-I and other cholesterol acceptors (Figure 8.15b). The first step is the formation of a tight complex between ABCA1 and its ligands. The second step is lipidation of apoA-I and the dissociation of the complex. The first step is strongly supported by the crosslinking data between WT and mutant forms of ABCA1 and apoA-I forms.[18,345,346] Lack of association between ABCA1 and apoA-I variants, or the formation of a weak complex, may prevent lipidation of apoA-I and cholesterol efflux. Formation of a weak complex may, for instance, occur in the case of the carboxy-terminal mutants of apoA-I which were shown to have reduced affinity for ABCA1, as well as in the case of

the various ABCA1 mutants that are associated with Tangier disease and fail to crosslink to ABCA1.[345,346]

The second step in cholesterol efflux is supported by the binding and dissociation studies between WT and mutant forms of apoA-I and ABCA1. It has been shown that WT and mutant forms of apoA-I crosslink with different efficiencies to WT ABCA1 and the W590S mutant.[345] In addition, WT apoA-I forms a complex with ABCA1[W590S] but is released lipid-free.[347] Overall, *in vitro* and *in vivo* analysis of several apoA-I mutants showed that the central helices, along with the 220–231 region, of apoA-I are required for cholesterol efflux *in vitro* and HDL biogenesis *in vivo*. The studies favor direct binding of apoA-I to ABCA1 and provide a molecular explanation for Tangier disease and HDL deficiencies (Figure 8.15b).

Functional interactions between lipid-bound apoA-I and the HDL receptor/scavenger receptor class B type I

SRBI is a membrane protein with two transmembrane regions and two short amino- and carboxy-terminal cytosolic regions (see Figure 8.7). Initial studies involving direct binding and competition experiments established that SRBI is a multiligand receptor that binds HDL, LDL, and modified lipoproteins. SRBI binds to HDL and reconstituted HDL, at least in part by apoA-I.[17,351] On binding to HDL, SRBI mediates selective uptake of both cholesteryl esters and other lipids from HDL to cells, bidirectional movement of unesterified cholesterol, and net efflux of excess cholesterol.[315] Binding of HDL and selective lipid uptake is preserved when purified SRBI is reconstituted into phospholipid/cholesterol liposomes.[351] SRBI has been purified from lysates of cells expressing epitope-tagged SRBI, and was reconstituted into phospholipid/cholesterol liposomes. The reconstituted receptors displayed high-affinity binding and selective lipid uptake.[351] It has recently been shown that interaction of HDL with SRBI activates eNOS.[64] It was proposed that binding of HDL to SRBI initiates tyrosine kinase (Src)-mediated signaling, which leads to parallel activation of protein kinase B (PKB) and mitogen-activated protein (MAP) kinases via phosphatidylinositol 3 (PI3) kinases. These signaling cascades activated the phosphorylation of eNOS and promoted the release of NO.[64] Another study suggested that eNOS activation following binding of HDL to SRBI is not mediated by an increase in the intracellular calcium concentration or by activation of PKB, but rather results from a reversible increase in the intracellular ceramide levels.[352]

Overexpression of SRBI protects mice from atherosclerosis despite the reduction of plasma HDL levels

The physiological importance of SRBI interaction with HDL (apoA-I) has been established by a variety of in vivo studies in mice (Table 8.8). SRBI expression in the liver of mice decreased HDL cholesterol and apoA-I in a dose-dependent manner, irrespective of diet, owing to the accelerated clearance of the HDL. It also decreased plasma VLDL and LDL levels.[353,354]

A deficiency of SRBI in SRBI–/– mice resulted in increased total plasma cholesterol, decreased stores of cholesteryl ester in steroidogenic tissues, and the generation of apoE-enriched HDL-like particles.[355] It also decreased cholesterol secretion without alterations in bile acid secretion, bile acid pool size, or fecal bile excretion.[355–357] The findings suggested that SRBI appears to mediate the transfer of cholesterol from plasma HDL to the bile for excretion, and the delivery of cholesterol to steroidogenic tissues for synthesis of steroid hormones.

Adenovirus-mediated gene transfer of SRBI in LDLr–/– mice with early or advanced lesions reduced plasma apoA-I and HDL levels, had small effects on non-HDL cholesterol levels, and protected the mice from diet-induced atherosclerosis.[358,359] Atherosclerosis was also reduced in SRBI transgenics heterozygous for LDLr background.[360] Using apoB-transgenic × SRBI-transgenic mice, atherosclerosis was reduced in mice that expressed low, but not high, levels of SRBI, suggesting that SRBI exerts a beneficial effect within a certain range.[361] The inactivation of the SRBI gene in mice dramatically accelerated the onset of atherosclerosis in the background of apoE–/– or LDLr–/– mice (Table 8.8).[356,363]

SRBI+/– × apoE–/– mice develop premature occlusive coronary atherosclerosis, spontaneous myocardial infarction, have cardiac hypertrophy and other severe cardiac dysfunctions, and die within 8 weeks of birth. These defects resemble those found in

human patients with coronary heart disease.[364] Remarkably, treatment of the SRBI–/– × apoE–/– mice with probucol extended their life by up to 60 weeks, and reversed most of their cardiac and red blood cell pathologies, as well as their lipid and lipoprotein profiles.[365]

Overall, the combination of in vivo and in vitro studies established that interactions of HDL with SRBI appear to control the structure and composition and concentration of plasma HDL,[315,353–355,359] and the cholesterol contents of the adrenal gland, the ovaries and the bile,[355,357,362] and to protect mice from atherosclerosis (Table 8.8).[356,360–363]

Effect of other proteins on HDL levels, composition, and functions

HDL is remodeled in the circulation by LCAT, CETP, PLTP, LPL, IIL, and EL.[366] CETP transgenic mice had a significant decrease in apoA-I and HDL levels.[367] The HDL and apoA-I levels were restored in human CETP × apoA-I double-transgenic mice.[368] In addition, plasma from these mice expressed in the background of apoE or LDL-receptor deficiency had a proatherogenic effect.[369]

Lecithin cholesterol acyltransferase-transgenic mice have increased atherosclerosis, possibly owing to the generation of an abnormal HDL species. Mice transgenic for human LCAT, or double transgenics for LCAT × apoA-I or LCAT × apoA-II, had increased apoA-I and HDL cholesterol levels.[371,372] Despite this increase, these transgenic animals display marked increases in atherosclerosis compared to controls.[371] Atherosclerosis was reduced by coexpression of LCAT and CETP in transgenic mice.[373] In contrast, the rabbits overexpressing the human LCAT gene had decreased levels of atherosclerotic lesions,[374] indicating the importance of species differences in the development of atherosclerosis (Table 8.8).

Mice transgenic for human PLTP did not have significant changes in plasma lipids and lipoprotein.[375] However, human PLTP × apoA-I transgenic mice increased apoA-I in pre-b HDL levels.[375] In contrast, PLTP–/– mice had a marked decrease in HDL and apoA-I.[376,377] Furthermore, PLTP–/– × apoB-transgenic and PLTP–/– × E–/– mice had markedly decreased atherosclerosis compared to apoB transgenic or apoE–/– mice (Table 8.8).[378]

LPL–/– mice had severe hypertriglyceridemia and very low HDL levels, and survived up to 18 hours after birth.[379] Mice expressing LPL in cardiac muscle had normal plasma triglycerides and HDL.[380] The overexpression of human LPL drastically lowered VLDL and increased HDL,[381] confirming the inverse relationship between hypertriglyceridemia and plasma HDL levels that was observed previously in clinical studies. Bone marrow transplantation of LPL-negative fetal liver cells in C57BL/6 mice resulted in a reduction in lesions in the proximal aorta as compared to mice transplanted with normal fetal liver cells, and had no effect on serum lipid levels (Table 8.8).[382]

HL-deficient mice had elevated levels of large HDL particles enriched in phospholipid and apoE.[383] HL × apoE–/– mice have reduced atherosclerosis compared to apoE–/– mice.[384] Rabbits and mice transgenic for human HL[385–387] have decreased levels of HDL-cholesterol in plasma and decreased HDL particle size. Reduction in aortic cholesterol has been reported in mice that express human HL (Table 8.8).[384] However, rabbits overexpressing HL do not have increased susceptibility to atherosclerosis.[386,387]

Mice deficient in EL have increased HDL levels,[29,30] whereas the EL knockout mice have decreased HDL levels.[30] The impact of EL on the development of atherosclerosis has not yet been determined (Table 8.8).

Acknowledgments

This work was supported by grants from the National Institutes of Health (HL33952, HL48739 and HL68216). We thank Anne Plunkett for preparing the manuscript.

References

1. Zannis VI, Kardassis D, Zanni EE. Genetic mutations affecting human lipoproteins, their receptors, and their enzymes. Adv Hum Genet 1993; 21:145–319.
2. Havel JH, Kane JP. Introduction: structure and metabolism of plasma lipoproteins. In: Scriver CR, Beaudet AL, Sly WS et al, eds. The metabolic and molecular bases of inherited disease. New York: McGraw-Hill, 2001: 2705–2716.
3. Utermann G. Lipoprotein(a). In: Scriver CR, Beaudet AL, Sly WS et al, eds. The metabolic and molecular bases of inherited disease. New York: McGraw-Hill, 2001: 2753–2787.
4. Tall AR, Breslow JL, Rubin EM. Genetic disorders affecting plasma high-density lipoproteins. In: Scriver CR, Beaudet AL, Valle D et al, eds. The metabolic and molecular bases of inherited disease. New York: McGraw-Hill, 2001: 2915–2936.
5. Kane JP, Havel RJ. Disorders of the biogenesis and secretion of lipoproteins containing the B apolipoproteins. In: Scriver CR, Beaudet AL, Valle D et al, eds. The metabolic and molecular bases of inherited disease. New York: McGraw-Hill, 2001: 2717–2752.
6. Brunzell JD, Deeb SS. Familial lipoprotein lipase deficiency, apoC-II deficiency, and hepatic lipase deficiency. In: Scriver CR, Beaudet AL, Valle D et al, eds. The metabolic and molecular bases of inherited disease. New York: McGraw-Hill, 2001: 2789–2816.
7. Mahley RW, Rall SC Jr. Type III hyperlipoproteinemia (dysbetalipoproteinemia): the role of apolipoprotein E in normal and abnormal lipoprotein metabolism. In: Scriver CR, Beaudet AL, Valle D et al, eds. The metabolic and molecular bases of inherited disease. New York: McGraw-Hill, 2001: 2835–2862.
8. Fredrickson DS, Lees RS. Familial hyperlipoproteinemia. In: Stanbury JB, Wyngaarden JB, Fredrickson DS, eds. The metabolic and molecular bases of inherited disease. New York: McGraw-Hill, 1966: 429.
9. Greenberg BH, Blackwelder WC, Levy RI. Primary type V hyperlipoproteinemia. A descriptive study in 32 families. Ann Intern Med 1977; 87:526–534.
10. Anderson KM, Wilson PW, Odell PM et al. An updated coronary risk profile. A statement for health professionals. Circulation 1991; 83:356–362.
11. Goldstein JL, Hobbs HH, Brown MS. Familial hypercholesterolemia. In: Scriver CR, Beaudet AL, Valle D et al, eds. The metabolic and molecular bases of inherited disease. New York: McGraw Hill, 2001: 2863–2913.
12. Santamarina-Fojo S, Hoeg JM, Assmann G et al. Lecithin cholesterol acyltransferase deficiency and fish eye disease. In: Scriver CR, Beaudet AL, Sly WS et al, eds. The metabolic and molecular bases of inherited disease. New York: McGraw-Hill, 2001: 2817–2834.
13. Assmann G, von Eckardstein A, Brewer HB. Familial analphalipoproteinemia: Tangier disease. In: Scriver CR, Beaudet AL, Sly WS et al, eds. The Metabolic and Molecular Basis of Inherited Disease. New York: McGraw-Hill, 2001: 2937–2960.
14. Allan CM, Walker D, Segrest JP et al. Identification and characterization of a new human gene (APOC4) in the apolipoprotein E, C-I, and C-II gene locus. Genomics 1995; 28:291–300.
15. Nolte RT, Atkinson D. Conformational analysis of apolipoprotein A-I and E-3 based on primary sequence and circular dichroism. Biophys J 1992; 63:1221–1239.
16. Segrest JP, Jones MK, Mishra VK et al. apoB-100 has a pentapartite structure composed of three amphipathic alpha-helical domains alternating with two amphipathic beta-strand domains. Detection by the computer program LOCATE. Arterioscler Thromb 1994; 14:1674–1685.

17. Liadaki KN, Liu T, Xu S et al. Binding of high density lipoprotein (HDL) and discoidal reconstituted HDL to the HDL receptor scavenger receptor class B type I. Effect of lipid association and APOA-I mutations on receptor binding. J Biol Chem 2000; 275:21262–21271.

18. Chroni A, Liu T, Gorshkova I et al. The central helices of apoA-I can promote ATP-binding cassette transporter A1 (ABCA1)-mediated lipid efflux. Amino acid residues 220–231 of the wild-type apoA-I are required for lipid efflux in vitro and high density lipoprotein formation in vivo. J Biol Chem 2003; 278:6719–6730.

19. Moestrup SK, Kozyraki R. Cubilin, a high-density lipoprotein receptor. Curr Opin Lipidol 2000; 11:133–140.

20. Fielding CJ, Shore VG, Fielding PE. A protein cofactor of lecithin: cholesterol acyltransferase. Biochem Biophys Res Commun 1972; 46:1493–1498.

21. Chen CH, Albers JJ. Activation of lecithin: cholesterol acyltransferase by apolipoproteins E-2, E-3, and A-IV isolated from human plasma. Biochim Biophys Acta 1985; 836:279–285.

22. Krauss RM, Herbert PN, Levy RI et al. Further observations on the activation and inhibition of lipoprotein lipase by apolipoproteins. Circ Res 1973; 33:403–411.

23. Kowal RC, Herz J, Weisgraber KH et al. Opposing effects of apolipoproteins E and C on lipoprotein binding to low density lipoprotein receptor-related protein. J Biol Chem 1990; 265:10771–10779.

24. Marais AD. Therapeutic modulation of low-density lipoprotein size. Curr Opin Lipidol 2000; 11:597–602.

25. Zambon A, Austin MA, Brown BG et al. Effect of hepatic lipase on LDL in normal men and those with coronary artery disease. Arterioscler Thromb 1993; 13:147–153.

26. Jaye M, Lynch KJ, Krawiec J et al. A novel endothelial-derived lipase that modulates HDL metabolism. Nature Genet 1999; 21:424–428.

27. Hirata K, Dichek HL, Cioffi JA et al. Cloning of a unique lipase from endothelial cells extends the lipase gene family. J Biol Chem 1999; 274:14170–14175.

28. Rader DJ, Jaye M. Endothelial lipase: a new member of the triglyceride lipase gene family. Curr Opin Lipidol 2000; 11:141–147.

29. Ma K, Cilingiroglu M, Otvos JD et al. Endothelial lipase is a major genetic determinant for high-density lipoprotein concentration, structure, and metabolism. Proc Natl Acad Sci USA 2003; 100:2748–2753.

30. Ishida T, Choi S, Kundu RK et al. Endothelial lipase is a major determinant of HDL level. J Clin Invest 2003; 111:347–355.

31. Funke H, von Eckardstein A, Pritchard PH et al. A molecular defect causing fish eye disease: an amino acid exchange in lecithin-cholesterol acyltransferase (LCAT) leads to the selective loss of alpha-LCAT activity. Proc Natl Acad Sci USA 1991; 88:4855–4859.

32. Drayna D, Jarnagin AS, McLean J et al. Cloning and sequencing of human cholesteryl ester transfer protein cDNA. Nature 1987; 327:632–634.

33. Chajek T, Fielding CJ. Isolation and characterization of a human serum cholesteryl ester transfer protein. Proc Natl Acad Sci USA 1978; 75:3445–3449.

34. van Tol A. Phospholipid transfer protein. Curr Opin Lipidol 2002; 13:135–139.

35. Huuskonen J, Olkkonen VM, Jauhiainen M et al. The impact of phospholipid transfer protein (PLTP) on HDL metabolism. Atherosclerosis 2001; 155:269–281.

36. Gimbrone MA Jr. Vascular endothelium, hemodynamic forces, and atherogenesis. Am J Pathol 1999; 155:1–5.

37. Cybulsky MI, Gimbrone MA Jr. Endothelial expression of a mononuclear leukocyte adhesion molecule during atherogenesis. Science 1991; 251:788–791.

38. Peters W, Charo IF. Involvement of chemokine receptor 2 and its ligand, monocyte chemoattractant protein-1, in the development of atherosclerosis: lessons from knockout mice. Curr Opin Lipidol 2001; 12:175–180.

39. Han KH, Han KO, Green SR et al. Expression of the monocyte chemoattractant protein-1 receptor CCR2 is increased in hypercholesterolemia. Differential effects of plasma lipoproteins on monocyte function. J Lipid Res 1999; 40:1053–1063.

40. Yamada Y, Doi T, Hamakubo T et al. Scavenger receptor family proteins: roles for atherosclerosis, host defence and disorders of the central nervous system. Cell Mol Life Sci 1998; 54:628–640.

41. Horkko S, Binder CJ, Shaw PX et al. Immunological responses to oxidized LDL. Free Radical Biol Med 2000; 28:1771–1779.

42. Ross R. Atherosclerosis – an inflammatory disease. N Engl J Med 1999; 340:115–126.

43. Virmani R, Kolodgie FD, Burke AP et al. Lessons from sudden coronary death: a comprehensive morphological classification scheme for atherosclerotic lesions. Arterioscler Thromb Vasc Biol 2000; 20:1262–1275.

44. Getz GS. When is atherosclerosis not atherosclerosis? Arterioscler Thromb Vasc Biol 2000; 20:1694.

45. Reardon CA, Getz GS. Mouse models of atherosclerosis. Curr Opin Lipidol 2001; 12:167–173.

46. Glass CK, Witztum JL. Atherosclerosis. the road ahead. Cell 2001; 104:503–516.

47. Curtiss LK, Boisvert WA. Apolipoprotein E and atherosclerosis. Curr Opin Lipidol 2000; 11:243–251.

48. Hansson GK. Cell-mediated immunity in atherosclerosis. Curr Opin Lipidol 1997; 8:301–311.

49. Colles SM, Irwin KC, Chisolm GM. Roles of multiple oxidized LDL lipids in cellular injury: dominance of 7 beta-hydroperoxycholesterol. J Lipid Res 1996; 37:2018–2028.

50. Lee RT, Libby P. The unstable atheroma. Arterioscler Thromb Vasc Biol 1997; 17:1859–1867.

51. Faber BC, Heeneman S, Daemen MJ et al. Genes potentially involved in plaque rupture. Curr Opin Lipidol 2002; 13:545–552.

52. Kolodgie FD, Gold HK, Burke AP et al. Intraplaque hemorrhage and progression of coronary atheroma. N Engl J Med 2003; 349:2316–2325.

53. Lusis AJ. Atherosclerosis. Nature 2000; 407:233–241.

54. Knowles JW, Reddick RL, Jennette JC et al. Enhanced atherosclerosis and kidney dysfunction in eNOS(–/–)Apoe(–/–) mice are ameliorated by enalapril treatment. J Clin Invest 2000; 105:451–458.

55. Tamminen M, Mottino G, Qiao JH et al. Ultrastructure of early lipid accumulation in ApoE-deficient mice. Arterioscler Thromb Vasc Biol 1999; 19:847–853.

56. Boren J, Gustafsson M, Skalen K et al. Role of extracellular retention of low density lipoproteins in atherosclerosis. Curr Opin Lipidol 2000; 11:451–456.

57. Hurt-Camejo E, Camejo G, Sartipy P. Phospholipase A2 and small, dense low-density lipoprotein. Curr Opin Lipidol 2000; 11:465–471.

58. Ivandic B, Castellani LW, Wang XP et al. Role of group II secretory phospholipase A2 in atherosclerosis: 1. Increased atherogenesis and altered lipoproteins in transgenic mice expressing group IIa phospholipase A2. Arterioscler Thromb Vasc Biol 1999; 19:1284–1290.

59. Leitinger N, Watson AD, Hama SY et al. Role of group II secretory phospholipase A2 in atherosclerosis: 2. Potential involvement of biologically active oxidized phospholipids. Arterioscler Thromb Vasc Biol 1999; 19:1291–1298.

60. Febbraio M, Hajjar DP, Silverstein RL. CD36: a class B scavenger receptor involved in angiogenesis, atherosclerosis, inflammation, and lipid metabolism. J Clin Invest 2001; 108:785–791.

61. Navab M, Hama SY, Anantharamaiah GM et al. Normal high density lipoprotein inhibits three steps in the formation of mildly oxidized low density lipoprotein: steps 2 and 3. J Lipid Res 2000; 41:1495–1508.

62. Schmitz G, Langmann T. Structure, function and regulation of the ABC1 gene product. Curr Opin Lipidol 2001; 12:129–140.

63. Mineo C, Yuhanna IS, Quon MJ et al. High density lipoprotein-induced endothelial nitric-oxide synthase activation is mediated by Akt and MAP kinases. J Biol Chem 2003; 278:9142–9149.

64. Yuhanna IS, Zhu Y, Cox BE et al. High-density lipoprotein binding to scavenger receptor-BI activates endothelial nitric oxide synthase. Nature Med 2001; 7:853–857.

65. Shi W, Wang NJ, Shih DM et al. Determinants of atherosclerosis susceptibility in the C3H and C57BL/6 mouse model: evidence for involvement of endothelial cells but not blood cells or cholesterol metabolism. Circ Res 2000; 86:1078–1084.

66. Grimsditch DC, Penfold S, Latcham J et al. C3H apoE(–/–) mice have less atherosclerosis than C57BL apoE(–/–) mice despite having a more atherogenic serum lipid profile. Atherosclerosis 2000; 151:389–397.

67. Dansky HM, Charlton SA, Sikes JL et al. Genetic background determines the extent of atherosclerosis in ApoE-deficient mice. Arterioscler Thromb Vasc Biol 1999; 19:1960–1968.

68. Mehrabian M, Wong J, Wang X et al. Genetic locus in mice that blocks development of atherosclerosis despite extreme hyperlipidemia. Circ Res 2001; 89:125–130.

69. Sjoland H, Eitzman DT, Gordon D et al. Atherosclerosis progression in LDL receptor-deficient and apolipoprotein E-deficient mice is independent of genetic alterations in plasminogen activator inhibitor-1. Arterioscler Thromb Vasc Biol 2000; 20:846–852.

70. Breslow JL. Mouse models of atherosclerosis. Science 1996; 272:685–688.

71. Powell-Braxton L, Veniant M, Latvala RD et al. A mouse model of human familial hypercholesterolemia: markedly elevated low density lipoprotein cholesterol levels and severe atherosclerosis on a low-fat chow diet. Nature Med 1998; 4:934–938.

72. Sanan DA, Newland DL, Tao R et al. Low density lipoprotein receptor-negative mice expressing human apolipoprotein B-100 develop complex atherosclerotic lesions on a chow diet: no accentuation by apolipoprotein(a). Proc Natl Acad Sci USA 1998; 95:4544–4549.

73. Napoli C, Glass CK, Witztum JL et al. Influence of maternal hypercholesterolaemia during pregnancy on progression of early atherosclerotic lesions in childhood: Fate of Early Lesions in Children (FELIC) study. Lancet 1999; 354:1234–1241.

74. Napoli C, Witztum JL, Calara F et al. Maternal hypercholesterolemia enhances atherogenesis in normocholesterolemic rabbits, which is inhibited by antioxidant or lipid-lowering intervention during pregnancy: an experimental model of atherogenic mechanisms in human fetuses. Circ Res 2000; 87:946–952.

75. Napoli C, de Nigris F, Welch JS et al. Maternal hypercholesterolemia during pregnancy promotes early atherogenesis in LDL receptor-deficient mice and alters aortic gene expression determined by microarray. Circulation 2002; 105:1360–1367.

76. Tsimikas S, Shortal BP, Witztum JL et al. In vivo uptake of radiolabeled MDA2, an oxidation-specific monoclonal antibody, provides an accurate measure of atherosclerotic lesions rich in oxidized LDL and is highly sensitive to their regression. Arterioscler Thromb Vasc Biol 2000; 20:689–697.

77. Walsh A, Ito Y, Breslow JL. High levels of human apolipoprotein A-I in transgenic mice result in increased plasma levels of small high density lipoprotein (HDL) particles comparable to human HDL3. J Biol Chem 1989; 264:6488–6494.

78. Chiesa G, Johnson DF, Yao Z et al. Expression of human apolipoprotein B100 in transgenic mice. Editing of human apolipoprotein B100 mRNA. J Biol Chem 1993; 268:23747–23750.

79. Rubin EM, Krauss RM, Spangler EA et al. Inhibition of early atherogenesis in transgenic mice by human apolipoprotein AI. Nature 1991; 353:265–267.

80. Purcell-Huynh DA, Farese RV Jr, Johnson DF et al. Transgenic mice expressing high levels of human apolipoprotein B develop severe atherosclerotic lesions in response to a high-fat diet. J Clin Invest 1995; 95:2246–2257.

81. Boisfer E, Lambert G, Atger V et al. Overexpression of human apolipoprotein A-II in mice induces

hypertriglyceridemia due to defective very low density lipoprotein hydrolysis. J Biol Chem 1999; 274:11564–11572.

82. Warden CH, Hedrick CC, Qiao JH et al. Atherosclerosis in transgenic mice overexpressing apolipoprotein A-II. Science 1993; 261:469–472.

83. Kalopissis AD, Pastier D, Chambaz J. Apolipoprotein A-II: beyond genetic associations with lipid disorders and insulin resistance. Curr Opin Lipidol 2003; 14:165–172.

84. Shimano H, Yamada N, Katsuki M et al. Overexpression of apolipoprotein E in transgenic mice: marked reduction in plasma lipoproteins except high density lipoprotein and resistance against diet-induced hypercholesterolemia. Proc Natl Acad Sci USA 1992; 89:1750–1754.

85. Huang Y, Liu XQ, Rall SC Jr et al. Overexpression and accumulation of apolipoprotein E as a cause of hypertriglyceridemia. J Biol Chem 1998; 273:26388–26393.

86. Zannis VI, Chroni A, Kypreos KE et al. Probing the pathways of chylomicron and HDL metabolism using adenovirus-mediated gene transfer. Curr Opin Lipidol 2004; 15:151–166.

87. Plump AS, Smith JD, Hayek T et al. Severe hypercholesterolemia and atherosclerosis in apolipoprotein E-deficient mice created by homologous recombination in ES cells. Cell 1992; 71:343–353.

88. Ito Y, Azrolan N, O'Connell A et al. Hypertriglyceridemia as a result of human apo CIII gene expression in transgenic mice. Science 1990; 249:790–793.

89. Duverger N, Tremp G, Caillaud JM et al. Protection against atherogenesis in mice mediated by human apolipoprotein A-IV. Science 1996; 273:966–968.

90. Cohen RD, Castellani LW, Qiao JH et al. Reduced aortic lesions and elevated high density lipoprotein levels in transgenic mice overexpressing mouse apolipoprotein A-IV. J Clin Invest 1997; 99:1906–1916.

91. Knowles JW, Maeda N. Genetic modifiers of atherosclerosis in mice. Arterioscler Thromb Vasc Biol 2000; 20:2336–2345.

92. Dong ZM, Brown AA, Wagner DD. Prominent role of P-selectin in the development of advanced atherosclerosis in ApoE-deficient mice. Circulation 2000; 101:2290–2295.

93. Dong ZM, Chapman SM, Brown AA et al. The combined role of P- and E-selectins in atherosclerosis. J Clin Invest 1998; 102:145–152.

94. Collins RG, Velji R, Guevara NV et al. P-Selectin or intercellular adhesion molecule (ICAM)-1 deficiency substantially protects against atherosclerosis in apolipoprotein E-deficient mice. J Exp Med 2000; 191:189–194.

95. Cushing SD, Berliner JA, Valente AJ et al. Minimally modified low density lipoprotein induces monocyte chemotactic protein 1 in human endothelial cells and smooth muscle cells. Proc Natl Acad Sci USA 1990; 87:5134–5138.

96. Rajavashisth TB, Andalibi A, Territo MC et al. Induction of endothelial cell expression of granulocyte and macrophage colony-stimulating factors by modified low-density lipoproteins. Nature 1990; 344:254–257.

97. Berliner JA, Territo MC, Sevanian A et al. Minimally modified low density lipoprotein stimulates monocyte endothelial interactions. J Clin Invest 1990; 85:1260–1266.

98. Boring L, Gosling J, Cleary M et al. Decreased lesion formation in CCR2−/− mice reveals a role for chemokines in the initiation of atherosclerosis. Nature 1998; 394:894–897.

99. Gu L, Okada Y, Clinton SK et al. Absence of monocyte chemoattractant protein-1 reduces atherosclerosis in low density lipoprotein receptor-deficient mice. Mol Cell 1998; 2:275–281.

100. Gosling J, Slaymaker S, Gu L et al. MCP-1 deficiency reduces susceptibility to atherosclerosis in mice that overexpress human apolipoprotein B. J Clin Invest 1999; 103:773–778.

101. Boisvert WA, Santiago R, Curtiss LK et al. A leukocyte homologue of the IL-8 receptor CXCR-2 mediates the accumulation of macrophages in atherosclerotic lesions of LDL receptor-deficient mice. J Clin Invest 1998; 101:353–363.

102. Smith JD, Trogan E, Ginsberg M et al. Decreased atherosclerosis in mice deficient in both macrophage colony-stimulating factor (op) and apolipoprotein E. Proc Natl Acad Sci USA 1995; 92:8264–8268.

103. Qiao JH, Tripathi J, Mishra NK et al. Role of macrophage colony-stimulating factor in atherosclerosis: studies of osteopetrotic mice. Am J Pathol 1997; 150:1687–1699.

104. Herijgers N, Van Eck M, Groot PH et al. Low density lipoprotein receptor of macrophages facilitates atherosclerotic lesion formation in C57Bl/6 mice. Arterioscler Thromb Vasc Biol 2000; 20:1961–1967.

105. Cyrus T, Witztum JL, Rader DJ et al. Disruption of the 12/15-lipoxygenase gene diminishes atherosclerosis in apo E-deficient mice. J Clin Invest 1999; 103:1597–1604.

106. Harats D, Shaish A, George J et al. Overexpression of 15-lipoxygenase in vascular endothelium accelerates early atherosclerosis in LDL receptor-deficient mice. Arterioscler Thromb Vasc Biol 2000; 20:2100–2105.

107. Dwyer JH, Allayee H, Dwyer KM et al. Arachidonate 5-lipoxygenase promoter genotype, dietary arachidonic acid, and atherosclerosis. N Engl J Med 2004; 350:29–37.

108. Mehrabian M, Allayee H, Wong J et al. Identification of 5-lipoxygenase as a major gene contributing to atherosclerosis susceptibility in mice. Circ Res 2002; 91:120–126.

109. Brennan ML, Penn MS, Van Lente F et al. Prognostic value of myeloperoxidase in patients with chest pain. N Engl J Med 2003; 349:1595–1604.

110. Brennan ML, Anderson MM, Shih DM et al. Increased atherosclerosis in myeloperoxidase-deficient mice. J Clin Invest 2001; 107:419–430.

111. Detmers PA, Hernandez M, Mudgett J et al. Deficiency in inducible nitric oxide synthase results in reduced atherosclerosis in apolipoprotein E-deficient mice. J Immunol 2000; 165:3430–3435.

112. Behr-Roussel D, Rupin A, Simonet S et al. Effect of chronic treatment with the inducible nitric oxide synthase inhibitor N-iminoethyl-L-lysine or with L-arginine on progression of coronary and aortic atherosclerosis in hypercholesterolemic rabbits. Circulation 2000; 102:1033–1038.

113. Nicoletti A, Paulsson G, Caligiuri G et al. Induction of neonatal tolerance to oxidized lipoprotein reduces

atherosclerosis in ApoE knockout mice. Mol Med 2000; 6:283–290.

114. Schonbeck U, Sukhova GK, Shimizu K et al. Inhibition of CD40 signaling limits evolution of established atherosclerosis in mice. Proc Natl Acad Sci USA 2000; 97:7458–7463.

115. Cladaras C, Hadzopoulou-Cladaras M, Nolte RT et al. The complete sequence and structural analysis of human apolipoprotein B-100: relationship between apoB-100 and apoB-48 forms. EMBO J 1986; 5:3495–3507.

116. Anant S, Davidson NO. Molecular mechanisms of apolipoprotein B mRNA editing. Curr Opin Lipidol 2001; 12:159–165.

117. Goldstein JL, Brown MS. The low-density lipoprotein pathway and its relation to atherosclerosis. Annu Rev Biochem 1977; 46:897–930.

118. Soria LF, Ludwig EH, Clarke HR et al. Association between a specific apolipoprotein B mutation and familial defective apolipoprotein B-100. Proc Natl Acad Sci USA 1989; 86:587–591.

119. Pullinger CR, Hennessy LK, Chatterton JE et al. Familial ligand-defective apolipoprotein B. Identification of a new mutation that decreases LDL receptor binding affinity. J Clin Invest 1995; 95:1225–1234.

120. Shelness GS, Sellers JA. Very-low-density lipoprotein assembly and secretion. Curr Opin Lipidol 2001; 12:151–157.

121. Wetterau JR, Aggerbeck LP, Bouma ME et al. Absence of microsomal triglyceride transfer protein in individuals with abetalipoproteinemia. Science 1992; 258:999–1001.

122. Haffner SM, D'Agostino R Jr, Goff D et al. LDL size in African Americans, Hispanics, and non-Hispanic whites : the insulin resistance atherosclerosis study. Arterioscler Thromb Vasc Biol 1999; 19:2234–2240.

123. Stampfer MJ, Krauss RM, Ma J et al. A prospective study of triglyceride level, low-density lipoprotein particle diameter, and risk of myocardial infarction. J Am Med Assoc 1996; 276:882–888.

124. Okumura K, Matsui H, Kawakami K et al. Relationship between the apolipoprotein E and angiotensin-converting enzyme genotypes and LDL particle size in Japanese subjects. Clin Chim Acta 1999; 285:91–103..

125. Friedlander Y, Kark JD, Sinnreich R et al. Inheritance of LDL peak particle diameter: results from a segregation analysis in Israeli families. Genet Epidemiol 1999; 16:382–396..

126. Austin MA, Stephens K, Walden CE et al. Linkage analysis of candidate genes and the small, dense low-density lipoprotein phenotype. Atherosclerosis 1999; 142:79–87.

127. Kazumi T, Kawaguchi A, Hozumi T et al. Low density lipoprotein particle diameter in young, nonobese, normolipidemic Japanese men. Atherosclerosis 1999; 142:113–119.

128. Festa A, D'Agostino R Jr, Mykkanen L et al. Low-density lipoprotein particle size is inversely related to plasminogen activator inhibitor-1 levels. The Insulin Resistance Atherosclerosis Study. Arterioscler Thromb Vasc Biol 1999; 19:605–610.

129. Hokanson JE, Brunzell JD, Jarvik GP et al. Linkage of low-density lipoprotein size to the lipoprotein lipase gene in heterozygous lipoprotein lipase deficiency. Am J Hum Genet 1999; 64:608–618.

130. Allayee H, Dominguez KM, Aouizerat BE et al. Contribution of the hepatic lipase gene to the atherogenic lipoprotein phenotype in familial combined hyperlipidemia. J Lipid Res 2000; 41:245–252.

131. Liu ML, Bergholm R, Makimattila S et al. A marathon run increases the susceptibility of LDL to oxidation in vitro and modifies plasma antioxidants. Am J Physiol 1999; 276:E1083–E1091.

132. Dreon DM, Fernstrom HA, Williams PT et al. A very low-fat diet is not associated with improved lipoprotein profiles in men with a predominance of large, low-density lipoproteins. Am J Clin Nutr 1999; 69:411–418.

133. Tinker LF, Parks EJ, Behr SR et al. (n-3) fatty acid supplementation in moderately hypertriglyceridemic adults changes postprandial lipid and apolipoprotein B responses to a standardized test meal. J Nutr 1999; 129:1126–1134.

134. Brown MS, Goldstein JL. A receptor-mediated pathway for cholesterol homeostasis (Nobel Lecture). Angew Chem Int Ed Engl 1986; 25:583–602.

135. Dwyer JH, Allayee H, Dwyer KM et al. Arachidonate 5-lipoxygenase promoter genotype, dietary arachidonic acid, and atherosclerosis. N Engl J Med 2004; 350:29–37.

136. Hobbs HH, Russell DW, Brown MS et al. The LDL receptor locus in familial hypercholesterolemia: mutational analysis of a membrane protein. Annu Rev Genet 1990; 24:133–170.

137. Krieger M, Herz J. Structures and functions of multiligand lipoprotein receptors: macrophage scavenger receptors and LDL receptor-related protein (LRP). Annu Rev Biochem 1994; 63:601–637.

138. Herz J, Hamann U, Rogne S et al. Surface location and high affinity for calcium of a 500-kd liver membrane protein closely related to the LDL-receptor suggest a physiological role as lipoprotein receptor. EMBO J 1988; 7:4119–4127.

139. Chappell DA, Fry GL, Waknitz MA et al. The low density lipoprotein receptor-related protein/alpha 2-macroglobulin receptor binds and mediates catabolism of bovine milk lipoprotein lipase. J Biol Chem 1992; 267:25764–25767.

140. Takahashi S, Kawarabayasi Y, Nakai T et al. Rabbit very low density lipoprotein receptor: a low density lipoprotein receptor-like protein with distinct ligand specificity. Proc Natl Acad Sci USA 1992; 89:9252–9256.

141. Sakai J, Hoshino A, Takahashi S et al. Structure, chromosome location, and expression of the human very low density lipoprotein receptor gene. J Biol Chem 1994; 269:2173–2182.

142. Kim DH, Iijima H, Goto K et al. Human apolipoprotein E receptor 2. A novel lipoprotein receptor of the low density lipoprotein receptor family predominantly expressed in brain. J Biol Chem 1996; 271:8373–8380.

143. Bersot TP, Mahley RW, Brown MS et al. Interaction of swine lipoproteins with the low density lipoprotein receptor in human fibroblasts. J Biol Chem 1976; 251:2395–2398.

144. Pitas RE, Innerarity TL, Mahley RW. Cell surface receptor binding of phospholipid . protein complexes containing different ratios of receptor-active and -inactive E apoprotein. J Biol Chem 1980; 255:5454–5460.

145. Goldstein JL, Anderson RG, Brown MS. Coated pits, coated vesicles, and receptor-mediated endocytosis. Nature 1979; 279:679–685.

146. Maxfield FR. Weak bases and ionophores rapidly and reversibly raise the pH of endocytic vesicles in cultured mouse fibroblasts. J Cell Biol 1982; 95:676–681.

147. Brown MS, Anderson RG, Goldstein JL. Recycling receptors: the round-trip itinerary of migrant membrane proteins. Cell 1983; 32:663–667.

148. Brown MS, Dana SE, Goldstein JL. Regulation of 3-hydroxy-3-methylglutaryl coenzyme A reductase activity in cultured human fibroblasts. Comparison of cells from a normal subject and from a patient with homozygous familial hypercholesterolemia. J Biol Chem 1974; 249:789–796.

149. Goldstein JL, Dana SE, Brown MS. Esterification of low density lipoprotein cholesterol in human fibroblasts and its absence in homozygous familial hypercholesterolemia. Proc Natl Acad Sci USA 1974; 71:4288–4292.

150. Basu SK, Goldstein JL, Brown MS. Characterization of the low density lipoprotein receptor in membranes prepared from human fibroblasts. J Biol Chem 1978; 253:3852–3856.

151. Schneider WJ, Beisiegel U, Goldstein JL et al. Purification of the low density lipoprotein receptor, an acidic glycoprotein of 164,000 molecular weight. J Biol Chem 1982; 257:2664–2673.

152. Tolleshaug H, Goldstein JL, Schneider WJ et al. Posttranslational processing of the LDL receptor and its genetic disruption in familial hypercholesterolemia. Cell 1982; 30:715–724.

153. Russell DW, Yamamoto T, Schneider WJ et al. cDNA cloning of the bovine low density lipoprotein receptor: feedback regulation of a receptor mRNA. Proc Natl Acad Sci USA 1983; 80:7501–7505.

154. Sudhof TC, Goldstein JL, Brown MS et al. The LDL receptor gene: a mosaic of exons shared with different proteins. Science 1985; 228:815–822.

155. Esser V, Limbird LE, Brown MS et al. Mutational analysis of the ligand binding domain of the low density lipoprotein receptor. J Biol Chem 1988; 263:13282–13290.

156. Russell DW, Brown MS, Goldstein JL. Different combinations of cysteine-rich repeats mediate binding of low density lipoprotein receptor to two different proteins. J Biol Chem 1989; 264:21682–21688.

157. Cummings RD, Kornfeld S, Schneider WJ et al. Biosynthesis of N- and O-linked oligosaccharides of the low density lipoprotein receptor. J Biol Chem 1983; 258:15261–15273.

158. Goldstein JL, Kita T, Brown MS. Defective lipoprotein receptors and atherosclerosis. Lessons from an animal counterpart of familial hypercholesterolemia. N Engl J Med 1983; 309:288–296.

159. Schneider WJ, Brown MS, Goldstein JL. Kinetic defects in the processing of the low density lipoprotein receptor in fibroblasts from WHHL rabbits and a family with familial hypercholesterolemia. Mol Biol Med 1983; 1:353–367.

160. Tolleshaug H, Hobgood KK, Brown MS et al. The LDL receptor locus in familial hypercholesterolemia: multiple mutations disrupt transport and processing of a membrane receptor. Cell 1983; 32:941–951.

161. Davis CG, van Driel IR, Russell DW et al. The low density lipoprotein receptor. Identification of amino acids in cytoplasmic domain required for rapid endocytosis. J Biol Chem 1987; 262:4075–4082.

162. Miyake Y, Tajima S, Funahashi T et al. Analysis of a recycling-impaired mutant of low density lipoprotein receptor in familial hypercholesterolemia. J Biol Chem 1989; 264:16584–16590.

163. Davis CG, Goldstein JL, Sudhof TC et al. Acid-dependent ligand dissociation and recycling of LDL receptor mediated by growth factor homology region. Nature 1987; 326:760–765.

164. Zuliani G, Arca M, Signore A et al. Characterization of a new form of inherited hypercholesterolemia: familial recessive hypercholesterolemia. Arterioscler Thromb Vasc Biol 1999; 19:802–809.

165. Cohen JC, Kimmel M, Polanski A et al. Molecular mechanisms of autosomal recessive hypercholesterolemia. Curr Opin Lipidol 2003; 14:121–127.

166. Arca M, Zuliani G, Wilund K et al. Autosomal recessive hypercholesterolaemia in Sardinia, Italy, and mutations in ARH: a clinical and molecular genetic analysis. Lancet 2002; 359:841–847.

167. Gagne C, Bays HE, Weiss SR et al. Efficacy and safety of ezetimibe added to ongoing statin therapy for treatment of patients with primary hypercholesterolemia. Am J Cardiol 2002; 90:1084–1091.

168. Bilheimer DW, Grundy SM, Brown MS et al. Mevinolin and colestipol stimulate receptor-mediated clearance of low density lipoprotein from plasma in familial hypercholesterolemia heterozygotes. Proc Natl Acad Sci USA 1983; 80:4124–4128.

169. Krieger M. Metabolism and movement of lipids. In: Lodish HF, ed. Molecular cell biology. New York: WH Freeman and Co, 2003: 743–777.

170. Hua X, Yokoyama C, Wu J et al. SREBP-2, a second basic–helix–loop–helix–leucine zipper protein that stimulates transcription by binding to a sterol regulatory element. Proc Natl Acad Sci USA 1993; 90:11603–11607.

171. Wang X, Sato R, Brown MS et al. SREBP-1, a membrane-bound transcription factor released by sterol-regulated proteolysis. Cell 1994; 77:53–62.

172. Oliner JD, Andresen JM, Hansen SK et al. SREBP transcriptional activity is mediated through an interaction with the CREB-binding protein. Genes Dev 1996; 10:2903–2911.

173. Brown MS, Goldstein JL. The SREBP pathway: regulation of cholesterol metabolism by proteolysis of a membrane-bound transcription factor. Cell 1997; 89:331–340.

174. Wang X, Pai JT, Wiedenfeld EA et al. Purification of an interleukin-1 beta converting enzyme-related cysteine protease that cleaves sterol regulatory element-binding proteins between the leucine zipper and transmembrane domains. J Biol Chem 1995; 270:18044–18050.

175. Wang X, Zelenski NG, Yang J et al. Cleavage of sterol regulatory element binding proteins (SREBPs) by CPP32 during apoptosis. EMBO J 1996; 15:1012–1020.

176. Hofmann SL, Russell DW, Brown MS et al. Overexpression of low density lipoprotein (LDL) receptor eliminates LDL from plasma in transgenic mice. Science 1988; 239:1277–1281.

177. Yokode M, Hammer RE, Ishibashi S et al. Diet-induced hypercholesterolemia in mice: prevention by overexpression of LDL receptors. Science 1990; 250:1273–1275.

178. Ishibashi S, Brown MS, Goldstein JL et al. Hypercholesterolemia in low density lipoprotein receptor knockout mice and its reversal by adenovirus-mediated gene delivery. J Clin Invest 1993; 92:883–893.

179. Ishibashi S, Herz J, Maeda N et al. The two-receptor model of lipoprotein clearance: tests of the hypothesis in 'knockout' mice lacking the low density lipoprotein receptor, apolipoprotein E, or both proteins. Proc Natl Acad Sci USA 1994; 91:4431–4435.

180. Strickland DK, Ashcom JD, Williams S et al. Sequence identity between the alpha 2-macroglobulin receptor and low density lipoprotein receptor-related protein suggests that this molecule is a multifunctional receptor. J Biol Chem 1990; 265:17401–17404.

181. Herz J, Kowal RC, Goldstein JL et al. Proteolytic processing of the 600 kDa low density lipoprotein receptor-related protein (LRP) occurs in a trans-Golgi compartment. EMBO J 1990; 9:1769–1776.

182. Weisgraber KH, Mahley RW, Kowal RC et al. Apolipoprotein C-I modulates the interaction of apolipoprotein E with beta-migrating very low density lipoproteins (beta-VLDL) and inhibits binding of beta-VLDL to low density lipoprotein receptor-related protein. J Biol Chem 1990; 265:22453–22459.

183. Willnow TE, Goldstein JL, Orth K et al. Low density lipoprotein receptor-related protein and gp330 bind similar ligands, including plasminogen activator–inhibitor complexes and lactoferrin, an inhibitor of chylomicron remnant clearance. J Biol Chem 1992; 267:26172–26180.

184. Herz J, Clouthier DE, Hammer RE. LDL receptor-related protein internalizes and degrades uPA–PAI-1 complexes and is essential for embryo implantation. Cell 1992; 71:411–421..

185. Raychowdhury R, Niles JL, McCluskey RT et al. Autoimmune target in Heymann nephritis is a glycoprotein with homology to the LDL receptor. Science 1989; 244:1163–1165.

186. Kerjaschki D, Farquhar MG. Immunocytochemical localization of the Heymann nephritis antigen (GP330) in glomerular epithelial cells of normal Lewis rats. J Exp Med 1983; 157:667–686.

187. Frykman PK, Brown MS, Yamamoto T et al. Normal plasma lipoproteins and fertility in gene-targeted mice homozygous for a disruption in the gene encoding very low density lipoprotein receptor. Proc Natl Acad Sci USA 1995; 92:8453–8457.

188. Kim DH, Magoori K, Inoue TR et al. Exon/intron organization, chromosome localization, alternative splicing, and transcription units of the human apolipoprotein E receptor 2 gene. J Biol Chem 1997; 272:8498–8504.

189. Li X, Kypreos K, Zanni EE et al. Domains of apoE required for binding to apoE receptor 2 and to phospholipids: iImplications for the functions of apoE in the brain. Biochemistry 2003; 42:10406–10417.

190. Herz J, Beffert U. Apolipoprotein E receptors: linking brain development and Alzheimer's disease. Nat Rev Neurosci 2000; 1:51–58.

191. Fogelman AM, Shechter I, Seager J et al. Malondialdehyde alteration of low density lipoproteins leads to cholesteryl ester accumulation in human monocyte-macrophages. Proc Natl Acad Sci USA 1980; 77:2214–2218.

192. Esterbauer H, Jurgens G, Quehenberger O et al. Autoxidation of human low density lipoprotein: loss of polyunsaturated fatty acids and vitamin E and generation of aldehydes. J Lipid Res 1987; 28:495–509.

193. Brown MS, Goldstein JL. Lipoprotein metabolism in the macrophage: implications for cholesterol deposition in atherosclerosis. Annu Rev Biochem 1983; 52:223–261.

194. Brown MS, Ho YK, Goldstein JL. The cholesteryl ester cycle in macrophage foam cells. Continual hydrolysis and re-esterification of cytoplasmic cholesteryl esters. J Biol Chem 1980; 255:9344–9352.

195. Brown MS, Goldstein JL, Krieger M et al. Reversible accumulation of cholesteryl esters in macrophages incubated with acetylated lipoproteins. J Cell Biol 1979; 82:597–613.

196. Kodama T, Reddy P, Kishimoto C et al. Purification and characterization of a bovine acetyl low density lipoprotein receptor. Proc Natl Acad Sci USA 1988; 85:9238–9242.

197. Kodama T, Freeman M, Rohrer L et al. Type I macrophage scavenger receptor contains alpha-helical and collagen-like coiled coils. Nature 1990; 343:531–535.

198. Rohrer L, Freeman M, Kodama T et al. Coiled-coil fibrous domains mediate ligand binding by macrophage scavenger receptor type II. Nature 1990; 343:570–572.

199. Matsumoto A, Naito M, Itakura H et al. Human macrophage scavenger receptors: primary structure, expression, and localization in atherosclerotic lesions. Proc Natl Acad Sci USA 1990; 87:9133–9137.

200. de Winther MP, Van Dijk KW, Havekes LM et al. Macrophage scavenger receptor class A: a multifunctional receptor in atherosclerosis. Arterioscler Thromb Vasc Biol 2000; 20:290–297.

201. Babaev VR, Gleaves LA, Carter KJ et al. Reduced atherosclerotic lesions in mice deficient for total or macrophage-specific expression of scavenger receptor-A. arterioscler Thromb Vasc Biol 2000; 20:2593–2599.

202. Herijgers N, de Winther MP, Van Eck M et al. Effect of human scavenger receptor class A overexpression in bone

marrow-derived cells on lipoprotein metabolism and atherosclerosis in low density lipoprotein receptor knockout mice. J Lipid Res 2000; 41:1402–1409.

203. Van Eck M, de Winther MP, Herijgers N et al. Effect of human scavenger receptor class A overexpression in bone marrow-derived cells on cholesterol levels and atherosclerosis in ApoE- deficient mice. Arterioscler Thromb Vasc Biol 2000; 20:2600–2606.

204. de Winther MP, Gijbels MJ, Van Dijk KW et al. Scavenger receptor deficiency leads to more complex atherosclerotic lesions in APOE3Leiden transgenic mice. Atherosclerosis 1999; 144:315–321.

205. Oquendo P, Hundt E, Lawler J et al. CD36 directly mediates cytoadherence of *Plasmodium falciparum* parasitized erythrocytes. Cell 1989; 58:95–101.

206. Silverstein RL, Febbraio M. CD36 and atherosclerosis. Curr Opin Lipidol 2000; 11:483–491.

207. Endemann G, Stanton LW, Madden KS et al. CD36 is a receptor for oxidized low density lipoprotein. J Biol Chem 1993; 268:11811–11816.

208. Platt N, Da Silva RP, Gordon S. Recognizing death: the phagocytosis of apoptotic cells. Trends Cell Biol 1998; 8:365–372.

209. Krieger M. The other side of scavenger receptors: pattern recognition for host defense. Curr Opin Lipidol 1997; 8:275–280.

210. Podrez EA, Febbraio M, Sheibani N et al. Macrophage scavenger receptor CD36 is the major receptor for LDL modified by monocyte-generated reactive nitrogen species. J Clin Invest 2000; 105:1095–1108.

211. Ibrahimi A, Bonen A, Blinn WD et al. Muscle-specific overexpression of FAT/CD36 enhances fatty acid oxidation by contracting muscle, reduces plasma triglycerides and fatty acids, and increases plasma glucose and insulin. J Biol Chem 1999; 274:26761–26766.

212. Nozaki S, Tanaka T, Yamashita S et al. CD36 mediates long-chain fatty acid transport in human myocardium: complete myocardial accumulation defect of radiolabeled long-chain fatty acid analog in subjects with CD36 deficiency. Mol Cell Biochem 1999; 192:129–135.

213. Jimenez B, Volpert OV, Crawford SE et al. Signals leading to apoptosis-dependent inhibition of neovascularization by thrombospondin-1. Nature Med 2000; 6:41–48.

214. Yehualaeshet T, O'Connor R, Green-Johnson J et al. Activation of rat alveolar macrophage-derived latent transforming growth factor beta-1 by plasmin requires interaction with thrombospondin-1 and its cell surface receptor, CD36. Am J Pathol 1999; 155:841–851.

215. Fadok VA, Bratton DL, Konowal A et al. Macrophages that have ingested apoptotic cells in vitro inhibit proinflammatory cytokine production through autocrine/paracrine mechanisms involving TGF-beta, PGE2, and PAF. J Clin Invest 1998; 101:890–898.

216. Aitman TJ, Glazier AM, Wallace CA et al. Identification of Cd36 (Fat) as an insulin-resistance gene causing defective fatty acid and glucose metabolism in hypertensive rats. Nature Genet 1999; 21:76–83.

217. Febbraio M, Abumrad NA, Hajjar DP et al. A null mutation in murine CD36 reveals an important role in fatty acid and lipoprotein metabolism. J Biol Chem 1999; 274:19055–19062.

218. Febbraio M, Podrez EA, Smith JD et al. Targeted disruption of the class B scavenger receptor CD36 protects against atherosclerotic lesion development in mice. J Clin Invest 2000; 105:1049–1056.

219. Utermann G. Lipoprotein(a): a genetic risk factor for premature coronary heart disease. Curr Opin Lipidol 1995; 1:404–410.

220. McLean JW, Tomlinson JE, Kuang WJ et al. cDNA sequence of human apolipoprotein(a) is homologous to plasminogen. Nature 1987; 330:132–137.

221. Callow MJ, Stoltzfus LJ, Lawn RM et al. Expression of human apolipoprotein B and assembly of lipoprotein(a) in transgenic mice. Proc Natl Acad Sci USA 1994; 91:2130–2134.

222. Linton MF, Farese RV Jr, Chiesa G et al. Transgenic mice expressing high plasma concentrations of human apolipoprotein B100 and lipoprotein(a). J Clin Invest 1993; 92:3029 3037.

223. Chiesa G, Hobbs HH, Koschinsky ML et al. Reconstitution of lipoprotein(a) by infusion of human low density lipoprotein into transgenic mice expressing human apolipoprotein(a). J Biol Chem 1992; 267:24369–24374.

224. Lawn RM, Wade DP, Hammer RE et al. Atherogenesis in transgenic mice expressing human apolipoprotein(a). Nature 1992; 360:670–672.

225. Krempler F, Kostner GM, Bolzano K et al. Turnover of lipoprotein (a) in man. J Clin Invest 1980; 65:1483–1490.

226. Salonen EM, Jauhiainen M, Zardi L et al. Lipoprotein(a) binds to fibronectin and has serine proteinase activity capable of cleaving it. EMBO J 1989; 8:4035–4040

227. Gavish D, Azrolan N, Breslow JL. Plasma Ip(a) concentration is inversely correlated with the ratio of Kringle IV/Kringle V encoding domains in the apo(a) gene. J Clin Invest 1989; 84:2021–2027.

228. Harpel PC, Gordon BR, Parker TS. Plasmin catalyzes binding of lipoprotein (a) to immobilized fibrinogen and fibrin. Proc Natl Acad Sci USA 1989; 86:3847–3851.

229. Loscalzo J, Weinfeld M, Fless GM et al. Lipoprotein(a), fibrin binding, and plasminogen activation. Arteriosclerosis 1990; 10:240–245.

230. Edelberg JM, Gonzalez-Gronow M, Pizzo SV. Lipoprotein a inhibits streptokinase-mediated activation of human plasminogen. Biochemistry 1989; 28:2370–2374.

231. Edelberg JM, Gonzalez-Gronow M, Pizzo SV. Lipoprotein(a) inhibition of plasminogen activation by tissue-type plasminogen activator. Thromb Res 1990; 57:155–162.

232. Clemmensen I, Petersen LC, Kluft C. Purification and characterization of a novel, oligomeric, plasminogen kringle 4 binding protein from human plasma: tetranectin. Eur J Biochem 1986; 156:327–333.

233. Etingin OR, Hajjar DP, Hajjar KA et al. Lipoprotein (a) regulates plasminogen activator inhibitor-1 expression in

endothelial cells. A potential mechanism in thrombogenesis. J Biol Chem 1991; 266:2459–2465.

234. Rath M, Niendorf A, Reblin T et al. Detection and quantification of lipoprotein(a) in the arterial wall of 107 coronary bypass patients. Arteriosclerosis 1989; 9:579–592.

235. Borth W, Chang V, Bishop P et al. Lipoprotein (a) is a substrate for factor XIIIa and tissue transglutaminase. J Biol Chem 1991; 266:18149–18153.

236. Klezovitch O, Edelstein C, Zhu L et al. Apolipoprotein(a) binds via its C-terminal domain to the protein core of the proteoglycan decorin. Implications for the retention of lipoprotein(a) in atherosclerotic lesions. J Biol Chem 1998; 273:23856–23865.

237. Harpel PC, Chang TS, Verderber E. Tissue plasminogen activator and urokinase mediate the binding of Glu-plasminogen to plasma fibrin I. Evidence for new binding sites in plasmin-degraded fibrin I. J Biol Chem 1985; 260:4432–4440.

238. Zioncheck TF, Powell LM, Rice GC et al. Interaction of recombinant apolipoprotein(a) and lipoprotein(a) with macrophages. J Clin Invest 1991; 87:767–771.

239. Syrovets T, Thillet J, Chapman MJ et al. Lipoprotein(a) is a potent chemoattractant for human peripheral monocytes. Blood 1997; 90:2027–2036.

240. Poon M, Zhang X, Dunsky KG et al. Apolipoprotein(a) induces monocyte chemotactic activity in human vascular endothelial cells. Circulation 1997; 96:2514–2519.

241. Kojima S, Harpel PC, Rifkin DB. Lipoprotein (a) inhibits the generation of transforming growth factor beta: an endogenous inhibitor of smooth muscle cell migration. J Cell Biol 1991; 113:1439–1445.

242. Yano Y, Seishima M, Tokoro Y et al. Stimulatory effects of lipoprotein(a) and low-density lipoprotein on human umbilical vein endothelial cell migration and proliferation are partially mediated by fibroblast growth factor-2. Biochim Biophys Acta 1998; 1393:26–34.

243. Grainger DJ, Kemp PR, Liu AC et al. Activation of transforming growth factor-beta is inhibited in transgenic apolipoprotein(a) mice. Nature 1994; 370:460–462.

244. Takami S, Yamashita S, Kihara S et al. Lipoprotein(a) enhances the expression of intercellular adhesion molecule-1 in cultured human umbilical vein endothelial cells. Circulation 1998; 97:721–728.

245. Allen S, Khan S, Tam S et al. Expression of adhesion molecules by lp(a): a potential novel mechanism for its atherogenicity. FASEB J 1998; 12:1765–1776.

246. Liu AC, Lawn RM, Verstuyft JG et al. Human apolipoprotein A-I prevents atherosclerosis associated with apolipoprotein[a] in transgenic mice. J Lipid Res 1994; 35:2263–2267.

247. Boonmark NW, Lou XJ, Yang ZJ et al. Modification of apolipoprotein(a) lysine binding site reduces atherosclerosis in transgenic mice. J Clin Invest 1997; 100:558–564.

248. Callow MJ, Verstuyft J, Tangirala R et al. Atherogenesis in transgenic mice with human apolipoprotein B and lipoprotein (a). J Clin Invest 1995; 96:1639–1646.

249. Seed M, Hoppichler F, Reaveley D et al. Relation of serum lipoprotein(a) concentration and apolipoprotein(a) phenotype to coronary heart disease in patients with familial hypercholesterolemia. N Engl J Med 1990; 322:1494–1499.

250. Dahlen GH, Guyton JR, Attar M et al. Association of levels of lipoprotein Lp(a), plasma lipids, and other lipoproteins with coronary artery disease documented by angiography. Circulation 1986; 74:758–765.

251. Kronenberg F, Steinmetz A, Kostner GM et al. Lipoprotein(a) in health and disease. Crit Rev Clin Lab Sci 1996; 33:495–543.

252 Carlson LA, Hamsten A, Asplund A. Pronounced lowering of serum levels of lipoprotein Lp(a) in hyperlipidaemic subjects treated with nicotinic acid. J Intern Med 1989; 226:271–276..

253 Palabrica TM, Liu AC, Aronovitz MJ et al. Antifibrinolytic activity of apolipoprotein(a) in vivo: human apolipoprotein(a) transgenic mice are resistant to tissue plasminogen activator-mediated thrombolysis. Nature Med 1995; 1:256–259.

254. Garcia Frade LJ, Alvarez JJ, Rayo I et al. Fibrinolytic parameters and lipoprotein (a) levels in plasma of patients with coronary artery disease. Thromb Res 1991; 63:407–418.

255. Kochl S, Fresser F, Lobentanz E et al. Novel interaction of apolipoprotein(a) with beta-2 glycoprotein I mediated by the kringle IV domain. Blood 1997; 90:1482–1489.

256. Harpel PC, Chang VT, Borth W. Homocysteine and other sulfhydryl compounds enhance the binding of lipoprotein(a) to fibrin: a potential biochemical link between thrombosis, atherogenesis, and sulfhydryl compound metabolism. Proc Natl Acad Sci USA 1992; 89:10193–10197.

257. Bjorkhem I, Boberg KM, Leitersdorf E. Inborn errors in bile acid biosynthesis and storage of sterols other than cholesterol. In: Scriver CR, Beaudet AL, Valle D et al eds. The metabolic and molecular bases of inherited disease. New York: McGraw-Hill, 2001: 2961–2988.

258. Russell DW, Setchell KD. Bile acid biosynthesis. Biochemistry 1992; 31:4737–4749.

259. Bjorkhem I, Eggertsen G. Genes involved in initial steps of bile acid synthesis. Curr Opin Lipidol 2001; 12:97–103.

260. Lee MH, Lu K, Patel SB. Genetic basis of sitosterolemia. Curr Opin Lipidol 2001; 12:141–149.

261. Fayard E, Schoonjans K, Auwerx J. Xol INXS: role of the liver X and the farnesol X receptors. Curr Opin Lipidol 2001; 12:113–120.

262. Figge A, Lammert F, Paigen B et al. Hepatic overexpression of murine abcb11 increases hepatobiliary lipid secretion and reduces hepatic steatosis. J Biol Chem 2004; 279:2790–2799.

263. Wang R, Lam P, Liu L et al. Severe cholestasis induced by cholic acid feeding in knockout mice of sister of P-glycoprotein. Hepatology 2003; 38:1489–1499.

264. Rosmorduc O, Hermelin B, Boelle PY et al. ABCB4 gene mutation-associated cholelithiasis in adults. Gastroenterology 2003; 125:452–459.

265. Mangelsdorf DJ, Thummel C, Beato M et al. The nuclear receptor superfamily: the second decade. Cell 1995; 83:835–839.

266. Repa JJ, Mangelsdorf DJ. Nuclear receptor regulation of cholesterol and bile acid metabolism. Curr Opin Biotechnol 1999; 10:557–563.

267. Willy PJ, Umesono K, Ong ES et al. LXR, a nuclear receptor that defines a distinct retinoid response pathway. Genes Dev 1995; 9:1033–1045.

268. Makishima M, Okamoto AY, Repa JJ et al. Identification of a nuclear receptor for bile acids. Science 1999; 284:1362–1365.

269. Parks DJ, Blanchard SG, Bledsoe RK et al. Bile acids: natural ligands for an orphan nuclear receptor. Science 1999; 284:1365–1368.

270. Wang H, Chen J, Hollister K et al. Endogenous bile acids are ligands for the nuclear receptor FXR/BAR. Mol Cell 1999; 3:543–553.

271. Herz J, Willnow TE. Lipoprotein and receptor interactions in vivo. Curr Opin Lipidol 1995; 6:97–103.

272. Schaefer EJ, Gregg RE, Ghiselli G et al. Familial apolipoprotein E deficiency. J Clin Invest 1986; 78:1206–1219.

273. Huang Y, von Eckardstein A, Wu S et al. A plasma lipoprotein containing only apolipoprotein E and with gamma mobility on electrophoresis releases cholesterol from cells. Proc Natl Acad Sci USA 1994; 91:1834–1838.

274. Shimano H, Ohsuga J, Shimada M et al. Inhibition of diet-induced atheroma formation in transgenic mice expressing apolipoprotein E in the arterial wall. J Clin Invest 1995; 95:469–476.

275. Linton MF, Fazio S. Macrophages, lipoprotein metabolism, and atherosclerosis: insights from murine bone marrow transplantation studies. Curr Opin Lipidol 1999; 10:97–105.

276. Zannis VI, Just PW, Breslow JL. Human apolipoprotein E isoprotein subclasses are genetically determined. Am J Hum Genet 1981; 33:11–24.

277. Breslow JL, Zannis VI, SanGiacomo TR et al. Studies of familial type III hyperlipoproteinemia using as a genetic marker the apoE phenotype E2/2. J Lipid Res 1982; 23:1224–1235.

278. Corder EH, Saunders AM, Strittmatter WJ et al. Gene dose of apolipoprotein E type 4 allele and the risk of Alzheimer's disease in late onset families. Science 1993; 261:921–923.

279. Corder EH, Saunders AM, Strittmatter WJ et al. Gene dose of apolipoprotein E type 4 allele and the risk of Alzheimer's disease in late onset families. Science 1993; 261:921–923.

280. Wilson C, Wardell MR, Weisgraber KH et al. Three-dimensional structure of the LDL receptor-binding domain of human apolipoprotein E. Science 1991; 252:1817–1822.

281. Zannis VI, Zanni EE, Makrides SC et al. Role of apolipoprotein E in Alzheimer's disease. In: Catravas JD ed. NATO ASI Series, Life Sciences. New York: Plenum Press, 1998: 179–209.

282. Havel RJ, Kotite L, Vigne JL et al. Radioimmunoassay of human arginine-rich apolipoprotein, apoprotein E. Concentration in blood plasma and lipoproteins as affected by apoprotein E-3 deficiency. J Clin Invest 1980; 66:1351–1362.

283. Lalazar A, Weisgraber KH, Rall SC Jr, et al. Site-specific mutagenesis of human apolipoprotein E. Receptor binding activity of variants with single amino acid substitutions. J Biol Chem 1988; 263:3542–3545.

284. Ghiselli G, Schaefer EJ, Gascon P et al. Type III hyperlipoproteinemia associated with apolipoprotein E deficiency. Science 1981; 214:1239–1241.

285. Cladaras C, Hadzopoulou-Cladaras M, Felber BK et al. The molecular basis of a familial apoE deficiency. An acceptor splice site mutation in the third intron of the deficient apoE gene. J Biol Chem 1987; 262:2310–2315.

286. Rosenfeld ME, Polinsky P, Virmani R et al. Advanced atherosclerotic lesions in the innominate artery of the ApoE knockout mouse. Arterioscler Thromb Vasc Biol 2000; 20:2587–2592.

287. Knouff C, Hinsdale ME, Mezdour H et al. Apo E structure determines VLDL clearance and atherosclerosis risk in mice. J Clin Invest 1999; 103:1579–1586.

288. Tsukamoto K, Tangirala R, Chun SH et al. Rapid regression of atherosclerosis induced by liver-directed gene transfer of ApoE in ApoE-deficient mice. Arterioscler Thromb Vasc Biol 1999; 19:2162–2170.

289. Desurmont C, Caillaud JM, Emmanuel F et al. Complete atherosclerosis regression after human ApoE gene transfer in ApoE-deficient/nude mice. Arterioscler Thromb Vasc Biol 2000; 20:435–442.

290. Tangirala RK, Pratico D, FitzGerald GA et al. Reduction of isoprostanes and regression of advanced atherosclerosis by apolipoprotein E. J Biol Chem 2001; 276:261–266.

291. Tsukamoto K, Tangirala RK, Chun S et al. Hepatic expression of apolipoprotein E inhibits progression of atherosclerosis without reducing cholesterol levels in LDL receptor-deficient mice. Mol Ther 2000; 1:189–194.

292. Boisvert WA, Curtiss LK. Elimination of macrophage-specific apolipoprotein E reduces diet-induced atherosclerosis in C57BL/6J male mice. J Lipid Res 1999; 40:806–813.

293. Van Eck M, Herijgers N, Vidgeon-Hart M et al. Accelerated atherosclerosis in C57Bl/6 mice transplanted with ApoE-deficient bone marrow. Atherosclerosis 2000; 150:71–80.

294. Hasty AH, Linton MF, Brandt SJ et al. Retroviral gene therapy in ApoE-deficient mice: ApoE expression in the artery wall reduces early foam cell lesion formation. Circulation 1999; 99:2571–2576.

295. Van Eck M, Zimmermann R, Groot PH et al. Role of macrophage-derived lipoprotein lipase in lipoprotein metabolism and atherosclerosis. Arterioscler Thromb Vasc Biol 2000; 20:E53–E62.

296. Thorngate FE, Rudel LL, Walzem RL et al. Low levels of extrahepatic nonmacrophage ApoE inhibit atherosclerosis without correcting hypercholesterolemia in ApoE-deficient mice. Arterioscler Thromb Vasc Biol 2000; 20:1939–1945.

297. Kim IH, Jozkowicz A, Piedra PA et al. Lifetime correction of genetic deficiency in mice with a single injection of helper-dependent adenoviral vector. Proc Natl Acad Sci USA 2001; 98:13282–13287.

298. Huang Y, Liu XQ, Rall SC Jr et al. Apolipoprotein E2 reduces the low density lipoprotein level in transgenic mice by impairing lipoprotein lipase-mediated lipolysis of triglyceride-rich lipoproteins. J Biol Chem 1998; 273:17483–17490.

299. Kypreos KE, Morani P, Van Dijk KW et al. The amino-terminal 1-185 domain of apoE promotes the clearance of lipoprotein remnants in vivo. The carboxy-terminal domain is required for induction of hyperlipidemia in normal and apoE-deficient mice. Biochemistry 2001; 40:6027–6035.

300. Kypreos KE, Van Dijk KW, van Der ZA et al. Domains of apolipoprotein E contributing to triglyceride and cholesterol homeostasis in vivo. Carboxyl-terminal region 203-299 promotes hepatic very low density lipoprotein-triglyceride secretion. J Biol Chem 2001; 276:19778–19786.

301. Kypreos KE, Teusink B, Van Dijk KW et al. Analysis of the structure and function relationship of the human apolipoprotein E in vivo, using adenovirus-mediated gene transfer. FASEB J 2001; 15:1598–1600.

302. Kypreos KE, Li X, Van Dijk KW et al. Molecular mechanisms of type III hyperlipoproteinemia: the contribution of the carboxy-terminal domain of apoE can account for the dyslipidemia that is associated with the E2/E2 phenotype. Biochemistry 2003; 42:9841–9853.

303. Gerritsen G, Kypreos KE, van Der ZA et al. Hyperlipidemia in APOE2 transgenic mice is ameliorated by a truncated apoE variant lacking the C-terminal domain. J Lipid Res 2003; 44:408–414.

304. Rall SC Jr, Weisgraber KH, Innerarity TL et al. Structural basis for receptor binding heterogeneity of apolipoprotein E from type III hyperlipoproteinemic subjects. Proc Natl Acad Sci USA 1982; 79:4696–4700.

305. Hazzard WR, Warnick GR, Utermann G et al. Genetic transmission of isoapolipoprotein E phenotypes in a large kindred: relationship to dysbetalipoproteinemia and hyperlipidemia. Metabolism 1981; 30:79–88.

306. Reardon CA, Kan HY, Cabana V et al. In vivo studies of HDL assembly and metabolism using adenovirus-mediated transfer of ApoA-I mutants in ApoA-I-deficient mice. Biochemistry 2001; 40:13670–13680.

307. Matsunaga T, Hiasa Y, Yanagi H et al. Apolipoprotein A-I deficiency due to a codon 84 nonsense mutation of the apolipoprotein A-I gene. Proc Natl Acad Sci USA 1991; 88:2793–2797.

308. McNeish J, Aiello RJ, Guyot D et al. High density lipoprotein deficiency and foam cell accumulation in mice with targeted disruption of ATP-binding cassette transporter-1. Proc Natl Acad Sci USA 2000; 97:4245–4250.

309. Williamson R, Lee D, Hagaman J et al. Marked reduction of high density lipoprotein cholesterol in mice genetically modified to lack apolipoprotein A-I. Proc Natl Acad Sci USA 1992; 89:7134–7138.

310. Borhani DW, Rogers DP, Engler JA et al. Crystal structure of truncated human apolipoprotein A-I suggests a lipid-bound conformation. Proc Natl Acad Sci USA 1997; 94:12291–12296.

311. Marcel YL, Kiss RS. Structure-function relationships of apolipoprotein A-I: a flexible protein with dynamic lipid associations. Curr Opin Lipidol 2003; 14:151–157.

312. Segrest JP, Li L, Anantharamaiah GM et al. Structure and function of apolipoprotein A-I and high-density lipoprotein. Curr Opin Lipidol 2000; 11:105–115.

313. Soutar AK, Garner CW, Baker HN et al. Effect of the human plasma apolipoproteins and phosphatidylcholine acyl donor on the activity of lecithin: cholesterol acyltransferase. Biochemistry 1975; 14:3057–3064.

314. Acton S, Rigotti A, Landschulz KT et al. Identification of scavenger receptor SRBI as a high density lipoprotein receptor. Science 1996; 271:518–520.

315. Krieger M. Scavenger receptor class B type I is a multiligand HDL receptor that influences diverse physiologic systems. J Clin Invest 2001; 108:793–797.

316. Gordon DJ, Probstfield JL, Garrison RJ et al. High-density lipoprotein cholesterol and cardiovascular disease. Four prospective American studies. Circulation 1989; 79:8–15.

317. Miyazaki A, Sakuma S, Morikawa W et al. Intravenous injection of rabbit apolipoprotein A-I inhibits the progression of atherosclerosis in cholesterol-fed rabbits. Arterioscler Thromb Vasc Biol 1995; 15:1882–1888.

318. Nissen SE, Tsunoda T, Tuzcu EM et al. Effect of recombinant ApoA-I Milano on coronary atherosclerosis in patients with acute coronary syndromes: a randomized controlled trial. J Am Med Assoc 2003; 290:2292–2300.

319. Paszty C, Maeda N, Verstuyft J et al. Apolipoprotein AI transgene corrects apolipoprotein E deficiency-induced atherosclerosis in mice. J Clin Invest 1994; 94:899–903.

320. Dansky HM, Charlton SA, Barlow CB et al. Apo A-I inhibits foam cell formation in Apo E-deficient mice after monocyte adherence to endothelium. J Clin Invest 1999; 104:31–39.

321. Hughes SD, Verstuyft J, Rubin EM. HDL deficiency in genetically engineered mice requires elevated LDL to accelerate atherogenesis. Arterioscler Thromb Vasc Biol 1997; 17:1725–1729.

322. Voyiaziakis E, Goldberg IJ, Plump AS et al. ApoA-I deficiency causes both hypertriglyceridemia and increased atherosclerosis in human apoB transgenic mice. J Lipid Res 1998; 39:313–321.

323. Li H, Reddick RL, Maeda N. Lack of apoA-I is not associated with increased susceptibility to atherosclerosis in mice. Arterioscler Thromb 1993; 13:1814–1821.

324. Benoit P, Emmanuel F, Caillaud JM et al. Somatic gene transfer of human ApoA-I inhibits atherosclerosis progression in mouse models. Circulation 1999; 99:105–110.

325. Tangirala RK, Tsukamoto K, Chun SH et al. Regression of atherosclerosis induced by liver-directed gene transfer of apolipoprotein A-I in mice. Circulation 1999; 100:1816–1822.

326. Boisvert WA, Black AS, Curtiss LK. ApoA1 reduces free cholesterol accumulation in atherosclerotic lesions of ApoE-deficient mice transplanted with ApoE-expressing macrophages. Arterioscler Thromb Vasc Biol 1999; 19:525–530.

327. Belalcazar LM, Merched A, Carr B et al. Long-term stable expression of human apolipoprotein A-I mediated by helper-dependent adenovirus gene transfer inhibits atherosclerosis progression and remodels atherosclerotic plaques in a mouse model of familial hypercholesterolemia. Circulation 2003; 107:2726–2732.

328. Shaul PW. Endothelial nitric oxide synthase, caveolae and the development of atherosclerosis. J Physiol 2003; 547:21–33.

329. Rader DJ. High-density lipoproteins and atherosclerosis. Am J Cardiol 2002; 90:62i–70i.

330. Navab M, Imes SS, Hama SY et al. Monocyte transmigration induced by modification of low density lipoprotein in cocultures of human aortic wall cells is due to induction of monocyte chemotactic protein 1 synthesis and is abolished by high density lipoprotein. J Clin Invest 1991; 88:2039–2046.

331. Navab M, Hama SY, Cooke CJ et al. Normal high density lipoprotein inhibits three steps in the formation of mildly oxidized low density lipoprotein: step 1. J Lipid Res 2000; 41:1481–1494.

332. Mackness MI, Arrol S, Durrington PN. Paraoxonase prevents accumulation of lipoperoxides in low-density lipoprotein. FEBS Lett 1991; 286:152–154.

333. Watson AD, Navab M, Hama SY et al. Effect of platelet activating factor-acetylhydrolase on the formation and action of minimally oxidized low density lipoprotein. J Clin Invest 1995; 95:774–782.

334. Watson AD, Berliner JA, Hama SY et al. Protective effect of high density lipoprotein associated paraoxonase. Inhibition of the biological activity of minimally oxidized low density lipoprotein. J Clin Invest 1995; 96:2882–2891.

335. Bart DG, Stengel D, Landeloos M et al. Effect of overexpression of human apo A-I in C57BL/6 and C57BL/6 apo E- deficient mice on 2 lipoprotein-associated enzymes, platelet-activating factor acetylhydrolase and paraoxonase. Comparison of adenovirus- mediated human apo A-I gene transfer and human apo A-I transgenesis. Arterioscler Thromb Vasc Biol 2000; 20:E68–E75.

336. Theilmeier G, De Geest B, Van Veldhoven PP et al. HDL-associated PAF-AH reduces endothelial adhesiveness in apoE–/– mice. FASEB J 2000; 14:2032–2039.

337. Shih DM, Xia YR, Wang XP et al. Combined serum paraoxonase knockout/apolipoprotein E knockout mice exhibit increased lipoprotein oxidation and atherosclerosis. J Biol Chem 2000; 275:17527–17535.

338. Bisoendial RJ, Hovingh GK, Levels JH et al. Restoration of endothelial function by increasing high-density lipoprotein in subjects with isolated low high-density lipoprotein. Circulation 2003; 107:2944–2948.

339. Joyce CW, Amar MJ, Lambert G et al. The ATP binding cassette transporter A1 (ABCA1) modulates the development of aortic atherosclerosis in C57BL/6 and apoE-knockout mice. Proc Natl Acad Sci USA 2002; 99:407–412.

340. Orso E, Broccardo C, Kaminski WE et al. Transport of lipids from golgi to plasma membrane is defective in tangi-er disease patients and Abc1-deficient mice. Nature Genet 2000; 24:192–196.

341. Haghpassand M, Bourassa PA, Francone OL et al. Monocyte/macrophage expression of ABCA1 has minimal contribution to plasma HDL levels. J Clin Invest 2001; 108:1315–1320.

342. Van Eck M, Bos IS, Kaminski WE et al. Leukocyte ABCA1 controls susceptibility to atherosclerosis and macrophage recruitment into tissues. Proc Natl Acad Sci USA 2002; 99:6298–6303.

343. Groen AK, Bloks VW, Bandsma RH et al. Hepatobiliary cholesterol transport is not impaired in Abca1-null mice lacking HDL. J Clin Invest 2001; 108:843–850.

344. Vaisman BL, Lambert G, Amar M et al. ABCA1 overexpression leads to hyperalphalipoproteinemia and increased biliary cholesterol excretion in transgenic mice. J Clin Invest 2001; 108:303–309.

345. Chroni A, Liu T, Fitzgerald ML et al. Cross-linking and lipid efflux properties of apoA-I mutants direct association between apoA-I helices and ABCA1. Biochemistry 2004; 43:2126–2139.

346. Fitzgerald ML, Morris AL, Rhee JS et al. Naturally occurring mutations in the largest extracellular loops of ABCA1 can disrupt its direct interaction with apolipoprotein A-I. J Biol Chem 2002; 277:33178–33187.

347. Fitzgerald ML, Morris AL, Chroni A et al. ABCA1 and amphipathic apolipoproteins form high affinity molecular complexes required for cholesterol efflux. J Lipid Res 2004; 45:287–294.

348. Chambenoit O, Hamon Y, Marguet D et al. Specific docking of apolipoprotein A-I at the cell surface requires a functional ABCA1 transporter. J Biol Chem 2001; 276:9955–9960.

349. Rigot V, Hamon Y, Chambenoit O et al. Distinct sites on ABCA1 control distinct steps required for cellular release of phospholipids. J Lipid Res 2002; 43:2077–2086.

350. Panagotopulos SE, Witting SR, Horace EM et al. The role of apolipoprotein A-I helix 10 in apolipoprotein-mediated cholesterol efflux via the ATP-binding cassette transporter ABCA1. J Biol Chem 2002; 277:39477–39484.

351. Liu B, Krieger M. Highly purified scavenger receptor class B, type I reconstituted into phosphatidylcholine/cholesterol liposomes mediates high affinity high density lipoprotein binding and selective lipid uptake. J Biol Chem 2002; 277:34125–34135..

352. Li XA, Titlow WB, Jackson BA et al. High density lipoprotein binding to scavenger receptor, Class B, type I activates endothelial nitric-oxide synthase in a ceramide-dependent manner. J Biol Chem 2002; 277:11058–11063..

353. Wang N, Arai T, Ji Y et al. Liver-specific overexpression of scavenger receptor BI decreases levels of very low density lipoprotein ApoB, low density lipoprotein ApoB, and high density lipoprotein in transgenic mice. J Biol Chem 1998; 273:32920–32926..

354. Ueda Y, Royer L, Gong E et al. Lower plasma levels and accelerated clearance of high density lipoprotein (HDL) and

non-HDL cholesterol in scavenger receptor class B type I transgenic mice. J Biol Chem 1999; 274:7165–7171..

355. Rigotti A, Trigatti BL, Penman M et al. A targeted mutation in the murine gene encoding the high density lipoprotein (HDL) receptor scavenger receptor class B type I reveals its key role in HDL metabolism. Proc Natl Acad Sci USA 1997; 94:12610–12615.

356. Trigatti B, Rayburn H, Vinals M et al. Influence of the high density lipoprotein receptor SRBI on reproductive and cardiovascular pathophysiology. Proc Natl Acad Sci USA 1999; 96:9322–9327.

357. Mardones P, Quinones V, Amigo L et al. Hepatic cholesterol and bile acid metabolism and intestinal cholesterol absorption in scavenger receptor class B type I-deficient mice. J Lipid Res 2001; 42:170–180.

358. Kozarsky KF, Donahee MH, Glick JM et al. Gene transfer and hepatic overexpression of the HDL receptor SRBI reduces atherosclerosis in the cholesterol-fed LDL receptor-deficient mouse. Arterioscler Thromb Vasc Biol 2000; 20:721–727.

359. Webb NR, de Beer MC, Yu J et al. Overexpression of SRBI by adenoviral vector promotes clearance of apoA-I, but not apoB, in human apoB transgenic mice. J Lipid Res 2002; 43:1421–1428.

360. Arai T, Wang N, Bezouevski M et al. Decreased atherosclerosis in heterozygous low density lipoprotein receptor-deficient mice expressing the scavenger receptor BI transgene. J Biol Chem 1999; 274:2366–2371.

361. Ueda Y, Gong E, Royer L et al. Relationship between expression levels and atherogenesis in scavenger receptor class B, type I transgenics. J Biol Chem 2000; 275:20368–20373.

362. Ji Y, Wang N, Ramakrishnan R et al. Hepatic scavenger receptor BI promotes rapid clearance of high density lipoprotein free cholesterol and its transport into bile. J Biol Chem 1999; 274:33398–33402.

363. Huszar D, Varban ML, Rinninger F et al. Increased LDL cholesterol and atherosclerosis in LDL receptor-deficient mice with attenuated expression of scavenger receptor B1. Arterioscler Thromb Vasc Biol 2000; 20:1068–1073.

364. Braun A, Trigatti BL, Post MJ et al. Loss of SRBI expression leads to the early onset of occlusive atherosclerotic coronary artery disease, spontaneous myocardial infarctions, severe cardiac dysfunction, and premature death in apolipoprotein E-deficient mice. Circ Res 2002; 90:270–276.

365. Braun A, Zhang S, Miettinen HE et al. Probucol prevents early coronary heart disease and death in the high-density lipoprotein receptor SRBI/apolipoprotein E double knock-out mouse. Proc Natl Acad Sci USA 2003; 100:7283–7288..

366. Rye KA, Clay MA, Barter PJ. Remodelling of high density lipoproteins by plasma factors. Atherosclerosis 1999; 145:227–238.

367. Melchior GW, Castle CK, Murray RW et al. Apolipoprotein A-I metabolism in cholesteryl ester transfer protein transgenic mice. Insights into the mechanisms responsible for low plasma high density lipoprotein levels. J Biol Chem 1994; 269:8044–8051.

368. Francone OL, Royer L, Haghpassand M. Increased prebeta-HDL levels, cholesterol efflux, and LCAT-mediated esterification in mice expressing the human cholesteryl ester transfer protein (CETP) and human apolipoprotein A-I (apoA-I) transgenes. J Lipid Res 1996; 37:1268–1277.

369. Plump AS, Masucci-Magoulas L, Bruce C et al. Increased atherosclerosis in ApoE and LDL receptor gene knock-out mice as a result of human cholesteryl ester transfer protein transgene expression. Arterioscler Thromb Vasc Biol 1999; 19:1105–1110.

370. Seguret S, Emmanuel F, Aubailly N et al. Effect of human LCAT on LpA-I and LpA-I:A-II metabolism after adenovirus mediated human LCAT gene transfer in human apoA-I and apoA-I/A-II transgenic mice. Circulation 1996; 94:I–275.

371. Berard AM, Foger B, Remaley A et al. High plasma HDL concentrations associated with enhanced atherosclerosis in transgenic mice overexpressing lecithin-cholesteryl acyltransferase. Nature Med 1997; 3:744–749.

372. Mehlum A, Muri M, Hagve TA et al. Mice overexpressing human lecithin: cholesterol acyltransferase are not protected against diet-induced atherosclerosis. APMIS 1997; 105:861–868.

373. Foger B, Chase M, Amar MJ et al. Cholesteryl ester transfer protein corrects dysfunctional high density lipoproteins and reduces aortic atherosclerosis in lecithin cholesterol acyltransferase transgenic mice. J Biol Chem 1999; 274: 36912–36920.

374. Hoeg JM, Vaisman BL, Demosky SJ Jr et al. Lecithin:cholesterol acyltransferase overexpression generates hyperalphalipoproteinemia and a nonatherogenic lipoprotein pattern in transgenic rabbits. J Biol Chem 1996; 271:4396–4402.

375. Jiang X, Francone OL, Bruce C et al. Increased prebeta-high density lipoprotein, apolipoprotein AI, and phospholipid in mice expressing the human phospholipid transfer protein and human apolipoprotein AI transgenes. J Clin Invest 1996; 98:2373–2380.

376. Jiang XC, Bruce C, Mar J et al. Targeted mutation of plasma phospholipid transfer protein gene markedly reduces high-density lipoprotein levels. J Clin Invest 1999; 103:907–914.

377. Qin S, Kawano K, Bruce C et al. Phospholipid transfer protein gene knock-out mice have low high density lipoprotein levels, due to hypercatabolism, and accumulate apoA-IV-rich lamellar lipoproteins. J Lipid Res 2000; 41:269–276.

378. Jiang XC, Qin S, Qiao C et al. Apolipoprotein B secretion and atherosclerosis are decreased in mice with phospholipid-transfer protein deficiency. Nature Med 2001; 7:847–852.

379. Weinstock PH, Bisgaier CL, Aalto-Setala K et al. Severe hypertriglyceridemia, reduced high density lipoprotein, and neonatal death in lipoprotein lipase knockout mice. Mild hypertriglyceridemia with impaired very low density lipoprotein clearance in heterozygotes. J Clin Invest 1995; 96:2555–2568.

380. Levak-Frank S, Hofmann W, Weinstock PH et al. Induced mutant mouse lines that express lipoprotein lipase in cardiac

muscle, but not in skeletal muscle and adipose tissue, have normal plasma triglyceride and high-density lipoprotein-cholesterol levels. Proc Natl Acad Sci USA 1999; 96:3165–3170.

381. Shimada M, Shimano H, Gotoda T et al. Overexpression of human lipoprotein lipase in transgenic mice. Resistance to diet-induced hypertriglyceridemia and hypercholesterolemia. J Biol Chem 1993; 268:17924–17929.

382. Babaev VR, Fazio S, Gleaves LA et al. Macrophage lipoprotein lipase promotes foam cell formation and atherosclerosis in vivo. J Clin Invest 1999; 103:1697–1705.

383. Homanics GE, de Silva HV, Osada J et al. Mild dyslipidemia in mice following targeted inactivation of the hepatic lipase gene. J Biol Chem 1995; 270:2974–2980.

384. Mezdour H, Jones R, Dengremont C et al. Hepatic lipase deficiency increases plasma cholesterol but reduces susceptibility to atherosclerosis in apolipoprotein E-deficient mice. J Biol Chem 1997; 272:13570–13575.

385. Busch SJ, Barnhart RL, Martin GA et al. Human hepatic triglyceride lipase expression reduces high density lipoprotein and aortic cholesterol in cholesterol-fed transgenic mice. J Biol Chem 1994; 269:16376–16382.

386. Fan J, Wang J, Bensadoun A et al. Overexpression of hepatic lipase in transgenic rabbits leads to a marked reduction of plasma high density lipoproteins and intermediate density lipoproteins. Proc Natl Acad Sci USA 1994; 91:8724–8728.

387. Barbagallo CM, Fan J, Blanche PJ et al. Overexpression of human hepatic lipase and ApoE in transgenic rabbits attenuates response to dietary cholesterol and alters lipoprotein subclass distributions. Arterioscler Thromb Vasc Biol 1999; 19:625–632.

388. Zannis VI, Breslow JL. Genetic mutations affecting human lipoprotein metabolism. Adv Hum Genet 1985; 14:125–126.

389. Allan CM, Walker D, Segrest JP et al. Identification and characterization of a new human gene (APOC4) in the apolipoprotein E, C-I, and C-II gene locus. Genomics 1995; 28:291–300.

390. Allan CM, Taylor JM. Expression of a novel human apolipoprotein (apoC-IV) causes hypertriglyceridemia in transgenic mice. J Lipid Res 1996; 37:1510–1518.

391. Pennacchio LA, Olivier M, Hubacek JA et al. An apolipoprotein influencing triglycerides in humans and mice revealed by comparative sequencing. Science 2001; 294:169–173.

392. Greaves DR, Gough PJ, Gordon S. Recent progress in defining the role of scavenger receptors in lipid transport, atherosclerosis and host defence. Curr Opin Lipidol 1998; 9:425–432.

393. Webb NR, Connell PM, Graf GA et al. SRBII, an isoform of the scavenger receptor BI containing an alternate cytoplasmic tail, mediates lipid transfer between high density lipoprotein and cells. J Biol Chem 1998; 273:15241–15248.

394. Jong MC, Gijbels MJ, Dahlmans VE et al. Hyperlipidemia and cutaneous abnormalities in transgenic mice overexpressing human apolipoprotein C1. J Clin Invest 1998; 101:145–152.

395. Shachter NS, Ebara T, Ramakrishnan R et al. Combined hyperlipidemia in transgenic mice overexpressing human apolipoprotein C1. J Clin Invest 1996; 98:846–855.

396. Shachter NS, Hayek T, Leff T et al. Overexpression of apolipoprotein CII causes hypertriglyceridemia in transgenic mice. J Clin Invest 1994; 93:1683–1690.

397. de Silva HV, Lauer SJ, Wang J et al. Overexpression of human apolipoprotein C-III in transgenic mice results in an accumulation of apolipoprotein B48 remnants that is corrected by excess apolipoprotein E. J Biol Chem 1994; 269:2324–2335.

398. Maeda N, Li H, Lee D et al. Targeted disruption of the apolipoprotein C-III gene in mice results in hypotriglyceridemia and protection from postprandial hypertriglyceridemia. J Biol Chem 1994; 269:23610–23616.

399. Hayek T, Azrolan N, Verdery RB et al. Hypertriglyceridemia and cholesteryl ester transfer protein interact to dramatically alter high density lipoprotein levels, particle sizes, and metabolism. Studies in transgenic mice. J Clin Invest 1993; 92:1143–1152.

400. Hayek T, Masucci-Magoulas L, Jiang X et al. Decreased early atherosclerotic lesions in hypertriglyceridemic mice expressing cholesteryl ester transfer protein transgene. J Clin Invest 1995; 96:2071–2074.

401. Raabe M, Flynn LM, Zlot CH et al. Knockout of the abetalipoproteinemia gene in mice: reduced lipoprotein secretion in heterozygotes and embryonic lethality in homozygotes. Proc Natl Acad Sci USA 1998; 95:8686–8691.

402. Ishibashi S, Goldstein JL, Brown MS et al. Massive xanthomatosis and atherosclerosis in cholesterol-fed low density lipoprotein receptor-negative mice. J Clin Invest 1994; 93:1885–1893.

403. Duverger N, Kruth H, Emmanuel F et al. Inhibition of atherosclerosis development in cholesterol-fed human apolipoprotein A-I-transgenic rabbits. Circulation 1996; 94:713–717.

404. Weng W, Breslow JL. Dramatically decreased high density lipoprotein cholesterol, increased remnant clearance, and insulin hypersensitivity in apolipoprotein A-II knockout mice suggest a complex role for apolipoprotein A-II in atherosclerosis susceptibility. Proc Natl Acad Sci USA 1996; 93:14788–14794.

405. Schultz JR, Verstuyft JG, Gong EL et al. Protein composition determines the anti-atherogenic properties of HDL in transgenic mice. Nature 1993; 365:762–764.

406. Aiello RJ, Brees D, Bourassa PA et al. Increased atherosclerosis in hyperlipidemic mice with inactivation of ABCA1 in macrophages. Arterioscler Thromb Vasc Biol 2002; 22:630–637.

407. Holm TM, Braun A, Trigatti BL et al. Failure of red blood cell maturation in mice with defects in the high-density lipoprotein receptor SRBI. Blood 2002; 99:1817–1824.

408. Sakai N, Vaisman BL, Koch CA et al. Targeted disruption of the mouse lecithin:cholesterol acyltransferase (LCAT) gene. Generation of a new animal model for human LCAT deficiency. J Biol Chem 1997; 272:7506–7510.

409. Sakai N, Vaisman BL, Koch CA et al. Lecithin:cholesterol acyltransferase (LCAT) knockout mice: A new animal

model for human LCAT-deficiency. Circulation 1996; 94(Suppl):I-274.

410. Hoeg JM, Santamarina-Fojo S, Berard AM et al. Overexpression of lecithin:cholesterol acyltransferase in transgenic rabbits prevents diet-induced atherosclerosis. Proc Natl Acad Sci USA 1996; 93:11448–11453.

411. Brousseau ME, Wang J, Demosky SJ Jr et al. Correction of hypoalphalipoproteinemia in LDL receptor-deficient rabbits by lecithin:cholesterol acyltransferase. J Lipid Res 1998; 39:1558–1567.

412. Brousseau ME, Kauffman RD, Herderick EE et al. LCAT modulates atherogenic plasma lipoproteins and the extent of atherosclerosis only in the presence of normal LDL receptors in transgenic rabbits. Arterioscler Thromb Vasc Biol 2000; 20:450–458.

413. Amar MJ, Vaisman BL, Foger B et al. The effect of hepatic lipase deficiency on the plasma lipids, lipoproteins and diet-induced atherosclerosis in LCAT transgenic mice. Circulation 1997; 96(Suppl):I-109.

414. Amar MJA, Shamburek RD, Foger B et al. Adenovirus-mediated expression of LCAT in non-human primates leads to an antiatherogenic lipoprotein profile with increased HDL and decreased LDL. Circulation 1998;98(Suppl):I-35.

415. Marotti KR, Castle CK, Boyle TP et al. Severe atherosclerosis in transgenic mice expressing simian cholesteryl ester transfer protein. Nature 1993; 364:73–75.

416. Jaari S, Van Dijk KW, Olkkonen VM et al. Dynamic changes in mouse lipoproteins induced by transiently expressed human phospholipid transfer protein (PLTP): importance of PLTP in prebeta-HDL generation. Comp Biochem Physiol B Biochem Mol Biol 2001; 128:781–792.

417. Accad M, Smith SJ, Newland DL et al. Massive xanthomatosis and altered composition of atherosclerotic lesions in hyperlipidemic mice lacking acyl CoA:cholesterol acyltransferase 1. J Clin Invest 2000; 105:711–719.

418. Brennan M, Gaur A, Pahuja A et al. Mice lacking myeloperoxidase are more susceptible to experimental autoimmune encephalomyelitis. J Neuroimmunol 2001; 112:97–105.

419. Emmanuel F, Caillaud JM, Hennuyer N, et al. Overexpression of human apolipoprotein A-I inhibits atherosclerosis development in Watanabe reabbits. Circulation 1996; 94(Suppl):I-632.

9

Diabetes mellitus as an atherogenic factor

Claudia Panzer, Yasuo Ido, Neil Ruderman

Introduction

Since the advent of insulin therapy, macrovascular disease affecting large and medium-sized arteries has become the principal cause of mortality in individuals with diabetes.[1-3] Coronary heart disease, stroke, and especially peripheral vascular disease, are all two to six times more common in patients with both types 1 and 2 diabetes than in the general population, and they occur at an earlier age (Table 9.1).[1] In addition, diabetes substantially eliminates the relative protection of women, and particularly premenopausal women, from these diseases. The principal cause of this macrovascular disease is atherosclerosis, which is morphologically indistinguishable from that in non-diabetic individuals, but occurs at an earlier age.[4-6] What is also clear is that the relative impact of diabetes on atherosclerosis varies with environmental factors.[1] Thus, as reported by Kawate and colleagues[7] nearly 40 years ago, the prevalence of ischemic heart disease at autopsy is two to three times greater in Japanese with diabetes living in Hawaii, a region with a high prevalence of atherosclerotic vascular disease, than in people with a similar genetic background living in Japan,

where the prevalence of coronary heart disease in the general population is low (Table 9.2).

The reasons why diabetes accelerates atherosclerosis are incompletely understood; however, a large array of evidence – both clinical and basic – has suggested that an early event may be endothelial cell dysfunction. For this reason, the endothelium will be a major focus of this review. The chapter is divided into four parts:

(1) A brief description of atherosclerotic vascular disease in types 1 and 2 diabetes and prediabetic states (i.e. impaired glucose tolerance and the metabolic syndrome);

(2) An examination of the evidence, largely based on studies with cultured cells, that high glucose and free fatty acid (FFA) levels initiate changes in endothelial cell metabolism that lead to inflammation and dysfunction (early events in atherogenesis), as do other risk factors, such as an excess of low-density lipoprotein (LDL);

(3) A review of the evidence suggesting that accelerated atherosclerosis and insulin resistance in the liver and muscle of patients with type 2 diabetes and the

Table 9.1 Age-adjusted incidence per 100 patient years of cardiovascular events according to sex and diabetic status. (Adapted from data of Kannel and McGee[114] for Framingham cohorts aged 45–74. From Ruderman and Haudenschild, 1984.[1])

Type of arterial disease	Men		Women	
	Diabetic	Non-diabetic	Diabetic	Non-diabetic
Cerebrovascular	4.7	1.9	6.2	1.7
Claudication	12.6	3.3	8.4	1.3
Coronary	24.8	14.9	17.8	6.9

Table 9.2 Prevalence (per cent affected) of vascular disease in diabetic populations. Adapted from Kawate et al.[7] Patients with retinopathy had diabetes of 10–19 years' duration. The prevalence of ischemic heart disease in Japan and Hawaii were based on studies in patients at least 40 years of age. Data from Hawaii are based on death certificates, and from Japan autopsy studies (*) or clinical diagnosis (+). (From Ruderman and Haudenschild, 1984.[1])

Population	Country	Ischemic heart disease	Retinopathy
Japanese	Japan	13.5* 9.7+	57.4
	Hawaii	32.7	
Caucasians	Hawaii	32.8	50.0
	US or England	39.8 (US)	54.7 (England)

metabolic syndrome could be due to similar mechanisms; and

(4) A discussion of the prevention of coronary heart disease in patients with types 1 and 2 diabetes: who should be treated, when, and how?

Atherosclerotic vascular disease in patients with types 1 and 2 diabetes and impaired glucose tolerance: common factors and differences

As already noted, it has long been appreciated that ischemic heart disease due to accelerated atherosclerosis is more common in patients with both types 1 and 2 diabetes, but that the factors responsible for this process in the two disorders are not identical. Thus, in patients with type 2 diabetes, macrovascular disease is associated with an increased prevalence of obesity, hypertension, dyslipidemia (hypertriglyceridemia, low high-density lipoprotein (HDL) cholesterol, increased small dense LDL), hyperinsulinemia, and insulin resistance, all of which are associated with increased coronary risk (Table 9.3). This clustering of risk factors, now referred to as the metabolic syndrome (Table 9.4),[8] is also found in most people with impaired glucose tolerance (which usually antedates type 2 diabetes), and it may account for the high prevalence of clinically significant ischemic heart disease in these individuals, as well as in individuals with type 2 diabetes at the time of diagnosis.[9]

Patients with type 1 diabetes, in contrast, are characterized by insulin deficiency, caused by autoimmune destruction of pancreatic β cells. If they develop the metabolic syndrome, it is typically related to intensive insulin therapy and increased adiposity.[10] Only rarely does the metabolic syndrome precede the onset of hyperglycemia in these patients. Whether this is relevant to the observation that individuals with type 1 diabetes develop clinically significant atherosclerotic vascular disease only many years after diagnosis remains to be determined. In many individuals with type 1 diabetes, nephropathy and hypertension may accelerate macrovascular disease; however, an increase in atherogenesis has also been observed in patients without these abnormalities.[11,12]

Molecular mechanisms that increase atherogenesis in diabetes

Diabetes appears to increase the risk of atherosclerotic vascular disease for several reasons. Thus, such coronary disease risk factors as hypertension, hypercholesterolemia, low HDL cholesterol, and hyperhomocysteinemia are more common in patients with type 2 diabetes, impaired glucose tolerance, and the metabolic syndrome than in the general population (Table 9.3). As discussed in earlier chapters, these factors influence inflammatory and other aspects of the atherogenic process, and their presence may account for the beneficial antiatherogenic effects of statins, fibric acid compounds, and antihypertensive agents in diabetic as well

Table 9.3 Prevalence of atherogenic and potentially atherogenic factors in patients with types 1 and 2 diabetes and impaired glucose tolerance (IGT)

Factor	Type 1		Type 2	IGT
	NRF	IRF		
Dyslipidemia	+	+ + +	+ + +	+ +
Hypertension	0	+ + +	+ +	+
Hypercholesterolemia	0–+	+ + +	+	+
Obesity	0–+	0	+ + +	+ +
Insulin resistance	+	+ +	+ + +	+ +
Elevated plasma FFA	+	+	+ +	+ +
Hyperhomocysteinemia	0	+–+ + +	+ + +	+ + +

+, increased prevalence; +++ the greatest increase in prevalence; 0, prevalence not different from that of the general population. NRF, normal renal function; IRF, impaired renal function; FFA, free fatty acids

as non-diabetic populations (see below). These risk factors, however, only partially account for the increased prevalence of macrovascular disease in patients with type 2 diabetes. In patients with type 1 diabetes, in the absence of renal dysfunction and hypertension, or possibly a metabolic syndrome secondary to intensive insulin therapy, they are probably of little significance.[1,13]

Endothelium

Glucose

One abnormality unique to patients with diabetes and impaired glucose tolerance that has been extensively studied as an atherogenic factor is hyperglycemia itself. Infusions of glucose that produce moderate hyperglycemia have been shown to cause endothelial cell dysfunction and increases in circulating nitrotyrosine levels, suggesting increased nitrosative and oxidative stress.[14] Similar findings have been described in patients with type 2 diabetes.[14] Likewise, the magnitude of hyperglycemia has been shown to correlate with the incidence of new vascular events in diabetic patients (mainly type 2) in some studies.[15–17] In addition, a continuous and graded relationship between cardiovascular events and glucose concentration across the range of non-diabetic glucose values has been noted.[18,19] In contrast, intervention studies in which glycemic control was moderately improved over an extended period have yielded only borderline benefits

Table 9.4 Definition of the metabolic syndrome. According to the Executive Summary of the Third Report of the National Cholesterol Education Program (NCEP) Expert Panel on Detection, Evaluation, and Treatment of High Blood Cholesterol in Adults (Adult Treatment Panel III)[115]

Three or more of the following criteria:

Abdominal obesity: waist circumference > 35 inches (women) or 40 inches (men)

Triglycerides ≥ 150 mg/dl

HDL cholesterol < 50 mg/dl (women) or < 40 mg/dl (men)

Blood pressure ≥ 130/85 mmHg

Fasting plasma glucose ≥ 110 mg/dl

HDL, high-density lipoprotein

in both type 2 (UK Prospective Diabetes Study (UKPDS), 1998) and type 1 (Diabetes Control and Complication Trial (DCCT), 1994) patients; however, the fact that the interventions used in these studies (e.g. insulin and sulfonylureas in the UKPDS) often increased obesity and probably tended to create a metabolic syndrome makes an evaluation of the effect of glucose lowering difficult. Moreover, in the initial DCCT study, perhaps because of the youth of the patients and their brief duration of diabetes, the incidence of myocardial disease was very low (see below).

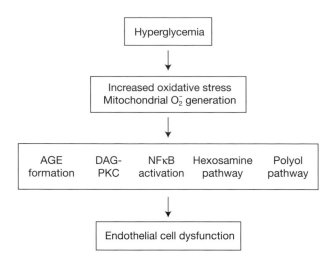

Figure 9.1 Hyperglycemia-induced endothelial cell dysfunction as a response to an increase in oxidative stress. AGE, advanced glycosylation end-product; DAG, 1,2-diacylglycerol; PKC, protein kinase C. (Adapted from reference 29)

Studies with cultured cells strongly suggest that exposure of endothelium to a high-glucose medium causes the same dysfunctional and biochemical changes observed after exposure to excess LDL and other atherogenic factors[20] (see Chapter 8). Thus, incubation of aortic endothelial cells with a high-glucose medium increases oxidant stress,[21] 1,2-diacylglycerol (DAG) synthesis and PKC activation,[22] NFκB translocation to the nucleus and NFκB-mediated gene expression (e.g. vascular cell adhesion molecule (VCAM) expression),[23] and apoptosis.[24] In addition, elevated concentrations of glucose have been found to cause inhibition of glucose-6-phosphate dehydrogenase (G6PD) by activating cyclic AMP-dependent protein kinase A in aortic endothelial cells.[25,26] Inhibition of G6PD, an important antioxidant enzyme in vascular cells, resulted in decreased NADPH, the main intracellular reductant, increased reactive oxygen species, and subsequent cell damage and death.[25,26] Hyperglycemia also increases the formation of hexosamines, polyols, and advanced glycosylation endproducts (AGE),[27] and enhances the adhesion of endothelium to mononuclear cells.[28] It has recently been suggested by Brownlee[29] that the primary effect of a high glucose concentration is to increase mitochondrial superoxide generation and oxidant stress, and that most of the changes listed above are secondary to this process (Figure 9.1). They recently also demonstrated that hyperglycemia-induced mitochondrial

superoxide generation inhibits G6PD activity,[30] confirming the work by Leopold and co-workers[25] and Zhang and associates.[26] By contrast, the observation that activation of PKC[21] and increased hexosamine[31] and AGE formation, as well as NFκB-mediated cytokine formation, can by themselves lead to oxidant stress,[32] suggests that the interrelations between oxidant stress and glucose-induced changes in the endothelium may be more complex. Also, when excess glucose or fatty acids are the stimulus, the increase in superoxide generation observed in both cultured endothelial and vascular smooth muscle cells may be mediated by cytoplasmic NAD(P)H oxidases.[21] Thus, despite its attractions, several elements of Brownlee's theory are open to question (Figure 9.2).

Most of the glucocentric theories of atherosclerosis in diabetes are built on the long-held assumption that glucose is the dominant fuel of the endothelial cell, and that most of the ATP generated is derived from glycolysis and, possibly, glucose oxidation.[29] This may not, however, be correct. In recent studies we have found that fatty acid oxidation can be a major source of ATP generation in endothelial cells (HUVEC); indeed, in endothelium deprived of glucose for several hours, cellular ATP levels were totally maintained and fatty acid oxidation was increased more than three-fold.[33] Conversely, in separate studies we found that incubation with a hyperglycemic medium for 24 hours led to an increase in the concentration of malonyl CoA (an

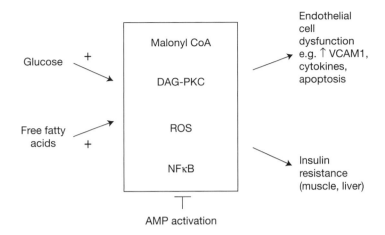

Figure 9.2 Changes caused by exposure of endothelial cells to excess glucose and/or free fatty acids (FFA) that lead to dysfunction are prevented by AMP-activated protein kinase (AMPK) activation. As reviewed in the text, similar events occur in skeletal muscle, liver, and the pancreatic β cell in the setting of the metabolic syndrome and in endothelial cells exposed to the proinflammatory cytokine TNF-α. DAG, 1,2-diacylglycerol; PKC, protein kinase C; ROS, reactive oxygen species; VACM, vascular cell adhesion molecules. (Adapted from reference 46)

allosteric inhibitor of carnitine palmitoyl transferase 1 (CPT1), a key enzyme controlling fatty acid uptake by mitochondria), a decrease in fatty acid oxidation, an increase in diacylglycerol synthesis, mitochondrial dysfunction, insulin resistance, and apoptosis[24] (Figure 9.3). An intriguing finding was that all of these changes were inhibited by incubation of the cells with AICAR (5-aminoimidazole-4-carboxamide riboside), an agent that activates the fuel-sensing enzyme AMP-activated protein kinase (AMPK) and secondarily lowers the concentration of malonyl CoA and increases fatty acid oxidation. Furthermore, a similar inhibition of apoptosis (caspase-3 activation) was obtained by overexpressing a constitutively active AMPK in the cells prior to placing them in a high-glucose medium. As will be discussed, a number of factors have been shown to diminish macrovascular disease or risk factors for it in patients with type 2 diabetes, impaired glucose tolerance (IGT), and the metabolic syndrome activate AMPK (see below).

Free fatty acids

A second factor often elevated in the plasma of patients with diabetes, IGT, and the metabolic syndrome that could contribute to increased atherogenesis is the concentration of free fatty acids (FFA). As initially shown by Steinberg and Baron and co-workers,[34] elevation of plasma FFA in humans, achieved by infusing a fat emulsion, causes impaired vasodilation, at least in part by inhibiting the stimulation of nitric oxide synthesis by insulin. Incubation of both endothelial cells[21] and vascular smooth muscle cells[21,35] with fatty acids has been shown to increase oxidative stress; indeed, in a head-to-head comparison in cultured endothelium, 0.5 mM palmitate caused much greater increases in both lipid peroxide production and DCHF fluorescence (a measure of cellular H_2O_2) than did 20 mM glucose[36] (Cacicedo et al., unpublished data). Likewise, we have found that incubation of HUVEC with palmitate increases NFκB activation, and the expression of NFκB-mediated genes, including VCAM-1 (vascular cell adhesion molecule). As with glucose incubation, these changes, as well as an increase in apoptosis caused by palmitate, were markedly inhibited by co-incubation with AICAR or a constitutively active AMPK. Likewise, AMPK activation had similar effects on the actions of the inflammatory cytokine, tumor necrosis factor-α (TNF-α)[37] (Cacicedo and Ido, unpublished). Overall, these findings are consistent with the notion that excesses of glucose and fatty acids account for, or at least contribute to, the 'unique' atherogenic effects of diabetes on the endothelium. They also suggest that increases in oxidant stress and NFκB activation play a pathogenetic role, as they appear to do when atherogenesis is stimulated by LDL cholesterol and other factors not specific for diabetes or the metabolic syndrome.[38]

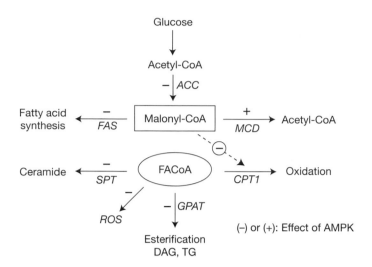

Figure 9.3 Regulation of malonyl CoA and cytosolic fatty acid CoA (FACoA) by AMP-activated protein kinase (AMPK). By inhibiting carnitine palmitoyl transferase 1 (CPT1), malonyl CoA, which is derived from glucose, diminishes FACoA entrance into mitochondria where they are oxidized, thereby making more cytosolic FACoA available for triglyceride (TG), 1,2-diacylglycerol (DAG) and ceramide synthesis, and possibly for lipid peroxidation. AMPK could inhibit these events and increase fatty acid oxidation, acutely by phosphorylating or otherwise inhibiting acetyl CoA carboxylase (ACC), glycerophosphate acyltransferase (GPAT), and malonyl CoA decarboxylase (MCD), and chronically by diminishing the expression of sterol response element binding protein (SREBP1c) and activating PPARγ co-activator 1α (PGI-α) and peroxisome proliferator-activated receptor-α (PPAR-α) (not shown). The basis for its ability to diminish oxidant stress (reactive O_2 species) is not known). FAS, fatty acid synthase; SPT, serine palmitoyltransferase; ROS, reactive oxygen species. (Adapted from reference 50)

Other players in the atherogenic process

Although we have emphasized the role of endothelial cell dysfunction in the pathogenesis of diabetic complications, it is highly likely that glucose, FFA, and other abnormalities associated with diabetes (e.g. increased cytokines) affect macrophages, vascular smooth muscle, platelets, lipoproteins, and other determinants of the atherogenic process. Thus, elevated concentrations of glucose and FFA have been shown to increase oxidant stress in vascular smooth muscle cells as well as in endothelial cells,[21] and glycated LDL is increased both in the circulation and the vascular wall of patients with diabetes.[39] Perhaps, in keeping with this view, LDL from the plasma of patients with diabetes appears to be more proinflammatory than LDL from non-diabetic individuals.[40]

One factor that has been linked to increased oxidant stress and to multiple components of the atherogenic process is AGE. AGE are glycated proteins, lipids, or nucleic acids that have been oxidatively modified (glycoxidized) as a function of glucose concentration and oxidative stress.[41] It has long been known that

they accumulate and cause dysfunction to a greater extent in tissues in patients with diabetes than in non-diabetic individuals,[29,41] and that their concentration in plasma increases, sometimes dramatically, in the presence of renal failure.[42] Schmidt and co-workers[43] have presented evidence that AGE bind to a specific receptor present in many cells of the vascular wall, including macrophages, smooth muscle cells, and endothelium. Engagement of this receptor (commonly referred to as RAGE) by AGE and other ligands leads to increases in oxidative stress and activation of inflammatory responses in all types of vascular cells. In macrophages it also causes an increased release of various proteases and growth factors. It has been shown that the administration of a soluble RAGE antibody (which acts as a decoy to bind circulating AGE) can both prevent the formation of new atheroma[43] and arrest the progression of established atheroma in diabetic mice.[44] Such 'inhibition of RAGE signaling' has also been shown to decrease levels of matrix-degrading proteinases and increase interstitial collagen, 'a crucial protector of the integrity of the plaque's fibrous cap'.[45] Whether AMPK activation prevents AGE formation or

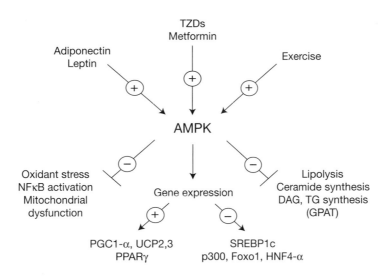

Figure 9.4   AMP-activated protein kinase (AMPK) activation and its effects on events that could contribute to or protect against endothelial cell dysfunction. By similar actions, AMPK appears to prevent dysfunction of muscle, liver, and the pancreatic β cell in situations associated with ectopic lipid accumulation and proinflammatory changes. TZD, thiazolidinediones; DAG, 1,2-diacylglycerol; TG, triglyceride; GPAT, glycerophosphate acyltransferase; SREBP1c, sterol response element binding protein; HNF, hepatocyte nuclear factor; PGC1-α, PPARγ co-activator 1α; UCP2,3, uncoupling protein 2 and 3; PPAR, peroxisome proliferator-activated receptor. (Adapted from reference 50)

alters the RAGE-mediated responses of cells involved in the atherogenic process has not, to our knowledge been studied.

Atherosclerosis and insulin resistance in liver and muscle in type 2 diabetes and the metabolic syndrome: is dysregulation of the malonyl Co/AMPK fuel-sensing network a common factor?

Premature atherosclerosis in patients with the metabolic syndrome is typically associated with pancreatic β-cell dysfunction and insulin resistance in both liver and muscle. Studies in experimental animals, and to some extent humans, suggest that a common feature in all of these tissues is a disturbance in intracellular lipid metabolism leading to increases in DAG-PKC signaling, oxidative stress, and increased NFκB activation.[46–49] A commonly found marker of these changes in muscle and liver may be an increase in intracellular

triglycerides. As reviewed elsewhere,[50] dysregulation of the AMPK malonyl CoA fuel-sensing network could be both a cause of these abnormalities and a target for their therapy.

Malonyl CoA is an intermediate in the de novo synthesis of fatty acids and an allosteric inhibitor of carnitine palmitoyl transferase 1 (CPT1), the enzyme that regulates the transfer of long-chain fatty acyl CoA molecules from the cytosol to the mitochondria, where they are oxidized. AMPK is an enzyme that responds to changes in the energy state of the cell, as reflected by the ratio AMP/ATP and perhaps other factors (Figure 9.4) Among its targets are acetyl CoA carboxylase (ACC), the rate-limiting enzyme for malonyl CoA synthesis; malonyl CoA decarboxylase, a key enzyme that degrades malonyl CoA; and glycerophosphate acyltransferase (GPAT), the first committed enzyme in the synthesis of diacylglycerol and triglycerides. When cells, including vascular cells, sense they are energy deprived (e.g. owing to glucose deprivation), the resultant increase in AMP relative to ATP activates AMPK. The activated AMPK, in turn, phosphorylates ACC and malonyl CoA decarboxylase, leading respectively to their inhibition and activation and, by unknown mechanisms, the inhibition of GPAT (see Figure 9.3). The net result of these changes is a decrease in the concentration of malonyl CoA, which enhances ATP generation by increasing fatty acid oxidation, and a diminution of ATP utilization caused by a partial inhibition of the synthesis of triglyceride and other glycerolipids (e.g. DAG, phospholipid), and other ATP-consuming processes.[50] Conversely, when many cells sense they have an excess of glucose, AMPK activity is diminished, the oxidation of fatty acids is decreased, and their esterification to form triglyceride and diacylglycerol is enhanced.

Increases in DAG and triglyceride concentration, accompanied by a decrease in AMPK activity, have been demonstrated in the liver and/or muscle of rats infused with glucose and insulin, and are associated with increases in PKC activity.[51,52] Similar phenomena, including a decrease in AMPK activity, have been observed in obese rodents deficient in leptin or a functional leptin receptor (Wu et al., submitted) and are associated with insulin resistance.[53] Other effects of AMPK activation that could contribute to its protective action on endothelial cells exposed to an excess of fatty acids (palmitate), glucose, or inflammatory cytokines are shown in Figures 9.3 and 9.4; among these (Figure 9.4) are a wide variety of transcription factors or coactivators that could contribute to its long-term biological effects.

Direct measurements of AMPK have not yet been systematically performed in insulin-resistant humans; however, it is noteworthy that a number of therapies known to increase insulin sensitivity, decrease ectopic lipid accumulation in patients with type 2 diabetes and/or the metabolic syndrome, and delay or prevent the development of type 2 diabetes, have been shown to increase AMPK activity in experimental animals. They include exercise,[54,55] diminished caloric intake (Saha and Ruderman, unpublished data) metformin,[56] and thiazolidinediones (TZD).[57] Likewise, the fat cell-derived hormone adiponectin, which appears to increase insulin sensitivity and protect against developing diabetes and atherosclerosis,[58,59] is an AMPK activator.[58,60] These therapies have also been shown to diminish endothelial cell dysfunction and circulating inflammatory markers (C-reactive protein, IL6) in insulin-resistant individuals.[50,61] Furthermore, adiponectin, like AICAR, diminishes TNF-α-induced NFκB activation in cultured endothelial cells.[62,63] Finally, factors that activate AMPK, such as exercise, and treatment with TZD and metformin, have been linked to a decrease in atherosclerotic vascular disease or an improvement of early vascular changes in patients with type 2 diabetes or those at risk for developing it.[64–67]

Prevention of coronary heart disease in patients with types 1 and 2 diabetes and impaired glucose tolerance: who should be treated, when and how?

As discussed earlier (see previous section), endothelial cell dysfunction, like insulin resistance, increased intracellular lipid accumulation in liver and muscle, and pancreatic β-cell abnormalities, is observed in humans with the metabolic syndrome, and a dysregulation of the AMPK–malonyl CoA fuel-sensing network could contribute to its occurrence and be a target for its therapy. In support of such a central role for this network, exercise, pharmacological agents, and hormones that activate it have been reported to diminish the development of both type 2 diabetes and atherosclerotic vascular disease. These findings raise the question: do we have sufficient evidence to use these and other therapeutic modalities that activate AMPK or attack other specific risk factors to prevent atherosclerotic heart disease in patients with types 1 and 2 diabetes, IGT, or the metabolic syndrome; and, if so, when should this therapy be initiated?

Type 2 diabetes

Patients with established type 2 diabetes demonstrate a spectrum of clinical abnormalities, including hyperglycemia, hypertension, and dyslipidemias, and increases in a wide variety of non-traditional risk factors for cardiovascular disease, including C-reactive protein (CRP), homocysteine, plasminogen-activator inhibitor 1 (PAI-1), and fibrinogen levels.[68] The available evidence clearly demonstrates that intervention targeted at a single risk factor, such as hypertension (Table 9.5) or dyslipidemia (Table 9.6), improves cardiovascular outcomes in these patients, as do exercise,[69]

Table 9.5 Primary prevention of cardiovascular events in patients with diabetes: hypertension trials

Study	Intervention	Outcome	Relative risk reduction
UKPDS Hypertension Study[116]	Blood pressure < 150/80 mmHg with captopril or atenolol versus blood pressure < 180/105 mmHg	Myocardial infarction	11% for each 10 mmHg decrease in SBP
HOT[117]	Felodipine and ACE-I or β-blocker with three diastolic blood pressures	Cardiovascular events	51% in target group ≤ 80 mmHg DBP
Syst-Eur[118]	Nitrendipin, enalapril ± HCTZ	Myocardial infarction, congestive heart failure, or sudden cardiac death	63%
MICRO-HOPE[119]	Ramipril or placebo	Myocardial infarction	22%

UKPDS, UK Prospective Diabetes Study; HOT, Hypertension Optimal Treatment randomized study; Syst-Eur, Systolic Hypertension in Europe trial; MICRO-HOPE, substudy of Heart Outcomes Prevention Evaluation study; ACE-I, angiotensin converting enzyme inhibitor; HCTZ, hydrochlorothiazide; SBP, systolic blood pressure; DBP, diastolic blood pressure

Table 9.6 Primary and secondary prevention of cardiovascular events in patients with diabetes: lipid trials

Study	Intervention	Endpoint	Relative risk reduction (%)
4S[120]	Simvastatin	CHD death or non-fatal MI	48
CARE[121]	Pravastatin	Coronary disease death, non-fatal MI or revascularization	21
VaHIT[122]	Gemfibrozil	CHD death or non-fatal MI	21
HPS[123]	Simvastatin	CHD, stroke, revascularization	33

4S, Scandinavian Simvastatin Survival Study; CARE, Cholesterol and Recurrent Events trial; VaHIT, Veterans Affairs High-density lipoprotein cholesterol Intervention Trial; HPS, Heart Protection Study; CHD, coronary heart disease; MI, myocardial infarction

metformin,[64] and statins.[70] The importance of glycemic control per se in the prevention of macrovascular disease is less clear, and the effect of lowering plasma free fatty acids has not been studied. With respect to hyperglycemia, elevations of HbA1c have been demonstrated to correlate both with oxidant stress markers (N^ε-carboxymethyl-lysine),[71] and with the incidence of new macrovascular events in patients with type 2 diabetes (see previous references). On the other hand, improved glycemic control with insulin or sulfonylurea therapy has yielded only a marginal improvement in macrovascular disease outcomes. Thus,

in the UK Prospective Diabetes Study,[9] only a trend toward the reduction of fatal and non-fatal myocardial infarction ($p = 0.052$) in intensively treated patients (mean decrease in HbA1c 0.9%) was seen in the primary analysis. A subanalysis of the patients, however, revealed a significant correlation between the magnitude of the decrease in HbA1c and the reduction in myocardial infarction (14% decrease in incidence of myocardial infarction for each 1% reduction in HbA1c).[72]

A decrease in cardiovascular events has been observed in patients treated with pharmacologic agents

Table 9.7   Multifactorial intervention and cardiovascular disease in patients with type 2 diabetes: treatment goals for the intensive-therapy group[80]

	Intensive therapy goals	
Variable	1993–1999	2000–2001
Systolic blood pressure (mmHg)	< 140	< 130
Diastolic blood pressure (mmHg)	< 85	< 80
Glycosylated hemoglobin (%)	< 6.5	< 6.5
Fasting serum cholesterol (mg/dl)	< 190	< 175
Fasting serum triglycerides (mg/dl)	< 150	< 150
ACE inhibitor irrespective of blood pressure	Yes	Yes
Aspirin therapy for patients		
With known ischemia	Yes	Yes
With peripheral vascular disease	Yes	Yes
Without coronary heart disease or peripheral vascular disease	No	Yes

ACE, angiotensin converting enzyme

that activate AMPK, such as metformin and thiazolidinediones, as well as by exercise. The Nurses' Health Study provided evidence that increased physical activity is associated with a substantial reduction in risk for cardiovascular events in diabetic women.[69] In addition, in the UKPDS study a subgroup of 342 obese patients, randomized to monotherapy with the insulin sensitizer and AMPK activator metformin, showed a significant reduction in the risk of myocardial infarction of 39%.[64] TZD, another class of insulin-sensitizing agents that activate AMPK in cultured cells[73] and in rodents,[57] also appear to improve cardiovascular outcomes.[74] Thus these drugs have been shown both to diminish neointimal tissue proliferation after coronary stent implantation in patients with type 2 diabetes[75] and to decrease non-classic risk factors for coronary artery disease (CAD) in diabetic patients.[76] Ongoing studies are assessing the ability of TZD to prevent atherosclerotic vascular disease.[77–79]

In light of the effectiveness of treatments aimed at specific risk factors in diminishing macrovascular events in patients with type 2 diabetes, the effect of multiple risk factor intervention was examined in the Steno-2 trial (Table 9.7).[80] In patients with established diabetes and microalbuminuria, a 50% reduction in cardiovascular events was demonstrated after a mean of 7.8 years in response to pharmacologic therapy and

behavioral modification (diet and exercise) targeted at modifiable risk factors (glycemia, blood pressure, dyslipidemia).[80] Although the benefits of multiple risk factor intervention were clearly demonstrated, morbidity and mortality rates in the Steno-2 trial were still high compared to those of non-diabetic individuals. Based on this and the fact that approximately 20% of the newly diagnosed patients in the UKPDS already had evidence of macrovascular complications,[9] one obvious possibility is that interventions aimed at preventing these complications need to be initiated in the prediabetic state.

Does treatment designed to prevent or delay the onset of diabetes prevent macrovascular disease?

The efficacy of therapy designed to prevent progression from impaired glucose tolerance to overt type 2 diabetes has been demonstrated (25–58% reduction in the incidence of diabetes) in a number of well-designed, randomized, controlled trials (Table 9.8).[81–84] The most impressive results were seen in the US Diabetes Prevention Program (USDPP), in which lifestyle modification with diet and exercise or metformin diminished progression to diabetes by 58% and

Table 9.8 Diabetes prevention trials

Study	Population	Duration (years/design)	Intervention group	Control	Reduction of incidence of diabetes (%)
Malmö Prevention Trial[88]	IGT 181	5 NR	Exercise and diet	Diet and exercise recommendations	50
DaQuing[124]	577 m/w with IGT	6 R	Three arms: 1. Diet only 2. Exercise only 3. Diet and exercise	General counseling on exercise and diet	Diet: 1 Exercise: 46 Diet and exercise: 42
Finnish Diabetes Prevention Study[82]	522 m/w with IGT	3.2 RC	Weight loss ≥ 5% Total fat intake ≤ 30% Saturated fat intake ≤ 10% Fiber intake ≥ 15 g/1000 kcal Exercise ≥ 30 min/day	General counseling on exercise and diet	58
USDPP[81]	3234 m/w with IGT	2.8 RC	Lifestyle modification including weight loss ≥ 7% Exercise of ≥ 150 min/week Low-fat, low-calorie diet OR Metformin + standard lifestyle recommendations	Standard lifestyle recommendations + placebo	Lifestyle modification: 58 Metformin: 31
TRIPOD[84]	266 w with h/o gestational diabetes 70% IGT	2.5 RC	Troglitazone	Placebo	56
STOP-NIDDM[83]	1429 m/w with IGT	3.3 RC	Acarbose	Placebo	25

N, non-randomized; RC, randomized controlled; IGT, impaired glucose tolerance; USDPP, US Diabetes Program; TRIPOD, Troglitazone in Prevention of Diabetes study; NIDDM, non-insulin-dependent diabetes mellitus

31%, respectively.[81] Cardiovascular outcome data from the USDPP are still lacking; however, early lifestyle intervention in this study was shown to diminish many cardiovascular risk factors. Thus over 1 year it decreased LDL cholesterol and triglyceride levels and systolic and diastolic blood pressure significantly more than did placebo or even metformin.[85] The need for additional therapy to control dyslipidemia and hypertension was also reduced. In a later report from this study beneficial effects on novel markers of cardiovascular disease, such as C-reactive protein, tissue plasminogen activator, and fibrinogen, were also noted. Once again, the effects of lifestyle change were greater

than those of metformin.[86] Whether or not these benefits result in a decrease in cardiovascular events remains to be determined. A significant reduction in cardiovascular events as a result of treatment with the α-glucosidase inhibitor acarbose was observed in the Study to Prevent Non-Insulin-Dependent Diabetes Mellitus (Stop-NIDDM).[87] In this trial 1429 participants with IGT, characterized by moderate postprandial hyperglycemia (mean age 55, BMI 31 kg/m^2) were randomized to receive either acarbose or placebo. After a mean follow-up of 3.3 years, a 49% relative risk reduction in the development of cardiovascular events was seen in the acarbose group, with the major

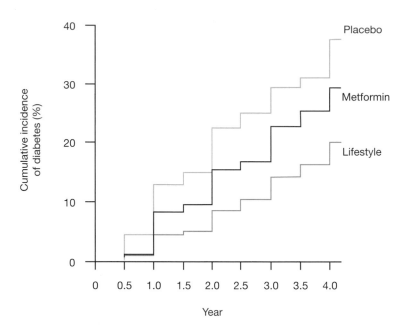

Figure 9.5   Cumulative incidence of diabetes according to study group in the US Diabetes Prevention Program Trial[81]

reduction found in the risk of myocardial infarction. Interestingly, the study subjects also showed a significant decrease in blood pressure. A marked decrease in myocardial infarction has also been reported in patients treated with lifestyle modification in the Malmö Study;[88] however, because the patients were not randomized, the significance of this finding remains unclear.

Should we be treating people with the metabolic syndrome even prior to the onset of impaired glucose tolerance?

The effects of preventing or delaying the onset of diabetes on atherosclerotic vascular disease in patients with IGT are not yet known; nevertheless, in light of the observation that CAD is already more prevalent in patients with IGT than in the general population,[17] the possibility that preventive therapy should be initiated earlier, i.e. in normoglycemic people with the metabolic syndrome or at high risk for developing it,[89] needs to be considered. An additional factor is that even though treatment of IGT with lifestyle changes and metformin decreases progression to type

2 diabetes, the incidence of diabetes in such individuals is still higher than in the general population (Figure 9.5). Another consideration is that the prevalence of the metabolic syndrome, which usually antedates even impaired glucose tolerance,[89,90] is rapidly increasing, and along with the obesity that accompanies it, is approaching epidemic proportions. Using the Adult Treatment Panel III report definitions, the age-adjusted prevalence of obesity is now estimated to be 23.7%, and increases to 43.5% in adults aged 60–69 years.[91] Individuals at high risk for developing diabetes and associated atherosclerotic disease can often be identified easily using the Adult Treatment Panel III criteria,[92] by family history of diabetes and macrovascular disease, and by taking into account factors such as birth weight, adult-onset weight gain, physical activity status, and the presence of associated diseases.[89] As noted above, at least two goals of treatment of the metabolic syndrome, namely, prevention of diabetes and prevention of cardiovascular disease, can possibly be achieved by therapies that activate AMPK, such as exercise, calorie reduction, metformin, and TZD (Table 9.9). The role of interventions against specific risk factors using antihypertensive therapy and statins remains to be determined.

Table 9.9 Effects of AMPK-activating modalities and pharmacological agents on the markers of the metabolic syndrome

Intervention	Obesity (abdominal)	Triglycerides	HDL cholesterol	Blood pressure	Glucose
Calorie/weight reduction	(–)	(–)	(+)	(–)	(–)
Exercise	(–)	(–)	(+)	(–)	(–)
Metformin	(–)	?	?	0	(–)
TZD	(–)	(–)	(+)	(–)	(–)

AMPK, AMP-activated protein kinase; HDL, high-density lipoprotein; TZD, thiazolidinediones; +, increased; –, decreased; 0, no effect

Exercise and calorie restriction

The level of physical fitness has been shown to be inversely associated with an increased clustering of the markers of the metabolic syndrome.[93] The DPP research group was able to demonstrate a 41% reduction in the prevalence of the metabolic syndrome in individuals treated with diet and exercise,[94] but could not distinguish the effects of these modalities. Regular physical activity has been shown both to improve individual markers of the metabolic syndrome and to decrease mortality in patients with the metabolic syndrome and diabetes.[95,96] Calorie restriction similarly induces weight loss, improves lipid profiles, reduces ectopic lipid deposition, lowers blood pressure, and improves insulin sensitivity.[53,97] Data regarding the effect of dietary interventions on the incidence of diabetes, again taken from the diabetes prevention trials, have shown reductions in the incidence of diabetes of nearly 60% in people who achieved a mean weight loss of 7% on a low-fat, low-calorie diet and moderate exercise (DPP), or a low-fat, low saturated fat, high-fiber diet and moderate exercise (Finnish Diabetes Prevention Study).[81,82] Thus far, no specific dietary recommendations for the treatment of the metabolic syndrome have been issued by health organizations, but results from the recently published Framingham Offspring Cohort on carbohydrate nutrition and insulin resistance suggest that wholegrain food, cereal fiber, and diets with a lower glycemic index are associated with a lower prevalence of the metabolic syndrome.[98]

Pharmacologic treatment with metformin or thiazolidinediones

Thiazolidinediones (TZD) and metformin, both of which are insulin sensitizers and AMPK activators, are widely used in the treatment of diabetes.[99] They exert their glucose-lowering effects mainly by decreasing insulin resistance in skeletal muscle (TZD and metformin) and liver (metformin). In addition, TZD may inhibit atherosclerosis by reducing endothelial cell dysfunction, vascular inflammation, cell growth and migration, and increasing reverse cholesterol transport[61,74] (Table 9.10). Their effects include an activation of the PPAR-γ receptor in adipose tissue, liver, vascular cells and muscle, that leads to changes in gene expression and adipocyte differentiation, and to decreased ectopic lipid deposition and increased insulin sensitivity.[53,100–102] The latter could be related to a lowering of plasma free fatty acid levels,[103,104] and/or an increase in adiponectin (see next section).

A reduction in endogenous insulin requirements, associated with the preservation of pancreatic β-cell function and subsequent protection from diabetes, was demonstrated in the Troglitazone in the Prevention of Diabetes (TRIPOD) Study, in which high-risk Hispanic women with a history of gestational diabetes (the majority with impaired glucose tolerance) were randomly treated with troglitazone or placebo. The cumulative incidence of diabetes dropped to zero after more than 3 years of treatment with troglitazone in a subset of the cohort, and persisted 8 months after the study medication was stopped because of hepatotoxicity in a small percentage of patients.[84,105]

Table 9.10   Actions of peroxisome proliferator-activated receptor-γ ligands to inhibit atherosclerosis

↑ Insulin-mediated glucose uptake	↑ Endothelial function
↓ Triglycerides	↓ Cell growth
↑ HDL-cholesterol	↓ Cell migration
↓ Small, dense LDL cholesterol	↓ Inflammation
↑ Reverse cholesterol transport	↓ Circulating PAI-1
↓ Free fatty acids and alter adipokines	↓ Blood pressure
↓ TNF-α	↑ Adiponectin
↓ NF-kB activity	

HDL, high-density lipoprotein; LDL, low-density lipoprotein; PAI, plasminogen activator inhibitor, TNF, tumor necrosis factor

Few studies have examined the effects of TZD in high-risk patients with normal glucose tolerance. A recent investigation in young, obese, normoglycemic first-degree relatives of patients with type 2 diabetes demonstrated that troglitazone markedly reduced insulin resistance without changing glucose tolerance. The improved insulin sensitivity was associated with a decrease in circulating triglyceride levels and a slightly increased suppression of plasma free fatty acids by insulin.[104] Although it remains to be determined whether TZD reduce the risk of atherosclerosis, they have been shown to increase endothelium-dependent and -independent vascular reactivity, and to reduce blood pressure and fasting insulin or CRP levels without significantly altering the fasting plasma glucose concentration.[106]

The use of metformin in non-diabetic patients with the metabolic syndrome has also received little attention. In a study of morbidly obese non-diabetic men, metformin has been shown to reduce weight, fasting insulin levels, leptin, LDL cholesterol and central obesity when administered for 28 weeks.[107]

Adiponectin

Cytokines released from adipose tissue have several effects on carbohydrate and lipid metabolism, nutritional intake, and energy expenditure. The plasma concentration of one of these cytokines, adiponectin, is negatively correlated with BMI, glucose intolerance, insulin resistance, and hyperinsulinemia. Indeed, low circulating levels of adiponectin, and polymorphisms in the gene that encode for it, antedate the development of diabetes, the metabolic syndrome, and even atherosclerotic vascular disease in some populations.[50] Adiponectin administration has also been shown to decrease insulin resistance in obese and lipoatrophic mice, and to attenuate the severity of atherosclerosis in apo-E-deficient mice.[58,106] Adiponectin synthesis by the fat cell and its concentration in plasma are increased by treatment with TZD. Several reports suggest that the insulin-sensitizing effect of adiponectin is linked to its ability to activate AMPK.[50,60]

Prevention of macrovascular disease in patients with type 1 diabetes

Endothelial dysfunction and accelerated atherosclerosis occur at an early age and may progress rapidly in some people with type 1 diabetes.

New data from the UK Diabetes Cohort, essentially all from patients with type 1 diabetes, have demonstrated that the risk of ischemic heart disease in these individuals is probably much higher than previously thought.[12] An exceptionally high risk of mortality was observed in adult women with type 1 diabetes. Thus, women in the 20–29-year age group were 45 times more likely to die of cardiovascular disease in the average 17 years of follow-up. In addition, their mortality risk was equal to that of men the same age, indicating a loss of the cardioprotection seen in premenopausal women in the general population.[12] Macrovascular disease in patients with type 1 diabetes may be secondary to nephropathy and hypertension, and in some patients autonomic neuropathy, dyslipidemia, and microvascular cardiac disease could play a role.[109–111] Whether hyperglycemia per se is a pathogenetic factor is unclear. As noted earlier, the DCCT trial did not provide definitive evidence on this issue; however, recent findings from the Epidemiology of Diabetes Interventions and Complications (EDIC) – the long-term follow-up of the DCCT – showed less progression of atherosclerosis, based on measurements of carotid intima-media thickness by ultrasound, in patients in whom blood glucose had previously been intensively controlled.[112] Interestingly, the difference was observed well beyond the 6.5 years of the initial clinical trial at a time when glycemic control in the previously intensively managed and control groups was the same. Progression of carotid intima-media thickness was associated with age, systolic blood pressure, smoking, and dyslipidemia, the conventional cardiovascular risk factors in type 2 diabetes, and a positive family history for type 2 diabetes. These findings, plus the observation that intensively treated DCCT individuals who had gained excessive weight developed changes in lipid levels and blood pressure similar to those of patients with the metabolic syndrome,[10] suggests that targeting insulin resistance in this setting is a reasonable approach. In this context, a recent randomized placebo-controlled trial of metformin therapy in normal-weight adolescents with poorly controlled type 1 diabetes and insulin requirements of > 1 U/kg/day showed improved glycemic control and decreased insulin dosage over a 3-month study period.[113] Whether this reflects an effect of metformin on insulin resistance or some other action (e.g. diminished desire to eat) remains to be determined.

Conclusions

Therapies aimed at AMPK and specific risk factors both appear to provide some benefit in protecting people with type 2 diabetes against the development of coronary heart disease. Despite this, the incidence of cardiovascular morbidity and mortality even with multiple interventions still appears to be higher than in non-diabetic populations. This may relate to the fact that ischemic heart disease is already present in many people with type 2 diabetes at the time of diagnosis. For this reason, treatment prior to the onset of diabetes is a logical next step. Whether it is sufficient to initiate therapy

when these individuals have impaired glucose tolerance, or whether therapy should be started earlier to obtain optimal results (e.g. when they show early evidence of the metabolic syndrome), remains to be determined. It is likely that aiming at the metabolic syndrome will be necessary, as the available data suggest that CAD is already more prevalent in people with impaired glucose tolerance than in the general population.[17] Why atherosclerotic vascular disease is more prevalent in people with type 1 diabetes is less clear. One factor is undoubtedly the presence of nephropathy and hypertension. Another is the development of the metabolic syndrome, which may be more common in patients intensively treated with insulin or with a family history of type 2 diabetes. Whether therapies that activate AMPK will prove useful in people with type 1 diabetes remains to be determined.

References

1. Ruderman NB, Haudenschild C. Diabetes as an atherogenic factor. Prog Cardiovasc Dis 1984; 26:373–412
2. Steinberg D. Diabetes and Atherosclerosis. In: Porte D ed. Ellenberg and Rifkin's diabetes mellitus. New York: McGraw-Hill Professional, 2002: 193–206
3. Nesto R, Zarich SW, Jacoby RM, Kamalesh M. Heart disease in diabetes. In: Kahn CR ed. Joslin's diabetes mellitus. Baltimore, MD: Williams & Wilkins, 1994: 836–851
4. Rao SV, McGuire DK. Epidemiology of diabetes mellitus and cardiovascular disease. In: Marso SP, Stern DM eds. Diabetes and cardiovascular disease: integrating science and clinical medicine. Baltimore, MD: Lippincott Williams & Wilkins, 2004, 153–178
5. Guzman MA, McMahan CA, McGill HC Jr et al. Selected methodologic aspects of the International Atherosclerosis Project. Lab Invest 1968; 18:479–497
6. Robertson WB, Strong JP. Atherosclerosis in persons with hypertension and diabetes mellitus. Lab Invest 1968; 18:538–551
7. Kawate R, Yamakido M, Nishimoto Y et al. Diabetes mellitus and its vascular complications in Japanese migrants on the Island of Hawaii. Diabetes Care 1979; 2:161–170
8. Reaven G. Syndrome X. Curr Treat Options Cardiovasc Med 2001; 3:323–332
9. UK Prospective Diabetes Study (UKPDS) VIII. Study design, progress and performance. Diabetologisa 1991; 34:877–890
10. Purnell JQ, Hokanson JE, Marcovina SM et al. Effect of excessive weight gain with intensive therapy of type 1 diabetes on lipid levels and blood pressure: results from the

DCCT. Diabetes Control and Complications Trial. J Am Med Assoc 1998; 280:140–146

11. Krolewski AS, Kosinski EJ, Warram JH et al. Magnitude and determinants of coronary artery disease in juvenile-onset, insulin-dependent diabetes mellitus. Am J Cardiol 1987; 59:750–755

12. Laing SP, Swerdlow AJ, Slater SD et al. Mortality from heart disease in a cohort of 23,000 patients with insulin-treated diabetes. Diabetologia 2003; 46:760–765

13. Olefsky JM, Revers RR, Prince M et al. Insulin resistance in non-insulin dependent (type II) and insulin dependent (type I) diabetes mellitus. Adv Exp Med Biol 1985; 189:176–205

14. Marfella R, Quagliaro L, Nappo F et al. Acute hyperglycemia induces an oxidative stress in healthy subjects. J Clin Invest 2001; 108:635–636

15. Pyorala K, Savolainen E, Lehtovirta E et al. Glucose tolerance and coronary heart disease: Helsinki policemen study. J Chronic Dis 1979; 32:729–745

16. Rodriguez BL, Curb JD, Burchfiel CM et al. Impaired glucose tolerance, diabetes, and cardiovascular disease risk factor profiles in the elderly. The Honolulu Heart Program. Diabetes Care 1996; 19:587–590

17. Jarrett RJ, McCartney P, Keen H. The Bedford survey: ten year mortality rates in newly diagnosed diabetics, borderline diabetics and normoglycaemic controls and risk indices for coronary heart disease in borderline diabetics. Diabetologia 1982; 22:79–84

18. Coutinho M, Gerstein HC, Wang Y et al. The relationship between glucose and incident cardiovascular events. A metaregression analysis of published data from 20 studies of 95,783 individuals followed for 12.4 years. Diabetes Care 1999; 22:233–240

19. Hoogwerf BJ, Sprecher DL, Pearce GL et al. Blood glucose concentrations < or = 125 mg/dl and coronary heart disease risk. Am J Cardiol 2002; 89:596–599

20. Libby P, Ridker PM, Maseri A. Inflammation and atherosclerosis. Circulation 2002; 105:1135–1143

21. Inoguchi T, Li P, Umeda F et al. High glucose level and free fatty acid stimulate reactive oxygen species production through protein kinase C-dependent activation of NAD(P)H oxidase in cultured vascular cells. Diabetes 2000; 49:1939–1945

22. Koya D, King GL. Protein kinase C activation and the development of diabetic complications. Diabetes 1998; 47:859–866

23. Nishikawa T, Edelstein D, Brownlee M. The missing link: a single unifying mechanism for diabetic complications. Kidney Int 2000; 77 (Suppl):S26–30

24. Ido Y, Carling D, Ruderman N. Hyperglycemia-induced apoptosis in human umbilical vein endothelial cells: inhibition by the AMP-activated protein kinase activation. Diabetes 2002; 51:159–167

25. Leopold JA, Cap A, Scribner AW et al. Glucose-6-phosphate dehydrogenase deficiency promotes endothelial oxidant stress and decreases endothelial nitric oxide bioavailability. FASEB J 2001; 15:1771–1773

26. Zhang Z, Apse K, Pang J et al. High glucose inhibits glucose-6-phosphate dehydrogenase via cAMP in aortic endothelial cells. J Biol Chem 2000; 275:40042–40047

27. Brownlee M. Negative consequences of glycation. Metabolism 2000; 49 (Suppl 1):9–13

28. Honda HM, Leitinger N, Frankel M et al. Induction of monocyte binding to endothelial cells by MM-LDL: role of lipoxygenase metabolites. Arterioscler Thromb Vasc Biol 1999; 19:680–686

29. Brownlee M. Biochemistry and molecular cell biology of diabetic complications. Nature 2001; 414:813–820

30. Du XL, Edelstein D, Brownlee M. Hyperglycemia-induced mitochondrial superoxide production inhibits glucose-6-phosphate dehydrogenase activity by inhibition of phosphotyrosine phosphatase. Diabetes 2003; 52(Suppl 1):A173

31. Kaneto H, Xu G, Song KH et al. Activation of the hexosamine pathway leads to deterioration of pancreatic beta-cell function through the induction of oxidative stress. J Biol Chem 2001; 276:31099–31104

32. Schmidt AM, Hori O, Chen JX et al. Advanced glycation endproducts interacting with their endothelial receptor induce expression of vascular cell adhesion molecule-1 (VCAM-1) in cultured human endothelial cells and in mice. A potential mechanism for the accelerated vasculopathy of diabetes. J Clin Invest 1995; 96:1395–1403

33. Dagher Z, Ruderman N, Tornheim K, et al. Acute regulation of fatty acid oxidation and amp-activated protein kinase in human umbilical vein endothelial cells. Circ Res 2001; 88:1276–1282

34. Steinberg HO, Paradisi G, Hook G, et al. Free fatty acid elevation impairs insulin-mediated vasodilation and nitric oxide production. Diabetes 2000; 49:1231–1238

35. Lu G, Greene EL, Nagai T, et al. Reactive oxygen species are critical in the oleic acid-mediated mitogenic signaling pathway in vascular smooth muscle cells. Hypertension 1998; 32:1003–1010

36. Ido Y, Zou M, Chen K, et al. The AMP-kinase (AMPK) activator, AICAR, inhibits the increase in oxidative stress induced by hyperglycemia and palmitate. Diabetes 2002; 51(Suppl 2):A396

37. Ido Y, Yagihashi N, Cacicedo JM et al. AMP-kinase activation prevents TNF-alpha induced ICAM expression by inhibiting NF-KB transactivation but not by inhibiting their translocation or DNA binding. Diabetes 2002; 51(Suppl 2):A458

38. Libby P. Inflammation in atherosclerosis. Nature 2002; 420:868–874

39. Witztum JL, Steinberg D. The oxidative modification hypothesis of atherosclerosis: does it hold for humans? Trends Cardiovasc Med 2001; 11:93–102

40. Artwohl M, Graier WF, Roden M et al. Diabetic LDL triggers apoptosis in vascular endothelial cells. Diabetes 2003; 52:1240–1247

41. Baynes JW. Chemical modification of proteins by lipids in diabetes. Clin Chem Lab Med 2003; 41:1159–1165

42. Makita Z, Radoff S, Rayfield EJ et al. Advanced glycosylation end products in patients with diabetic nephropathy. N Engl J Med 1991; 325:836–842

43. Schmidt AM, Yan SD, Wautier JL et al. Activation of receptor for advanced glycation end products: a mechanism for chronic vascular dysfunction in diabetic vasculopathy and atherosclerosis. Circ Res 1999; 84:489–497

44. Bucciarelli LG, Wendt T, Qu W et al. RAGE blockade stabilizes established atherosclerosis in diabetic apolipoprotein E-null mice. Circulation 2002; 106:2827–2835

45. Libby P, Plutzky J. Diabetic macrovascular disease: the glucose paradox? Circulation 2002; 106:2760–2763

46. Ruderman NB, Cacicedo JM, Itani S et al. Malonyl-CoA and AMP-activated protein kinase (AMPK): possible links between insulin resistance in muscle and early endothelial cell damage in diabetes. Biochem Soc Trans 2003; 31:202–206

47. Itani SI, Ruderman NB, Schmieder F et al. Lipid-induced insulin resistance in human muscle is associated with changes in diacylglycerol, protein kinase C, and IkappaB-alpha. Diabetes 2002; 51:2005–2011

48. Idris I, Gray S, Donnelly R. Protein kinase C activation: isozyme-specific effects on metabolism and cardiovascular complications in diabetes. Diabetologia 2001; 44:659–673

49. Evans JL, Goldfine ID, Maddux BA et al. Are oxidative stress-activated signaling pathways mediators of insulin resistance and beta-cell dysfunction? Diabetes 2003; 52:1–8

50. Ruderman N, Prentki M. AMP kinase and malonyl CoA: targets for therapy of the metabolic syndrome. Nat Rev Drug Discov 2004; 3:340–351.

51. Laybutt DR, Schmitz-Peiffer C, Saha AK et al. Muscle lipid accumulation and protein kinase C activation in the insulin-resistant chronically glucose-infused rat. Am J Physiol 1999; 277:E1070–E1076

52. Kraegen EW, Saha A, Preston E et al. Insulin resistance by glucose infusion is associated temporally with reduced muscle and liver AMPK activity. Diabetes 2003; S1:A330

53. Unger RH. Lipotoxic diseases. Annu Rev Med 2002; 53:319–336

54. Park H, Kaushik VK, Constant S et al. Coordinate regulation of malonyl-CoA decarboxylase, sn-glycerol-3-phosphate acyltransferase, and acetyl-CoA carboxylase by AMP-activated protein kinase in rat tissues in response to exercise. J Biol Chem 2002; 277:32571–32577

55. Winder WW, Hardie DG. Inactivation of acetyl-CoA carboxylase and activation of AMP-activated protein kinase in muscle during exercise. Am J Physiol 1996; 270:E299–E304

56. Zhou G, Myers R, Li Y et al. Role of AMP-activated protein kinase in the mechanism of metformin action. J Clin Invest 2001; 108:1167–1174

57. Saha AK, Avilucea PR, Ye JM et al. Pioglitazone treatment activates AMP-activated protein kinase in rat liver and adipose tissue in vivo. Biochem Biophys Res Commun 2004; 314:580–585

58. Yamauchi T, Kamon J, Waki H et al. Globular adiponectin protected ob/ob mice from diabetes and ApoE-deficient mice from atherosclerosis. J Biol Chem 2003; 278:2461–2468

59. Okamoto Y, Kihara S, Ouchi N et al. Adiponectin reduces atherosclerosis in apolipoprotein E-deficient mice. Circulation 2002; 106:2767–2770

60. Tomas E, Tsao TS, Saha AK et al. Enhanced muscle fat oxidation and glucose transport by ACRP30 globular domain: acetyl-CoA carboxylase inhibition and AMP-activated protein kinase activation. Proc Natl Acad Sci USA 2002; 99:16309–16313

61. Haffner SM. Insulin resistance, inflammation, and the prediabetic state. Am J Cardiol 2003; 92:18J–26J

62. Ouchi N, Kihara S, Arita Y et al. Adiponectin, an adipocyte-derived plasma protein, inhibits endothelial NF-kappaB signaling through a cAMP-dependent pathway. Circulation 2000; 102:1296–1301

63. Matsuzawa Y, Funahashi T, Kihara S et al. Adiponectin and metabolic syndrome. Arterioscler Thromb Vasc Biol 2004; 24:29–33

64. UK Prospective Diabetes Study (UKPDS) Group. Effect of intensive blood-glucose control with metformin on complications in overweight patients with type 2 diabetes (UKPDS 34). Lancet 1998; 352:854–865

65. Eriksson KF, Lindgarde F. No excess 12-year mortality in men with impaired glucose tolerance who participated in the Malmo Preventive Trial with diet and exercise. Diabetologia 1998; 41:1010–1016

66. Koshiyama H, Shimono D, Kuwamura N et al. Rapid communication: inhibitory effect of pioglitazone on carotid arterial wall thickness in type 2 diabetes. J Clin Endocrinol Metab 2001; 86:3452–3456

67. Manson JE, Hu FB, Rich-Edwards JW et al. A prospective study of walking as compared with vigorous exercise in the prevention of coronary heart disease in women. N Engl J Med 1999; 341:650–658

68. Saito I, Folsom AR, Brancati FL et al. Nontraditional risk factors for coronary heart disease incidence among persons with diabetes: the Atherosclerosis Risk in Communities (ARIC) Study. Ann Intern Med 2000; 133:81–91

69. Hu FB, Stampfer MJ, Solomon C et al. Physical activity and risk for cardiovascular events in diabetic women. Ann Intern Med 2001; 134:96–105

70. Pyorala K, Pedersen TR, Kjekshus J et al. Cholesterol lowering with simvastatin improves prognosis of diabetic patients with coronary heart disease. A subgroup analysis of the Scandinavian Simvastatin Survival Study (4S). Diabetes Care 1997; 20:614–620

71. Schleicher ED, Wagner E, Nerlich AG. Increased accumulation of the glycoxidation product N(epsilon)-(carboxymethyl)lysine in human tissues in diabetes and aging. J Clin Invest 1997; 99:457–468

72. Stratton IM, Adler AI, Neil HA et al. Association of glycaemia with macrovascular and microvascular complications of type 2 diabetes (UKPDS 35): prospective observational study. Br Med J 2000; 321:405–412

73. Fryer LG, Parbu-Patel A, Carling D. The anti-diabetic drugs rosiglitazone and metformin stimulate AMP-activated protein kinase through distinct signaling pathways. J Biol Chem 2002; 277:25226–25232

74. Hsueh WA, Law R. The central role of fat and effect of peroxisome proliferator-activated receptor-gamma on

progression of insulin resistance and cardiovascular disease. Am J Cardiol 2003; 92:3J–9J

75. Takagi T, Yamamuro A, Tamita K et al. Pioglitazone reduces neointimal tissue proliferation after coronary stent implantation in patients with type 2 diabetes mellitus: an intravascular ultrasound scanning study. Am Heart J 2003; 146:E5

76. Haffner SM, Greenberg AS, Weston WM et al. Effect of rosiglitazone treatment on nontraditional markers of cardiovascular disease in patients with type 2 diabetes mellitus. Circulation 2002; 106:679–684.

77. Viberti G, Kahn SE, Greene DA et al. A diabetes outcome progression trial (ADOPT): an international multicenter study of the comparative efficacy of rosiglitazone, glyburide, and metformin in recently diagnosed type 2 diabetes. Diabetes Care 2002; 25:1737–1743

78. Diabetes Reduction Approaches with Ramipril and Rosiglitazone Medications (DREAM) Trial. In: www.dream-ctn.org

79. Action to Control Cardiovascular Risk in Diabetes (ACCORD) Trial. In: www.accord.ne.org

80. Gaede P, Vedel P, Larsen N et al. Multifactorial intervention and cardiovascular disease in patients with type 2 diabetes. N Engl J Med 2003; 348:383–393

81. Knowler WC, Barrett-Connor E, Fowler SE et al. Reduction in the incidence of type 2 diabetes with lifestyle intervention or metformin. N Engl J Med 2002; 346:393–403

82. Tuomilehto J, Lindstrom J, Eriksson JG et al. Prevention of type 2 diabetes mellitus by changes in lifestyle among subjects with impaired glucose tolerance. N Engl J Med 2001; 344:1343–1350

83. Chiasson JL, Josse RG, Gomis R et al. Acarbose for prevention of type 2 diabetes mellitus: the STOP-NIDDM randomised trial. Lancet 2002; 359:2072–2077

84. Buchanan TA, Xiang AH, Peters RK et al. Preservation of pancreatic beta-cell function and prevention of type 2 diabetes by pharmacological treatment of insulin resistance in high-risk Hispanic women. Diabetes 2002; 51:2796–2803

85. Diabetes Prevention Program Research Group. Impact of lifestyle and metformin therapy on cardiovascular (CVD) risk factors and events in the diabetes prevention program. Diabetes 2003; 52 (Suppl 1):A169

86. Diabetes Prevention Program Research Group. The effects of intensive lifestyle intervention (ILS) and metformin (MET) on C-reactive protein (CRP), tissue plasminogen activator (TPA) and fibrinogen (FIB) in the Diabetes Prevention Program (DPP). Diabetes 2003; 52(Suppl 1):A18

87. Chiasson JL, Josse RG, Gomis R et al. Acarbose treatment and the risk of cardiovascular disease and hypertension in patients with impaired glucose tolerance: the STOP NIDDM trial. J Am Med Assoc 2003; 290:486-494.

88. Eriksson KF, Lindgarde F. Prevention of type 2 (non-insulin-dependent) diabetes mellitus by diet and physical exercise. The 6-year Malmo feasibility study. Diabetologia 1991; 34:891–898

89. Ruderman N, Chisholm D, Pi-Sunyer X et al. The metabolically obese, normal-weight individual revisited. Diabetes 1998; 47:699–713

90. Reaven GM. Banting lecture 1988. Role of insulin resistance in human disease. Diabetes 1988; 37:1595–1607

91. Ford ES, Giles WH, Dietz WH. Prevalence of the metabolic syndrome among US adults: findings from the third National Health and Nutrition Examination Survey. J Am Med Assoc 2002; 287:356–359

92. Executive Summary of the Third Report of the National Cholesterol Education Program (NCEP) Expert Panel on Detection, Evaluation, and Treatment of High Blood Cholesterol In Adults (Adult Treatment Panel III). J Am Med Assoc 2001; 285:2486–2497

93. Whaley MH, Kampert JB, Kohl HW III et al. Physical fitness and clustering of risk factors associated with the metabolic syndrome. Med Sci Sports Exerc 1999; 31:287–293

94. Diabetes Prevention Program Research Group. The effect of intensive lifestyle intervention (ILS) and metformin (MET) on the incidence of the metabolic syndrome among participants in the Diabetes Prevention Program (DPP). Diabetes 2003; 52 (Suppl 1):A58

95. Church TS, Cheng YJ, Earnest CP et al. Exercise capacity and body composition as predictors of mortality among men with diabetes. Diabetes Care 2004; 27:83–88

96. Katzmarzyk PT, Leon AS, Wilmore JH et al. Targeting the metabolic syndrome with exercise: evidence from the HERITAGE Family Study. Med Sci Sports Exerc 2003; 35:1703–1709

97. Mulrow CD, Chiquette E, Angel L et al. Dieting to reduce body weight for controlling hypertension in adults. Cochrane Database Syst Rev 2000(2):CD000484

98. McKeown NM, Meigs JB, Liu S et al. Carbohydrate nutrition, insulin resistance, and the prevalence of the metabolic syndrome in the Framingham Offspring Cohort. Diabetes Care 2004; 27:538–546

99. Bell DS. Beneficial effects resulting from thiazolidinediones for treatment of type 2 diabetes mellitus. Postgrad Med 2003; 8:35–44

100. Olefsky JM, Saltiel AR. PPAR gamma and the treatment of insulin resistance. Trends Endocrinol Metab 2000; 11:362–368

101. Unger RH, Orci L. Diseases of liporegulation: new perspective on obesity and related disorders. FASEB J 2001; 15:312–321

102. Fonseca VA. Management of diabetes mellitus and insulin resistance in patients with cardiovascular disease. Am J Cardiol 2003; 92:50J–60J

103. Olefsky JM. Treatment of insulin resistance with peroxisome proliferator-activated receptor gamma agonists. J Clin Invest 2000; 106:467–472

104. Levin K, Hother-Nielsen O, Henriksen JE et al. Effects of troglitazone in young first-degree relatives of patients with type 2 diabetes. Diabetes Care 2004; 27:148–154

105. Buchanan TA. Prevention of type 2 diabetes: what is it really? Diabetes Care 2003; 26:1306–1308

106. Wang TD, Chen WJ, Lin JW, et al. Effects of rosiglitazone on endothelial function, C-reactive protein, and components of the metabolic syndrome in nondiabetic patients with the metabolic syndrome. Am J Cardiol 2004; 93:362–365

107. Glueck CJ, Fontaine RN, Wang P, et al. Metformin reduces weight, centripetal obesity, insulin, leptin, and low-density lipoprotein cholesterol in nondiabetic, morbidly obese subjects with body mass index greater than 30. Metabolism 2001; 50:856–861

108. Yamauchi T, Kamon J, Waki H et al. The fat-derived hormone adiponectin reverses insulin resistance associated with both lipoatrophy and obesity. Nature Med 2001; 7:941–946

109. Burger AJ, Weinrauch LA, D'Elia JA et al. Effect of glycemic control on heart rate variability in type I diabetic patients with cardiac autonomic neuropathy. Am J Cardiol 1999; 84:687–691

110. Koivisto VA, Stevens LK, Mattock M et al. Cardiovascular disease and its risk factors in IDDM in Europe. EURO-DIAB IDDM Complications Study Group. Diabetes Care 1996; 19:689–697

111. Standl E, Schnell O. A new look at the heart in diabetes mellitus: from ailing to failing. Diabetologia 2000; 43:1455–1469

112. Nathan DM, Lachin J, Cleary P et al. Intensive diabetes therapy and carotid intima-media thickness in type 1 diabetes mellitus. N Engl J Med 2003; 348:2294–2303

113. Hamilton J, Cummings E, Zdravkovic V et al. Metformin as an adjunct therapy in adolescents with type 1 diabetes and insulin resistance: a randomized controlled trial. Diabetes Care 2003; 26:138–143

114. Kannel WB, McGee DL. Diabetes and cardiovascular disease. The Framingham study. J Am Med Assoc 1979; 241:2035–2038

115. Third report of the National Cholesterol Education Program (NCEP) expert panel on detection evaluation, and treatment of high blood cholesterol in adults (Adult Treatment Panel III) final report. Circulation 2002; 106:3143–1421

116. Adler AI, Stratton IM, Neil HA et al. Association of systolic blood pressure with macrovascular and microvascular complications of type 2 diabetes (UKPDS 36): prospective observational study. Br Med J 2000; 321:412–419

117. Hansson L, Zanchetti A, Carruthers SG et al. Effects of intensive blood-pressure lowering and low-dose aspirin in patients with hypertension: principal results of the Hypertension Optimal Treatment (HOT) randomised trial. HOT Study Group. Lancet 1998; 351:1755–1762

118. Tuomilehto J, Rastenyte D, Birkenhager WH et al. Effects of calcium-channel blockade in older patients with diabetes and systolic hypertension. Systolic Hypertension in Europe Trial Investigators. N Engl J Med 1999; 340:677–684

119. Heart Outcomes Prevention Evaluation Study Investigators. Effects of ramipril on cardiovascular and microvascular outcomes in people with diabetes mellitus: results of the HOPE study and MICRO-HOPE substudy. Lancet 2000; 355:253–259

120. Haffner SM, Alexander CM, Cook TJ et al. Reduced coronary events in simvastatin-treated patients with coronary heart disease and diabetes or impaired fasting glucose levels: subgroup analyses in the Scandinavian Simvastatin Survival Study. Arch Intern Med 1999; 159:2661–2667

121. Sacks FM, Pfeffer MA, Moye LA et al. The effect of pravastatin on coronary events after myocardial infarction in patients with average cholesterol levels. Cholesterol and Recurrent Events Trial Investigators. N Engl J Med 1996; 335:1001–1009

122. Rubins HB, Robins SJ, Collins D et al. Gemfibrozil for the secondary prevention of coronary heart disease in men with low levels of high-density lipoprotein cholesterol. Veterans Affairs High-Density Lipoprotein Cholesterol Intervention Trial Study Group. N Engl J Med 1999; 341:410–418

123. Collins R, Armitage J, Parish S et al. MRC/BHF Heart Protection Study of cholesterol-lowering with simvastatin in 5963 people with diabetes: a randomised placebo-controlled trial. Lancet 2003; 361:2005–2016

124. Pan XR, Li GW, Hu YH et al. Effects of diet and exercise in preventing NIDDM in people with impaired glucose tolerance. The Da Qing IGT and Diabetes Study. Diabetes Care 1997; 20:537–544

10

Hypertension and atherogenesis

Diane E. Handy, Haralambos Gavras

Introduction

It has been estimated that more than 40 million adults in the USA over the age of 25 have hypertension and that, of these, only about half are currently treated with medications.[1] The vascular effects of elevated blood pressure promote atherothrombotic disease, with consequences for cardiac, cerebral, and renal function. Large epidemiological studies, such as the Framingham Heart Study, have shown that increasing systolic or diastolic blood pressure increases the likelihood of coronary events and mortality from coronary artery disease.[2] The Cardiovascular Health Study confirmed a linear relationship between cardiovascular disease (CVD) risk and blood pressure in subjects ≥ 65 years of age.[3] Similarly, the Multiple Risk Factor Intervention Trial (MRFIT) found a significant increase in the relative risk for coronary heart disease with increased blood pressure in a younger cohort of men (aged 35–47).[4] Overall, these studies found the lowest CVD risk to be in patients with the lowest blood pressure. In numerous studies, treatments with antihypertensive agents have been found to decrease morbidity and mortality from cardiovascular disease,[5] suggesting that optimal blood pressure control can contribute to improved quality of life. Notably, the decrease in stroke, renal failure, and heart failure rate is more pronounced than the decrease in the incidence of myocardial infarction (MI) accompanying a reduction in blood pressure.

This chapter summarizes the current understanding of the link between hypertension and atherosclerosis by reviewing major clinical studies that have established hypertension as a risk factor for CVD, and discussing recent experimental evidence that illuminates some of the pathophysiological mechanisms by which hypertension may promote vascular disease. In linking atherosclerotic predisposition with hypertension, it is important to consider not only the mechanical effects of elevated intra-arterial pressure, but also the cluster of clinical characteristics known as the metabolic syndrome. Decreased insulin sensitivity is characteristic of essential hypertension, even in non-obese subjects, and is further aggravated by obesity, especially visceral adiposity. In the metabolic syndrome, insulin resistance may contribute to hypertension and a predisposition to develop type 2 diabetes, which is also associated with an abnormal lipid profile. Each one of these characteristics is atherogenic and can augment CVD risk. This chapter will discuss these disorders, especially the latter, as diabetes accelerates the risk of adverse CVD outcomes. In addition, this chapter summarizes some of the major studies that have shown the effectiveness of antihypertensive therapies in reducing CVD risk, and will also discuss whether these protective effects are due to lowering of blood pressure or to other effects of these pharmacological agents.

Epidemiology: the link between hypertension and atherosclerosis

The prospective and ongoing analysis in the Framingham Heart Study has provided invaluable information regarding CVD risk factors. A 12-year follow-up of 2489 men and 2856 women in the Framingham cohort, who were 30–74 years of age at baseline, showed that 28% of coronary events in men and 29% of coronary events in women were attributable to blood pressure levels over the high normal range (i.e. blood pressure $\geq 130/85$ mmHg).[2] Analysis of Framingham outcomes revealed that higher levels of blood pressure are associated with abnormal cholesterol levels, increased body mass index, and an increased prevalence of diabetes. Furthermore, in the Atherosclerosis Risk in Communities (ARIC) study, the incidence rates of new-onset diabetes were higher in hypertensives not receiving antihypertensive therapies than in those treated with antihypertensives. In the ARIC cohort, change in intima-media thickness was found to correlate with LDL cholesterol, triglycerides, and the development of diabetes and hypertension.[6]

A common clustering of hypertension and diabetes has been found in numerous studies. In the Cardiovascular Health Study, 5888 adults aged 65 and over were recruited from four US centers. Participants had no prior MI, congestive heart failure (CHF), or stroke, and were followed for up to 4 years.[3] Baseline systolic blood pressure (SBP) was associated with age, carotid intima-media thickness, and a prevalence of diabetes. The adjusted model hazard ratio for MI associated with 1-SD increases in adjusted SBP was 1.24 (95% CI 1.15–1.35) and for diastolic pressure was 1.13 (95% CI 1.04–1.35). The adjusted model hazard ratio for pulse pressure was 1.21 (95% CI 1.12–1.31), reflecting the fact that a wide pulse pressure is a marker for loss of arterial wall elasticity. The associated hazard ratios for stroke were even higher: SBP 1.34 (95% CI 1.21–1.47); DBP 1.29 (95% CI 1.17–1.42), and pulse pressure 1.21 (95% CI 1.10–1.34). Furthermore, in treated hypertensives the risks for MI and stroke were lower than in untreated hypertensives; however, even at the same blood pressure level, treated hypertensives apparently had more risk at a given blood pressure than normotensives. Thus, better blood pressure control or earlier treatment may be necessary to reverse completely the increased cardiovascular risk associated with elevated blood pressure. MRFIT, which analyzed risk factors in over 340 000 men without a prior MI, concluded that there was an increase in mortality with risk factors such as diabetes, hypercholesterolemia, smoking, and elevated blood pressure.[4] Based on the analysis of these and numerous other published studies, the National Cholesterol Education Program Adult Treatment Panel III (NCEP ATP III) has determined that hypertension, obesity, and dislipidemia (i.e. the components of the metabolic syndrome), along with smoking, are major modifiable risk factors for atherosclerotic disease.[7]

Normotension and hypertension

Fundamentally, blood pressure is defined by the Poiseuille equation: BP = cardiac output X total peripheral resistance. The dynamic physiological control of blood pressure involves central and peripheral systems that influence cardiac output, blood volume, and vascular tone. Major contributors to blood pressure control include the sympathetic nervous system (SNS) and the renin–angiotensin–aldosterone (RAAS) system. Dysregulation of either of these systems contributes to hypertension and can promote atherosclerosis.

The SNS influences both acute and long-term blood pressure homeostasis by the actions of catecholamines (primarily norepinephrine, and to a lesser extent epinephrine) on adrenergic receptors in the vasculature of target organs (Figure 10.1). There are many different types of adrenergic receptor, including β_1, β_2, β_3, α_{1A}, α_{1B}, α_{1C}, α_{2A}, α_B, and α_{2C}. Adrenergic receptors are members of the 7-transmembrane family of G-protein-coupled receptors.[8] Depending on the receptor type and the cell location, agonist binding to these receptors can activate or inhibit various effector systems, for example adenylyl cyclase to regulate cAMP levels, or phospholipase C, which controls calcium mobilization.[9] Stimulation of presynaptic central α_2-adrenergic receptors by α_2-agonists such as clonidine is sympathoinhibitory and reduces blood pressure. Studies in different lines of knockout mice that lack each of the three α_2-adrenergic receptor subtypes indicate that, in the central nervous system, the α_{2A}-subtype of adrenergic receptors is responsible for mediating the central sympathoinhibitory function of norepinephrine,[10] whereas the α_{2B} subtype is sympathoexcitatory and responsible for the hyperadrenergic state of salt-induced hypertension.[11] The outflow of catecholamines can directly affect blood pressure by altering cardiac function and vascular resistance via postsynaptic receptor action: via β_1-adrenergic receptors in the heart that regulate heart rate, and β_2-adrenergic receptors in the vasculature, which have a vasodilatory function;[12] and via α-adrenergic receptors in the vessels. In the endothelium, α_{2A}-adrenergic receptor stimulation can promote the production of endothelium-derived relaxing factor (EDRF), which is nitric oxide (NO) or a related derivative. In contrast, activation of α-adrenergic receptors on vascular smooth muscle cells causes contraction, with α_1-adrenergic

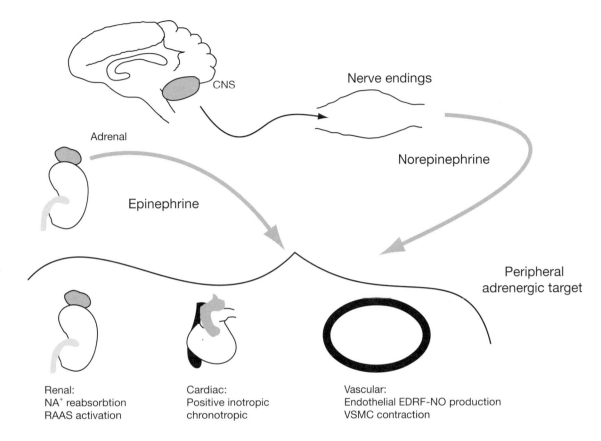

Figure 10.1 Effects of the sympathetic nervous system on blood pressure. Catecholamines, primarily norepinephrine (with some epinephrine), released from nerve endings, and epinephrine, (with some norepinephrine) released from the adrenal gland, activate peripheral adrenergic receptors. In the kidney, stimulation of adrenergic receptors increases sodium reabsorption and activates the renin–angiotensin–aldosterone system (RAAS). Adrenergic receptors in the heart regulate contractility. Adrenergic receptors in vessels contribute to vascular tone by offsetting pressor actions on vascular smooth muscle cells and dilator actions through the release of endothelium-derived relaxing factor (EDRF) (or nitric oxide, NO) from endothelial cells. Importantly, stimulation of α_{2A}-subtype adrenergic receptors in the central nervous system (CNS) causes sympathoinhibition, whereas the centrally located α_{2B}-adrenergic receptors are sympathoexcitatory. VSMC, vascular smooth muscle cell

receptors responsible for as much as 68% of the norepinephrine-induced vasconstriction and α_{2A}-adrenergic receptors responsible for the remainder of norepinephrine's vasoconstrictor effects.[13] The SNS has other, indirect effects on blood pressure, by stimulating Na^+ reabsorption in the proximal tubules and stimulating renin release in the kidney.[12] Younger hypertensives in the earlier stages of the disease often have a rapid heart rate, high cardiac output, and elevation in circulating catecholamines, indicating dysregulation of the SNS.

RAAS plays a most important role in regulating blood pressure. Angiotensin II (AII) is the end-product of this system (Figure 10.2). It is formed by cleavage of angiotensinogen by the enzyme renin to produce AI, an inactive decapeptide which is a substrate for the angiotensin-converting enzyme (ACE). The ACE cleaves off two amino acids to produce the octapeptide AII, a potent vasoconstrictor acting on angiotensin type 1 (AT$_1$) receptors on smooth muscle cells. It has been proposed that AT$_2$ receptors counteract some of the effects of AII binding to AT$_1$ receptors, but most of the cardiovascular effects of AII are due to binding to the higher-affinity AT$_1$ receptors.[14] Similar to the adrenergic receptors, the AT$_1$ receptors are members of the 7-transmembrane family of G-protein-coupled receptors. AII acting as a systemic hormone stimulates adrenal

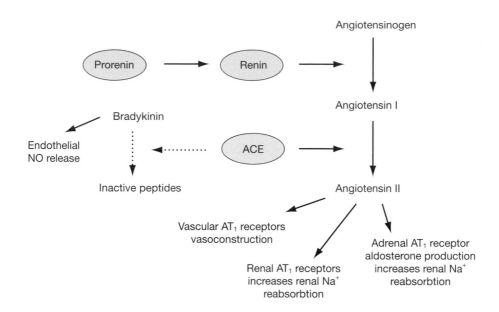

Figure 10.2 The role of the renin–angiotensin–aldosterone system (RAAS) in hypertension. Renin is formed as a proenzyme, prorenin, in the juxtaglomerular cells of the kidney. The active renin enzyme, released by adrenergic stimulation, cleaves angiotensinogen to produce angiotensin I (AI), an inactive decapeptide, which is a substrate for the angiotensin-converting enzyme (ACE). ACE cleaves off two amino acids to produce the octapeptide angiotensin II (AII), a potent vascular constrictor acting on angiotensin II type 1 (AT$_1$) receptors on vascular smooth muscle cells. ACE also inactivates bradykinin, a potent vasodilator, by enzymatic digestion to inactive peptides. It has been proposed that some of the benefits of ACE inhibition stem from blocking the inactivation of bradykinin. AII can increase blood pressure by stimulating an increase in renal sodium reabsorption, indirectly by increasing aldosterone production in the adrenal glands, and directly by activating receptors in the kidney. AII can also increase blood pressure by activating the sympathetic nervous system

production of aldosterone which, together with AII, regulates renal salt and water retention. AII can also influence the SNS by stimulating catecholamine release, thereby raising blood pressure. The RAAS system can modulate the effects of the nitric oxide-dependent vasodilator bradykinin, which is inactivated by the proteolytic actions of ACE. In addition to its systemic actions, AII can also act as a local tissue hormone, whose effects depend on the type of cells affected. Thus, it has positive inotropic, chronotropic, and trophic effects on cardiomyocytes, affects ion exchange in renal cells, and stimulates vascular smooth muscle cell hypertrophy and proliferation. The multiple effects of ACE and AII promote increases in blood pressure, and any dysregulation of the systems that normally keep these actions in check can promote hypertension, cardiac and vascular wall hypertrophy, ischemia, and damage to vital organs. Proinflammatory, proliferative, and pro-oxidant effects of AII may also contribute to the

vascular remodeling and endothelial damage found in atherosclerosis, as discussed later in the chapter.

Pathogenic links between hypertension and atherosclerosis

Vascular remodeling, endothelial dysfunction and AII

Ross[15] hypothesized that atherosclerosis is an inflammatory disease. The earliest vascular lesions, fatty streaks, consist of adherent macrophages and T lymphocytes. Increased SBP has been shown to be associated with increased intima-media thickness,[6,16,17] an early clinical measure of preatherosclerotic changes.

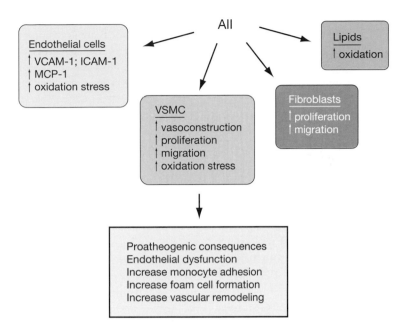

Figure 10.3 The proatherogenic consequences of angiotensin II (AII). AII has pleiotrophic effects on many target cells. AII activation of the AII receptor type 1 (AT_1) increases NAD(P)H oxidase activity, cellular production of superoxide, and oxidative stress in vascular smooth muscle cells (VSMC) and endothelial cells, contributing to endothelial dysfunction. Loss of bioavailable nitric oxide (NO) further augments the damaging effects of AII, by causing an increase in vascular AT_1 receptors. Expression of vascular cellular adhesion molecules (VCAM-1), intercellular adhesion molecules (ICAM-1), and monocyte chemoattractant protein (MCP-1) increases monocyte adhesion to the endothelium. AII effects on the growth and migration of VSMC and fibroblasts contribute to vascular remodeling, whereas the AII-mediated increase in lipid oxidation contributes to foam cell development and lesion formation

Hypertension has been shown to stimulate the development of aortic atherosclerosis in animal models of dyslipidemia. For example, in the Watanabe Heritable Hyperlipidemic (WHHL) rabbit, which has dyslipidemia due to a genetic defect in the low-density lipoprotein receptor, experimental renovascular hypertension caused a marked increase in lesion area and the severity of lesions in the aorta.[18] Similarly, New Zealand White rabbits fed an atherogenic diet showed increased monocyte adhesion to the aorta when blood pressure was increased by aortic coarctation.[19] Other studies in the WHHL rabbit, however, suggest that even in the absence of hypertension, ACE inhibitors and AT_1 receptor inhibitors can decrease atherosclerotic lesions.[20,21] It was suggested that the slight decrease in blood pressure caused by treatment with antihypertensive agents in these studies may be partly responsible for the reduction in lesion area and complexity, although direct inhibition of AII within the vascular wall must also have contributed to the observed changes.

The relationship between the RAAS system and atherosclerotic changes in the vasculature may be explained in part by the local tissue actions of AII, such as its proliferative, proinflammatory, and oxidative effects (Figure 10.3). In cell culture models, AII has been shown to increase leukocyte adhesion,[22] an early and important step in fatty streak formation.

The importance of endothelial dysfunction in hypertension and atherosclerosis is controversial, but the changes caused by AII can also promote superoxide generation,[23] which may lead to a reduction in bioactive NO, oxidative stress, and subsequent endothelial dysfunction.[24–27] Alterations in NO-mediated vasorelaxation can be found in hypertensive subjects.[25–28] Alterations in vascular function are considered to be an early marker of atherosclerotic changes.[29] These changes may reflect an imbalance between vasodilator and constrictor systems. For example, endothelin-1 (ET-1), a potent vasoconstrictor, blunts acetylcholine-mediated vasodilation in hypertensives but not in normotensives, as blocking the ET-1 receptor appears to correct the endothelial dysfunction in hypertensives but has no effect in normotensives, where there is no endothelial dysfunction.[30] ET-1 has been shown to stimulate leukocyte activation,[31] suggesting that increased levels of this factor may contribute to atherogenic changes and hypertension, even if it does not contribute to sustained elevation of systemic blood pressure. Improvements in acetylcholine-mediated vasodilation of the femoral artery were found after blockade of AT_1 receptors in patients with atherosclerosis,[32] indicating that an excess of vasoconstrictor activity may alter vascular function in atherosclerosis.

AII, acting via the AT_1 receptor, has many proatherogenic actions, such as increasing lipid oxidation, which feeds fatty streak formation, uptake of oxidized LDL by macrophages, and subsequent foam cell formation.[33] AII-mediated signaling has also been linked to increases in endothelial cell production of cytokines, such as monocyte chemoattractant protein (MCP-1), and activation of vascular cellular adhesion molecules (VCAM-1) and intercellular adhesion molecules (ICAM-1) that contribute to the adhesion of monocytes and plaque formation. In addition, AII can stimulate the growth and migration of smooth muscle cells and fibroblasts, thereby contributing to vascular remodeling. These multiple effects are reviewed in the work of Nickenig and colleagues.[34] Thus, increased AII production in hypertensives may promote atherogenic changes via both the mechanical stress of its vasoconstricting action and the local effects within vulnerable tissues.

NO production may keep the vascular actions of AII in check, thereby preventing the endothelial damage that leads to atherogenic changes. In the cholesterol-fed rabbit, the nitric oxide synthase inhibitor N-nitro-L-arginine methyl ester (L-NAME) accelerates atherosclerosis.[35] In the rat, the effect of L-NAME treatment, which in addition to blood pressure elevation resulted also in increased monocyte infiltration in coronary vessels and myocardial interstitial areas, MCP-1 expression, NFκB activation, and superoxide production could be prevented by either an AT_1 receptor antagonist or a thiol antioxidant.[36] A combination of AII and L-NAME was shown to increase the proinflammatory and proliferative effects of AII in the rat aorta.[37] NO has been shown to downregulate the AT_1 receptor, and it is this receptor that mediates the vasoconstrictor, cell growth, and superoxide generating effects of AII.[38] Specifically, AT_1 receptor

activation increases the expression of gp91-phox (or homologs), which are key components of the NADPH oxidase, a major cellular source of superoxide. *In vivo*, AT_1 receptor blockade decreased gp91-phox in mammary arteries from patients with coronary artery disease.[39] These data suggest that antihypertensive treatments targeting the ACE or the AT_1 receptors may have the added benefit of reducing oxidative stress in vessels. It should be noted, however, that pure antioxidant therapies have had mixed results in preventing atherosclerosis. For example, probucol was found to attenuate atherosclerosis in WHHL rabbits,[40,41] but had no effect on vascular pathology in apoE knockout (apoE–/–) mice.[42] Thus, most likely, the ability of ACE inhibitors or AT_1 receptor blockers to prevent or attenuate cardiovascular damage is attributable to their systemic hemodynamic and metabolic effects. The inhibition of proatherogenic and proinflammatory effects of AII may, however, also contribute to the effectiveness of these drugs in reducing cardiovascular disease risk.

A substudy of the Anglo-Scandinavian Outcomes Trial (ASCOT) determined that hypertensives had an increase in circulating plasma markers indicative of a prothrombotic, proangiogenic state with endothelial activation and dysfunction (as measured by increases in von Willebrand factor, tissue factor, and vascular endothelial growth factor).[43] Furthermore, this study reported alterations in flow-mediated vasodilation in hypertensives. Six months of intensive treatment to lower blood pressure and control lipids decreased tissue factor, vascular endothelial growth factor, and von Willebrand factor levels and improved flow-mediated vasodilation. These patients were either treated with calcium channel blockers (with or without an ACE inhibitor) or β-blockers (with or without diuretics), suggesting that numerous treatments that lower blood pressure and correct metabolic aberrations can potentially improve vascular outcomes.

Sympathetic nervous system dysfunction

Recent studies, such as the β-Blocker Cholesterol Lowering Asymptomatic Plaque Study and the Effects of Long-Term Treatment of Metoprolol on Surrogate Variables for Atherosclerotic Disease Trial, demonstrated that the addition of β-blockers to treatments reduces plaque thickness,[44] suggesting a role for the SNS in vascular lesion formation. Increased plasma norepinephrine levels have been found in hypertensives compared to normotensives with enhanced vascular α-adrenergic tone.[45,46] Experimentally, excessive dietary salt intake was shown to produce hypertension characterized by a hyperadrenergic state.[11]

Activation of the SNS can contribute to atherosclerosis in many ways (Figure 10.4).[47] *In vivo*, catecholamine infusion in the rabbit or monkey was found to increase vascular remodeling and atherosclerotic lesion formation.[48,49] Adrenergic stimulation, acting through α₁-adenergic receptors, causes the proliferation of vascular smooth muscle cells in cell culture[50] as well as in rat arteries in a carotid balloon injury model.[42,51] Adrenergic stimulation may also increase cytokine

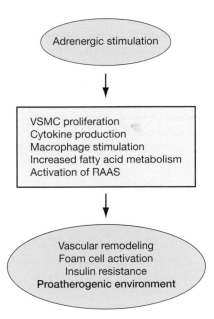

Figure 10.4 The proatherogenic consequences of adrenergic stimulation. Adrenergic stimulation has been shown to increase vascular smooth muscle cell (VSMC) proliferation, increase cytokine production in endothelial cells and macrophages, increase macrophage activation, and activate the renin–angiotensin–aldosterone system (RAAS), through which angiotensin II has many proatherogenic effects. Thus, adrenergic stimulation can contribute to vascular remodeling and foam cell activation. In addition, the lipolytic effects of adrenergic stimulation increases free fatty acids, which contribute to obesity and insulin resistance. The feedback between the sympathetic nervous system (SNS) and insulin resistance, which will in turn stimulate the SNS, serves to promote hypertension, dyslipidemia, diabetes, and vascular disease

production in endothelial cells[52] and increase lipolysis, causing an overall increase in free fatty acids,[53] thereby contributing to obesity, diabetes, and cardiovascular disease.[54] Directly, stimulation of postsynaptic α₂-adenergic receptors on macrophages can activate these inflammatory cells.[55] In the atherosclerotic WHHL rabbits, the level of circulating norepinephrine was nearly three times higher than in non-atherogenic New Zealand White rabbits.[56] Along with this apparent sympathetic dysregulation, abundant α₂ₐ-adenergic receptors were found in macrophage-rich lesions in the aorta. It is difficult to determine whether the increase in norepinephrine levels preceded the vascular lesion changes; however, the presence of excessive levels of norepinephrine may enhance lesion progression by acting on the foam cells in the vessel wall. Finally, increases in SNS activity may promote vascular damage indirectly by activating the RAAS. In the atherogenic apoE–/– mice, only the combination of an α₁-blocker and an AT₁ receptor blocker decreased atherosclerosis,[57] suggesting a role for both the SNS and the RAAS in atherosclerosis.

The metabolic syndrome: hypertension and type 2 diabetes

Hypertension is twice as common in diabetics as in nondiabetics, and essential hypertension is characterized by various degrees of insulin resistance and hyperinsulinemia. Insulin resistance, hyperinsulinemia, dyslipidemia, obesity, and hypertension are all atherogenic and are independent coronary risk factors. They are also the components of what has been labeled the metabolic syndrome, reviewed in the work of Scott.[58] Many individuals with the metabolic syndrome eventually develop type 2 diabetes. The prevalence of this syndrome has been increasing considerably throughout the world: the age-adjusted prevalence being 23.7% in the USA and increasing to 43.5% in those 60 years of age or older.[59] These rates are higher in African-Americans and appear to be rising with the increase in obesity and sedentary lifestyle in the USA, and to a greater extent in developing countries.

A common underlying factor in diabetes and hypertension is insulin resistance. Insulin normally has a vasodilatory effect, but in patients with insulin resistance this effect is lacking. It has been suggested that sympathetic stimulation may underlie insulin resistance.[60] Insulin resistance can contribute to hypertension, obesity, hyperinsulinemia, hypercoagulability, diabetes, and dyslipidemia.[61,62] As discussed below, certain antihypertensive medications that are important in controlling blood pressure may further improve disease risk outcomes in individuals with the metabolic syndrome, perhaps by preventing the development and progression of diabetes. Statins can also control the dyslipidemia found in individuals with the metabolic syndrome. Another important class of drugs, the γ-peroxisome proliferator activator receptor (PPAR-γ) agonists, appear to improve insulin resistance in obese subjects and diabetic subjects, and in animal models of atherosclerosis.[63–65]

PPAR are nuclear factor receptors that act as transcription factors on numerous gene targets after heterodimerization with the retinoid X-receptors. Three subtypes of PPAR, α, β, and γ, have been described, but it is the γ subtype that modulates the actions of insulin in adipocytes and other tissues.[66] The PPAR-γ agonists (thiazolidinediones) that improve tissue sensitivity to insulin appear also to antagonize AII actions and decrease blood pressure.[65,67] These agents are also anti-inflammatory: in macrophages, they reduce iNOS and cytokine production.[68] In endothelial cells, PPAR-γ ligands have been shown to stimulate basal expression of adhesion molecules but can downregulate adhesion molecule expression, and subsequent monocyte attachment, in endothelial cells activated by tumor necrosis factor-α (TNF-α), phorbol 12-myristate 13-acetate (PMA) or lipopolysaccharide.[69,70] Overall, PPAR-γ ligands have a positive effect on vascular wall remodeling.

Treatment strategies that lower blood pressure reduce disease risk

Several large clinical studies have examined the effects of antihypertensive agents on reducing blood pressure risk. ASCOT assessed primary prevention in high-risk patients without pre-existing coronary heart disease. In this study, blood pressure control combined with atorvastatin treatment provided a 36% reduction in the combined primary endpoints of death and MI after 3.3 years of follow-up.[71] Experimental studies in rat models

indicate that statins alone can improve vascular hemodynamics and reduce blood pressure in some models of hypertension.[72]

All antihypertensive treatments have been shown to improve outcomes, and invariably the benefits are more pronounced in diabetics, who are at increased risk. In the Systolic Blood Pressure in the Elderly (SHEP) study blood pressure lowering was protective, with 36% fewer strokes and 27% fewer non-fatal MI, and there was a greater benefit of treatment in diabetic hypertensives than non-diabetic hypertensives (RR 0.44 vs 0.81).[73] Furthermore, the United Kingdom Prospective Diabetes (UKPD) and the Appropriate Blood Pressure Control in Diabetes (ABCD) trials suggest that intensive therapy to reduce diastolic blood pressure (DBP < 80 mmHg in UKPD and < 77 mmHg in ABCD) can decrease adverse cardiovascular outcomes in this high-risk population. Importantly, the UKPD used ACE inhibitors or β-blockers, and either treatment improved both microvascular and macrovascular complications,[74] suggesting that the decisive factor was the degree of blood pressure control. In ABCD, either nisoldipine or enalapril was used, and both showed a reduction in stroke risk with tight blood pressure control and a reduction in risk of microvascular diabetic complications.[75] In an analysis of a secondary endpoint of fatal and non-fatal MI, however, the calcium channel blocker was found to have a greater relative risk than the ACE inhibitor (9.5, 95% CI 2.6–33).[76] It was proposed that this difference was due to the cardioprotective effects of ACE inhibitors, and not because the calcium antagonist was detrimental.[75]

The Losartan Intervention For Endpoint (LIFE) reduction in hypertension study recruited over 9100 hypertensives with electrocardiographically defined left ventricular hypertrophy from Scandinavia, the UK, and the USA. Participants were randomized to either the AT$_1$ receptor blocker or a β-blocker (atenolol), with additional drugs used as necessary to achieve optimal blood pressure control, so that by the end of the study many subjects were taking multiple drugs to control blood pressure. The composite endpoint of cardiovascular events, including death, stroke, and MI, was significantly lower with the losartan treatment (RR 0.87, 95% CI 0.77–0.81). There was no difference in relative risk of MI or overall cardiovascular disease mortality, but losartan treatment provided a significant reduction in the fatal and non-fatal incidence of stroke (RR 0.75, 95% CI 0.63–0.89).[77] It also protected subjects from new-onset type 2 diabetes, whose incidence was one-third less in the losartan than in the atenolol arm. Moreover, a separate analysis of diabetic participants, who were at inherently higher risk, showed a far more impressive benefit from losartan than in the general study population.

ALLHAT, the Antihypertensive and Lipid Lowering Treatment to Prevent Heart Attack Trial, is notable because of its large size: over 33 000 older individuals with high risk for CVD (because they had hypertension and another risk factor, such as diabetes or atherosclerosis) participated in this study. Initially, there were four arms: amlodipine, a dihydropyridine calcium channel blocker; lisinopril, an ACE inhibitor; doxazosin, an α-blocker; or chlorthalidone, a thiazide diuretic. The primary outcomes were fatal coronary heart disease or non-fatal MI and stroke. Owing to an increased occurrence of heart failure in the doxazosin arm compared with the diuretic arm, this treatment was stopped early. Additional treatments were given to control blood pressure as necessary, such that a large percentage of participants were on at least two medications by the end of the study. Even with multiple treatments, the decreases in blood pressure among the various arms of the study was not equivalent. Overall, at the end of 3.6 years of average follow-up there were no significant differences in primary outcomes between the diuretic treatment or the ACE inhibitor or calcium channel blocker arms.[78] In keeping with other studies, the lisinopril subjects had one-third less new-onset type 2 diabetes, and because of the high percentage of African-Americans, who are notoriously resistant to ACE inhibition, they had a lesser blood pressure response, and, as a consequence, a higher incidence of stroke.

Many of these studies compare one antihypertensive treatment against another, making it difficult to assess an overall benefit of lowering blood pressure per se. The Hypertension Optimal Treatment Trial (HOT) included over 18 790 patients for 26 countries, who were randomized into three therapeutic groups with the goal of achieving a diastolic blood pressure ≤ 90 mmHg, ≤ 85 mmHg, or ≤ 80 mmHg to assess the relationship between target diastolic blood pressure and major cardiovascular events.[79] All subjects were treated at baseline with the calcium antagonist felodipine to control blood pressure, with additional antihypertensive therapy added according to a set protocol in a stepwise manner. This study found that the lowest incidence of major adverse

cardiovascular events occurred in the group with the lowest target diastolic blood pressure. The decrease in risk for a change in diastolic blood pressure was even more striking in diabetics, who had a 51% reduction of risk with an approximately 10 mmHg drop in diastolic blood pressure,[80] suggesting that tight blood pressure control per se is beneficial. By contrast, the African-American Study of Kidney Disease and Hypertension (AASK) study found the progression to end-stage renal disease in hypertensive patients with chronic renal failure is decelerated more by ACE inhibitors than by calcium channel blockers, whereas a more aggressive blood pressure lowering strategy did not offer additional advantage.[81] This study contrasts with experimental studies that suggest calcium channel blockers are protective against atherosclerosis.[82]

The Heart Outcomes Prevention Evaluation Study (HOPE) enrolled over 9000 patients 55 years of age or over who were at high risk for mortality and morbidity owing to a history of coronary artery disease, stroke, peripheral artery disease, or diabetes, and at least one other risk factor, such as hypertension, hypercholesterolemia, lower HDL, smoking, or microalbuminuria.[83] Subjects had no known heart failure or left ventricular dysfunction. They were randomized to receive the ACE inhibitor ramipril, or placebo, added to conventional therapy. This study found that treatment with 10 mg/day ramipril decreased CVD incidence by 26%, MI by 20%, stroke by 32%, and all-cause mortality by 16%. Other vascular and microvascular complications were reduced with this treatment, as was the risk for developing new-onset diabetes. Interestingly, the changes in blood pressure with ramipril treatment were modest (as half the subjects were not hypertensive), with decreases in systolic blood pressure of 3.3 mmHg and decreases in diastolic blood pressure of 1.4 mmHg. This has led to the suggestion that the ACE inhibitor's effects act not only by decreasing blood pressure but also through blockade of other effects of AII on vascular function.[83] As with all recent outcome trials, an important feature of HOPE is that all patients were on an active treatment that included a variety of other drugs, such as β-blockers, diuretics, calcium channel blockers, and lipid-lowering agents.

Analysis of subgroups of the HOPE trial revealed, not surprisingly, that diabetics with microalbuminuria had the greatest benefit from ACE inhibition. And, in line with other trials of ACE inhibitors or AII receptor blockers, the ramipril arm had about one-third less new-onset diabetes during the brief period of follow-up. Other interesting pieces of information from this study included a substudy with vitamin E which, as in other studies in the past, failed to show a benefit attributable to the antioxidant properties of this vitamin; and the SECURE (Study to Evaluate Carotid UltRrasound changEs) substudy, which showed that ramipril treatment decreased the progression of atherosclerotic changes as measured by the intima-media thickness index.[84] All of these data support the notion that AII blockade offers benefits beyond blood pressure control, and that antioxidant supplements have no perceptible benefits.

By contrast, in the ELSA (European Lacidipine on Atherosclerosis Study), a 4-year treatment with a calcium channel blocker was able to decrease intima-media thickness progression by 40% in mild to moderate hypertensives compared to β-blocker (atenolol) treatment, even though clinical blood pressure measurements were equivalent in these groups.[85] This could explain the repeatedly documented observation that dihydropyridines offer better protection from stroke than do β-blockers, as the incidence of stroke is more closely correlated to blood pressure levels than the incidence of coronary disease and MI.

Summary

Several lines of experimental and clinical evidence indicate that elevated blood pressure promotes atherothrombotic disease. AII acting via the AT_1 receptor has many systemic and tissue-specific actions that contribute to vascular remodeling and lesion formation. Dysregulation of the SNS may also contribute to atherosclerosis in many ways, by promoting vascular smooth muscle cell proliferation and activation of macrophage foam cells. Both the RAAS and the SNS may contribute to insulin resistance in the metabolic syndrome, in which the concurrence of hypertension, obesity, dyslipidemia, and type 2 diabetes, all consequences of insulin resistance, contributes to increased risk for adverse cardiovascular events. Treatments that lower blood pressure and those that increase insulin sensitivity can improve measures of vascular function and slow the progression of atherosclerosis. In general, the cerebrovascular complications of hypertension are more closely correlated to blood pressure levels than the cardiovascular and renal complications, for which the metabolic effects of antihypertensive drugs also play an important role.

Acknowledgments

The authors thank Dr Irene Gavras for her insightful guidance and invaluable assistance. The authors also thank Mary Graves and Stephanie Tribuna for expert secretarial assistance.

References

1. Hyman DJ, Pavlik VN. Characteristics of patients with uncontrolled hypertension in the United States. N Engl J Med 2001; 345:479–486

2. Wilson PW, D'Agostino RB, Levy D et al. Prediction of coronary heart disease using risk factor categories. Circulation 1998; 97:1837–1847

3. Psaty BM, Furberg CD, Kuller LH et al. Association between blood pressure level and the risk of myocardial infarction, stroke, and total mortality: the cardiovascular health study. Arch Intern Med 2001; 161:1183–1192

4. Domanski M, Mitchell G, Pfeffer M et al. Pulse pressure and cardiovascular disease-related mortality: follow-up study of the Multiple Risk Factor Intervention Trial (MRFIT). J Am Med Assoc 2002; 287:2677–2683

5. Ogden LG, He J, Lydick E et al. Long-term absolute benefit of lowering blood pressure in hypertensive patients according to the JNC VI risk stratification. Hypertension 2000; 35:539–543

6. Chambless LE, Folsom AR, Davis V et al. Risk factors for progression of common carotid atherosclerosis: the Atherosclerosis Risk in Communities Study, 1987–1998. Am J Epidemiol 2002; 155:38–47

7. Linton MF, Fazio S. A practical approach to risk assessment to prevent coronary artery disease and its complications. Am J Cardiol 2003; 92:19i–26i

8. Guimaraes S, Moura D. Vascular adrenoceptors: an update. Pharmacol Rev 2001; 53:319–356

9. Piascik MT, Soltis EE, Piascik MM et al. Alpha-adrenoceptors and vascular regulation: molecular, pharmacologic and clinical correlates. Pharmacol Ther 1996; 72:215–241

10. Makaritsis KP, Johns C, Gavras I et al. Sympathoinhibitory function of the alpha(2A)-adrenergic receptor subtype. Hypertension 1999; 34:403–407

11. Gavras I, Gavras H. Role of alpha2-adrenergic receptors in hypertension. Am J Hypertens 2001; 14:171S–177S

12. Wenzel RR, Bruck H, Noll G et al. Antihypertensive drugs and the sympathetic nervous system. J Cardiovasc Pharmacol 2000; 35(Suppl 4):S43–S52

13. Duka I, Gavras I, Johns C et al. Role of the postsynaptic alpha(2)-adrenergic receptor subtypes in catecholamine-induced vasoconstriction. Gen Pharmacol 2000; 34:101–106

14. Weir MR, Dzau VJ. The renin-angiotensin-aldosterone system: a specific target for hypertension management. Am J Hypertens 1999; 12:205S–213S

15. Ross R. Atherosclerosis – an inflammatory disease. N Engl J Med 1999; 340:115–126

16. Csanyi A, Egervari A, Nagy Z. Influence of hypertension and smoking as the single vascular risk factors on the intima-media thickness. Eur J Epidemiol 2001; 17:855–861

17. Mancia G, Parati G, Hennig M et al. Relation between blood pressure variability and carotid artery damage in hypertension: baseline data from the European Lacidipine Study on Atherosclerosis (ELSA). J Hypertens 2001; 19:1981–1989

18. Chobanian AV, Lichtenstein AH, Nilakhe V et al. Influence of hypertension on aortic atherosclerosis in the Watanabe rabbit. Hypertension 1989; 14:203–209

19. Tropea BI, Huie P, Cooke JP et al. Hypertension-enhanced monocyte adhesion in experimental atherosclerosis. J Vasc Surg 1996; 23:596–605

20. Chobanian AV, Haudenschild CC, Nickerson C et al. Antiatherogenic effect of captopril in the Watanabe heritable hyperlipidemic rabbit. Hypertension 1990; 15:327–331

21. Hope S, Brecher P, Chobanian AV. Comparison of the effects of AT1 receptor blockade and angiotensin converting enzyme inhibition on atherosclerosis. Am J Hypertens 1999; 12:28–34

22. Tayeh MA, Scicli AG. Angiotensin II and bradykinin regulate the expression of P-selectin on the surface of endothelial cells in culture. Proc Assoc Am Phys 1998; 110:412–421

23. Griendling KK, Minieri CA, Ollerenshaw JD et al. Angiotensin II stimulates NADH and NADPH oxidase activity in cultured vascular smooth muscle cells. Circ Res 1994; 74:1141–1148

24. Warnholtz A, Nickenig G, Schulz E et al. Increased NADH-oxidase-mediated superoxide production in the early stages of atherosclerosis: evidence for involvement of the renin-angiotensin system. Circulation 1999; 99:2027–2033

25. Treasure CB, Manoukian SV, Klein JL et al. Epicardial coronary artery responses to acetylcholine are impaired in hypertensive patients. Circ Res 1992; 71:776–781

26. Muiesan ML, Salvetti M, Monteduro C et al. Effect of treatment on flow-dependent vasodilation of the brachial artery in essential hypertension. Hypertension 1999; 33:575–580

27. Panza JA, Garcia CE, Kilcoyne CM et al. Impaired endothelium-dependent vasodilation in patients with essential hypertension. Evidence that nitric oxide abnormality is not localized to a single signal transduction pathway. Circulation 1995; 91:1732–1738

28. Park JB, Charbonneau F, Schiffrin EL. Correlation of endothelial function in large and small arteries in human essential hypertension. J Hypertens 2001; 19:415–420

29. Mano T, Masuyama T, Yamamoto K et al. Endothelial dysfunction in the early stage of atherosclerosis precedes appearance of intimal lesions assessable with intravascular ultrasound. Am Heart J 1996; 131:231–238

30. Cardillo C, Campia U, Kilcoyne CM et al. Improved endothelium-dependent vasodilation after blockade of endothelin receptors in patients with essential hypertension. Circulation 2002; 105:452–456

31. Zouki C, Baron C, Fournier A et al. Endothelin-1 enhances neutrophil adhesion to human coronary artery endothelial cells: role of ET(A) receptors and platelet-activating factor. Br J Pharmacol 1999; 127:969–979

32. Prasad A, Tupas-Habib T, Schenke WH et al. Acute and chronic angiotensin-1 receptor antagonism reverses endothelial dysfunction in atherosclerosis. Circulation 2000; 101:2349–2354

33. Singh BM, Mehta JL. Interactions between the renin–angiotensin system and dyslipidemia: relevance in the therapy of hypertension and coronary heart disease. Arch Intern Med 2003; 163:1296–1304

34. Nickenig G, Harrison DG. The AT(1)-type angiotensin receptor in oxidative stress and atherogenesis: part I: oxidative stress and atherogenesis. Circulation 2002; 105:393–396

35. Cayatte AJ, Palacino JJ, Horten K et al. Chronic inhibition of nitric oxide production accelerates neointima formation and impairs endothelial function in hypercholesterolemic rabbits. Arterioscler Thromb 1994; 14:753–759

36. Usui M, Egashira K, Tomita H et al. Important role of local angiotensin II activity mediated via type 1 receptor in the pathogenesis of cardiovascular inflammatory changes induced by chronic blockade of nitric oxide synthesis in rats. Circulation 2000; 101:305–310

37. Kato H, Hou J, Chobanian AV et al. Effects of angiotensin II infusion and inhibition of nitric oxide synthase on the rat aorta. Hypertension 1996; 28:153–158

38. Raij L. Workshop: hypertension and cardiovascular risk factors: role of the angiotensin II-nitric oxide interaction. Hypertension 2001; 37:767–773

39. Rueckschloss U, Quinn MT, Holtz J et al. Dose-dependent regulation of NAD(P)H oxidase expression by angiotensin II in human endothelial cells: protective effect of angiotensin II type 1 receptor blockade in patients with coronary artery disease. Arterioscler Thromb Vasc Biol 2002; 22:1845–1851

40. Braesen JH, Beisiegel U, Niendorf A. Probucol inhibits not only the progression of atherosclerotic disease, but causes a different composition of atherosclerotic lesions in WHHL-rabbits. Virchows Arch 1995; 426:179–188

41. Oshima R, Ikeda T, Watanabe K et al. Probucol treatment attenuates the aortic atherosclerosis in Watanabe heritable hyperlipidemic rabbits. Atherosclerosis 1998; 137:13–22

42. Zhang SH, Reddick RL, Avdievich E et al. Paradoxical enhancement of atherosclerosis by probucol treatment in apolipoprotein E-deficient mice. J Clin Invest 1997; 99:2858–2866

43. Felmeden DC, Spencer CG, Chung NA et al. Relation of thrombogenesis in systemic hypertension to angiogenesis and endothelial damage/dysfunction (a substudy of the Anglo-Scandinavian Cardiac Outcomes Trial [ASCOT]). Am J Cardiol 2003; 92:400–405

44. Wikstrand J, Berglund G, Hedblad B et al. Antiatherosclerotic effects of beta-blockers. Am J Cardiol 2003; 91:25H–29H

45. Egan B, Panis R, Hinderliter A et al. Mechanism of increased alpha adrenergic vasoconstriction in human essential hypertension. J Clin Invest 1987; 80:812–817

46. de Champlain J, Petrovich M, Gonzalez M et al. Abnormal cardiovascular reactivity in borderline and mild essential hypertension. Hypertension 1991; 17(Suppl):III22–III28

47. Remme WJ. The sympathetic nervous system and ischaemic heart disease. Eur Heart J 1998; (Suppl F):F62–F71

48. Kukreja RS, Datta BN, Chakravarti RN. Catecholamine-induced aggravation of aortic and coronary atherosclerosis in monkeys. Atherosclerosis 1981; 40:291–298

49. Pauletto P, Scannapieco G, Pessina AC. Sympathetic drive and vascular damage in hypertension and atherosclerosis. Hypertension 1991; 17(Suppl 4):III75–III81

50. Yu SM, Tsai SY, Guh JH et al. Mechanism of catecholamine-induced proliferation of vascular smooth muscle cells. Circulation 1996;94:547–554

51. deBlois D, Schwartz SM, van Kleef EM et al. Chronic alpha 1-adrenoreceptor stimulation increases DNA synthesis in rat arterial wall. Modulation of responsiveness after vascular injury. Arterioscler Thromb Vasc Biol 1996; 16:1122–1129

52. Gornikiewicz A, Sautner T, Brostjan C et al. Catecholamines up-regulate lipopolysaccharide-induced IL-6 production in human microvascular endothelial cells. FASEB J 2000; 14:1093–1100

53. Large V, Arner P. Regulation of lipolysis in humans. Pathophysiological modulation in obesity, diabetes, and hyperlipidaemia. Diabetes Metab 1998; 24:409–418

54. Saleh J, Sniderman AD, Cianflone K. Regulation of Plasma fatty acid metabolism. Clin Chim Acta 1999; 286:163–180

55. Spengler RN, Allen RM, Remick DG et al. Stimulation of alpha-adrenergic receptor augments the production of macrophage-derived tumor necrosis factor. J Immunol 1990; 145:1430–1434

56. Handy DE, Johns C, Bresnahan MR et al. Expression of alpha2-adrenergic receptors in normal and atherosclerotic rabbit aorta. Hypertension 1998; 32:311–317

57. Makaritsis KP, Gavras H, Du Y et al. Alpha1-adrenergic plus angiotensin receptor blockade reduces atherosclerosis in apolipoprotein E-deficient mice. Hypertension 1998; 32:1044–1048

58. Scott CL. Diagnosis, prevention, and intervention for the metabolic syndrome. Am J Cardiol 2003; 92:35i–42i

59. Kereiakes DJ, Willerson JT. Metabolic syndrome epidemic. Circulation 2003; 108:1552–1553

60. Supiano MA, Hogikyan RV, Morrow LA et al. Hypertension and insulin resistance: role of sympathetic nervous system activity. Am J Physiol 1992; 263:E935–E942

61. Ginsberg HN, Stalenhoef AF. The metabolic syndrome: targeting dyslipidaemia to reduce coronary risk. J Cardiovasc Risk 2003; 10:121–128

62. Fonseca VA. Management of diabetes mellitus and insulin resistance in patients with cardiovascular disease. Am J Cardiol 2003; 92:50J–60J

63. Nolan JJ, Ludvik B, Beerdsen P et al. Improvement in glucose tolerance and insulin resistance in obese subjects treated with troglitazone. N Engl J Med 1994; 331:1188–1193

64. Suter SL, Nolan JJ, Wallace P et al. Metabolic effects of new oral hypoglycemic agent CS-045 in NIDDM subjects. Diabetes Care 1992; 15:193–203

65. Saku K, Zhang B, Ohta T et al. Troglitazone lowers blood pressure and enhances insulin sensitivity in Watanabe heritable hyperlipidemic rabbits. Am J Hypertens 1997; 10:1027–1033

66. Plutzky J. The potential role of peroxisome proliferator-activated receptors on inflammation in type 2 diabetes mellitus and atherosclerosis. Am J Cardiol 2003; 92:34J–41J

67. Diep QN, El Mabrouk M, Cohn JS et al. Structure, endothelial function, cell growth, and inflammation in blood vessels of angiotensin II-infused rats: role of peroxisome proliferator-activated receptor-gamma. Circulation 2002; 105:2296–2302

68. Chen CW, Chang YH, Tsi CJ et al. Inhibition of IFN-gamma-mediated inducible nitric oxide synthase induction by the peroxisome proliferator-activated receptor gamma agonist, 15-deoxy-delta 12,14-prostaglandin J2, involves inhibition of the upstream Janus kinase/STAT1 signaling pathway. J Immunol 2003; 171:979–988

69. Jackson SM, Parhami F, Xi XP et al. Peroxisome proliferator-activated receptor activators target human endothelial cells to inhibit leukocyte-endothelial cell interaction. Arterioscler Thromb Vasc Biol 1999; 19:2094–2104

70. Chen NG, Han X. Dual function of troglitazone in ICAM-1 gene expression in human vascular endothelium. Biochem Biophys Res Commun 2001; 282:717–722

71. Sever PS, Dahlof B, Poulter NR et al. Prevention of coronary and stroke events with atorvastatin in hypertensive patients who have average or lower-than-average cholesterol concentrations, in the Anglo-Scandinavian Cardiac Outcomes Trial – Lipid Lowering Arm (ASCOT-LLA): a multicentre randomised controlled trial. Lancet 2003; 361:1149–1158

72. Susic D, Varagic J, Ahn J et al. Beneficial pleiotropic vascular effects of rosuvastatin in two hypertensive models. J Am Coll Cardiol 2003; 42:1091–1097

73. Systolic Hypertension in the Elderly Program Cooperative Research Group. Prevention of stroke by antihypertensive drug treatment in older persons with isolated systolic hypertension. Final results of the Systolic Hypertension in the Elderly Program (SHEP). J Am Med Assoc 1991; 265:3255–3264

74. Leslie RD. United Kingdom prospective diabetes study (UKPDS): what now or so what? Diabetes Metab Res Rev 1999; 15:65–71

75. Estacio RO, Jeffers BW, Gifford N et al. Effect of blood pressure control on diabetic microvascular complications in patients with hypertension and type 2 diabetes. Diabetes Care 2000; 23 (Suppl 2):B54–B64

76. Estacio RO, Jeffers BW, Hiatt WR et al. The effect of nisoldipine as compared with enalapril on cardiovascular outcomes in patients with non-insulin-dependent diabetes and hypertension. N Engl J Med 1998; 338:645–652

77. Dahlof B, Devereux RB, Kjeldsen SE et al. Cardiovascular morbidity and mortality in the Losartan Intervention For Endpoint reduction in hypertension study (LIFE): a randomised trial against atenolol. Lancet 2002; 359:995–1003

78. Antihypertensive and Lipid-Lowering Treatment to prevent Heart Attack Trail Collaborative Research Group. Major outcomes in high-risk hypertensive patients randomized to angiotensin-converting enzyme inhibitor or calcium channel blocker vs diuretic: The Antihypertensive and Lipid-Lowering Treatment to Prevent Heart Attack Trial (ALL-HAT). J Am Med Assoc 2002; 288:2981–2997

79. The Hypertension Optimal Treatment Study (the HOT Study). Blood Press 1993; 2:62–68

80. Hansson L, Zanchetti A, Carruthers SG et al. Effects of intensive blood-pressure lowering and low-dose aspirin in patients with hypertension: principal results of the Hypertension Optimal Treatment (HOT) randomised trial. HOT Study Group. Lancet 1998; 351:1755–1762

81. Agodoa LY, Appel L, Bakris GL et al. Effect of ramipril vs amlodipine on renal outcomes in hypertensive nephrosclerosis: a randomized controlled trial. J Am Med Assoc 2001; 285:2719–2728

82. Henry PD. Calcium antagonists as antiatherogenic agents. Ann NY Acad Sci 1988; 522:411–419

83. Yusuf S, Sleight P, Pogue J et al. Effects of an angiotensin-converting-enzyme inhibitor, ramipril, on cardiovascular events in high-risk patients. The Heart Outcomes Prevention Evaluation Study Investigators. N Engl J Med 2000; 342:145–153.

84. Lonn E, Yusuf S, Dzavik V et al. Effects of ramipril and vitamin E on atherosclerosis: the study to evaluate carotid ultrasound changes in patients treated with ramipril and vitamin E (SECURE). Circulation 2001; 103:919–925

85. Zanchetti A, Bond MG, Henning M et al. Calcium antagonist lacidipine slows down progression of asymptomatic carotid atherosclerosis: principal results of the European Lacidipine Study on Atherosclerosis (ELSA), randomized, double-blind, long-term trail. Circulation 2002; 106:2422–2427.

11

Smoking and the molecular mechanisms of atherogenesis

Aran Kadar, Avrum Spira

Introduction

Although cigarette smoke appears to be associated with atherogenesis, the details of this relationship remain incompletely defined. Cigarette smoke contains over 4000 compounds, at least 40 of which are carcinogens.[1] Not surprisingly, the intersection of a complex biological chain of events with an inhalation that amounts to thousands of concurrent exposures generates many potential mechanisms of pathogenesis (Table 11.1). Given that an estimated 47 million people – one in four adults in the USA – are current smokers, the relationship between tobacco exposure and atherosclerosis has significant public health implications.

Evidence linking smoking and atherosclerosis originates from population, genetic, and molecular studies. Epidemiological surveys have drawn a clear association between smoking and an increased risk of coronary heart disease (CHD), peripheral vascular disease (PVD), and stroke. Smokers have almost twice the lifetime risk of developing CHD; furthermore, smoking accounts for 90% of PVD and 20–30% of CHD among non-diabetics.[1] At a genetic level, a growing number of single nucleotide polymorphisms exhibit a link between smoking and atherogenesis. Dysregulation of enzymes involved in detoxification causes a maladaptive response to the oxidant stress of smoking. In addition, polymorphisms in a number of genes involved in inflammation, endothelial function, and fat metabolism have been associated with increased risk of atherosclerosis in smokers.[2,3]

Histologically, the earliest lesions associated with atherosclerosis appear in the form of fatty streaks. The precise local conditions determining lipid entry into

Table 11.1 Selected list of major toxic compounds of cigarette smoke obtained from Surgeon General's Report on Smoking (1989). Chemicals in bold type have been linked to atherogenesis

Carbon monoxide[99]
Carbonyl sulfide
Benzene[100]
Formaldehyde[101]
3-Vinylpyridine
Hydrogen cyanide
Hydrazine
Nitrogen oxides
N-Nitrosodimethylamine
N-Nitrosopyrrolidine
Tar[96]
Nicotine[80]
Phenol
Catechol
o-Toluidine
2-Naphthylamine
4-Aminobiphenyl
Benz(a)anthracene[95]
Benzo(a)pyrene[95]
Quinoline
(4-methylnitrosamino)-1-(3-pyridyl)-1-butanone (NNN)
N′-nitrosonornicotine (NNK)
N-Nitrosodiethanolamine
Cadmium[102]
Nickel[103]
Polonium-210

the endothelium remain unclear.[4] Smoke exposure impairs endothelial vasodilatory function and disrupts endovascular integrity by altering the junctions between endothelial cells, both of which may affect permeability.[5] Blood viscosity increases and the capacity of the vascular bed to handle alterations in flow diminishes, leading to turbulence. Additionally, broad molecular changes occur in response to smoke exposure. Lipids and proteins undergo quantitative and qualitative oxidative changes when exposed to the free radicals and reactive oxygen species present in smoke. Procoagulant proteins and platelets appear to function at heightened levels, contributing to atherothrombosis. Cigarette smoke also activates numerous inflammatory pathways, which are emerging contributors to atherogenesis.

The goal of this chapter is to describe in further detail the mechanisms underlying the pathological states outlined above. The biological mechanisms at the intersection of smoking and atherogenesis fall into five overlapping categories: oxidant stress, lipid and glucose metabolism, endothelial function, thrombogenesis, and inflammation. Whereas myriad toxins in smoke contribute to the disease process, nicotine stands out as one of the most readily studied individual compounds and will be discussed in a separate section.

Smoking-induced oxidant stress

Oxidative stress and free radical formation represent a wide-ranging pathogenic contribution to atherogenesis. Cigarette smoke, in addition to supplying free radicals and reactive oxygen species, stimulates the subsequent generation of these species.[6] The component of smoke responsible for this oxidant stress is unknown. Of interest are the polyaromatic hydrocarbons, ubiquitous constituents of cigarette smoke that interact with the aryl hydrocarbon receptor to increase the transcription of P450 enzyme isoforms CYP1A1 and CYP1B1.[7] These enzymes oxygenate hydrocarbons in smoke to create more reactive species. Although smoking produces a large amount of free radicals *in vitro*, these moieties are short-lived, presenting a difficult challenge for *in vivo* study. Consequently, investigators have relied on various indirect markers of oxidation to draw mechanistic conclusions.[6]

Research on the interaction among smoking, oxidation, and atherogenesis focuses largely on endothelial dysfunction and the generation and consequences of oxidized low-density lipoproteins (LDL), which makes numerous pathogenic contributions to athero-

genesis (Figure 11.1). Several experimental models demonstrate impaired endothelial vasodilation after smoke exposure.[8] Their relevance to oxidant stress stems from measurements of vascular reactivity in the presence of supplemental antioxidants.[9] A potential oxidant-induced mechanism of diminished arterial wall relaxation in the face of active or passive smoke exposure is interference with cellular messengers mediating endothelium-dependent relaxation: in a human umbilical vein endothelial model, smoke exposure impaired the ability of endothelial cells to synthesize both prostacyclins and nitric oxide.[10,11]

Smoking also has far-reaching effects on atherogenic lipid species. Cigarette smoke not only results in a more atherogenic lipid profile by altering the absolute concentrations of the component lipids (see Lipid and glucose metabolism, below), but also generates oxidized LDL with its greater propensity for atheroma formation.[12] These oxidized LDL particles potentially contribute to atheroma progression by promoting monocyte adhesion to the endothelium, decreasing nitric oxide (NO)-mediated endothelial vasodilation, activating macrophage phagocytosis and foam cell formation, and acting as a mitogen for smooth muscle and endothelial cells (Figure 11.1).[13] Several studies in humans have shown that LDL isolated from smokers oxidizes with greater ease than do samples from non-smokers.[12] Additionally, oxidized LDL levels measured 90 minutes after smoking were demonstrated to be significantly higher compared with those measured after 24 hours of abstinence.[14]

Protein oxidation contributes to the process of atherogenesis. Insofar as a prothrombotic state is thought to contribute to the progression of atherosclerotic lesions, smoking not only correlates with absolute levels of fibrinogen[15] (see section on Hematological effects of smoking), but also appears to increase the amount of oxidized fibrinogen,[16] which exhibits a greater propensity for coagulation. Nitrated fibrinogen acquires a twofold increase in thrombin-induced clotting compared to normal fibrinogen.[17]

Smoking appears to deplete natural reserves of antioxidants. Population studies of smokers demonstrate lower levels of vitamin C and other antioxidants,[18] an effect noted even when adjusted for the dietary variations of smokers.[19] As little as one cigarette produces a measurable, transient decrease in the serum levels of nitrate and vitamin C.[20]

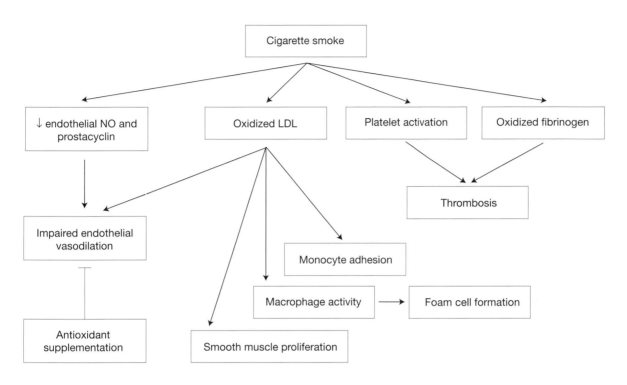

Figure 11.1 Contribution of smoking-induced oxidant stress to atherogenesis. Reactive oxygen species from cigarette smoke generate oxidized low-density lipoproteins (LDL), contributing to atherogenesis through the activation of macrophages, the promotion of monocyte adhesion, and acceleration of smooth muscle proliferation. The generation of oxidized fibrinogen and activation of platelets lower the threshold for thrombosis. Additionally, reactive oxygen species impair endothelial vasodilation secondary to a decreased expression of NO and prostacyclin. Antioxidant supplementation attenuates the effect of smoking on endothelial function. ↓, facilitates; ⊥, inhibits

Several investigators have provided indirect evidence of the significance of oxidant stress by measuring the ability of antioxidants to attenuate the component pathogenic effects of smoking. *In vitro* and guinea pig models provide evidence that vitamin C protects against smoking-induced oxidation.[21,22] Whether this effect translates into a decreased rate of atherogenesis has not yet been established. In a human model, 20 smokers received vitamin C supplementation and exhibited a short-lived improvement in endothelial function noted at 2 hours, an effect that was no longer present at 8 weeks.[23] Studies with vitamin E yielded similar results.[24] Attempts to demonstrate a decrease in the secondary markers of oxidation mentioned above have led to more conflicting data. Urinary levels of markers such as F_2-isoprostanes and 3-nitrotyrosine do not consistently decrease with supplemental antioxidant therapy.[25] A 6-month trial of combined vitamin C and E

supplementation failed to show an effect on levels of oxidized LDL or antibodies to oxidized LDL,[26] whereas F_2-isoprostanes showed a tendency to decrease.[27]

Lipid and glucose metabolism

The majority of the data linking smoking, lipids, and atherosclerosis originate from epidemiological studies. Smokers exhibit a proatherogenic lipid profile, including elevated total cholesterol, very low-density lipoprotein (VLDL), LDL, and triglycerides, as well as reduced high-density lipoprotein (HDL) levels.[28,29] Smokers with hyperlipidemia tend to have more marked abnormalities in their lipid profiles than do non-smokers with hyperlipidemia;[30] a reduction in or abstinence from smoking eventually eliminates these differences.[29] It is important to note that smoking-induced hyperlipidemia does not account for all of the increased risk of CHD in smokers.[31]

Lipid intolerance correlates with smoking, as evidenced by the abnormal levels of triglycerides measured in fasting subjects, which may be as much as 50% higher than those of non-smoking subjects.[28] The dyslipidemia of smoking exhibits dose–response characteristics.[32] Despite the weight gain commonly seen with smoking cessation, an increase in HDL and a decrease in LDL appear as early as 8 weeks after the last cigarette.[33,34]

Smoking has also shown pathological effects on glucose homeostasis. Diabetes mellitus, an independent risk factor for CHD and hyperlipidemia, is more common among smokers, and appears to be dose-related to the smoking habit. Even in smokers without a diagnosis of diabetes, glucose tolerance is impaired. Smokers with diabetes using insulin for glucose control demonstrate significantly higher insulin requirements than do non-smoking diabetics.[35–37]

The mechanism by which smoking increases LDL or impairs lipid and glucose tolerance remains unknown. Many of the metabolic effects appear to be mediated by the effect of nicotine on catecholamines, which is discussed further below. Smoking reduces the activity of paraoxonase, an antioxidant enzyme found associated with HDL that is involved in metabolizing organophosphate and other reactive oxygen substrates. Polymorphisms in this gene have correlated with CHD and stroke risk; additionally, smoking cessation restores paraoxonase activity within 2 years.[2]

Endovascular effects of smoking

Contrary to early views of the endothelium as the inert lining of a passive conduit, these cells have been re-envisaged as a dynamic participant in a complex set of interactions between peripheral blood components and the vascular wall.[4] Smoking hampers normal endothelial function through several mechanisms. Endothelial dysfunction represents a vascular phenotype that evolves early and persists throughout the development of the atheroma, affecting not only pathogenesis but also clinical prognosis.[38]

Despite not being directly implicated in atheroma formation, intimal thickness disrupts the fluid mechanics of the artery and leads to turbulent flow, which has been proposed as an early determinant of fatty streak location.[39] The paucity of atheroma in arterial sections with few branches supports this theory.[4] Alternatively, laminar shear forces may play a protective role by inducing genes for superoxide dismutase, nitric oxide synthase, tissue plasminogen activator (t-PA), and prostacyclin synthase.[40–42] In a human model, smoking has shown an association with carotid intimal thickness as assessed by ultrasound in 42 smokers and 40 control subjects.[43]

Smoking impairs endothelium-dependent relaxation, as measured by response to acetylcholine (which promotes nitric oxide release) or the ability of vessels to accommodate altered flow. The catecholamine release associated with nicotine in cigarette smoke increases vascular tone and impairs dilation.[44] An additional mechanism of impaired relaxation is free radical exposure, as evidenced by the reduced vasodilation seen in directly exposed microcirculation.[45,46] Xanthine oxidase creates free radicals that appear to be involved in smoking-induced dysfunction. Acetylcholine-mediated vasodilation is impaired in human smokers; however, subjects given allopurinol, a xanthine oxidase inhibitor, demonstrated improved vasodilation.[47] Other mechanisms by which smoking potentially impairs endothelium-mediated vasodilation include an inhibitory effect on nitric oxide synthesis or enhanced nitric oxide inactivation after release from endothelial cells.[48] Aqueous smoke extract has also been shown to inhibit the synthesis of prostacyclin, another potent vasodilator and platelet inhibitor produced by the endothelium.[49]

Lipid infiltration of the endothelium appears early in the course of atherogenesis as the fatty streak. Lipids putatively enter the endothelium after an alteration in membrane permeability[39] or disruption in the normal ratio of proteoglycans in the extracellular matrix of the intima.[4] Smoking-related endothelial damage may alter permeability. Electron microscopy of the aorta from rats exposed to nicotine or smoke demonstrated no change with nicotine, whereas smoke exposure led to bleb formation, microvillus projections, and a more frequent appearance of plasmalemma vesicles, suggesting a mechanism for increased transport of extraluminal substances.[50]

Endothelial surface proteins altered by smoking may participate in atherogenesis by recruiting peripheral blood cells into the local environment of the arterial intima. Cell surface adhesion molecules thought to play the most significant role in atherogenesis include the P-selectins and vascular cell adhesion molecule-1 (VCAM-1).[51,52] Smoking leads to activation of several adhesion molecules by phosphorylating protein kinase C, which subsequently activates NFκB and leads to a downstream increase in cell adhesion molecule expression.[53,54] Nitric oxide antagonizes the expression of cell surface adhesion molecules by interfering with NFκB activation. Smoking may also indirectly influence adhesion molecules through its effect on the lipid profile. Mice deficient in apolipoprotein E and on a high-cholesterol diet expressed higher levels of VCAM-1 and tissue factor and more macrophages on the plaque surface when exposed to smoke than did control mice.[55]

Analogous to the effects on airway epithelial cells, the mitogenic influence of smoking appears to interfere with the normal cell cycle of arterial smooth muscle cells.[56] Proliferation of smooth muscle cells thickens the arterial walls, interfering with normal vasodilation and local rheology. Cultured endothelial cells inhibit smooth muscle proliferation, in part through a heparin-like glycosaminoglycan, which has been shown to inhibit a protein kinase C-dependent pathway of cell cycle progression.[57] Inflammation at the site of the endothelium potentially depletes this oligosaccharide and promotes unchecked proliferation.[58] Smoking also appears to promote endothelial apoptosis, leading to increased tissue factor expression and thrombogenesis.[59] The increase in thrombosis results not only in the less stable plaques associated with acute coronary events, but possibly also in preclinical thrombotic events that contribute to plaque growth as they heal.

Hematological effects of smoking

The proposed interactions among smoking, atherosclerosis, and blood components stem from associations of increased thrombogenesis and altered fluid mechanics with atheroma progression. Whereas thrombosis is commonly associated with plaque rupture and subsequent acute coronary syndromes, small preclinical thrombotic events in the arterial wall contribute to the development of plaques by promoting matrix accumulation and smooth muscle cell proliferation during the healing process. Rather than a linear evolution from healthy intima to unstable plaque, the vessel wall undergoes a succession of injuries that promote the growth of the atheromatous lesion.[4]

Cigarette smoke promotes pathological changes in platelet function, fibrinogen, and blood viscosity. A single cigarette can produce measurable effects on platelet activation state.[60] Platelet samples from nonsmokers exposed to plasma from smokers displayed increased aggregation, an effect eliminated when plasma donors were given an antioxidant prior to smoking.[61] Additional *in vivo* evidence of platelet activity comes from increased levels of urinary metabolites of thromboxane A_2 in smokers. A decrease in platelet-derived NO observed in chronic smokers increases the activation of those platelets.[28]

Smokers are twice as likely to have elevated fibrinogen levels.[62] Viscosity and fibrinogen increase in relation to age in smokers, exhibiting a dose–response effect that is greater in men.[56] Both act as independent risk factors for CHD.[63] Fibrinogen serves as the substrate for thrombosis in the arterial wall. The subsequent fibrinolytic degradation products stimulate local smooth muscle cell proliferation and promote uptake of lipids by macrophages.[64,65]

Inflammatory mediators of smoking

An increasing number of investigators have described a role for acute-phase reactants in the pathogenesis and prognosis of CHD. Suggesting a generalized inflammatory state, smokers exhibit elevated levels of peripheral leukocytes.[66] The increased relative fraction of circulating monocytes correlates with atherogenic progression.[67] Among various indices of inflammation, C-reactive protein (CRP) has emerged as a predictor of risk for a first cardiovascular event in women,[68] and has been known to rise in smokers for some time. Whether this increase proceeds from or contributes to underlying coronary artery disease remains to be seen. CRP can interfere directly with endothelial function by decreasing prostacyclin release, and activates the NFκB pathway in saphenous vein endothelial cells.[69]

Several other observations strengthen the argument for smoking as a proinflammatory stimulus. Mice exposed to smoke develop elevated levels of pro-inflammatory cytokines, including interleukin-1 (IL-1), IL-6, and tumor necrosis factor-α (TNF-α).[70] Oxidized LDL plays a prominent proinflammatory role by binding CD14 and CRP, and by activating macrophage Toll-like receptors.[71] Statins, long thought to reduce risk strictly by improving the lipid profile, demonstrate an anti-inflammatory effect independent of their effects on atherosclerosis and cholesterol. The administration of atorvastatin to human CRP transgenic mice without atherosclerosis resulted in decreased absolute levels and transcriptional activity of huCRP, thought to result from a decrease in nuclear NFκB complexes.[72] Endothelial chemoattraction and adherence to monocytes and T lymphocytes plays a role early in atherogenesis. In hamsters, vitamin C prevents leukocytes from binding to endothelium or platelets.[73] Nitric oxide also appears to play a role in the adhesion of immune cells to the endothelium: L-arginine, the synthetic precursor of nitric oxide, blocks the ability of serum taken from smokers to increase monocyte adhesion to endothelial cells.[74]

There are emerging data suggesting a link between infection and atherosclerosis. Chronic infections, in particular with *Chlamydia pneumoniae*, may injure vessel walls directly or contribute systemic inflammatory mediators such as endotoxin or heat-shock protein 60.[75] Sustained endotoxemia has been shown to accelerate atherosclerosis in a rabbit model.[76] The Bruneck study offers an epidemiological association between smoking, atherosclerosis, and chronic infection. In this population study, the excess risk of atherosclerosis seen in current and former smokers resulted entirely from those with chronic infections, comprising mainly patients with chronic obstructive pulmonary disease (COPD) and recurrent infections or chronic bronchitis.[77]

Nicotine and atherogenesis

Of the many components of cigarette smoke, nicotine is one of the most easily studied. Numerous experiments have tested the effects of this compound as it relates to the biological systems discussed above. Many of those effects arise from the stimulation of catecholamines, which has already been described. This section characterizes the additional consequences of nicotine exposure as they relate to atherogenesis.

Gene expression profiling of endothelial cells exposed to nicotine shows activity in several regulatory pathways, including NFκB and the cAMP regulatory binding protein.[78] The downstream results of these changes lead to increased expression of the genes that code for nitric oxide synthase, plasminogen activator inhibitor-1 (PAI-1), von Willebrand factor (vWF), and VCAM-1.[79]

In the absence of free radicals supplied by cigarette smoke, nicotine continues to function as a pro-oxidant by facilitating the generation of reactive species. For example, LDL is oxidized by copper more rapidly in the presence of nicotine.[14]

Although smoking appears to have clear effects on cholesterol, the contribution from nicotine appears less consistent. Independently of cigarette smoke, nicotine can alter lipid profiles. Several animal models have verified that nicotine raises LDL and decreases HDL; however, experimental doses usually exceed those found in cigarettes. Furthermore, human subjects given oral nicotine did not demonstrate any change in LDL, HDL, or apolipoprotein A1 or B.[80]

Apart from catecholamine-induced vasoconstriction, nicotine exerts a variety of effects on the arterial wall. The two primary means by which blood-borne substances enter the endothelium are the intercellular clefts and plasmalemma vesicles. Nicotine induces a more rudimentary cleft formation and results in increased permeability to albumin, suggesting a possible mechanism by which LDL and inflammatory cells enter the endothelium.[5,50] Additionally, nicotine facilitates atherogenesis by promoting the conversion of smooth muscle cells from a contractile to a synthetic state, and inducing changes in the rate of apoptosis. During atherogenesis, endothelial cells lose their contractile function and begin to proliferate and synthesize substances that alter the extracellular matrix, leading to thickening of the arterial wall and entrapment of LDL and various inflammatory mediators.[81,82] Nicotine given in low doses promotes cytoskeleton protein synthesis, whereas higher doses lead to cessation of synthesis and increased cell destruction.[83] In normally functioning arterial tissue, injury to the lining causes cessation of endothelial contractile function and a shift of activity to synthesis. In the face of injury, nicotine potentiates the increased synthesis.[80] Finally, in contrast to the available gene expression data, nicotine interferes with endothelial function by inhibiting the synthesis and release of nitric oxide and stimulating endothelin-1 production.[84]

Data linking nicotine to thrombosis vary. Although it is thought to increase platelet activity and affect prostaglandin function, *in vitro* models have shown no effect of nicotine on platelet function;[85] however, *in vivo* exposure leads to small vessel contraction, a state that promotes turbulent flow and which may influence platelet activity. Intravenous nicotine appears to activate platelets, but standard nicotine supplements have failed to show any effect on *in vivo* platelet function assays. Nicotine alone does not influence the level of platelet breakdown products excreted in the urine of male smokers.[86,87] Attempts to find a thrombogenic effect of nicotine via fibrinogen or prostacyclin intermediates have not shown a prominent effect. There is increased uptake of labeled fibrinogen by the carotid artery in a canine model, but no effect was seen when the animals received inhaled nicotine.[88] Human studies have not verified any consistent alteration in coagulation factors, fibrinogen, or prostacyclin due to nicotine.[80]

Nicotine contributes to inflammation largely through its effects on dendritic cells. When given intravenous infusions of nicotine, mouse dendritic cells migrate into atherosclerotic plaques in mice without apolipoprotein E. Nicotine has also been observed to increase the secretion of IL-12 in dendritic cells, which subsequently increases the ability of these antigen-presenting cells to activate T cells.[89] Although nicotine affects several mediators of inflammation, when smokers switch to a transdermal patch, their leukocyte counts return to normal, arguing against nicotine as a sole or major determinant of inflammation.[86]

Genetic susceptibility to smoking-induced injury

Half of patients who smoke do not die prematurely from disease attributable to smoking,[90] suggesting a genetic component to the interaction that increases the risk of smoke exposure. Genes implicated in smoking-related atherosclerosis include representative genes from the various elements of the larger pathway of atherogenesis. This section describes polymorphisms in select genes from a number of these pathways.

Functional polymorphisms in genes involved in detoxification and redox stress would be expected to affect the risk of smoking. Patients with a null mutation in the gene coding for glutathione-*S*-transferase exhibit an increased baseline risk for CHD. As one would expect, smoking created a synergistic increase in that risk.[91] Additionally, a single nucleotide polymorphism in CYP1A1, one of the key detoxification enzymes for cigarette smoke, has been associated with an increased risk of three-vessel disease in light smokers (fewer than 20 pack-years).[92]

Apolipoprotein (a) (Apo(a))is a modified form of LDL that shares an area of homology with plasminogen, resulting in interference with plasmin formation and fibrinolysis.[93] Apo(a) polymorphisms in the e4 allele have been associated with an increased risk of CHD and appear to mediate their affect largely through susceptibility to smoking. Smokers with the e4 allele of apo(a) carry a threefold risk of developing CHD, whereas in non-smokers with the identical allele the baseline risk does not differ.[3]

Data regarding the transcription factor and tumor suppressor p53 have conflicted over its possible contribution to developing CHD. Wang and colleagues[94] reported an increased prevalence of disease among patients with both the HaeIII and MspI variants. Using logistic regression, they found a significant interactive effect of the two polymorphisms and cigarette smoking on CHD, but no association between CHD and either individual p53 polymorphic marker. Presumably a decrease in p53 would lead to unsuppressed smooth muscle proliferation, arterial wall thickening, and progression of atherosclerosis.[4] Other investigators have not confirmed a role for p53 in CHD risk in smokers.[90] The notion that carcinogens can promote atherosclerosis was also demonstrated in an experiment in which cockerels received carcinogens at doses below those associated with tumor development.[95] The exposed birds developed increased atherosclerotic plaques along their aortas. A similar effect occurred with birds exposed to inhaled butadiene.[96]

Given the role of chronic inflammation in atherosclerosis, polymorphisms in a number of inflammatory mediators have been associated with an increased risk for CHD in smokers. A functional polymorphism in the promoter region of CD14, an endotoxin receptor that enhances the endotoxin-neutralizing capacity of plasma, was associated with increased common carotid artery intima-media thickness in current and former smokers.[97] Endotoxin is a potent mediator of inflammation that demonstrates elevated levels in smokers. Additionally, an interleukin-6 promoter polymorphism has been associated with reduced flow-mediated dilation of the brachial artery in male smokers compared to non-smokers of the same genotype.[98]

The search for candidate genes that predispose to smoking-induced atherosclerosis has focused on the ability of individual genes or gene polymorphisms to account for the excessive burden of disease compared with controls. Notably lacking are genome-level studies casting a wider net in the search for a committee of responsible genes. As Wang and Mahaney[3] point out, given the complexity of the pathway involved, the 'one gene' approach will very likely provide instances of significant genetic involvement; however, this approach limits the ability to gain a wider, systemic view of the mechanisms involved.

Conclusion

Given the complex assembly of toxins in cigarette smoke, it is not surprising to find far-ranging effects within each of the major biological systems involved in the generation of atheroma. Smoking impairs endothelial function while concurrently promoting oxidant stress, inflammation, and a pathological lipid profile, elements that participate in the initiation and progression of atherosclerosis. A growing body of data points to the pathogenic synergism between smoke exposure and a variety of polymorphisms. Subtle alterations in the function of genes or gene products involved in detoxification, inflammation, lipoprotein synthesis, and carcinogenesis potentiate the effects of cigarette smoke on atherogenesis. Large-scale microarray analyses of smoking and CHD have just begun to bring into focus the biological pathways linking cigarette smoke exposure and endovascular disease. Future directions for research include experiments harnessing the technologies that have ushered in the postgenomic era, employing high-throughput platforms to approach the complex pathogenic system of smoking-induced atherogenesis.

References

1. Burns DM. Nicotine addiction. In: Braunwald E, Fauci AS, Kasper DL et al., eds. Harrison's principles of internal medicine. New York: McGraw Hill, 2004: 2574–2576.
2. Talmud PJ, Humphries SE. Gene–environment interaction in lipid metabolism and effect on coronary heart disease risk. Curr Opin Lipidol 2002; 13:149–154.
3. Wang XL, Mahaney MC. Genotype-specific effects of smoking on risk of CHD. Lancet 2001; 358:87–88.
4. Libby P. The vascular biology of atherosclerosis. In: Braunwald E, Zipes DP, Libby P, eds. Braunwald's heart disease: a textbook of cardiovascular medicine. Philadelphia: WB Saunders, 2004: 995–1009.
5. Zimmerman M, McGeachie J. Quantitation of the relationship between aortic endothelial intercellular cleft morphology and permeability to albumin. Atherosclerosis 1986; 59:277–582.
6. Burke A, Fitzgerald GA. Oxidative stress and smoking-induced vascular injury. Prog Cardiovasc Dis 2003; 46:79–90.
7. Kerzee JK, Ramos KS. Constitutive and inducible expression of Cyp1a1 and Cyp1b1 in vascular smooth muscle cells: role of the Ahr bHLH/PAS transcription factor. Circ Res 2001; 89:573–582.
8. Celermajer DS, Sorensen KE, Georgakopoulos D et al. Cigarette smoking is associated with dose-related and potentially reversible impairment of endothelium-dependent dilation in healthy young adults. Circulation 1993; 88:2149–2155.
9. Chisolm GM, Steinberg D. The oxidative modification hypothesis of atherogenesis: an overview. Free Radical Biol Med 2000; 28:1815–1826.
10. Ulm MR, Plockinger B, Pirich C et al. Umbilical arteries of babies born to cigarette smokers generate less prostacyclin and contain less arginine and citrulline compared with those of babies born to control subjects. Am J Obstet Gynecol 1995; 172:1485–1487.
11. Barua RS, Ambrose JA, Srivastava S et al. Reactive oxygen species are involved in smoking-induced dysfunction of nitric oxide biosynthesis and upregulation of endothelial nitric oxide synthase: an in vitro demonstration in human coronary artery endothelial cells. Circulation 2003; 107:2342–2344.
12. Scheffler E, Wiest E, Woehrle J et al. Smoking influences the atherogenic potential of low-density lipoprotein. Clin Invest 1992; 70:263–238.
13. Steinberg D. Low density lipoprotein oxidation and its pathobiological significance. J Biol Chem 1997; 272:20963–20966.
14. Gouaze V, Dousset N, Dousset JC et al. Effect of nicotine and cotinine on the susceptibility to in vitro oxidation of LDL in healthy non smokers and smokers. Clin Chim Acta 1998; 277:25–37.
15. Stec JJ, Silbershatz H, Tofler GH et al. Association of fibrinogen with cardiovascular risk factors and cardiovascular

disease in the Framingham Offspring Population. Circulation 2000; 102:1634–1638.

16. Pignatelli B, Li CQ, Boffetta P et al. Nitrated and oxidized plasma proteins in smokers and lung cancer patients. Cancer Res 2001; 61:778–784.

17. Gole MD, Souza JM, Choi I et al. Plasma proteins modified by tyrosine nitration in acute respiratory distress syndrome. Am J Physiol Lung Cell Mol Physiol 2000; 278:L961–L967.

18. Wei W, Kim Y, Boudreau N. Association of smoking with serum and dietary levels of antioxidants in adults: NHANES III, 1988-1994. Am J Public Health 2001; 91:258–264.

19. Dietrich M, Block G, Benowitz NL et al. Vitamin C supplementation decreases oxidative stress biomarker f2-isoprostanes in plasma of nonsmokers exposed to environmental tobacco smoke. Nutr Cancer 2003; 45:176–184.

20. Tsuchiya M, Asada A, Kasahara E et al. Smoking a single cigarette rapidly reduces combined concentrations of nitrate and nitrite and concentrations of antioxidants in plasma. Circulation 2002; 105:1155–1157.

21. Panda K, Chattopadhyay R, Chattopadhyay DJ et al. Vitamin C prevents cigarette smoke-induced oxidative damage in vivo. Free Radical Biol Med 2000; 29:115–124.

22. Panda K, Chattopadhyay R, Ghosh MK et al. Vitamin C prevents cigarette smoke induced oxidative damage of proteins and increased proteolysis. Free Radical Biol Med 1999; 27:1064–1079.

23. Raitakari OT, Adams MR, McCredie RJ et al. Oral vitamin C and endothelial function in smokers: short-term improvement, but no sustained beneficial effect. J Am Coll Cardiol 2000; 35:1616–1621.

24. Neunteufl T, Priglinger U, Heher S et al. Effects of vitamin E on chronic and acute endothelial dysfunction in smokers. J Am Coll Cardiol 2000; 35:277–283.

25. Mulholland CW, Strain JJ, Trinick TR. Serum antioxidant potential, and lipoprotein oxidation in female smokers following vitamin C supplementation. Int J Food Sci Nutr 1996; 47:227–231.

26. Porkkala-Sarataho E, Salonen JT, Nyyssonen K et al. Long-term effects of vitamin E, vitamin C, and combined supplementation on urinary 7-hydro-8-oxo-2'-deoxyguanosine, serum cholesterol oxidation products, and oxidation resistance of lipids in nondepleted men. Arterioscler Thromb Vasc Biol 2000; 20:2087–2093.

27. Kinlay S, Behrendt D, Fang JC et al. Long-term effect of combined vitamins E and C on coronary and peripheral endothelial function. J Am Coll Cardiol 2004; 43:629–634.

28. Tsiara S, Elisaf M, Mikhailidis DP. Influence of smoking on predictors of vascular disease. Angiology 2003; 54:507–530.

29. Brischetto CS, Connor WE, Connor SL et al. Plasma lipid and lipoprotein profiles of cigarette smokers from randomly selected families: enhancement of hyperlipidemia and depression of high-density lipoprotein. Am J Cardiol 1983; 52:675–680.

30. Schuitemaker GE, Dinant GJ, van der Pol GA et al. Relationship between smoking habits and low-density lipoprotein-cholesterol, high-density lipoprotein-cholesterol, and triglycerides in a hypercholesterolemic adult cohort, in relation to gender and age. Clin Exp Med 2002; 2:83–88.

31. Cullen P, Schulte H, Assmann G. Smoking, lipoproteins and coronary heart disease risk. Data from the Munster Heart Study (PROCAM). Eur Heart J 1998; 19:1632–1641.

32. Imamura H, Teshima K, Miyamoto N et al. Cigarette smoking, high-density lipoprotein cholesterol subfractions, and lecithin: cholesterol acyltransferase in young women. Metabolism 2002; 51:1313–1316.

33. Mikhailidis DP, Papadakis JA, Ganotakis ES. Smoking, diabetes and hyperlipidaemia. J R Soc Health 1998; 118:91–93.

34. Stamler J, Rains-Clearman D, Lenz-Litzow K et al. Relation of smoking at baseline and during trial years 1–6 to food and nutrient intakes and weight in the special intervention and usual care groups in the Multiple Risk Factor Intervention Trial. Am J Clin Nutr 1997; 65:374S–402S.

35. Madsbad S, McNair P, Christensen MS et al. Influence of smoking on insulin requirement and metbolic status in diabetes mellitus. Diabetes Care 1980; 3:41–43.

36. Lundman BM, Asplund K, Norberg A. Smoking and metabolic control in patients with insulin-dependent diabetes mellitus. J Intern Med 1990; 227:101–106.

37. Facchini FS, Hollenbeck CB, Jeppesen J et al. Insulin resistance and cigarette smoking. Lancet 1992; 339:1128–1130.

38. Puranik R, Celermajer DS. Smoking and endothelial function. Prog Cardiovasc Dis 2003; 45:443–458.

39. Tarbell JM. Mass transport in arteries and the localization of atherosclerosis. Annu Rev Biomed Eng 2003; 5:79–118.

40. Gimbrone MA Jr, Resnick N, Nagel T et al. Hemodynamics, endothelial gene expression, and atherogenesis. Ann NY Acad Sci 1997; 811:1–10.

41. Topper JN, Cai J, Falb D et al. Identification of vascular endothelial genes differentially responsive to fluid mechanical stimuli: cyclooxygenase-2, manganese superoxide dismutase, and endothelial cell nitric oxide synthase are selectively up-regulated by steady laminar shear stress. Proc Natl Acad Sci USA 1996; 93:10417–10422.

42. Diamond SL, Sharefkin JB, Dieffenbach C et al. Tissue plasminogen activator messenger RNA levels increase in cultured human endothelial cells exposed to laminar shear stress. J Cell Physiol 1990; 143:364–371.

43. Poredos P, Orehek M, Tratnik E. Smoking is associated with dose-related increase of intima-media thickness and endothelial dysfunction. Angiology 1999; 50:201–208.

44. Barua RS, Ambrose JA, Eales-Reynolds LJ et al. Heavy and light cigarette smokers have similar dysfunction of endothelial vasoregulatory activity: an in vivo and in vitro correlation. J Am Coll Cardiol 2002; 39:1758–1763.

45. Zhu BQ, Parmley WW. Hemodynamic and vascular effects of active and passive smoking. Am Heart J 1995; 130:1270–1275.

46. Pittilo RM, Bull HA, Gulati S et al. Nicotine and cigarette smoking: effects on the ultrastructure of aortic endothelium. Int J Exp Pathol 1990; 71:573–586.

47. Guthikonda S, Sinkey C, Barenz T et al. Xanthine oxidase inhibition reverses endothelial dysfunction in heavy smokers. Circulation 2003; 107:416–421.

48. Drexler H, Hornig B. Endothelial dysfunction in human disease. J Mol Cell Cardiol 1999; 31:51–60.

49. Jeremy JY, Mikhailidis DP, Dandona P. Cigarette smoke extracts, but not nicotine, inhibit prostacyclin (PGI2) synthesis in human, rabbit and rat vascular tissue. Prostaglandins Leuko Med 1985; 19:261–270.

50. Pittilo RM, Mackie IJ, Rowles PM et al. Effects of cigarette smoking on the ultrastructure of rat thoracic aorta and its ability to produce prostacyclin. Thromb Haemost 1982; 48:173–176.

51. Dong ZM, Chapman SM, Brown AA et al. The combined role of P- and E-selectins in atherosclerosis. J Clin Invest 1998; 102:145–152.

52. Li H, Cybulsky MI, Gimbrone MA Jr et al. Inducible expression of vascular cell adhesion molecule-1 by vascular smooth muscle cells in vitro and within rabbit atheroma. Am J Pathol 1993; 143:1551–1559.

53. Shen Y, Rattan V, Sultana C et al. Cigarette smoke condensate-induced adhesion molecule expression and transendothelial migration of monocytes. Am J Physiol 1996; 270:H1624–H1633.

54. Weber C, Erl W. Modulation of vascular cell activation, function, and apoptosis: role of antioxidants and nuclear factor-kappa B. Curr Top Cell Regul 2000; 36:217–235.

55. Matetzky S, Tani S, Kangavari S et al. Smoking increases tissue factor expression in atherosclerotic plaques: implications for plaque thrombogenicity. Circulation 2000; 102:602–604.

56. Fuster V, Gotto AM, Libby P et al. 27th Bethesda Conference: matching the intensity of risk factor management with the hazard for coronary disease events. Task Force 1. Pathogenesis of coronary disease: the biologic role of risk factors. J Am Coll Cardiol 1996; 27:964–976.

57. Castellot JJ Jr, Addonizio ML, Rosenberg R et al. Cultured endothelial cells produce a heparin like inhibitor of smooth muscle cell growth. J Cell Biol 1981; 90:372–379.

58. Castellot JJ Jr, Pukac LA, Caleb BL et al. Heparin selectively inhibits a protein kinase C-dependent mechanism of cell cycle progression in calf aortic smooth muscle cells. J Cell Biol 1989; 109:3147–3155.

59. Tedgui A, Mallat Z. Apoptosis, a major determinant of atherothrombosis. Arch Mal Coeur Vaiss 2003; 96:671–675.

60. Nair S, Kulkarni S, Camoens HM et al. Changes in platelet glycoprotein receptors after smoking – a flow cytometric study. Platelets 2001; 12:20–26.

61. Blache D. Involvement of hydrogen and lipid peroxides in acute tobacco smoking-induced platelet hyperactivity. Am J Physiol 1995; 268:H679–H685.

62. Bazzano LA, He J, Muntner P et al. Relationship between cigarette smoking and novel risk factors for cardiovascular disease in the United States. Ann Intern Med 2003; 138:891–897.

63. Sweetnam PM, Thomas HF, Yarnell JW et al. Fibrinogen, viscosity and the 10-year incidence of ischaemic heart disease. Eur Heart J 1996; 17:1814–1820.

64. Smith EB, Keen GA, Grant A et al. Fate of fibrinogen in human arterial intima. Arteriosclerosis 1990; 10:263–275.

65. Lowe GD, Wood DA, Douglas JT et al. Relationships of plasma viscosity, coagulation and fibrinolysis to coronary risk factors and angina. Thromb Haemost 1991; 65:339–343.

66. Blann AD, Kirkpatrick U, Devine C et al. The influence of acute smoking on leucocytes, platelets and the endothelium. Atherosclerosis 1998; 141:133–139.

67. Boyajian RA, Otis SM. Atherogenic progression of carotid stenosis associates selectively with monocyte fraction in circulating leukocytes. Eur J Neurol 2002; 9:307–310.

68. Ridker PM, Hennekens CH, Buring JE et al. C-reactive protein and other markers of inflammation in the prediction of cardiovascular disease in women. N Engl J Med 2000; 342:836–843.

69. Verma S, Badiwala MV, Weisel RD et al. C-reactive protein activates the nuclear factor-kappaB signal transduction pathway in saphenous vein endothelial cells: implications for atherosclerosis and restenosis. J Thorac Cardiovasc Surg 2003; 126:1886–1891.

70. Zhang J, Liu Y, Shi J et al. Side-stream cigarette smoke induces dose-response in systemic inflammatory cytokine production and oxidative stress. Exp Biol Med (Maywood) 2002; 227:823–829.

71. Miller YI, Chang MK, Binder CJ et al. Oxidized low density lipoprotein and innate immune receptors. Curr Opin Lipidol 2003; 14:437–445.

72. Kleemann R, Verschuren L, De Rooij BJ et al. Evidence for anti-inflammatory activity of statins and PPAR(alpha)-activators in human C-reactive protein transgenic mice in vivo and in cultured human hepatocytes in vitro. Blood 2004 (Epub ahead of print).

73. Lehr HA, Frei B, Arfors KE. Vitamin C prevents cigarette smoke-induced leukocyte aggregation and adhesion to endothelium in vivo. Proc Natl Acad Sci USA 1994; 91:7688–7692.

74. Adams MR, Jessup W, Celermajer DS. Cigarette smoking is associated with increased human monocyte adhesion to endothelial cells: reversibility with oral L-arginine but not vitamin C. J Am Coll Cardiol 1997; 29:491–497.

75. Pockley AG. Heat shock proteins in health and disease: therapeutic targets or therapeutic agents? Expert Rev Mol Med 2001; 3:1–21.

76. Lehr HA, Sagban TA, Ihling C et al. Immunopathogenesis of atherosclerosis: endotoxin accelerates atherosclerosis in rabbits on hypercholesterolemic diet. Circulation 2001; 104:914–920.

77. Kiechl S, Werner P, Egger G et al. Active and passive smoking, chronic infections, and the risk of carotid atherosclerosis: prospective results from the Bruneck Study. Stroke 2002; 33:2170–2176.

78. Zhang S, Day I, Ye S. Nicotine induced changes in gene expression by human coronary artery endothelial cells. Atherosclerosis 2001; 154:277–283.

79. Zhang S, Day IN, Ye S. Microarray analysis of nicotine-induced changes in gene expression in endothelial cells. Physiol Genomics 2001; 5:187–192.

80. Kilaru S, Frangos SG, Chen AH et al. Nicotine: a review of its role in atherosclerosis. J Am Coll Surg 2001; 193:538–546.

81. Williams KJ, Tabas I. The response-to-retention hypothesis of atherogenesis reinforced. Curr Opin Lipidol 1998; 9:471–474.

82. Camejo G, Hurt-Camejo E, Wiklund O et al. Association of zapo B lipoproteins with arterial proteoglycans: pathological significance and molecular basis. Atherosclerosis 1998; 139:205–222.

83. Csonka E, Somogyi A, Augustin J et al. The effect of nicotine on cultured cells of vascular origin. Virchows Arch A Pathol Anat Histopathol 1985; 407:441–447.

84. Lee WO, Wright SM. Production of endothelin by cultured human endothelial cells following exposure to nicotine or caffeine. Metabolism 1999; 48:845–848.

85. Pfueller SL, Burns P, Mak K et al. Effects of nicotine on platelet function. Haemostasis 1988; 18:163–169.

86. Benowitz NL, Fitzgerald GA, Wilson M et al. Nicotine effects on eicosanoid formation and hemostatic function: comparison of transdermal nicotine and cigarette smoking. J Am Coll Cardiol 1993; 22:1159–1167.

87. Mundal HH, Hjemdahl P, Gjesdal K. Acute effects of low dose nicotine gum on platelet function in non-smoking hypertensive and normotensive men. Eur J Clin Pharmacol 1995; 47:411–416.

88. Allen DR, Browse NL, Rutt DL. Effects of cigarette smoke, carbon monoxide and nicotine on the uptake of fibrinogen by the canine arterial wall. Atherosclerosis 1989; 77:83–88.

89. Aicher A, Heeschen C, Mohaupt M et al. Nicotine strongly activates dendritic cell-mediated adaptive immunity: potential role for progression of atherosclerotic lesions. Circulation 2003; 107:604–611.

90. Benowitz NL. Cigarette smoking and cardiovascular disease: pathophysiology and implications for treatment. Prog Cardiovasc Dis 2003; 46:91–111.

91. Wang XL, Raveendran M, Wang J. Genetic influence on cigarette-induced cardiovascular disease. Prog Cardiovasc Dis 2003; 45:361–382.

92. Wang XL, Greco M, Sim AS et al. Effect of CYP1A1 MspI polymorphism on cigarette smoking related coronary artery disease and diabetes. Atherosclerosis 2002; 162:391–367.

93. Loscalzo J, Weinfeld M, Fless GM et al. Lipoprotein(a), fibrin binding, and plasminogen activation. Arteriosclerosis 1990; 10:240–245.

94. Wang XL, Wang J, Wilcken DE. Interactive effect of the p53 gene and cigarette smoking on coronary artery disease. Cardiovasc Res 1997; 35:250–255.

95. Penn A, Snyder C. Arteriosclerotic plaque development is 'promoted' by polynuclear aromatic hydrocarbons. Carcinogenesis 1988; 9:2185–2189.

96. Penn A, Snyder CA. 1,3-Butadiene, a vapor phase component of environmental tobacco smoke, accelerates arteriosclerotic plaque development. Circulation 1996; 93:552–557.

97. Risley P, Jerrard-Dunne P, Sitzer M et al. Promoter polymorphism in the endotoxin receptor (CD14) is associated with increased carotid atherosclerosis only in smokers: the Carotid Atherosclerosis Progression Study (CAPS). Stroke 2003; 34:600–604.

98. Brull DJ, Leeson CP, Montgomery HE et al. The effect of the interleukin-6-174G > C promoter gene polymorphism on endothelial function in healthy volunteers. Eur J Clin Invest 2002; 32:153–157.

99. Smith CJ, Steichen TJ. The atherogenic potential of carbon monoxide. Atherosclerosis 1993; 99:137–149.

100. Reznik ND, Vaisman VD. Arteriosclerosis and hypertensive disease in patients with chronic poisoning with benzene derivatives at the remote period. Gig Tr Prof Zabol 1974; 18:13–16.

101. Yu PH, Deng YL. Endogenous formaldehyde as a potential factor of vulnerability of atherosclerosis: involvement of semicarbazide-sensitive amine oxidase-mediated methylamine turnover. Atherosclerosis 1998; 140:357–363.

102. Subramanyam G, Bhaskar M, Govindappa S. The role of cadmium in induction of atherosclerosis in rabbits. Indian Heart J 1992; 44:177–180.

103. Hopfer SM, Sunderman FW Jr, Morse EE et al. Effects of intrarenal injection of nickel subsulfide in rodents. Ann Clin Lab Sci 1980; 10:54–64.

12

Homocysteine and atherogenesis

Diane E. Handy, Joseph Loscalzo

Introduction

Hyperhomocysteinemia is a known risk factor for cardiovascular disease. The link between homocysteine and atherosclerosis was first recognized in 1969 by McCully,[1] who found similar atherothrombotic sequelae in patients with hyperhomocysteinemia arising from different genetic defects. Subsequently, Wilcken and Wilcken[2] reported that homocysteine levels were higher in patients with coronary artery disease than in normal subjects. Several population-based studies have provided evidence that modest elevations of plasma homocysteine correlate with increased cardiovascular disease risk in a graded manner. Furthermore, the magnitude of risk was found to be similar to that of other conventional risk factors, such as dyslipidemia or smoking.[3]

Many environmental and genetic factors can influence homocysteine concentrations.[4,5] This chapter summarizes the current knowledge of factors that regulate plasma homocysteine concentrations, discusses the molecular mechanisms by which homocysteine may contribute to atherosclerosis, and provides an overview of recent clinical studies on homocysteine and cardiovascular risk, and therapies to reduce homocysteine levels.

Plasma homocysteine measurements

Homocysteine is found in multiple forms in plasma. Only approximately 1% of total homocysteine (tHcy) exists as free thiol; the remainder of circulating homocysteine is oxidized. Approximately 20–30% of this amino acid exists as homocystine or mixed low-molecular weight disulfides (20–30%). The remaining 70–80% is disulfide bound to plasma proteins.[6]

High-performance liquid chromatography (HPLC)-based methods that rely on either electrochemical or fluorescent detection of derivatized thiols are most commonly used to quantify homocysteine concentrations.[7] Other methods that involve enzymatic conversion of homocysteine to S-adenosyl-homocysteine (SAH) followed by immunodetection of SAH have also been developed, but are not widely used. Plasma tHcy measurements are most reliable on samples obtained after fasting, as dietary intake of protein-rich meals can increase tHcy. Normal tHcy levels range from 5 to 15 µM;[8,9] however, high-normal levels have been associated with cardiovascular disease risk in many studies (see below). Moderately elevated levels are defined as 15–30 µM, intermediate levels as 31–100 µM, and severe levels as > 100 µM.[10] Usually, only individuals with either renal insufficiency or an underlying genetic defect in homocysteine metabolism have intermediate or severe hyperhomocysteinemia, respectively.

Metabolism of homocysteine

Homocysteine is a byproduct of the biochemistry of methylation (Figure 12.1).[11] A multitude of transmethylase reactions produce SAH as a result of the transfer of a methyl group from S-adenosyl methionine (SAM) to acceptor molecules, such as proteins, phospholipids, small-molecule metabolites, and nucleic acids. The hydrolysis of SAH by SAH-hydrolase in turn yields homocysteine. The action of the SAH hydrolase is reversible, but the rapid cellular export of excess

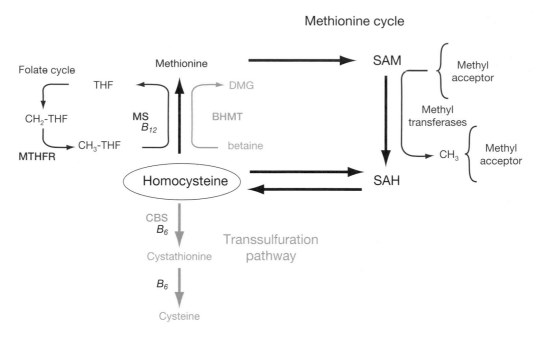

Figure 12.1 Homocysteine metabolism. Homocysteine is produced as a byproduct of methylation pathways that use *S*-adenosylmethionine (SAM) as a methyl donor to produce *S*-adenosylhomocysteine (SAH), which is rapidly hydrolyzed to form homocysteine. Homocysteine is remethylated to methionine either by methionine synthase (MS) or by betaine-homocysteine methyl transferase (BHMT), using the methyl donors 5-methyltetrahydrofolate (CH$_3$-THF) or betaine, respectively. The latter enzyme is only found in liver and kidney. MS is a vitamin B$_{12}$-dependent enzyme. Methylenetetrahydrofolate reductase (MTHFR) is involved in the synthesis of CH$_3$-THF. Homocysteine is further catabolized to form cysteine and other sulfur-containing compounds, including glutathione, in the transsulfuration pathway. The enzymes cystathionine-ß-synthase (CBS) and γ-cystathionase (not shown in the figure) are both vitamin B$_6$-containing enzymes in the transsulfuration pathway

homocysteine limits SAH reformation. The usual metabolic fate of intracellular homocysteine is remethylation to methionine, or conversion, via the transsulfuration pathway, to cystathionine and other sulfur-containing metabolites, such as cysteine or glutathione.

Vitamins B$_{12}$, B$_6$, and folate are necessary for adequate intracellular processing of homocysteine. In all cells, the primary remethylation pathway involves methionine synthase (MS), a vitamin B$_{12}$-dependent enzyme that catalyzes a methyl group transfer from the folate-containing methyl donor, 5-methyltetrahydrofolate (CH$_3$-THF), to homocysteine yielding methionine. Methylenetetrahydrofolate reductase (MTHFR) is a key enzyme involved in synthesizing CH$_3$-THF. In liver and kidney, there is an alternative remethylation pathway that relies on the enzyme betaine-homocysteine methyl transferase (BHMT), with betaine (trimethylglycine) serving as the methyl donor. The activity of this second pathway can be augmented by dietary betaine. In

severe hyperhomocysteinemic patients betaine is commonly used to increase homocysteine remethylation and, thereby, therapeutically reduce tHcy.[12]

Unlike the methionine cycle, transsulfuration is an irreversible process that results in the production of cysteine and glutathionine. This pathway involves cystathionine-β-synthase (CBS) and γ-cystathionase, two vitamin B$_6$-dependent enzymes. The transsulfuration pathway is only active in a few cell types and is an important pathway in hepatocytes, which produce most of the circulating homocysteine.[13]

Genetic defects that cause hyperhomocysteinemia

Severe hyperhomocysteinemia is inherited as a homozygous recessive disorder and is most commonly caused by mutations in the CBS gene. Thus far, over 100 such mutations have been characterized.[14] In addition to hyperhomocysteinemia, which, if untreated, results in severe vascular events by the age of 30, CBS-deficient individuals may have mental retardation, skeletal anomalies, and ectopia lentis. Tissue-specific deficiencies in cysteine production caused by the lack of the transsulfuration pathway may be the basis for some of the connective tissue disorders associated with many CBS mutations. Some CBS mutations located at the carboxy terminus of the CBS protein result in an enzyme that is catalytically active but which lacks the normal SAM-dependent increase in enzyme activity. These genetic variants apparently cause hyperhomocysteinemia and are associated with an increased risk of thrombotic events; however, there are no discernible connective tissue anomalies associated with these variants.[15]

Defects in the methionine cycle are not associated with connective tissue disorders; however, rare mutations that directly cause methionine synthase (MS) deficiency, or genetic defects that inhibit vitamin B_{12} metabolism and, subsequently, reduce MS activity, can also cause hyperhomocysteinemia. In addition, homozygous mutations in the MTHFR gene are associated with severe hyperhomocysteinemia accompanied by a phenotype of developmental delay, with a wide range of neurological disturbances.[16,17]

Common genetic polymorphisms may also contribute to tHcy levels. A mutation of the MTHFR gene that involves a 'T' substitution for a 'C' at position 677 (C677T) results in a valine substituted for an alanine and produces a thermolabile enzyme with reduced activity in *in vitro* studies.[18] High folate levels can stabilize this mutant form of the MTHFR enzyme. Furthermore, clinical studies have uncovered a gene–diet interaction between the C677T mutant and dietary folate, such that individuals with low folate and the mutation have higher levels of homocysteine; by contrast, in the presence of adequate folate the mutation has no effect on homocysteine levels.[19]

Other common mutations in genes involved in methionine remethylation may influence plasma levels of homocysteine. Mutations in MS, MS reductase, the enzyme that maintains the pool of activated cobalamin (vitamin B_{12}), and transcobalamin, a vitamin B_{12} transport protein, have been described to date.[20–22]

Recent studies suggest that vitamin B_{12} intake may modulate the effects of transcobalamin variants on tHcy levels: high vitamin B_{12} has a beneficial homocysteine-lowering effect in individuals with a proline at position 259, but did not influence tHcy levels in individuals with an arginine at position 259.[22]

Dietary and other factors that influence homocysteine

Nearly two-thirds of cases of mild hyperhomocysteinemia were proposed to be due to deficiencies in folate, vitamin B_{12} or, to a lesser extent, vitamin B_6.[23] Recent mandated folate supplementation in the USA and Canada may, however, have changed the frequency of this association.

Folate and vitamin B_6 utilization may be affected by many diverse pharmacological treatments.[24] Methotrexate and other folate antagonists used in cancer therapies can raise homocysteine levels. Drugs, such as theophylline, used for treating asthma, and isoniazid, used as an antimycobacterial agent, may inadvertently increase plasma homocysteine levels by interfering with vitamin B_6 metabolism. Similarly, cholestyramine and metformin can interfere with B-vitamin uptake from the gut, resulting in increases in tHcy levels. Fenofibrate and related compounds used to lower lipids increase homocysteine levels, perhaps by altering renal function.[25] In addition, certain dietary supplements or drugs, such as levodopa, niacin, and L-arginine, may also elevate tHcy by increasing methylation reactions that utilize SAM and increasing SAH production.[26–28] In a recent study of patients with Parkinson's disease it was found that those on levodopa therapy had significantly elevated tHcy levels compared with patients not receiving this treatment ($16.1 \pm 6.2\ \mu M$ versus $12.2 \pm 4.2\ \mu M$). Elevated homocysteine levels were associated with an increase in coronary artery disease in these patients,[29] suggesting that the therapeutic use of drugs or supplements that raise tHcy levels may have unwanted cardiovascular consequences.

Renal dysfunction, male sex, increased age, and the menopause are all associated with increased levels of plasma tHcy. These and other factors that influence tHcy have been reviewed by Schneede and colleagues.[5]

Hyperhomocysteinemia and atherothrombosis: a review of the clinical evidence

The 1995 meta-analysis by Boushey and co-workers[3] is often cited as proof that elevated tHcy increases the risk of coronary, peripheral, and cerebral vascular disease. In combining data from 27 observational studies, this meta-analysis concluded that a 5 µM elevation in tHcy increases coronary artery disease (CAD) risk 1.6-fold (95% CI 1.4–1.7) in men and 1.8-fold (95% CI 1.3–1.9) in women, increases peripheral arterial disease risk 6.8-fold (95% CI 2.9–15.8), and increases cerebrovascular disease risk 1.5-fold (95% CI 1.3–1.9). This modest incremental change in homocysteine was found to increase risk as much as a 20 mg/dl increase in plasma cholesterol. Subsequently, several large retrospective studies, such as the European Concerted Action Project,[30] also showed significantly higher levels of tHcy in patients with atherosclerosis compared to normal subjects. In contrast, results from prospective studies are less consistent. For example, the Physician's Health Study 5-year update[31] found an increase in relative risk for myocardial infarction (MI) in individuals with elevated tHcy, whereas the 7.5-year update[32] found no association between elevated tHcy and cardiovascular disease (CVD) events.

Most recent meta-analyses have concluded that there is a significant association between tHcy and CVD. For example, Bautista and colleagues[33] found a significant increase in the relative risk for elevated tHcy and coronary heart disease (CHD) of 1.34 (95% CI 1.17–1.54). Similarly, a meta-analysis of prospective studies by Wald and colleagues[34] calculated an odds ratio of 1.32 (1.19–1.45) for ischemic heart disease for each 5 µM increase in tHcy. Furthermore, the Homocysteine Studies Collaboration,[35] which analyzed studies from 1966 to 1999, found a 16% increase in risk for CVD in individuals in the top quintile of tHcy with no prior history of cardiovascular disease. Importantly, this study reported that individuals with lower tHcy levels had a lower risk for ischemic heart disease (OR 0.89, 95% CI 0.83–0.96) and stroke (OR 0.81, 95% CI 0.69–0.95).

Several large, population-based prospective studies, such as the Framingham Heart Study, have also found that modest hyperhomocysteinemia significantly increases the risk for all-cause mortality and CVD mortality, after adjustments for other cardiovascular risk factors.[36] AFCAPS/TexCAPS and the Women's Health Study[37] reported that modest elevations of tHcy can increase the risk of CVD even in otherwise healthy individuals.

The relationship between tHcy and adverse outcomes was especially strong in individuals with pre-existing CHD. In a Finnish population, both women and men with elevated tHcy and pre-existing CHD were found to have a significantly increased risk of coronary events.[38,39] In other recent studies of high-risk CHD patients,[40–44] modest elevations in tHcy (cutoffs as low as 14.1 µM) correlated with increased mortality or an increased risk of MI. In patients with angiographically defined CAD, the relative hazard ratio increased by 16% for each 5 µM incremental increase in tHcy level.[40] Nygard and colleagues[45] also reported a graded response between tHcy levels and mortality in patients with angiographically defined CAD.

tHcy levels are probably not a predictor of incident peripheral artery disease (PAD).[46] In patients with established PAD, however, there was a significant increase in relative risk reported for all-cause mortality in the highest quintile of tHcy (≥ 17.9 µM), and the risk of death from vascular disease increased 5.6% for each 1 µM increase in tHcy levels in this study.[47]

Recent studies have examined tHcy levels and restenosis risk after percutaneous coronary interventions (PCI). In one study that followed 183 patients after PCI, tHcy levels correlated with the restenosis rate:[48] individuals with tHcy levels < 9 µM were found to have lower rates of restenosis (25.3% vs 50%) and major adverse cardiovascular events (15.7% vs 28.4%).[49] Interestingly, when larger vessels were stented the association between tHcy and restenosis disappeared. This result is consistent with the findings of the Generation Study (Global Evaluation of New Events and Restenosis After Stent Implantation). In 483 patients with successful coronary stenting, tHcy was not a predictor for subsequent ischemic events.[50] In a much larger study of 504 patients, followed for a year after successful angioplasty, a graded relationship was found between tHcy levels and major adverse coronary events (MACE).[49]

MTHFR polymorphisms and cardiovascular disease

In 1995 Frosst and co-workers[51] suggested that the common C677T polymorphism in the MTHFR gene was a likely risk factor for CVD, as the resulting amino acid substitution in the protein altered enzyme function. Subsequent population studies have suggested that the effect of this polymorphism on homocysteine production is dependent on folate status.[19] Many studies have found no significant association between the TT genotype and CVD risk. For example, Klujtmans and colleagues[52] studied angiographically defined CAD patients and found that elevated tHcy correlated with the presence of the MTHFR variant; however, there was no increased occurrence of CAD in individuals with the TT genotype. In Physicians Health Study participants, no significant association was found between the MTHFR genotype and the risk of MI. An association was found, however, between tHcy levels and the TT genotype in the lowest quartile of plasma folate. In the high-folate group tHcy levels were the same regardless of MTHFR genotype.[53]

The controversy about the influence of the MTHFR genotype on CVD is still unresolved. A meta-analysis that included eight case–control studies for a total of 2476 CAD patients and 2481 controls, found a significant risk for CAD in homozygous TT individuals (OR 1.22, 95% CI 1.01–1.47), whereas another meta-analysis from 1998[54] reported that the TT genotype correlated with elevated tHcy (25% higher than in individuals with the CC genotype), even though this genotype had no association with CVD. The most recent meta-analysis performed by the MTHFR Studies Collaboration Group[55] suggested that folate fortification in North America and Canada minimized the effect of the TT genotype on CHD in North American studies performed after 1998. In support of a protective role for folate fortification, this study found that individuals with folate levels below the median and the TT genotype had a greater risk for CHD (OR 1.44, 95% CI 1.12–1.83) than individuals with the CC genotype and folate levels above the median.

Mechanism of homocysteine's pathobiological action

Homocysteine has pleiotrophic effects that contribute to a proatherogenic and prothrombotic state (Figure 12.2). It has been hypothesized that oxidative stress is responsible for many of these effects; however, other mechanisms that are independent of oxidative stress may be involved in mediating homocysteine's atherogenic actions. Clinical studies, such as those discussed in the previous sections of this chapter, suggest that modest increases in tHcy levels can contribute to CVD risk. In determining the mechanisms for homocysteine's pathobiological actions, investigators have studied the physiological and molecular effects of homocysteine both *in vivo* and in isolated cells. As discussed below, in *in vivo* studies a mere doubling of homocysteine levels is sufficient to cause some proatherogenic changes. In many animal studies, the atherogenic effects of homocysteine have been studied in combination with hyperlipidemia, at times under conditions that produce moderate hyperhomocysteinemia, i.e. levels of tHcy of approximately 50 μM, or 10–20 times-higher than normal. In contrast, in cell culture studies a wide variety of conditions have been used to study the deleterious consequences of exposure to homocysteine. Although some untoward effects of homocysteine are apparent at physiologically (10–50 μM) or pathophysiologically (100–300 μM) relevant concentrations, other adverse effects are only detected when cells are subjected to superphysiological (1–5 mM) levels of homocysteine. Thus, it has been debated as to whether or not some of the effects of homocysteine exposure identified in experimental systems are relevant to the *in vivo* consequences of modest increases in tHcy levels.

In vivo models: the proatherogenic actions of homocysteine

Experimental evidence in animal models confirms the role of homocysteine as a proatherogenic factor. This is most apparent in studies with the apoE knockout (apoE–/–) mice, which have severe hypercholesterolemia leading to the development of atherosclerotic lesion. In apoE–/– mice fed a high-methionine diet depleted in folate and vitamin B$_6$ for 8 weeks, lesion area

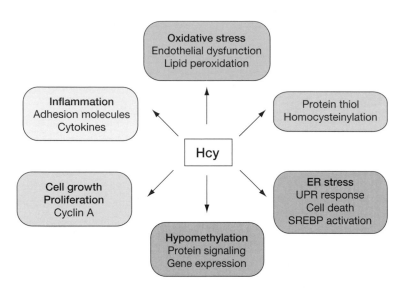

Figure 12.2 Mechanisms of homocysteine's pathobiological actions. Homocysteine (Hcy) has pleiotrophic effects that contribute to a proatherogenic environment. These mechanisms are not mutually exclusive. For example, oxidative stress, possibly via NFκB activation, contributes to the inflammatory response by increasing the expression of adhesion molecules and cytokines. Redox disturbances contribute to protein misfolding, endoplasmic reticulum (ER) stress, the unfolded protein response (UPR), and sterol-binding protein activation (SREBP). Activation of SREBP may increase the expression of genes involved in cholesterol biosynthesis. Oxidative stress, ER stress, and hypomethylation of genomic DNA may all alter gene expression. Hypomethylation of ras contributes to endothelial growth inhibition in cell culture. The relationship of protein or gene hypomethylation and protein cysteine homocysteinylation to atherogenesis is speculative

nearly doubled in size, concurrent with a substantial increase in tHcy (from 2.5 ± 0.3 μM to 47.3 ± 3.2 μM).[56] The addition of supplemental folate and B vitamins to the high-methionine diet partially mitigated the effect of methionine on tHcy levels (18.4 μM) and prevented the increase in atheroma size. Similarly, in another study, 18 weeks of dietary methionine or the administration of homocysteine increased aortic root atherosclerosis in apoE–/– mice.[57] Both of these regimens increased tHcy levels to a similar extent, from 9.46 ± 0.28 μM in untreated apoE–/– to 53.60 ± 8.68 μM with methionine treatment, and to 51.54 ± 2.92 μM with homocysteine treatment. Interestingly, oxidized homocysteine, in the form of homocystine, only increased tHcy levels to approximately 16 μM and had no effect on atherosclerotic lesion development. Modest elevations of tHcy levels (from 3.8 ± 0.9 μM to 7.4 ± 2.9 μM), achieved by crossing the heterozygous CBS-deficient mice into the apoE–/– strain, resulted in a significant increase in aortic lesion area at 12 months of age,[58] indicating that small changes in tHcy levels can

promote atherosclerosis, especially in combination with other risk factors (in the case of the apoE–/–, dyslipidemia).

One intriguing study used 3-deaza-adenosine, an adenosine analog known to inhibit SAH hydrolase, to reduce homocysteine levels in apoE–/– mice fed an atherogenic diet.[59] Twelve weeks of this treatment reduced the atheroma burden by over 60%. The authors suggested that the reduction of homocysteine by this therapy was responsible for the reduction in atherosclerosis in these mice; however, homocysteine levels are already low in this model (approximately 5.3 μM in this study), and although the treatment reduced tHcy by 35% after 12 weeks and by 45% after 24 weeks, 3-deaza-adenosine is also a known inflammatory suppressor.[60] Thus, it is not clear whether the antiatherogenic effects of this treatment are solely a consequence of reducing homocysteine levels or whether other effects of the SAH hydrolase inhibitor on SAH levels, adenosine levels, or other metabolites contributed to its action.

Endothelial dysfunction, oxidative stress and hyperhomocysteinemia

Endothelial dysfunction is considered to be an early marker of vascular injury in atherogenesis. In heterozygous CBS-deficient (CBS+/–) mice, the endothelium-dependent vasodilator substances methacholine and bradykinin have a paradoxical vasoconstrictor effect on mesenteric arteries that show normal endothelium-independent vasodilator responses.[61] Homocysteine levels in the CBS+/– mice are only approximately two-fold higher than that of their CBS+/+ wild-type siblings. The CBS+/– mice were found to have other signs of oxidative stress, including a deficiency in acetyl-choline-stimulated cGMP in isolated aorta, an increase in immunodetectable aortic 3-nitrotyrosine, and an increase in the levels of F_2-isoprostanes. Taken together, these data suggest a lack of bioavailable nitric oxide (NO) in these CBS-deficient mice. Other studies in endothelial cells and in the CBS-deficient mice suggest that homocysteine can decrease the activity of cellular glutathione peroxidase (GPx1), a major intracellular antioxidant enzyme,[62–64] thereby contributing to the accumulation of reactive oxygen species (ROS) and the subsequent inactivation of NO (Figure 12.3). A decrease in GPx1 activity was also found in hyper-homocysteinemia caused by folate depletion in the rat,[65] confirming the sensitivity of this antioxidant enzyme to inactivation by mild hyperhomocysteinemia.

An impairment of endothelium-dependent vasodi-lation was also found in monkeys that were made mildly hyperhomocysteinemic by dietary means.[66] Furthermore, an acute elevation in homocysteine levels caused by methionine infusion can also impair NO-dependent vasodilator function in normal subjects,[67] and endothelial dysfunction has also been found in adults with mild hyperhomocysteinemia.[68,69]

Recent studies have suggested that NO synthase (S) activity may be directly inhibited by an accumulation of asymmetric dimethyl arginine (ADMA) in the presence of elevated homocysteine levels.[70] Homocysteine apparently blocks dimethylarginine dimethylaminohy-drolase, an enzyme that metabolizes ADMA and prevents its accumulation. It has also been proposed that physiological levels of homocysteine can interfere with L-arginine uptake by the Y+ transporter, at least in platelets.[71] It is unclear whether homocysteine inter-feres with this transporter in endothelial cells;

nevertheless, this is another potential pathway by which homocysteine may decrease NO in biological systems.

Recent studies have shown that the oxidative stress and endothelial dysfunction caused by hyperhomocys-teinemia *in vivo* can be prevented by increasing the antioxidant capacity, either by increasing the levels of the protective enzyme GPx1 or by the use of antioxi-dants, such as L-2-oxothiazolidine-4-carboxylic acid (OTC), a precursor of glutathione.[63,64] These findings support the hypothesis that homocysteine causes endothelial dysfunction and damage, in part via oxidative stress.

Homocysteine and inflammation

The earliest vascular lesions, fatty streaks, consist of adherent macrophages and T lymphocytes. Oxidant stress caused by homocysteine may promote the expression of adhesion molecules and inflammatory cell mediators in the endothelium, contributing to a proatherogenic state by attracting monocytes to the vessel wall and facilitating fatty streak formation. Furthermore, high plasma tHcy is associated with an increase in lipid peroxidation: oxidative modifications of low-density lipoproteins (LDL) can contribute to enhanced LDL uptake by macrophages in the vessel wall and the formation of foam cells. Compared to con-trol mice, hyperhomocysteinemic CBS+/– mice have increased soluble and endothelial-bound P-selectin,[64] suggesting that the mild hyperhomocysteinemia in this model is sufficient to activate endothelial cells. In the general population and in other patient groups, elevat-ed plasma tHcy levels have also been associated with enhanced soluble adhesion molecule expression.[72,73] In the CBS+/– mice OTC treatment caused an increase in glutathione levels and glutathione peroxidase activity, with a concomitant decrease in soluble and membrane bound P-selectin,[64] suggesting that an increase in antioxidant capacity can attenuate homocysteine-induced adhesion molecule production. Another study has shown that *in vivo* elevation of homocysteine in apoE–/– mice can promote vascular cell adhesion mol-ecule-1 (VCAM-1) expression, and suggests that homocysteine promotes an inflammatory response in the vessel wall by enhancing NFκB activation.[56]

A consequence of enhanced adhesion molecule expression on the endothelium is increased inflamma-

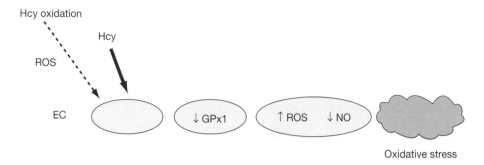

Figure 12.3   Homocysteine (Hcy) and endothelial dysfunction. Oxidation of homocysteine can cause reactive oxygen species (ROS) accumulation. ROS may also accumulate because homocysteine decreases the activity of the cellular glutathione peroxidase (GPx1), a major antioxidant enzyme. In the presence of reduced GPx1 cells accumulate ROS, which can inactivate nitric oxide (NO), leading to a reduced vasodilator response and endothelial dysfunction in endothelial cells. Treatments that enhance GPx1 activity have been shown to improve NO production and vascular responsiveness. EC, endothelial cells

tory cell recruitment to the vessel wall. Homocysteine, at levels from 20 to 100 μM, has been shown to induce adhesion molecule expression and promote monocyte and T-cell adhesion to cultured human aortic endothelial cells (HAEC).[74,75] Similarly, diet-induced hyperhomocysteinemia in rats increased VCAM-1 and E-selectin expression, resulting in a detectable increase in monocyte attachment to the endothelium[76] and contributing to a proatherogenic vascular environment.

In addition to promoting adhesion molecule expression, homocysteine also promotes expression of the monocyte chemoattractant protein-1 (MCP-1), which has been shown to be induced in cultured endothelial cells, vascular smooth muscle cells, and monocytes by levels of homocysteine as low as 10 μM.[77–79] Blocking MCP-1 recruitment of monocytes has been shown to attenuate atherosclerosis in apoE–/– mice.[80] Taken together, these data illustrate that enhanced inflammatory responses supported by homocysteine may also contribute to the progression of atherosclerotic lesions.

Homocysteine and cell growth

Homocysteine may also promote vascular lesion formation by inhibiting endothelial cell growth, while at the same time promoting vascular smooth muscle cell proliferation.[81,82] In cell culture, these effects on cell growth could be detected with micromolar levels of homocysteine. In human umbilical vein endothelial cells (HUVEC) the inhibitory actions of homocysteine can be traced to the suppression of cyclin A expression

and signaling,[83] whereas in vascular smooth muscle cells homocysteine can augment cyclin A and cyclin D1 gene expression.[81,84] Cyclins A and D1 are major regulators of the cell cycle.

Homocysteine and inhibition of transmethylases

Hyperhomocysteinemia may also cause hypomethylation of DNA and even some proteins, owing to the effect of increased SAH levels on transmethylases, most of which are inhibited by SAH. Theoretically, alterations in genomic DNA methylation can modify gene expression: DNA methylation is associated with an inhibition of gene transcription, whereas unmethylated DNA is more accessible to nuclear factor binding and transcription. In some proteins, such as ras and other GTPases, methylation is a key step in enzyme activation.[85]

Physiological levels (10–50 μM) of homocysteine have been shown to cause hypomethylation of ras and attenuate the ras/mitogen-activated protein (MAP) signaling pathway.[86] Recent studies suggest that increased cellular levels of SAH can inhibit the isoprenyl-cysteine carboxymethyltransferase which methylates ras and other proteins that undergo prenylation.[87] Thus, homocysteine may influence cellular function by modulating the methylation and activation of proteins.

Studies in homozygous CBS–/– mice reported that genomic DNA methylation was decreased in liver and kidney, tissues in which transsulfuration is important for modulating homocysteine levels.[88] Similarly, genomic DNA isolated from different tissues in hyper-homocysteinemic MTHFR-deficient mice was found to be hypomethylated.[89] In otherwise healthy female subjects, mildly elevated levels of tHcy were associated with global hypomethylation of lymphocyte DNA.[90] Global hypomethylation of human lymphocyte DNA has also been found to be influenced by folate levels and the MTHFR polymorphism.[91,92] Furthermore, in patients with hyperhomocysteinemia as a consequence of uremia, the alterations in DNA hypomethylation were found to be sufficient to promote the expression of genetic loci that are normally suppressed because of imprinting or sex-linked hypermethylation.[93] This latest study is the only one to have demonstrated homocysteine-induced DNA hypomethylation at specific genetic loci. Theoretically, modulation of gene methylation is another potential mechanism by which homocysteine can affect gene expression and modify cellular functions, however, the significance of this mechanism to atherosclerosis has yet to be elucidated. The causal link between methylation and atherosclerosis appears to be complex, with some studies suggesting that specific gene hypermethylation may be important for atherosclerotic lesion development.[94]

Gene expression, endoplasmic reticulum dysfunction, and homocysteine

Endoplasmic reticulum (ER) stress has also been proposed as a mechanism by which homocysteine alters gene expression to promote cellular dysfunction and cell death. The thiol-containing homocysteine has been proposed to disrupt disulfide bond formation, thereby activating the unfolded protein response (UPR) in cells as a means to alleviate the accumulation of misfolded proteins in the ER.[95] The accumulation of unfolded proteins in the ER promotes the dissociation of GRP78/BiP, an ER chaperone protein, from transmembrane ER sensor proteins, resulting in their activation. Subsequent downstream events induce the expression of a number of ER chaperone proteins and other stress-induced proteins.[96] The type 1 ER transmembrane kinase (IRE1), the activating transcription factor 6 (ATF6) and the double stranded (ds)RNA-dependent pancreatic elF2α (PKR)-like ER kinase (PERK) are the three known mammalian sensor proteins that regulate the cellular response to ER

stress by transmitting signals from the ER to the nucleus. The activation pathways involved in ER stress and the UPR are shown in more detail in Figure 12.4.

Homocysteine at millimolar concentrations has been shown to activate the IRE1 protein; this pattern of activation has been tied to apoptosis in HUVEC.[97] In other studies, differential display and microarray analysis of mRNA from HUVEC have shown that millimolar concentrations of homocysteine can also induce the expression of many ER stress markers, such as GRP78/BiP, GRP94, Herp, RTP, and GADD153.[98,99] GRP78 mRNA was also elevated in the livers of heterozygous CBS-deficient mice that have mild hyperhomocysteinemia.[98] Recent studies suggest that overexpression of GRP78 may protect cells from apoptosis.[100] Thus, overexpression of GRP78 in the liver of a hyperhomocysteinemic mouse may represent an adaptive response to homocysteine-induced cellular stress.

Treatment of cultured cells with millimolar concentrations of homocysteine was also found to increase the expression of the sterol response-binding protein (SREBP), a nuclear factor that regulates the expression of many genes involved in cholesterol biosynthesis. As expected, the increase in SREBP expression caused by homocysteine treatment resulted in an upregulation of mRNA levels of genes involved in cholesterol biosynthesis, such as HMG-CoA reductase, isopentenyl diphosphate (IPP) isomerase, and farnesyl diphosphate (FPP) synthase in hepatic cells, human endothelial cells, and human aortic smooth muscle cells.[101] Some of these transcripts were also elevated in livers from mice made hyperhomocysteinemic by dietary means. The authors of this study suggested that the alterations in cholesterol biosynthesis found in these mice may contribute to the development of hepatic steatosis and the progression of atherosclerotic lesions.

Another recent study used a combination of differential display and cDNA arrays of stress genes to compare the hepatic expresion of transcripts from CBS-deficient and wild-type mice.[102] Surprisingly few differences in gene expression were found; only five genes were identified by the initial differential display, and an additional eight genes were identified from experiments with the stress arrays. Several of these alterations were only apparent in the CBS−/− mouse and not in the mildly hyperhomocysteinemic CBS+/− mice; other alterations in transcript levels were apparent in only male or female CBS−/− mice. mRNA from genes encoding various

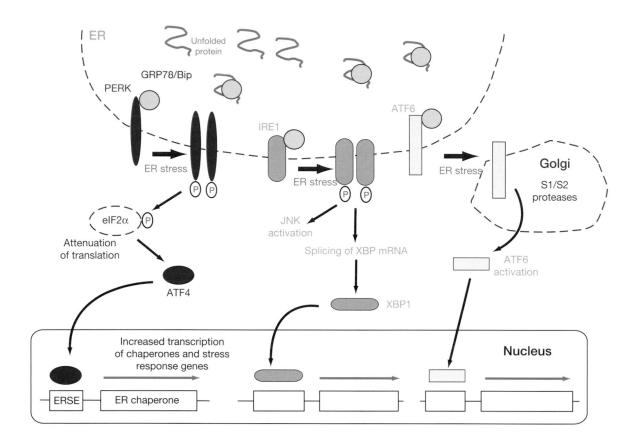

Figure 12.4 Endoplasmic reticulum (ER) stress response. Homocysteine has been proposed to disrupt disulfide bond formation and thereby activate the unfolded protein response (UPR) to alleviate the accumulation of misfolded proteins in the ER.[95] Many other metabolic, chemical, and genetic perturbations can activate the UPR. Three resident ER membrane proteins act as sensors for ER stress. Normally these sensor proteins bind to GRP78/Bip, an ER chaperone protein. Activation of the UPR occurs when the accumulation of misfolded proteins in the ER promotes the dissociation of GRP78/BiP from these sensor proteins. Activation of the ER stress response causes alterations in protein translation and an upregulation of ER chaperones and proteins involved in protein degradation and refolding. Activation of the double stranded (ds)RNA-dependent pancreatic eIF2α (PKR)-like ER kinase (PERK) and the type 1 ER transmembrane kinase (IRE1) leads to dimerization and subsequent autophosphorylation of serine/threonine kinase domains. Activated PERK phosphorylates and inactivates eIF2α, attenuating normal protein translation and allowing for translation of the nuclear factor activating transcription factor 4 (ATF4) and other transcripts that have special signals which allow for translation in the absence of functional eIF2α. IRE signaling activates the c-jun N-terminal kinase (JNK) pathway and promotes the splicing of a small intron from the XBP1 mRNA, leading to the expression of the X-box binding protein (XBP1) transcription factor. Activation of the activating transcription factor 6 (ATF6) involves translocation to the Golgi and cleavage by the S1/S2 proteases, which release the active ATF6 transcription factor. Binding of these transcription factors to ER stress elements induces the transcription of genes such as GRP78/BiP, GRP94, GADD153, and protein disulfide isomerase

cytochrome P450 proteins were found to be either up- or downregulated in the CBS-deficient mice, suggesting an alteration in the redox state of the cell. The cytochrome c oxidase subunit 1 transcript was also downregulated, suggesting mitochondrial dysfunction; and heme oxygenase mRNA and protein were upregulated, as has been shown in other models of oxidative

stress. In addition, there was a substantial decrease in the PON1 transcript that correlated with a decrease in hepatic paraoxonase activity. Paraoxonase is an esterase that is thought to protect LDL from oxidation. Furthermore, dietary treatments that modestly increased homocysteine levels twofold were able to decrease hepatic paraoxonase activity significantly in CBS+/− mice, suggesting that slight elevations in homocysteine could promote lipid oxidation. Thus, although it is difficult to determine the significance of all of these changes to atherosclerosis, these data generally support the hypothesis that homocysteine can promote oxidative stress.

Homocysteine and protein modifications

Most circulating homocysteine is disulfide bound to proteins, and it has been suggested that homocysteinylation of reactive cysteines may interfere with protein folding or function. *In vitro* studies have shown that several plasma proteins have available cysteine residues that can form mixed disulfides with homocysteine. Binding of homocysteine to factor Va or fibronectin has been shown to interfere with the normal activity of these proteins;[103,104] however, the *in vivo* association of homocysteine to these proteins has not been confirmed. Recent studies have determined that transthyretin, the thyroid hormone-binding plasma protein that is dysfunctional in familial amyloid polyneuropathy, can be modified by homocysteine binding in human plasma.[105,106] Furthermore, homocysteinylation occurs at a specific cysteine residue at amino acid position 10 in the transthyretin protein. Although the significance of this modification for the normal function of transthyretin is not apparent, these studies clearly illustrate that homocysteine binds to serum proteins other than albumin, and that the degree of homocysteinylation in human plasma correlates with the levels of circulating homocysteine. Homocysteine binding to free thiols in proteins may have no effect on protein function or may alter protein function by interfering with protein folding, protein–protein interactions, or other protein modifications at reactive cysteine residues. Many ongoing projects are focused on the significance of homocysteinylation or other oxidative post-translational modifications to protein structure and function in hyperhomocysteinemia.

Therapies for lowering total plasma homocysteine levels

Vitamin B_6 therapy successfully lowers homocysteine levels in approximately 50% of CBS-deficient, severely hyperhomocysteinemic patients. To lower homocysteine in other CBS-deficient patients, methionine restriction, combined with supplements of betaine and folate, is the recommended treatment. Lowering tHcy has been found to reduce atherothrombotic events greatly in this high-risk population.[107]

Homocysteine levels can be reduced by folate supplementation in individuals with normal to high-normal levels of tHcy.[108] For example, folic acid supplementation of 0.5–5 mg/day has been found to lower tHcy by 25% (95% CI 23–28%).[109] Homocysteine levels can be reduced by another 7% (95% CI 3–10%) by adding vitamin B_{12} (0.5 mg/day) to the folate supplementation, whereas vitamin B_6 supplementation had no additional benefit. In patients with high-normal tHcy levels, as little as 0.1 mg folic acid per day may lower tHcy.[110] In contrast, renal failure patients are resistant to the tHcy-lowering effects of folate, and may require levels up to 15 mg/day to reduce tHcy.[111]

In individuals with vitamin B_{12} insufficiency excess folic acid can mask the hematological symptoms of this deficiency. Thus, to avoid unwanted neurological complications in these patients, B_{12} supplements should be given as an adjunct to folate therapy.

Folic acid treatment has been associated with both a lowering of tHcy and an improvement in endothelial function. As discussed earlier, endothelial dysfunction can be caused by hyperhomocysteinemia. Acute infusions of folate or 5-methyltetrahydrofolate, the active form of folate, have been found to improve endothelial dysfunction.[67,112] Long-term treatment with folic acid supplements has also been shown to lower tHcy and improve endothelium-dependent vascular function in individuals with high-normal homocysteine levels.[113,114] Folic acid may also have antioxidant properties that can improve vascular function through mechanisms independent of its effect on tHcy levels.[115,116]

Many large prospective studies on the effects of folate in preventing CHD are ongoing. One recent study chronicled the protective effects of a combination of folic acid plus vitamin B_{12} and B_6 following PCI.[117] These supplements significantly lowered tHcy and the occurrence of major adverse effects after 6 months of treatment. The protective effect of the folate/vitamin B_6/vitamin B_{12} therapy persisted for 6 months after treatment was stopped.[118]

Other therapies

Another possible therapy to lower homocysteine levels is creatine supplementation. Creatine synthesis normally involves the methylation of guanidinoacetate by the SAM-dependent guanidinoacetate methyl transferase. This highly active hepatic pathway produces creatine (to maintain circulating levels of approximately 50 μM) and, as a byproduct, SAH, contributing to homocysteine production by the liver. Creatine actually downregulates the arginine–glycine–amidinotransferase (AGAT) found in the kidney, which is the first enzyme in creatine biosynthesis. In normal rats, dietary supplementation with creatine reduces tHcy by approximately 30%.[28] Another recent study determined that creatine treatment had no effect on tHcy levels in normal rats but could lower tHcy levels in a model of renal failure associated with mild hyperhomocysteinemia.[119] These studies are intriguing, but additional research is necessary to determine the effectiveness of creatine in reducing tHcy and improving CVD outcomes.

Summary

Homocysteine contributes to CVD through many mechanisms that promote atherogenesis. Notably, oxidative stress and a lack of bioavailable NO caused by a reduction in glutathione peroxidase and/or a decrease in NOS activity contributes to endothelial dysfunction, increased expression of inflammatory mediators and monocyte binding to the endothelium, and the oxidation of lipids and proteins. Alterations in cellular redox status may contribute to alterations in gene expression, ER stress, and activation of cholesterol biosynthesis. Inhibition of transmethylases, by the concomitant increase in SAH, can prevent methylation of genes and proteins, altering gene expression patterns and blocking protein signaling and cellular functions, such as proliferation. Theoretically, direct protein modification by homocysteine binding to free cysteines may disrupt protein folding and function.

Epidemiological studies implicate homocysteine as a risk factor for incidental cardiovascular disease and for secondary events in those with existing CVD. Experimental evidence suggests that lowering homocysteine or augmenting antioxidant status may slow the development of atherosclerotic lesions, improve endothelial function, and prevent endothelial activation and other changes associated with homocysteine-induced oxidative stress. Initial clinical trials suggest that folate therapy is a relatively inexpensive method to reduce tHcy levels and improve vascular function in many individuals. Additional studies of the mechanisms by which homocysteine contributes to vascular disease may reveal other effective therapies to improve cardiovascular disease outcomes.

References

1. McCully KS. Vascular pathology of homocysteinemia: implications for the pathogenesis of arteriosclerosis. Am J Pathol 1969; 56:111–128
2. Wilcken DE, Wilcken B. The pathogenesis of coronary artery disease. A possible role for methionine metabolism. J Clin Invest 1976; 57:1079–1082
3. Boushey CJ, Beresford SA, Omenn GS et al. A quantitative assessment of plasma homocysteine as a risk factor for vascular disease. Probable benefits of increasing folic acid intakes. J Am Med Assoc 1995; 274:1049–1057
4. Selhub J. Homocysteine metabolism. Annu Rev Nutr 1999; 19:217–246
5. Schneede J, Refsum H, Ueland PM. Biological and environmental determinants of plasma homocysteine. Semin Thromb Hemost 2000; 26:263–279
6. Ueland PM. Homocysteine species as components of plasma redox thiol status. Clin Chem 1995; 41:340–342
7. Ubbink JB. Assay methods for the measurement of total homocyst(e)ine in plasma. Semin Thromb Hemost 2000; 26:233–241
8. Ueland PM, Refsum H, Stabler SP et al. Total homocysteine in plasma or serum: methods and clinical applications. Clin Chem 1993; 39:1764–1779
9. Jacobsen DW, Gatautis VJ, Green R et al. Rapid HPLC determination of total homocysteine and other thiols in serum and plasma: sex differences and correlation with cobalamin and folate concentrations in healthy subjects. Clin Chem 1994; 40:873–881
10. Kang SS, Wong PW, Malinow MR. Hyperhomocyst(e)inemia as a risk factor for occlusive vascular disease. Annu Rev Nutr 1992; 12:279–298
11. Finkelstein JD, Kyle W, Harris BJ. Methionine metabolism in mammals. Regulation of homocysteine methyltransferases in rat tissue. Arch Biochem Biophys 1971; 146:84–92
12. Wilcken DE, Wilcken B. The natural history of vascular disease in homocystinuria and the effects of treatment. J Inherit Metab Dis 1997; 20:295–300
13. Mudd SH, Finkelstein JD, Irreverre F et al. Transsulfuration in mammals. Microassays and tissue distributions of three enzymes of the pathway. J Biol Chem 1965; 240:4382–4392

14. Kraus JP, Janosik M, Kozich V et al. Cystathionine beta-synthase mutations in homocystinuria. Hum Mutat 1999; 13:362–375

15. Maclean KN, Gaustadnes M, Oliveriusova J et al. High homocysteine and thrombosis without connective tissue disorders are associated with a novel class of cystathionine beta-synthase (CBS) mutations. Hum Mutat 2002; 19:641–655

16. Goyette P, Frosst P, Rosenblatt DS et al. Seven novel mutations in the methylenetetrahydrofolate reductase gene and genotype/phenotype correlations in severe methylenetetrahydrofolate reductase deficiency. Am J Hum Genet 1995; 56:1052–1059

17. Leclerc D, Campeau E, Goyette P et al. Human methionine synthase: cDNA cloning and identification of mutations in patients of the cblG complementation group of folate/cobalamin disorders. Hum Mol Genet 1996; 5:1867–1874

18. Kang SS, Zhou J, Wong PW et al. Intermediate homocysteinemia: a thermolabile variant of methylenetetrahydrofolate reductase. Am J Hum Genet 1988; 43:414–421

19. Jacques PF, Bostom AG, Williams RR et al. Relation between folate status, a common mutation in methylenetetrahydrofolate reductase, and plasma homocysteine concentrations. Circulation 1996; 93:7–9

20. Gaughan DJ, Kluijtmans LA, Barbaux S et al. The methionine synthase reductase (MTRR) A66G polymorphism is a novel genetic determinant of plasma homocysteine concentrations. Atherosclerosis 2001; 157:451–456

21. Harmon DL, Shields DC, Woodside JV et al. Methionine synthase D919G polymorphism is a significant but modest determinant of circulating homocysteine concentrations. Genet Epidemiol 1999; 17:298–309

22. Lievers KJ, Afman LA, Kluijtmans LA et al. Polymorphisms in the transcobalamin gene: association with plasma homocysteine in healthy individuals and vascular disease patients. Clin Chem 2002; 48:1383–1389

23. Selhub J, Jacques PF, Wilson PW et al. Vitamin status and intake as primary determinants of homocysteinemia in an elderly population. J Am Med Assoc 1993; 270:2693–2698

24. Desouza C, Keebler M, McNamara DB et al. Drugs affecting homocysteine metabolism: impact on cardiovascular risk. Drugs 2002; 62:605–616

25. Westphal S, Dierkes J, Luley C. Effects of fenofibrate and gemfibrozil on plasma homocysteine. Lancet 2001; 358:39–40

26. Basu TK, Mann S. Vitamin B-6 normalizes the altered sulfur amino acid status of rats fed diets containing pharmacological levels of niacin without reducing niacin's hypolipidemic effects. J Nutr 1997; 127:117–121

27. Allain P, Le Bouil A, Cordillet E et al. Sulfate and cysteine levels in the plasma of patients with Parkinson's disease. Neurotoxicology 1995; 16:527–529

28. Stead LM, Au KP, Jacobs RL et al. Methylation demand and homocysteine metabolism: effects of dietary provision of creatine and guanidinoacetate. Am J Physiol Endocrinol Metab 2001; 281:E1095–E1100

29. Rogers JD, Sanchez-Saffon A, Frol AB et al. Elevated plasma homocysteine levels in patients treated with levodopa: association with vascular disease. Arch Neurol 2003; 60:59–64

30. Graham IM, Daly LE, Refsum HM et al. Plasma homocysteine as a risk factor for vascular disease. The European Concerted Action Project. J Am Med Assoc 1997; 277:1775–1781

31. Stampfer MJ, Malinow MR, Willett WC et al. A prospective study of plasma homocyst(e)ine and risk of myocardial infarction in US physicians. J Am Med Assoc 1992; 268:877–881

32. Chasan-Taber L, Selhub J, Rosenberg IH et al. A prospective study of folate and vitamin B6 and risk of myocardial infarction in US physicians. J Am Coll Nutr 1996; 15:136–143

33. Bautista LE, Arenas IA, Penuela A et al. Total plasma homocysteine level and risk of cardiovascular disease: a meta-analysis of prospective cohort studies. J Clin Epidemiol 2002; 55:882–887

34. Wald DS, Law M, Morris JK. Homocysteine and cardiovascular disease: evidence on causality from a meta-analysis. Br Med J 2002; 325:1202

35. Homocysteine Studies Collaboration. Homocysteine and risk of ischemic heart disease and stroke: a meta-analysis. J Am Med Assoc 2002; 288:2015–2022

36. Bostom AG, Silbershatz H, Rosenberg IH et al. Nonfasting plasma total homocysteine levels and all-cause and cardiovascular disease mortality in elderly Framingham men and women. Arch Intern Med 1999; 159:1077–1080

37. Ridker PM, Manson JE, Buring JE et al. Homocysteine and risk of cardiovascular disease among postmenopausal women. J Am Med Assoc 1999; 281:1817–1821

38. Knekt P, Alfthan G, Aromaa A et al. Homocysteine and major coronary events: a prospective population study amongst women. J Intern Med 2001; 249:461–465

39. Knekt P, Reunanen A, Alfthan G et al. Hyperhomocystinemia: a risk factor or a consequence of coronary heart disease? Arch Intern Med 2001; 161:1589–1594

40. Anderson JL, Muhlestein JB, Horne BD et al. Plasma homocysteine predicts mortality independently of traditional risk factors and C-reactive protein in patients with angiographically defined coronary artery disease. Circulation 2000; 102:1227–1232

41. Omland T, Samuelsson A, Hartford M et al. Serum homocysteine concentration as an indicator of survival in patients with acute coronary syndromes. Arch Intern Med 2000; 160:1834–1840

42. Acevedo M, Pearce GL, Kottke-Marchant K et al. Elevated fibrinogen and homocysteine levels enhance the risk of mortality in patients from a high-risk preventive cardiology clinic. Arterioscler Thromb Vasc Biol 2002; 22:1042–1105

43. Whincup PH, Refsum H, Perry IJ et al. Serum total homocysteine and coronary heart disease: prospective study in middle aged men. Heart 1999; 82:448–454

44. Stubbs PJ, Al-Obaidi MK, Conroy RM et al. Effect of plasma homocysteine concentration on early and late events in patients with acute coronary syndromes. Circulation 2000; 102:605–610

45. Nygard O, Nordrehaug JE, Refsum H et al. Plasma homocysteine levels and mortality in patients with coronary artery disease. N Engl J Med 1997; 337:230–236

46. Ridker PM, Stampfer MJ, Rifai N. Novel risk factors for systemic atherosclerosis: a comparison of C-reactive protein, fibrinogen, homocysteine, lipoprotein(a), and standard cholesterol screening as predictors of peripheral arterial disease. J Am Med Assoc 2001; 285:2481–2485

47. Taylor LM Jr, Moneta GL, Sexton GJ et al. Prospective blinded study of the relationship between plasma homocysteine and progression of symptomatic peripheral arterial disease. J Vasc Surg 1999; 29:8–19, discussion 19–21

48. Schnyder G, Roffi M, Flammer Y et al. Association of plasma homocysteine with restenosis after percutaneous coronary angioplasty. Eur Heart J 2002; 23:726–733

49. Schnyder G, Flammer Y, Roffi M et al. Plasma homocysteine levels and late outcome after coronary angioplasty. J Am Coll Cardiol 2002; 40:1769–1776

50. Zairis MN, Ambrose JA, Manousakis SJ et al. The impact of plasma levels of C-reactive protein, lipoprotein (a) and homocysteine on the long-term prognosis after successful coronary stenting: The Global Evaluation of New Events and Restenosis After Stent Implantation Study. J Am Coll Cardiol 2002; 40:1375–1382

51. Frosst P, Blom HJ, Milos R et al. A candidate genetic risk factor for vascular disease: a common mutation in methylenetetrahydrofolate reductase. Nature Genet 1995; 10:111–113

52. Kluijtmans LA, Kastelein JJ, Lindemans J et al. Thermolabile methylenetetrahydrofolate reductase in coronary artery disease. Circulation 1997; 96:2573–2577

53. Ma J, Stampfer MJ, Hennekens CH et al. Methylenetetrahydrofolate reductase polymorphism, plasma folate, homocysteine, and risk of myocardial infarction in US physicians. Circulation 1996; 94:2410–2416

54. Brattstrom L, Wilcken DE, Ohrvik J et al. Common methylenetetrahydrofolate reductase gene mutation leads to hyperhomocysteinemia but not to vascular disease: the result of a meta-analysis. Circulation 1998; 98:2520–2526.

55. Klerk M, Verhoef P, Clarke R et al. MTHFR 677C→T polymorphism and risk of coronary heart disease: a meta-analysis. J Am Med Assoc 2002; 288:2023–2031.

56. Hofmann MA, Lalla E, Lu Y et al. Hyperhomocysteinemia enhances vascular inflammation and accelerates atherosclerosis in a murine model. J Clin Invest 2001; 107:675–683.

57. Zhou J, Moller J, Ritskes-Hoitinga M et al. Effects of vitamin supplementation and hyperhomocysteinemia on atherosclerosis in apoE-deficient mice. Atherosclerosis 2003; 168:255–262.

58. Wang H, Jiang X, Yang F et al. Hyperhomocysteinemia accelerates atherosclerosis in cystathionine beta-synthase and apolipoprotein E double knock-out mice with and without dietary perturbation. Blood 2003; 101:3901–3907.

59. Langheinrich AC, Braun-Dullaeus RC, Walker G, et al. Effects of 3-deazaadenosine on homocysteine and atherosclerosis in apolipoprotein E-deficient mice. Atherosclerosis 2003; 171:181–192.

60. Shankar R, de la Motte CA, DiCorleto PE. 3-Deazaadenosine inhibits thrombin-stimulated platelet-derived growth factor production and endothelial-leukocyte adhesion molecule-1-mediated monocytic cell adhesion in human aortic endothelial cells. J Biol Chem 1992; 267:9376–9382.

61. Eberhardt RT, Forgione MA, Cap A et al. Endothelial dysfunction in a murine model of mild hyperhomocyst(e)inemia. J Clin Invest 2000; 106:483–491.

62. Upchurch GR Jr, Welch GN, Fabian AJ et al. Homocyst(e)ine decreases bioavailable nitric oxide by a mechanism involving glutathione peroxidase. J Biol Chem 1997; 272:17012–17017.

63. Weiss N, Zhang YY, Heydrick S et al. Overexpression of cellular glutathione peroxidase rescues homocyst(e)ine-induced endothelial dysfunction. Proc Natl Acad Sci USA 2001; 98:12503–12508.

64. Weiss N, Heydrick S, Zhang YY et al. Cellular redox state and endothelial dysfunction in mildly hyperhomocysteinemic cystathionine beta-synthase-deficient mice. Arterioscler Thromb Vasc Biol 2002; 22:34–41.

65. Huang RF, Hsu YC, Lin HL et al. Folate depletion and elevated plasma homocysteine promote oxidative stress in rat livers. J Nutr 2001; 131:33–38.

66. Lentz SR, Malinow MR, Piegors DJ et al. Consequences of hyperhomocyst(e)inemia on vascular function in atherosclerotic monkeys. Arterioscler Thromb Vasc Biol 1997; 17:2930–2934.

67. Usui M, Matsuoka H, Miyazaki H et al. Endothelial dysfunction by acute hyperhomocyst(e)inaemia: restoration by folic acid. Clin Sci (London) 1999; 96:235–239.

68. Schlaich MP, John S, Jacobi J et al. Mildly elevated homocysteine concentrations impair endothelium dependent vasodilation in hypercholesterolemic patients. Atherosclerosis 2000; 153:383–389.

69. Virdis A, Ghiadoni L, Cardinal H et al. Mechanisms responsible for endothelial dysfunction induced by fasting hyperhomocystinemia in normotensive subjects and patients with essential hypertension. J Am Coll Cardiol 2001; 38:1106–1115.

70. Stuhlinger MC, Oka RK, Graf EE et al. Endothelial dysfunction induced by hyperhomocyst(e)inemia: role of asymmetric dimethylarginine. Circulation 2003; 108:933–938.

71. Leoncini G, Pascale R, Signorello MG. Effects of homocysteine on L-arginine transport and nitric oxide formation in human platelets. Eur J Clin Invest 2003; 33:713–719.

72. Becker A, Van Hinsbergh VW, Kostense PJ et al. Serum homocysteine is weakly associated with von Willebrand factor and soluble vascular cell adhesion molecule 1, but not with C-reactive protein in type 2 diabetic and non-diabetic subjects – The Hoorn Study. Eur J Clin Invest 2000; 30:763–770.

73. Brude IR, Finstad HS, Seljeflot I et al. Plasma homocysteine concentration related to diet, endothelial function and mononuclear cell gene expression among male hyperlipidaemic smokers. Eur J Clin Invest 1999; 29:100–108.

74. Silverman MD, Tumuluri RJ, Davis M et al. Homocysteine upregulates vascular cell adhesion molecule-1 expression in cultured human aortic endothelial cells and enhances monocyte adhesion. Arterioscler Thromb Vasc Biol 2002; 22:587–592.

75. Koga T, Claycombe K, Meydani M. Homocysteine increases monocyte and T-cell adhesion to human aortic endothelial cells. Atherosclerosis 2002; 161:365–374.

76. Wang G, Woo CW, Sung FL et al. Increased monocyte adhesion to aortic endothelium in rats with hyperhomocysteinemia: role of chemokine and adhesion molecules. Arterioscler Thromb Vasc Biol 2002; 22:1777–1783.

77. Poddar R, Sivasubramanian N, DiBello PM et al. Homocysteine induces expression and secretion of monocyte chemoattractant protein-1 and interleukin-8 in human aortic endothelial cells: implications for vascular disease. Circulation 2001; 103:2717–2723.

78. Zeng X, Dai J, Remick DG et al. Homocysteine mediated expression and secretion of monocyte chemoattractant protein-1 and interleukin-8 in human monocytes. Circ Res 2003; 93:311–320.

79. Desai A, Lankford HA, Warren JS. Homocysteine augments cytokine-induced chemokine expression in human vascular smooth muscle cells: implications for atherogenesis. Inflammation 2001; 25:179–186.

80. Ni W, Egashira K, Kitamoto S et al. New anti-monocyte chemoattractant protein-1 gene therapy attenuates atherosclerosis in apolipoprotein E-knockout mice. Circulation 2001; 103:2096–2101.

81. Tsai JC, Wang H, Perrella MA et al. Induction of cyclin A gene expression by homocysteine in vascular smooth muscle cells. J Clin Invest 1996; 97:146–153.

82. Chen C, Halkos ME, Surowiec SM et al. Effects of homocysteine on smooth muscle cell proliferation in both cell culture and artery perfusion culture models. J Surg Res 2000; 88:26–33.

83. Wang H, Jiang X, Yang F et al. Cyclin A transcriptional suppression is the major mechanism mediating homocysteine-induced endothelial cell growth inhibition. Blood 2002; 99:939–945.

84. Tsai JC, Perrella MA, Yoshizumi M et al. Promotion of vascular smooth muscle cell growth by homocysteine: a link to atherosclerosis. Proc Natl Acad Sci USA 1994; 91:6369–6373.

85. Rando RR. Chemical biology of protein isoprenylation/methylation. Biochim Biophys Acta 1996; 1300:5–16.

86. Wang H, Yoshizumi M, Lai K et al. Inhibition of growth and p21ras methylation in vascular endothelial cells by homocysteine but not cysteine. J Biol Chem 1997; 272:25380–25385.

87. Kramer K, Harrington EO, Lu Q et al. Isoprenylcysteine carboxyl methyltransferase activity modulates endothelial cell apoptosis. Mol Biol Cell 2003; 14:848–857.

88. Choumenkovitch SF, Selhub J, Bagley PJ et al. In the cystathionine beta-synthase knockout mouse, elevations in total plasma homocysteine increase tissue S-adenosylhomocysteine, but responses of S-adenosylmethionine and DNA methylation are tissue specific. J Nutr 2002; 132:2157–2160.

89. Chen Z, Karaplis AC, Ackerman SL et al. Mice deficient in methylenetetrahydrofolate reductase exhibit hyperhomocysteinemia and decreased methylation capacity, with neuropathology and aortic lipid deposition. Hum Mol Genet 2001; 10:433–443.

90. Yi P, Melnyk S, Pogribna M et al. Increase in plasma homocysteine associated with parallel increases in plasma S-adenosylhomocysteine and lymphocyte DNA hypomethylation. J Biol Chem 2000; 275:29318–29323.

91. Jacob RA, Gretz DM, Taylor PC et al. Moderate folate depletion increases plasma homocysteine and decreases lymphocyte DNA methylation in postmenopausal women. J Nutr 1998; 128:1204–1212.

92. Friso S, Choi SW, Girelli D et al. A common mutation in the 5,10-methylenetetrahydrofolate reductase gene affects genomic DNA methylation through an interaction with folate status. Proc Natl Acad Sci USA 2002; 99:5606–5611.

93. Ingrosso D, Cimmino A, Perna AF, et al. Folate treatment and unbalanced methylation and changes of allelic expression induced by hyperhomocysteinaemia in patients with uraemia. Lancet 2003; 361:1693–1699.

94. Dong C, Yoon W, Goldschmidt-Clermont PJ. DNA methylation and atherosclerosis. J Nutr 2002; 132(Suppl 8):2406S–2409S.

95. Lawrence de Koning AB, Werstuck GH, Zhou J et al. Hyperhomocysteinemia and its role in the development of atherosclerosis. Clin Biochem 2003; 36:431–441.

96. Rutkowski DT, Kaufman RJ. A trip to the ER: coping with stress. Trends Cell Biol 2004; 14:20–28.

97. Zhang C, Kawauchi J, Adachi MT et al. Activation of JNK and transcriptional repressor ATF3/LRF1 through the IRE1/TRAF2 pathway is implicated in human vascular endothelial cell death by homocysteine. Biochem Biophys Res Commun 2001; 289:718–724.

98. Outinen PA, Sood SK, Liaw PC et al. Characterization of the stress-inducing effects of homocysteine. Biochem J 1998; 332:213–221.

99. Kokame K, Kato H, Miyata T. Homocysteine-respondent genes in vascular endothelial cells identified by differential display analysis. GRP78/BiP and novel genes. J Biol Chem 1996; 271:29659–29665.

100. Reddy RK, Mao C, Baumeister P et al. Endoplasmic reticulum chaperone protein GRP78 protects cells from apoptosis induced by topoisomerase inhibitors: role of ATP binding site in suppression of caspase-7 activation. J Biol Chem 2003; 278:20915–20924.

101. Werstuck GH, Lentz SR, Dayal S et al. Homocysteine-induced endoplasmic reticulum stress causes dysregulation of the cholesterol and triglyceride biosynthetic pathways. J Clin Invest 2001; 107:1263–1273.

102. Robert K, Chasse JF, Santiard-Baron D et al. Altered gene expression in liver from a murine model of hyperhomocysteinemia. J Biol Chem 2003; 278:31504–31511.

103. Undas A, Williams EB, Butenas S et al. Homocysteine inhibits inactivation of factor Va by activated protein C. J Biol Chem 2001; 276:4389–4397.

104. Majors AK, Sengupta S, Willard B et al. Homocysteine binds to human plasma fibronectin and inhibits its interaction with fibrin. Arterioscler Thromb Vasc Biol 2002; 22:1354–13549.

105. Lim A, Sengupta S, McComb ME et al. In vitro and in vivo interactions of homocysteine with human plasma transthyretin. J Biol Chem 2003; 278:49707–49713.

106. Sass JO, Nakanishi T, Sato T et al. S-homocysteinylation of transthyretin is detected in plasma and serum of humans with different types of hyperhomocysteinemia. Biochem Biophys Res Commun 2003; 310:242–246.

107. Yap S, Boers GH, Wilcken B et al. Vascular outcome in patients with homocystinuria due to cystathionine beta-synthase deficiency treated chronically: a multicenter observational study. Arterioscler Thromb Vasc Biol 2001; 21:2080–2085.

108. Verhaar MC, Stroes E, Rabelink TJ. Folates and cardiovascular disease. Arterioscler Thromb Vasc Biol 2002; 22:6–13.

109. Clarke R, Armitage J. Vitamin supplements and cardiovascular risk: review of the randomized trials of homocysteine-lowering vitamin supplements. Semin Thromb Hemost 2000; 26:341–348.

110. Venn BJ, Mann JI, Williams SM et al. Assessment of three levels of folic acid on serum folate and plasma homocysteine: a randomised placebo-controlled double-blind dietary intervention trial. Eur J Clin Nutr 2002; 56:748–754.

111. van Guldener C, Robinson K. Homocysteine and renal disease. Semin Thromb Hemost 2000; 26:313–24.

112. Verhaar MC, Wever RM, Kastelein JJ et al. 5-methyltetrahydrofolate, the active form of folic acid, restores endothelial function in familial hypercholesterolemia. Circulation 1998; 97:237–241.

113. Bellamy MF, McDowell IF, Ramsey MW et al. Oral folate enhances endothelial function in hyperhomocysteinaemic subjects. Eur J Clin Invest 1999; 29:659–662.

114. Title LM, Cummings PM, Giddens K et al. Effect of folic acid and antioxidant vitamins on endothelial dysfunction in patients with coronary artery disease. J Am Coll Cardiol 2000; 36:758–765.

115. Doshi SN, McDowell IF, Moat SJ et al. Folic acid improves endothelial function in coronary artery disease via mechanisms largely independent of homocysteine lowering. Circulation 2002; 105:22–26.

116. Ashfield-Watt PA, Moat SJ, Doshi SN et al. Folate, homocysteine, endothelial function and cardiovascular disease. What is the link? Biomed Pharmacother 2001; 55:425–433.

117. Schnyder G, Roffi M, Pin R, et al. Decreased rate of coronary restenosis after lowering of plasma homocysteine levels. N Engl J Med 2001; 345:1593–1600.

118. Schnyder G, Roffi M, Flammer Y et al. Effect of homocysteine-lowering therapy with folic acid, vitamin B(12), and vitamin B(6) on clinical outcome after percutaneous coronary intervention: the Swiss Heart study: a randomized controlled trial. J Am Med Assoc 2002; 288:973–979.

119. Taes YE, Delanghe JR, De Vriese AS et al. Creatine supplementation decreases homocysteine in an animal model of uremia. Kidney Int 2003; 64:1331–1337.

13

Infection and atherogenesis

Caroline Attardo Genco, Frank C. Gibson III

Infection and inflammation in atherosclerosis – introduction

As many as 50% of patients with atherosclerosis lack currently identified risk factors, an observation suggesting that additional factors predisposing to atherosclerosis are as yet undetected.[1] Atherosclerosis, formerly considered a lipid storage disease, actually involves an ongoing inflammatory response. Inflammation in the arterial vessel wall is considered to play an important role in the pathogenesis of atherosclerosis.[2,3] Recent advances have established a fundamental role for inflammation in mediating all stages of this disease, from initiation through progression and, ultimately, the thrombotic complications of atherosclerosis.[3]

In humans, ongoing inflammatory reactions within coronary atherosclerotic plaques are increasingly thought to be crucial determinants of the clinical course of coronary artery diseases. Likewise, in a variety of animal models of atherosclerosis, signs of inflammation occur hand-in-hand with incipient lipid accumulation in the artery wall. The stimuli that initiate and sustain the inflammatory process, however, have not been fully identified. Modified lipoproteins and local or distant infections have been proposed to contribute to the inflammatory process in atherosclerosis.[3–5] Accumulating evidence has implicated specific infectious agents, including cytomegalovirus (CMV), *Chlamydia pneumoniae*, *Helicobacter pylori*, herpes simplex virus types 1 and 2 (HSV), and *Porphyromonas gingivalis* in the progression of atherosclerosis. These microorganisms are found in atherosclerotic lesions and can aggravate atherosclerosis in experimental models,[4,6–11] yet the mechanisms by which microbe recognition occurs in the artery wall are not clear. To date, the precise

molecular mechanisms by which infections contribute to the progression of atherosclerosis, and the links between lipids, microbial antigens, and innate immune and inflammatory responses are not well understood. The concept that specific infections represent a group of novel risk factors for the acceleration and/or initiation of cardiovascular disease (CVD) is controversial, as lifestyle issues such as poor hygiene, and lack of adequate health care can place patients at greater risk for other diseases, including CVD, through non-specific or unknown processes. In this chapter we review the current literature from human epidemiological and treatment studies, and from animal model studies, and discuss putative mechanisms by which infection accelerates and/or contributes to atherogenesis.

The role of infection and inflammation in atherosclerosis

Injury to the vessel wall and the associated inflammatory response are now generally recognized as the essential components of atherogenesis. The triggers that initiate and sustain the inflammatory process, however, have not been definitively identified. Among the candidate triggers are oxidized low-density lipoprotein (ox-LDL) and heat-shock proteins (HSP). These components of the atheroma are believed by some investigators to elicit an inflammatory response.[4] Patients with cardiovascular disease can develop antibodies to these proteins, and although controversial, some studies suggest that these antibodies may play a role in causing autoimmune-induced damage to the vessel wall.[4] Another candidate trigger of both inflammatory and autoimmune responses that leads to the

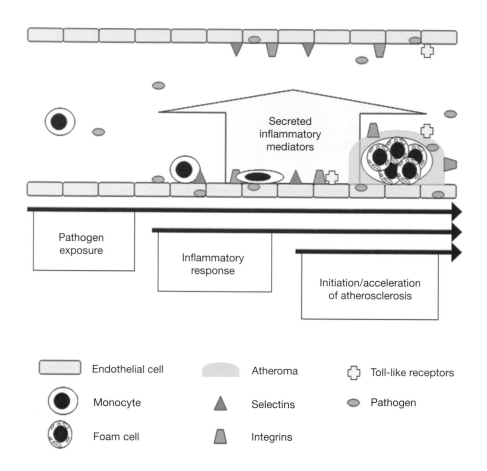

Figure 13.1 Infection-induced inflammation and initiation and acceleration of atherosclerosis. In this model invasion of the vascular endothelium by pathogenic bacteria or viruses results in the induction of a local inflammatory response which contributes to the initiation and/or acceleration of atherosclerosis

initiation and/or acceleration of atherosclerosis is infection (Figure 13.1).

Evidence in humans suggesting that infection predisposes to atherosclerosis is derived from studies demonstrating that infectious agents reside in the wall of atherosclerotic vessels, and seroepidemiological studies demonstrating an association between the pathogen-specific IgG antibodies and atherosclerosis.[4,5,8,10] Recently, it has been proposed that multiple infectious agents contribute to atherosclerosis, and that the risk of CVD posed by infection is related to the number of pathogens to which an individual has been exposed (the pathogen burden hypothesis).[5]

Specific infectious agents

Chlamydia pneumoniae

C. pneumoniae has been implicated in the pathogenesis of coronary artery disease by serological and pathological studies. The results of some of these seroepidemiologic studies, however, vary considerably.[12] A recent report describes the meta-analysis of seroepidemiologic studies of the relationship between *C. pneumoniae* and atherosclerosis.[13] The MEDLINE database was searched from January 1997 to December 2000 for studies describing the seroprevalence of IgG antibodies to *C. pneumoniae* in relation to clinically manifested atherosclerosis. These authors determined that the overall odds ratio of cross-sectional case–control studies was higher than that of prospective studies, and concluded that the results may have been influenced by the design of the individual studies.

A recent study[14] concluded that the presence of *C. pneumoniae* in coronary atherosclerotic plaques of patients with unstable angina undergoing coronary bypass grafting did not have prognostic significance. These authors also concluded that serology did not allow for the differentiation of those patients with plaque infection by *C. pneumoniae*, and did not provide any prognostic information in these patients. A separate study examined the joint effect of chronic *C. pneumoniae* infection, persistently elevated human HSP60 antibodies, and C-reactive protein (CRP) on coronary risk. The participants of this prospective nested control study were obtained from the Helsinki Heart Study, during which 241 non-fatal myocardial infarctions or coronary deaths occurred among 4081 dyslipidemic middle-aged men. It was concluded from this study that persistently – but not transiently – elevated immunocomplex-bound and serum IgA antibodies to *C. pneumoniae* and human HSP60 IgA antibodies, especially when present together with elevated CRP, predicted coronary events.[15] A separate study found that the presence of elevated anti-chlamydial HSP60 (cHSP60) IgG antibodies, but not anti-human or anti-*Escherichia coli* homologs, was independently associated with cardiovascular disease.[15]

Results from other studies support the theory that *C. pneumoniae* infection might contribute to early atherogenesis, which might be associated with chronic inflammation and atherosclerosis at an early stage even before clinical events occur.[16] Prager and colleagues[17] recently described studies on the detection of *C. pneumoniae* in the atherosclerotic plaques of the carotid artery, in samples of apparently healthy greater saphenous veins, and in circulating leukocytes from the same individual patients. The authors found that the presence of *C. pneumoniae*-specific DNA in leukocytes significantly coincided with the presence of the DNA in the plaques of carotid arteries. In contrast, the majority of apparently healthy saphenous veins were negative for *C. pneumoniae*.[17]

Cytomegalovirus and herpes viruses

Danesh and colleagues[18] have reported that the presence of antibodies to HSV types 1 and 2 has not been generally associated with CVD in epidemiological studies. In a more recent case–controlled study of elderly subjects, however, the presence of IgG antibodies for HSV-1 was associated with non-fatal myocardial infarction.[19] Several epidemiological studies have also reported a possible association of various forms of vascular disease with the presence and titer of cytomegalovirus (CMV) antibodies.[20–23] Other studies show the presence of the virus, viral antigens, or nucleic acid in atherosclerotic lesions.[24] Several studies have demonstrated CMV DNA particles in restenotic lesions in atherosclerotic coronary arteries.[25] In addition, high anti-CMV IgG titers in patient sera are associated with active coronary disease and with post-coronary angioplasty restenosis. In a recent study the anti-CMV antibody titer in patients with risk factors for atherosclerosis (but without documented clinical manifestations) was found to be associated with risk factors for disease. It was proposed that an immunological response against CMV could be a marker of long-standing immunological reaction causing an inflammatory response that would eventually cause advanced atherosclerosis, and it was suggested that anti-CMV antibody titers should be used as an early predictor of atherosclerosis.[26] As with the studies examining the presence of *C. pneumoniae* in plaque samples discussed above, results from these studies support an association between CMV infection and atherosclerosis at an early stage.

In a study of 75 patients with atherosclerosis the positive rate of CMV DNA in artery vascular tissue specimens was higher in atherosclerosis patients than in controls. CMV DNA was observed mainly in the nuclei of endothelial cells and the muscularis under the intima, as well as in smooth muscle of the atheroclerotic plaque area.[27] The authors of this study concluded that the artery could be the site of CMV latency. In addition, higher levels of CMV IgG and IgM were found to be associated with virus persistence, indicating that a periodically active latent infection or a continuously active infection is present in atherosclerosis patients.

Studies in animal models and cell culture studies present attractive mechanisms by which CMV may play a role in atherogenesis. It has been proposed that infection with CMV is associated with endothelial dysfunction. Endothelial dysfunction is an early marker for atherosclerosis. A recent study demonstrated that CMV-seropositive individuals have endothelial dysfunction and impaired responses to nitric oxide (NO). This association was independent of conventional risk factors, and was postulated to be associated with increased atherosclerosis burden.[28]

Helicobacter pylori

A number of epidemiological studies have reported on the association of *H. pylori* antibody titers and the risk for coronary heart disease and stroke.[29,30] A problem with some of these studies, however, is that some potential confounding factors seem to be associated with both *H. pylori* infection and coronary heart disease. A few studies have also reported that individuals who were seropositive for *H. pylori* had high plasma concentrations of markers of inflammation that could have been associated with an increased risk of vascular disease. *H. pylori* strains that possess the toxin CagA have been shown to be associated with atherosclerosis. A recent study demonstrated the presence of CagA antibodies in atherosclerotic vessel sections.[31] It was postulated that the binding of anti-CagA antibodies to antigens in injured arteries could influence the progression of atherosclerosis in CagA-positive *H. pylori*-infected patients. One recent study suggests that virulent strains of *H. pylori* may induce systemic inflammation, whereas avirulent strains do not and thus would not be associated with accelerated atherosclerosis.[32] These authors suggested that the association between *H. pylori* and atherosclerosis may be due to a higher prevalence of more virulent *H. pylori* strains in patients with atherosclerosis. The general view at this time is that the current studies do not provide convincing epidemiological evidence for or against a casual association between *H. pylori* infection and coronary heart disease.[33,34]

Porphyromonas gingivalis

There is evidence to support the relationship between human periodontal disease and an increased risk for acute myocardial infarction.[6,10,35] Periodontal disease is characterized by generalized alveolar bone resorption and, in severe cases, early loss of dentition.[36] Despite rigorous clinical intervention strategies, recent reports suggest that up to 30% of adults in the USA over the age of 40 have measurable periodontal bone loss.[37] Case–control studies have demonstrated a significant correlation between CVD and periodontal disease after adjusting for cholesterol, smoking, hypertension, social class, and body mass index.[6,10,38] Although some reports have not confirmed this association, this may be due to the fact that self-reported periodontal disease was used for the analysis of the patient population.[39] The primary bacterium associated with adult periodontal disease, *P. gingivalis*, has also been detected in atherosclerotic plaque.[35] It has been suggested that periodontal disease can lead to low-level bacteremia, an elevated white cell count, and systemic endotoxemias, which could affect endothelial integrity, the metabolism of plasma lipoproteins, blood coagulation, and platelet function. Patients with periodontal disease have higher systemic levels of CRP and interleukin-6 (IL-6).[40,41] Furthermore, it is well established that infection with *P. gingivalis* induces local inflammation. The induction of this inflammatory response can lead to gingival ulceration and local vascular changes, which have the potential to increase the incidence and severity of transient bacteremias. It has been proposed that the systemic consequences of periodontal infection increase the risk for vascular thromboembolic events, such as that seen with acute myocardial infarction and stroke.[42]

Multiple pathogens

The extent of atherosclerosis and the prognosis of patients with atherosclerosis seem to be correlated with the number of infections to which an individual has been exposed. In a prospective study the effects of eight pathogens and the aggregate pathogen burden on the progression of carotid atherosclerosis were evaluated in 504 patients.[5] Elevated IgA antibodies against *C. pneumoniae* and IgG antibodies to Epstein Barr virus (EBV) and HSV were associated with progression of atherosclerosis. Infectious burden was also significantly associated with progression of atherosclerosis. The authors concluded from this study that the number of infectious pathogens to which an individual has been exposed contributes independently to the progression of carotid atherosclerosis.[5] A more recent study also demonstrated a strong association between pathogen burden and CVD, independently of classic risk factors.[43] These authors suggested that the pathogen burden could also be a predictor of coronary complications, which are mainly the consequence of plaque rupture, as well as cardiovascular development, which could reflect the initiation and the development of the plaque itself. It is also important to point out that poor hygiene, inadequate health care, and poor nutrition and lifestyle may represent important complicating factors to the multiple burden hypothesis, as these issues may confound this hypothesis because individuals with these factors are commonly at risk for many diseases including the development of CVD.

It has been hypothesized that numerous infections may predispose patients to atherosclerosis by collectively inflicting endothelial injury. A recent study examined 375 patients undergoing coronary angiography for endothelial function and for IgG antibody titers to CMV, *C. pneumoniae, H. pylori*, and HSV. Pathogen burden was defined as the number of pathogens, as detected by antibody response to the different pathogens, and was correlated with the presence of coronary arteriosclerosis. Moreover, the disease severity was independently associated with pathogen burden. Interestingly, pathogen burden was also an independent predictor of endothelial dysfunction.[44] These authors concluded that endothelial dysfunction provides the crucial link by which pathogens may contribute to atherogenesis. Endothelial dysfunction may play a significant role in the mechanistic link between infection and the acceleration of atherosclerosis.

In a prospective population-based survey on the pathogenesis of atherosclerosis it was found that chronic infections amplified the risk for atherosclerosis.[45] In subjects with chronic infection, atherosclerosis risk was highest in those with a prominent inflammatory response, as defined by elevated soluble adhesion molecules and circulating bacterial endotoxin, and elevated levels of soluble human HSP60 and antibodies to mycobacterial HSP65. CRP levels and infectious burden have also been reported to be associated with atherosclerosis risk in young women.[46]

A recent study examined whether *C. pneumoniae* and/or *H. pylori* seropositivity was associated with ele-

vated levels of soluble endothelial cell adhesion molecules in 193 coronary heart disease patients. These studies found that the concentrations of soluble intercellular adhesion molecule-1 (sICAM-1) and E-selectin were higher in patients with positive rather than negative chlamydia lipopolysaccharide (LPS) IgA. However, *H. pylori* antibodies alone did not predict increased levels of sCAM. These authors concluded that *C. pneumoniae* contributes to increased inflammation in coronary heart disease, and that this contribution is even more pronounced when *C. pneumoniae* is present in combination with *H. pylori* IgA antibodies.

Neureiter and colleagues[47] evaluated the detection rate of *C. pneumoniae* and *H. pylori* in normal versus atherosclerotic carotids and compared these findings with serology, plaque morphology, and inflammatory cell infiltrates and apoptosis rate. The study was performed on 40 morphologically normal carotids from autopsy and 20 advanced atherosclerotic carotids from endarterectomy after stroke.[47] *C. pneumoniae* was found significantly more frequently in atherosclerotic than in normal carotids, and this correlated with elevated *C. pneumoniae* IgG antibody titers. Although *H. pylori* was not detected, elevated *H. pylori* antibody titers were significantly associated with the degree of atherosclerosis. *C. pneumoniae*-infected carotids exhibited enhanced infiltration of T cells, and the authors of this study concluded that an immune-mediated inflammatory process involving the vascular walls plays a role in *C. pneumoniae*-accelerated atherosclerosis.

A recent study provided epidemiological evidence that the proatherogenic effects of cigarette smoking are mediated in part by the chronic infections found in smokers.[48] Smoking, as well as systemic and peripheral infections, may produce endothelial irritation through noxious agents, antigenic effects, and/or stimulation of proinflammatory cytokines, and together these may adversely affect the host inflammatory response, thereby causing disease.

Treatment studies

A number of recent studies have examined the effects of antibiotic therapy in the prevention of atherosclerosis in humans.[49] A variety of small pilot studies have been reported and several multicenter trials are currently under way. The pilot studies have shown significant positive clinical effects and will need to be confirmed by large randomized trials. In addition, the choice of antibiotic and the time course of therapy will need to be addressed. In general, the majority of antibiotic studies have been secondary prevention studies that have targeted patients infected with *C. pneumoniae* and have utilized azithromycin or roxithromycin. The Weekly Intervention with Zithromax for Atherosclerosis and its Related Disorders (WIZARD) study has been the largest completed to date. In this study postmyocardial infarction patients were randomized to receive a 3-month course of azithromycin. Although these patients demonstrated a significant reduction in death and myocardial infarction by 6 months, the benefit was not sustained throughout the remaining follow-up period.

An earlier study of 272 patients with ischemic stroke evaluated the effect of roxithromycin therapy (twice daily for 30 days) on the progression of the intima-media thickness of the common carotid artery, with a follow-up of 2 years.[50] The levels of anti-*C. pneumoniae* antibodies were also examined. The results of this study demonstrated a positive impact of antibiotic therapy on early atherosclerosis progression in *C. pneumoniae*-seropositive patients with cerebrovascular disease. In a separate study, 872 patients were treated with roxithromycin or placebo daily for 6 weeks, and mortality was evaluated during a 12-month follow-up period.[51] Treatment of acute myocardial infarction patients with roxithromycin did not reduce event rates during the 12-month follow-up period. The authors of this study concluded that antibiotic therapy for successful secondary prevention of atherosclerosis could not be made based on the results of this study. However, it is important to note that the final outcome in this study was mortality. It appears that positive outcomes may have only been seen with early atherosclerosis progression, owing to the chronic nature of the infections associated with atherosclerosis. Two ongoing studies, the Azithromycin and Coronary Events (ACES) and Pravastatin or Atorvastatin Evaluation and Infections Therapy (PROVE-IT) trials, are currently under way and their results may help to confirm or refute the positive effects of antibiotic therapy on adverse cardiovascular events.

Sawayama and colleagues[52] recently compared the effect of lipid-lowering drugs on carotid intima-media thickness between patients who were seropositive and seronegative for antibodies to *C. pneumoniæ*. The authors observed that *C. pneumoniae* infection (as determined by seropositivity) reduced the effect of lipid-lowering therapy on carotid atherosclerosis. Several more recent studies have also begun to examine vaccination as a possible treatment for atherosclerosis.[53] Naghavi and colleagues[54] in a case–control study, reported that vaccination against influenza virus was negatively associated with the development of recurrent myocardial infarction. A separate study found a decrease in sudden cardiac death in patients receiving an influenza vaccine.[54,55] Results obtained from two additional epidemiological and one small clinical trial have suggested that influenza vaccination is associated with a 50% reduction in the incidence of sudden cardiac death.[56]

Limitations of human epidemiological and treatment studies

Although there have been numerous human studies published to date which have attempted to establish a link between infection and atherosclerosis, it is important to point out that there are limitations to these studies that affect the outcomes. For example, some studies have not utilized the appropriate methodology to establish definitively the diagnosis of cardiovascular disease, and often studies have not adequately adjusted for possible confounding factors. Thus, although associations were observed using univariate analysis, on multivariate analysis these associations disappeared. In many reports the total numbers of patients studied were small and thus the statistical significance of the results was marginal. In addition, many of the cross-sectional studies have been limited in scope owing to the lack of prospective follow-up data.

In seroepidemiological studies the proper choice of antigen is important in the detection of specific pathogens. In addition, IgG titers may not be the best serologic marker for assessing persistent infection. Inflammation following infection with various pathogens might contribute to the early stages of atherosclerosis, and infection may vary from acute to chronic. It is necessary to ascertain how long a chronic infection with the various pathogens has persisted in the vascular wall, and it is not known whether seropositivity may indicate a chronic active infection or simply reflect past exposure. Indeed, the high prevalence of antibodies to organisms that cause chronic infections can be explained simply by frequent reinfections. It is also important to note that different pathogens may act differently in regard to their ability to induce an inflammatory response, and hence the association with specific pathogens and atherosclerosis risk may vary. In addition, the capacity of the host to control the pathogen-induced inflammatory response may be influenced by genetic factors.

Animal studies

Although definitive proof of a causal role of infection in atherogenesis is lacking in humans (and may be due to limitations of human studies, as discussed above), numerous investigations have demonstrated that infectious agents evoke cellular and molecular changes supportive of such a role in *in vivo* model systems.[4,8] Initial studies were performed using dietary models to study the progression of atherosclerosis and have certainly demonstrated the importance of elevated lipid levels in the progression of this disease.[57–59] In addition to dietary supplementation, animals with defined mutations in genes that prevent proper lipid metabolism and result in hyperlipidemia have become indispensable to defining the mechanisms that underlie atheroma formation.[60,61] The experimental data regarding infection-accelerated atherosclerosis in animals is controversial; however, several pathogens, including *C. pneumoniae*, *C. trachomatis*, influenza virus, CMV, and *P. gingivalis*, have been reported to accelerate atheroma formation in genetically defined animals.

One-time *C. pneumoniae* infection at 5 months of age was demonstrated to accelerate the progression of overt coronary artery disease in a CVD Dahl salt-sensitive hypertensive rat model.[62] Furthermore, these authors found that infection with *C. pneumoniae* induced the acceleration of foam cell formation in hyperlipidemic recruited peritoneal macrophages. It was concluded that untreated *C. pneumoniae* infection could be a causal risk factor for CVD progression, and that this was most likely mediated by *C. pneumoniae*-induced accelerated macrophage foam cell formation.

Blessing and colleagues[63] demonstrated that *C. pneumoniae* did not accelerate lesion development in mice if a high-fat, high-cholesterol diet was started after infection in wild-type mice, indicating that *C. pneumoniae* is a co-risk factor with hyperlipidemia for CVD. In an apoE knockout mouse model of atherosclerosis *C. pneumoniae* infection was shown to enhance the inflammatory process by increasing T lymphocytes in the plaque and accelerating the formation of complex lesions.[64] Upregulation of proinflammatory endothelial cell adhesion molecules and decreased bioactivity of endothelial NO are important in the pathogenesis of atherosclerosis. Coinfection of apoE knockout mice with *C. pneumoniae* and *H. pylori* seems to be associated with impaired bioactivity of endothelial NO and increased expression of vascular cellular adhesion molecules-1 (VCAM-1) at branching sites.[65] Using an LDL-receptor apoE double knockout mouse, Ezzahiri and colleagues[66] demonstrated that *C. pneumoniae* infection induces an unstable atherosclerotic plaque phenotype and suggested that infection may predispose to plaque instability.

In a pig model of coronary artery disease preexisting coronary lesions were shown to be a prerequisite for *C. pneumoniae*-induced proliferation. Clarithromycin administration in a rabbit model was shown to modify *C. pneumoniae*-induced atherosclerotic lesions and reduced the ability to detect the organism in tissue. However, early treatment was more effective than delayed treatment.[67]

Infection with *P. gingivalis* has also recently been demonstrated to accelerate atherosclerosis in an apoE mouse model of disease.[7,11,68] Studies from our laboratory have established that oral challenge with *P. gingivalis* in apoE knockout mice results in enhanced atherosclerosis compared to unchallenged mice.[11] The mechanism involved in *P. gingivalis*-accelerated atherosclerotic plaque accumulation involved a specific immune response to invasive *P. gingivalis*, as aortic tissue from apoE knockout mice orally challenged with wild-type *P. gingivalis* presented with enhanced expression of the host innate immune system receptors Toll-like receptors (TLR)-2 and TLR-4 (see below). Importantly, prophylactic control of *P. gingivalis* oral infection by immunization prevented accelerated atherosclerotic plaque accumulation in response to *P. gingivalis* oral infection.

Inflammation and innate immunity

Blood leukocytes, mediators of host defense and inflammation, localize in the earliest lesions of atherosclerosis in both experimental animal models and humans. The normal endothelium does not in general support binding of leukocytes. However, early after initiation of an atherogenic diet some arterial endothelial cells begin to express on their surface selective adhesion molecules that bind to various classes of leukocytes. Once adherent to the endothelium, the leukocytes penetrate into the intima. Once resident in the arterial wall, the blood-derived inflammatory cells participate in and perpetuate a local inflammatory response. Inflammatory processes not only promote initiation and evolution of the atheroma, but also contribute decisively to precipitating the acute thrombotic complications of atheroma.[3]

Innate immunity is the inherent immune mechanisms of a host to prevent or control an infectious challenge, and is typically characterized by the activation and recruitment of monocytes and macrophages. Activation of monocytes and macrophages is an important initial step in the cascades of events leading to many acute and chronic inflammatory diseases. The immune system is capable of making qualitatively distinct responses against different microbial infections, and recent advances are starting to reveal how it manages this complex task. Genome-encoded innate immune systems target structurally conserved pathogen-associated microbial products (PAMP) there by allowing an immediate – and in most cases sufficient – response to eliminate invading pathogens.[69] The recently described TLR recognize a specific set of PAMP and appear to play a key role in detecting microbes and initiating inflammatory responses.

Currently 10 TLR have been identified. Ligation of these receptors initiates the activation of nuclear factor-κB (NFκB), resulting in the expression of a wide array of inflammatory genes.[70,71] The best-studied of the TLR are TLR-2 and TLR-4. As the receptor for Gram-negative bacterial LPS, TLR-4 is the best-characterized member of the TLR family. LPS is bound in serum by LPS-binding protein (LBP), which delivers LPS to CD14, a protein that exists both in soluble form and as a glycosylphatidylinositol (GPI)-linked outer membrane protein.[72] CD14 physically associates with a complex including TLR-4 and an extracellular accessory protein, MD-2. Each component of this complex is required for efficient LPS-induced signaling. HSP60 from both human and microbial sources has also been reported to activate inflammatory signaling through TLR-4.[73] Several other bacterial proteins have been suggested to activate immune cells through TLR-4, including teichuronic acid and bacterial fimbriae.[70,74,75]

An array of molecules has been reported to activate innate immune responses through TLR-2, including bacterial lipopeptides, peptidoglycan, and zymosan.[76–79] In addition, certain structural variants of LPS are detected by TLR-2, including LPS from *P. gingivalis*.[80,81] Some of the broad ligand specificity attributed to TLR-2 may be accounted for by the observation that TLR-2 must dimerize with other TLR to detect ligands and induce signaling. Expression of a chimeric CD14–TLR-4 fusion protein that induces dimerization of the cytoplasmic domain of TLR-4 activates intracellular signaling, suggesting that ligand-induced dimerization might be a mechanism of TLR-4 activation.[82] Similar dimerization of TLR-2 signaling domains fails to induce activation of proinflammatory responses, such as NFκB translocation to the nucleus and tumor necrosis factor-α (TNF-α), IL-12, or IL-1β secretion.[82] Instead, heterodimerization of TLR-2 with either TLR-6 or TLR-1 induces signaling. Whereas several microbial products appear capable of stimulating inflammatory responses through TLR-2 and TLR-4, to date only single microbial targets have been identified for TLR-3, TLR-5, and TLR-9. TLR-5 recognizes bacterial flagellin. Recently, TLR-9 was identified as the receptor for CpG DNA. TLR-3 recognizes double-stranded RNA.

Activation of proinflammatory responses through Toll-like receptors

Cellular activation through TLR sets in motion a chain of events that ultimately leads to the activation of proinflammatory cytokines. The intracellular signaling pathways activated by TLR share much in common with the IL-1R signaling, owing to their conserved TIR (Toll/IL-1R homology) domains.[71] Activation of signaling through TIR domains results in recruitment of the cytoplasmic adapter molecule MyD88 (which itself has a TIR domain), activation of serine/threonine kinases of the IRAK family, and ultimately degradation of IκB and translocation of NFκB to the nucleus.[83] Recently, an additional molecule, Tollip, has been proposed to interact with TIR signaling domains and to participate in signal propagation.[69] Another TLR signaling pathway is a MyD88-independent TLR-4 pathway. Recently two groups have identified a molecule called TIRAP or MAL that interacts specifically with TLR-4 and is likely to be responsible for this MyD88-independent signaling.[84,85]

The functions that have been described for several of the mammalian TLR published to date indicate that TLR play a central role in inflammation and innate immune defense, and are important regulators of adaptive immunity. It has been proposed that costimulation of more than one receptor would provide a more reliable signal and that small amounts of TLR ligands would not trigger a response, but that if several putative substances of microbial origin were encountered simultaneously the innate immune system would spring into action.[86] Maximal activation by any one TLR pathway does not preclude further activation by another, suggesting that common downstream regulatory components are not limiting.

Regulation of Toll receptor expression

There is increasing evidence for differential responses in cells activated with different TLR stimuli, indicating that the repertoire of TLR that detect a pathogen may coordinate a response tailored for defense against a class of organism.[87–89] *In vivo* the primary source of differential signaling through TLR might arise not from the expression of different intracellular signaling cascades, but from the expression of different TLR in different cell types. Consistent with their roles in immune surveillance, TLR mRNA are expressed at higher levels in tissues exposed to the external environment, such as lung and the gastrointestinal tract, as well as in immunologically important settings such as peripheral blood leukocytes and spleen.[90] TLR-3 and TLR-5, which share significant sequence homology,

are both expressed broadly at levels comparable with those in spleen (perhaps suggesting a general role in different tissues), and both are regulated by bacteria and their products. TLR-5, -7, -8, and -10 are stimulated by both Gram-positive and Gram-negative bacteria.[90] Bacterial LPS has also been shown to upregulate TLR-2, TLR-3, and TLR-4 mRNA in human and murine monocytes and macrophages.[91] Cytokines, which are induced by microbial products, can also alter TLR expression,[90] suggesting that differential production of cytokines in particular pathological contexts may affect the spectrum of TLR responses of which cells are capable in that setting.

Several recent reports have also appeared on the expression of TLR in response to bacterial challenge or to diseased states. For example, human intestinal epithelial cells constitutively express TLR-3; however, expression of TLR-3 is decreased in Crohn's disease but not in ulcerative colitis.[92] A separate study has shown that human bladder epithelial cells express high levels of TLR-4, which enables them to respond rapidly to bacterial infections *in vitro* and *in vivo*. In contrast, TLR-4 is not expressed on human proximal tubule cells isolated from the renal cortex, which may explain the cortical localization of bacteria in pyelonephritis.[93] TLR-2 is expressed at very low levels in unstimulated human epithelial cells and is greatly upregulated by infection with *Haemophilus influenzae*.[94] Likewise, infection of murine macrophages with *Mycobacterium avium* has been demonstrated to induce TLR-2 mRNA.[95]

Toll-like receptors and atherosclerosis

Recent reports indicate that expression of the TLR proinflammatory signaling receptors is enhanced in atherosclerotic lesions. Dybdahl and colleagues[96] recently reported on the expression of monocyte TLR-2 and TLR-4 following coronary artery bypass grafting in humans. Likewise, Frantz and colleagues[97] recently found that cardiac myocytes constitutively express TLR-4, and that this expression is upregulated in the hearts of humans with CVD. Edfeldt and colleagues[98] also reported that TLR-1, TLR-2, and TLR-4 were markedly augmented in human atherosclerotic lesions, and that this occurred preferentially by endothelial cells and macrophages. Significant proportions of these cells were activated, as shown by the nuclear translocation of NFκB. Another report has demonstrated TLR-2 expression within atherosclerotic plaques in humans.[99]

Xu and colleagues[100] have recently demonstrated that TLR-4 is expressed in lipid-rich, macrophage-infiltrated atherosclerotic lesions of mice and humans, and that TLR-4 mRNA in cultured macrophages is upregulated by oxidized ox-LDL but not native LDL. These findings raise the possibility that enhanced TLR-4 expression may play a role in inflammation in atherosclerosis. Furthermore, the findings of increased expression of TLR-4 induced by ox-LDL suggest a potential mechanism for the synergistic effects of hypercholesterolemia and infection in the acceleration of atherosclerosis observed in experimental models and human epidemiological observations. These findings provide additional new insights into the links between lipids, infection/inflammation, and atherosclerosis.

A recent study suggests that polymorphisms in the human TLR-4 gene which attenuates receptor signaling and diminishes the inflammatory response to Gram-negative pathogens is associated with low levels of certain circulating mediators of inflammation and a decreased risk for atherosclerosis in humans.[101] Likewise, a separate study found that the TLR-4 polymorphism was associated with the risk of cardiovascular events in men with documented coronary artery disease.[102] Another study reported that this TLR-4 polymorphism does not influence the predisposition to and progression of coronary artery disease.[103] As discussed by the authors of this study, however, the lack of association does not exclude the involvement of the TLR-4 gene in atherosclerotic plaque formation or plaque stability, as opposed to vessel stenosis. Clearly, understanding how intermediate phenotypes relate to complex disease phenotypes is critical when interpreting genotype/phenotype correlations in humans. Furthermore, these results from epidemiological studies illustrate how important it is to perform well-controlled animal studies to address the specific involvement of defined innate signaling molecules in the progression of atherosclerosis. In this regard, it was recently demonstrated that mice lacking expression of MyD88, which transduces cell signaling events downstream of TLR, exhibit reduced atherosclerotic lesion

development.[104] However, what is still unidentified is the impact of infection on TLR-mediated acceleration of atherosclerosis. Taken together, these recent studies collectively illustrate that an efficient innate immune defense and a repertoire of TLR are associated with inflammatory activation in human atherosclerotic lesions, and they encourage further exploration of innate immunity in the pathogenesis of atherosclerosis.

Putative mechanisms by which infection leads to atherosclerosis

The precise molecular mechanisms by which infection contributes to the progression of atherosclerosis and the links between lipids and innate immune and inflammatory responses, are not well understood. Because atherosclerosis is a chronic inflammatory response initiated at the vascular wall, interactions between infectious agents and endothelial cells, and the subsequent host cell response to infection, are clearly important in the pathogenesis of atherosclerosis. Indeed, the strength of the epidemiological associations of infectious agents with atherosclerosis can be increased by the demonstration that these organisms can initiate and sustain growth in human vascular cells.

The production of reactive oxygen species is fundamental to cell-mediated killing and eradication of microbial infection.[105] Additionally, antibody-catalyzed water-oxidative pathways can kill bacteria,[106] via the generation of peroxide[107] and, potentially, ozone.[106] Human atherosclerotic plaques possess inflammatory cells and the components necessary for antibody-catalyzed reactive oxygen species.[108] In light of the paradigm shift in our understanding of atherosclerosis and the contribution of leukocytes and antibodies to the inflammatory reaction underlying the pathogenesis of atherosclerosis, the importance of oxidative pathways to atheroma development must be defined. Reactive oxygen species generated as part of the inflammatory response that occurs during atherosclerosis may contribute to pathogenesis through the oxidation of cholesterol, as oxidized cholesterol derivatives are reported to stimulate atherogenesis[109] and can stimulate foam cell formation.[108] As *C. pneumoniae* and *P. gingivalis* have been detected in human atheroma, and high levels of circulating antibody to organisms such as *C. pneumonia* have been detected in patients with CVD, it is reasonable to hypothesize that these circulating antibodies could react with a microbe or antigens from this organism in the developing atheroma, and that this reaction could stimulate atheroma development. Future research in this area will unveil the role of these pathways in infection-accelerated atherosclerosis.

An overall assessment of the literature supports the view that three general mechanisms appear to govern infection-initiated/-accelerated atherosclerosis, these include: a direct consequence of systemic dissemination of a pathogen from a focus of local infection, probably via a hemotogenous route, with subsequent infection of arterial vasculature; molecular mimicry; and immunological sounding, whereby a local infection elicits a systemic response and the progression of atheroma is due to the activated host inflammatory response (Figure 13.2). These mechanisms are outlined below.

Pathogen-initiated/-accelerated stimulation of atherosclerosis: direct causality of vascular endothelial cell infection

A plethora of experimental data support the view that numerous pathogens possess the ability to adhere to, invade, and infect vascular endothelial cells; however, it appears that only a few of these organisms are associated with atherosclerosis.[1,4] Data from humans indicate that pathogens such as *C. pneumoniae*, *P. gingivalis* and others can be detected in atherosclerotic plaque by polymerase chain reaction (PCR). The finding of pathogens in atherosclerotic plaque, however, does not define the cause of the developing atheroma, as it is not possible to determine whether the DNA is associated with viable organisms, or whether the pathogen was present before the development of the atheroma or whether it simply localized within it.

Following infection of endothelial cells, myriad changes occur to the endothelium that could accelerate atherosclerosis (Figure 13.3). Normal endothelium is antithrombotic owing to expressed heparin sulfate, NO, plasminogen activator, prostacyclin, and thrombomodulin; however, upon infection the endothelium

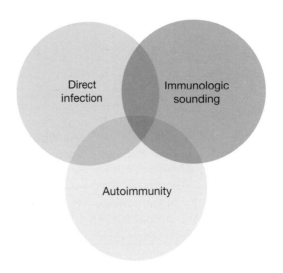

Figure 13.2 Mechanisms that govern infection-initiated/-accelerated atherosclerosis. Three putative mechanisms by which infection may contribute to accelerated atherosclerosis include direct consequences of systemic dissemination of a pathogen from a local infection, autoimmune reaction to defined human proteins, and immunological sounding, whereby a local infection elicits a systemic response. These pathways can occur concurrently and may not necessarily be mutually exclusive

shifts from being anti- to being prothrobotic.[110,111] One way that infection shifts this balance is via the expression of tissue factor (TF),[112] the primary initiator of inflammation-induced thrombin production.[113] In addition to infection,[110,114] a variety of inflammatory mediators have been shown to stimulate TF expression on endothelium, including cytokines and CRP.[112] There is an additional shift to a prothrombotic environment owing to relaxation of the endothelium in response to infection.[115] One of the earliest responses thought to occur during coronary artery disease is loss of vascular tone. It has been shown that loss of endothelium-mediated coronary vasodilator response occurs in patients infected with CMV. The precise mechanism by which infection affects vascular tonicity is not known, but appears to involve mechanisms that are both dependent and independent of NO.[4]

Numerous studies support that the organisms associated with atherosclerosis are capable of adhering to and infecting vascular endothelial cells. The identification and study of the TLR recently support the prospect that defined receptors are utilized for

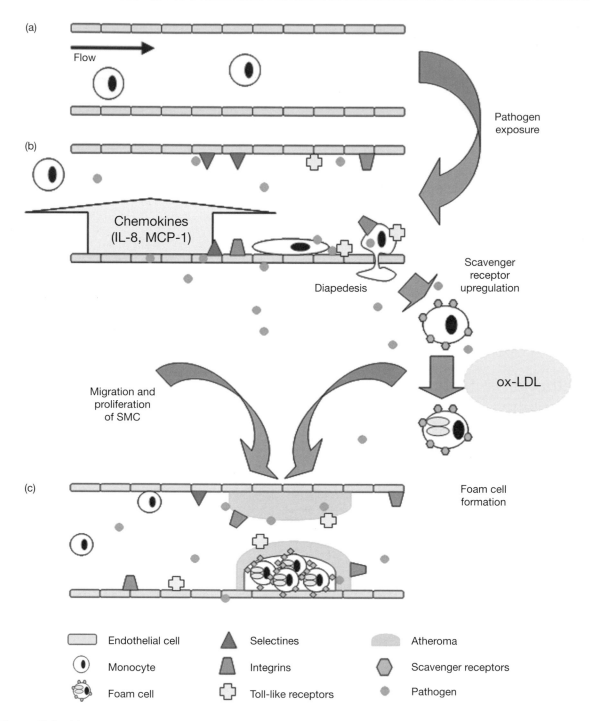

Figure 13.3 Atheroma development as a consequence of chronic infection. Once the vascular endothelium becomes activated in response to infection, endothelial cells produce a number of soluble mediators including interleukin-8 (IL-8), monocyte chemoattractant protein-1 (MCP-1), and IL-6 which function in recruiting mononuclear cells to the sites of infection. Ultimately these mononuclear cells develop into foam cells as a result of the uptake of oxidized low-density lipoprotein (ox-LDL). The resulting pathogen-infected chronic lesion thus may be similar in composition to atherosclerotic lesions induced by ox-LDL, but this has not been experimentally demonstrated. sCAM, soluble cellular adhesion molecules

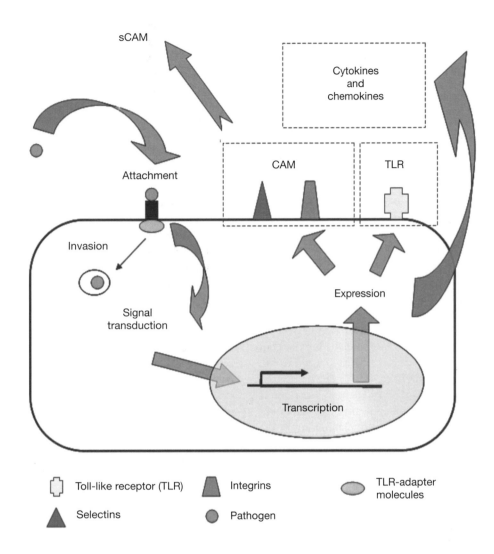

Figure 13.4 Response of the endothelium to local infection. Following infection of endothelial cells, numerous changes occur in the endothelium. This may be a direct result of both adherence to and invasion of the endothelium. In response, the endothelial cell expresses a group of innate immune receptors which signal for the expression of cytokines and chemokines, cell adhesion molecules, acute-phase mediators, and lipid-scavenging receptors

microbial parisitization of endothelial cells. Following binding and invasion by pathogenic microbes, endothelial cells respond by producing cell adhesion molecules (CAM) such as E-selectin, ICAM-1 and VCAM-1, as well as a vast array of cytokines including TNF-α, interferon-γ (IFN-γ), and chemokines including IL-8 and monocyte chemoattractant protein-1 (MCP-1). The expressed CAM play a role in arresting inflammatory cells such as monocytes that are honed

to the site of bacterially infected endothelium. Emerging data support that sICAM and sVCAM are released from endothelium, and that these molecules are associated with CVD.

As the host vascular endothelium becomes activated in response to infection, endothelial cells produce a variety of soluble mediators, including IL-8, MCP-1, and IL-6, which collectively support atherogenesis (Figure 13.4). Mononuclear cells are recruited to these sites of infection and respond by producing inflammatory mediators, savaging molecules, including ox-LDL and PAMPs, that facilitate the establishment of a closed loop whereby the host immune response, following initiation by a pathogen, is self-feeding, thus perpetuating atheroma development. Currently, it is not known which microbial structures play a direct role in the stimulation of atherosclerosis. Certainly it is established that HSP antigenic mimicry may play an important role in atheroma formation (discussed below).

P. gingivalis invasion of aortic, heart, and vein endothelial cells (HUVEC) induces the expression of the chemokines IL-8 and MCP-1, and the expression of cell-associated ICAM-1, VCAM-1, and P- and E-selectins.[116,117] We have recently shown that infection of human aortic endothelial cells (HAEC) with invasive *P. gingivalis* results in a significant stimulation of TLR-2 and TLR-4. However, we did not observe the stimulation of TLR-2 or TLR-4 when HAEC were co-cultured with a *P. gingivalis fimA* mutant that does not invade or signal for IL-8 or MCP-1 production. Likewise, *P. gingivalis* fimbriae or LPS did not stimulate the expression of these TLR. These studies support the hypothesis that invasive infection can either directly or indirectly increase local inflammation in the endothelium which is characteristic of the atherosclerotic lesion.

From the data currently available, it appears that only infectious agents that cause chronic infectious diseases, such as *C. pneumoniae*, HSV-1, CMV, and respiratory syncytial virus, and chronic disease such as gastritis (gastric ulcers and/or gastric carcinoma) and periodontal disease, are risk factors for accelerated atherosclerosis. The order in which these infections occur in a host susceptible to both chronic infection and atherosclerosis is not known. It is certainly arguable that humans can begin to develop atheroma early in life, and that this process continues throughout life. Thus it appears that infections might accelerate but not initiate atheroma formation. Alternatively, it is equally difficult to assess host colonization and infection with each of these pathogens, as most humans are also exposed to these organisms early in life. Thus it is equally (if not more) attractive to hypothesize that the infection initiates the inflammatory immune response in vascular endothelial cells, and that the area of activated endothelium then becomes prone to develop atheroma.

Effects on smooth muscle cells

Migration of smooth muscle cells (SMC) from the media and adventitia to the developing neointima, with subsequent SMC proliferation, is a critical step in atheroma formation.[4] Zhou and colleagues[118] demonstrated that direct infection of rat SMC with human CMV led to replication of the SMC. The mechanism by which CMV stimulates SMC proliferation is through suppression of p53. It is known that p53 plays an important role in cell replication.[119] Studies by Yonemitsu and colleagues[120] demonstrated that transfer of the p53 gene to SMC prevented SMC proliferation. As IE2-84, an immediate-early gene product of CMV binds to p53 and inhibits p53 gene transcription, it is possible that CMV infection could lead to SMC proliferation through downregulation of p53.[4] Additionally, it has been demonstrated that SMC proliferation can be driven by soluble components of the host innate immune response of *Chlamydia*-infected endothelial cells.[121] In these studies, HUVEC cells were challenged with live, heat-killed, or chloramphenicol-treated *C. pneumoniae*, and supernatant fluids were collected at various times following infection and applied to cultures of SMC. Dose- and time-dependent SMC proliferation was observed, and supernatant fluids collected from live or killed *C. pneumoniae*-challenged HUVEC elicited SMC proliferation, demonstrating that HUVEC were the source of the soluble factor that elicited SMC proliferation.[121] The direct mechanism of SMC proliferation is not known, but may involve platelet-derived growth factor[122,123] and transforming growth factor-β1,[123] whereas SMC migration may be linked to levels of RANTES and MCP-1.[124] In addition to stimulation of proliferation and migration, SMC have been shown to accumulate intracellular stores of lipids following infection, probably via scavenger receptor-1-dependent mechanisms.[125]

Interactions of mononuclear cells following infection

Infection of mononuclear cells has also been shown to set into motion a series of events that leads to monocyte adhesiveness, upregulation of receptors that

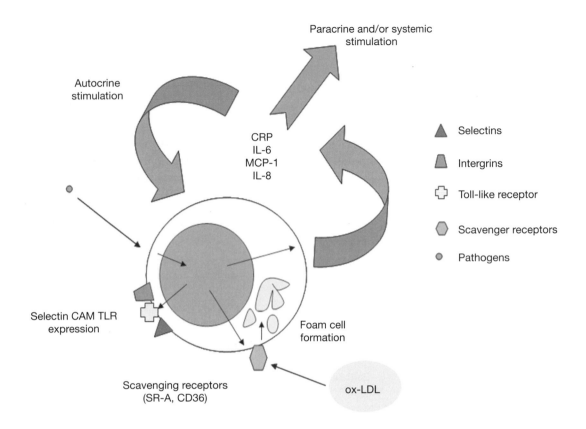

Figure 13.5 Stimulation of mononuclear cells to form foam cells. Infection of mononuclear cells sets in motion a series of events that leads to monocyte adhesiveness, upregulation of receptors that scavenge lipids (SR-A and CD36), and the production of cytokines and chemokines that can promote the initiation or acceleration of atherosclerotic plaque deposition. Stimulation may occur through autocrine, and paracrine/systemic pathways. CRP, C-reactive protein; IL-6, interleukin-6; MCP, monocyte chemoattractant protein; CAM, cellular adhesion molecules; ox-LDL, oxidized low-density lipoprotein

scavenge lipids, such as scavenger receptor A and CD36, as well as the production of cytokines and chemokines that could promote the initiation or acceleration of atherosclerotic plaque deposition (Figure 13.5). The purpose of this chapter is not to describe the innate immune response of macrophages to infection, as this is well documented. However, as the immune response of monocytes during atherosclerosis and infection possesses many similarities, we will focus on several plausible mechanisms by which infection leads to atherosclerosis. Foam cells – monocytes that have taken up quantities of ox-LDL via scavenger receptors such as SR-A or CD36 – are the predominant cells present in the fatty streak, the earliest characteristic lesion observed during the development of atherosclerosis.[3,4] The mechanism by which macrophages accumulate and form fatty streaks has not been fully elucidated; however, MCP-1, a potent monocyte chemoattractant, has been detected in atherosclerotic lesions.[126] Further supporting the role of MCP-1 in honing macrophages to atheroma, mice deficient in CCR2, the receptor for MCP-1, present with low levels of atherosclerosis compared to wild-type mice.[127] In addition, it has been demonstrated that mice deficient in CXCR-2 also present with reduced atherosclerosis, thus suggesting a role for chemokines other than MCP-1 in the development of atherosclerosis.[128] It is well documented that infectious agents can stimulate MCP-1 production from endothelium and thus may initiate monocyte recruitment to the infected endothelium. Additionally, direct infection of monocytes can stim-

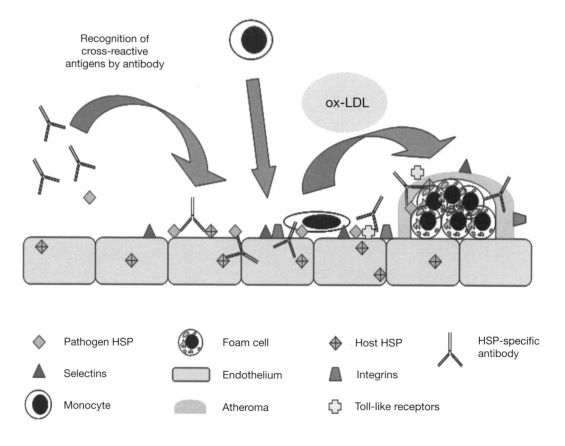

Figure 13.6 Infection-induced stimulation of accelerated atherosclerosis by molecular mimicry. Depicted is a mechanism for molecular mimicry to heat-shock proteins (HSP). Molecular mimicry requires infection by a pathogen that possesses a molecule with significant homology to a host molecule. Following a host response to the pathogen, the response presents as an autoimmune insult against those tissues with cross-reactive epitopes. The resulting inflammatory response leads ultimately to foam cell formation and to the acceleration of the atheroma. 0x-LDL, oxidized low-density lipoprotein

ulate cytokine, chemokine, and scavenger receptor expression, indicating that monocytes respond to infection in a manner that could promote atheroma formation.

Molecular mimicry

The hypothesis that infection can stimulate an autoimmune attack has been proposed as one mechanism by which infectious agents accelerate atherosclerosis.[3,4,129] The best-described mechanism is that for molecular mimicry of HSP (Figure 13.6). Bacteria and humans possess HSP with high degrees of sequence homology. It has been reported that serologic cross-reactivity exists between human and chlamydial HSP, as well as between *M. tuberculosis* and human HSP.[130,131] More recently, Chung and colleagues[132] have reported that patients with atherosclerosis and periodontal disease possess antibodies that react with *P. gingivalis* HSP. Interestingly, it was reported that patients with CVD presented with elevated levels of cross-reactive antibody that recognized both chlamydial HSP and human HSP.[130] Molecular mimicry requires infection by a pathogen that possesses a molecule with significant homology to a host molecule. The host response is initiated against the pathogen; however, the response then presents as an autoimmune insult against those host tissues that possess these cross-reactive epitopes.[129] At the site of infec-

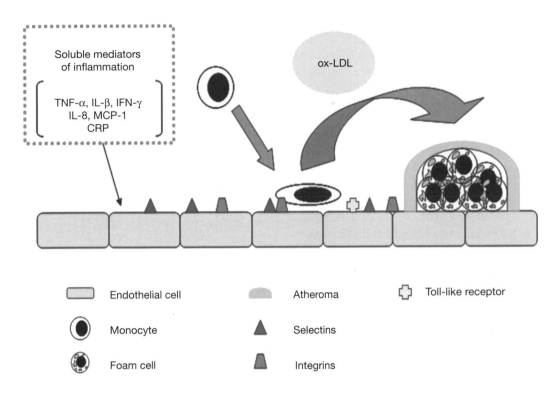

Figure 13.7 Infection-induced stimulation of accelerated atherosclerosis by immunological sounding. Persistent local infection may also promote atherosclerosis via chronic upregulation of inflammatory cascades involving tumor necrosis factor (TNF), interleukin-1 (IL-1), interferon (IFN), IL-8, monocyte chemoattractant protein-1 (MCP-1), and C-reactive protein (CRP). This results in the stimulation, migration, and proliferation of smooth muscle cells which, together with oxidized low-density lipoprotein (ox-LDL), ultimately results in acceleration of the atheroma

tion elevated cytokines, free radicals, homocysteine, hypercholesterolemia, and hypertension, as well as destruction of both endothelial cells and infiltrating phagocytic cells and the infectious agent would become a focus for elevated host HSP release, thereby generating a site of immunologic activity that would lead to subsequent immunologic activation and thus facilitate the progression of atherosclerosis.[4,130]

In addition to HSP, other molecules that share homology between pathogens associated with atherosclerosis and host proteins include IL-6, IL-10, and chemokine receptors.[4,133] Several classes of molecules present on pathogens resemble host molecules that have been associated with developing atherosclerotic lesions, indicating that molecular mimicry may be an important mechanism underlying pathogen-accelerated atherosclerosis. Recent data support that the injection of HSP into the circulation of hyperlipi-

demic mice aggravates atheroma development, suggesting that HSP are involved in accelerating atherosclerosis; however, direct evidence that it is in fact via molecular mimicry has not been confirmed. Future studies will shed light on this important area of study.

Immunological sounding

An additional mechanism that may play a role in infection-accelerated atherosclerosis could be via immunological sounding from the site of local infection throughout the host via secreted inflammatory mediators (Figure 13.7).[4] Indeed, it is well established that atherosclerosis is an inflammatory disease, and it is feasible that a persistent local infection could promote atherosclerosis via chronic upregulation of inflammatory cascades. It is well documented that animals deficient in chemokines such as MCP-1, as well as other soluble mediators, deposit atherosclerotic plaque much slower than do wild-type animals.[134] Chronic local infections, despite evidence of a specific upregulated inflammatory response, are not readily cleared by the host. Thus perpetuation of these infections may result in low-level long-term 'smoldering' immunological activation that could result in chronically upregulated cytokine and chemokine production. As it is known that cytokines and chemokines play a role in activation of endothelium, SMC, and the monocytes associated with developing atheroma, it is feasible that chronic infections promote a proatherogenic host environment. The systemic activation of the endothelium would shift the balance of the endothelium to procoagulant, and upregulate cell adhesion molecules that participate in localization of leukocytes. In addition, these soluble mediators could stimulate both the migration and the proliferation of SMC. To date, it has not been demonstrated experimentally that immunological sounding alone is a mechanism by which local infection can aggravate systemic diseases such as atherosclerosis. Despite this, intranasal challenge of mice with *Chlamydia*,[135] as well as oral challenge of mice with *P. gingivalis*,[7] presents with evidence of local infection and aggravation of atherosclerosis. In each of these studies there was evidence of pathogen localization in the site predisposed for atheroma development; however, pathogens were not cultivated from these sites. Although the data have many interpretations, it could be argued that inflammatory mediators released at the site of local infection initiated the activation of accelerated atherosclerosis, and that during the development of the atheroma, antigens or DNA from these pathogens became localized within it. Indeed, it has been demonstrated that in mice *P. gingivalis* enters the vasculature soon after oral challenge. It is feasible that upon the organism's entering this immunologically privileged site the host mounts a response while it is in the blood, independent of pathogen–endothelium interactions. It is well documented that both monocytes and polymorphonuclear leukocytes are activated and secrete proinflammatory cytokines and chemokines in response to infection. Additionally, these cells produce scavenger receptors and adhesion molecules. Thus, the immunological response to blood borne infection may be sufficient to activate the host immunologically in a manner that promotes

atherosclerosis. Future studies are needed to determine the impact of chronic local infection and the inflammatory response to these infections, and its relationship with the acceleration of atherosclerosis.

Trafficking of pathogens to privileged sites

Despite evidence of bacteremia, in many cases the precise mechanism by which a pathogen localizes within the endothelium in a manner that could initiate or accelerate atheroma development is not well defined. It is plausible that these pathogens do not migrate to the endothelium directly following entry into the blood. In the case of chronic infection the host is unable to remove the infecting organism effectively, despite evidence of an active immunological response. *C. pneumoniae* and *P. gingivalis* infections are both characterized by potent cellular inflammatory reactions. This is probably a result of local tissue destruction and the upregulation of proinflammatory cytokines and chemokines that signal for cellular migration to the site to clear the infection. In the case of an acute infection, either the infection is cured or the host dies. During chronic infection, the host is perpetually bombarded with a pathogen it is ill-equipped to eradicate. It is feasible that mononuclear cells infiltrating many of these sites of localized chronic infection could migrate back into the vasculature and impinge upon the endothelium, which would also be activated, expressing more elevated levels of cell adhesion molecules owing to the upregulated cytokine and chemokine response that would occur at the site of the chronic infection (Figure 13.8).

Conclusions

Cardiovascular disease is a major cause of morbidity and mortality in industrialized societies.[136] Evidence in humans suggesting that infection predisposes to atherosclerosis is derived from studies demonstrating that infectious agents reside in the wall of atherosclerotic vessels, and seroepidemiological studies demonstrating an association between the pathogen-specific IgG antibodies and atherosclerosis. It has recently been suggested that the number of infectious pathogens to which an individual has been exposed may be a more relevant marker of risk than seropositivity to individual viral or

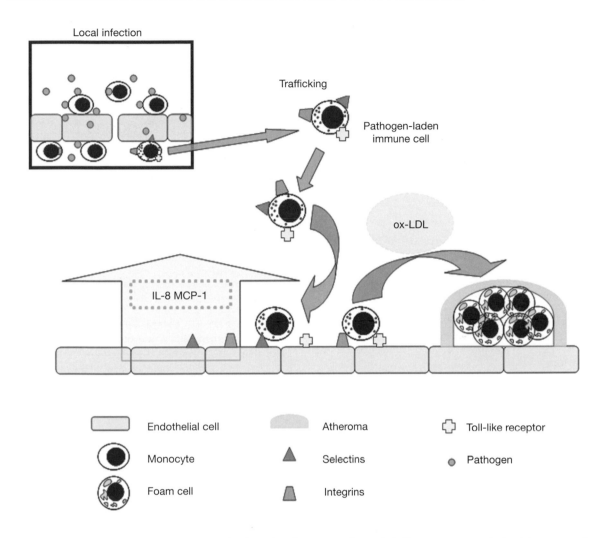

Figure 13.8 Trafficking of pathogens. Localization of pathogens to the endothelium may occur via host immune cells. Following uptake of pathogens by mononuclear cells, these cells may migrate back to the vasculature and further enhance the activation of the endothelium, ultimately resulting in acceleration of the atheroma. IL-8, interleukin-8; MCP-1, monocyte chemoattractant protein-1; ox-LDL, oxidized low-density lipoprotein

bacterial pathogens. Epidemiological studies on the relationship between infection and atherosclerosis have mainly used antibody titers against microorganisms to assess exposure status, instead of a history of clinical symptoms. The advantage of the latter approach is that clinical symptoms may be associated with the extent of the inflammatory reaction caused by the infection.

The available data highlight the current lack of a complete understanding of the molecular mechanisms that link infection to innate immunity and trigger the

signals for enhanced inflammation and atherogenesis. Recent studies have reported that polymorphisms in the human TLR-4 gene, which attenuates receptor signaling, is associated with a decreased risk for atherosclerosis. Expression of TLR has also been demonstrated to be markedly augmented in human atherosclerotic lesions. An improved understanding of the molecular mechanism driving TLR overexpression and signaling, and the role of the resulting chronic inflammation during atherosclerosis, may provide new targets for therapy. Large ongoing clinical trials of either anti-inflammatory drugs or vaccines and anti-biotics should ultimately elucidate the role of infection and inflammation in atherosclerosis.[136]

Acknowledgments

The authors are supported in part by Public Health Service grants PO1DE13191 (CAG) and R01DE14774 (FCG) from the National Institute of Dental and Craniofacial Research.

References

1. Vita JA, Loscalzo J. Shouldering the risk factor burden: infection, atherosclerosis, and the vascular endothelium. Circulation 2002; 106:164–166.
2. Ross R. Atherosclerosis – an inflammatory disease. N Engl J Med 1999; 340:115–126.
3. Libby P, Ridker PM, Maseri A. Inflammation and atherosclerosis. Circulation 2002; 105:1135–1143.
4. Epstein SE, Zhou YF, Zhu J. Infection and atherosclerosis: emerging mechanistic paradigms. Circulation 1999; 100:e20–28.
5. Espinola-Klein C, Rupprecht HJ, Blankenberg S et al. Impact of infectious burden on progression of carotid atherosclerosis. Stroke 2002; 33:2581–2586.
6. Beck J, Garcia R, Heiss G et al. Periodontal disease and cardiovascular disease. J Periodontol 1996; 67:1123–1137.
7. Lalla E, Lamster IB, Hofmann MA et al. Oral infection with a periodontal pathogen accelerates atherosclerosis early atherosclerosis in apolipoprotein e-null mice. Arterioscler Thromb Vasc Biol 2003; 23:1405–1411.
8. Liu L, Hu H, Ji H et al. *Chlamydia pneumoniae* infection significantly exacerbates aortic atherosclerosis in an LDLR⁻/⁻ mouse model within six months. Mol Cell Biochem 2000; 215:123–128.
9. Rothstein NM, Quinn TC, Madico G et al. Effect of azithromycin on murine arteriosclerosis exacerbated by *Chlamydia pneumoniae*. J Infect Dis 2001; 183:232–238.
10. Scannapieco FA, Genco RJ. Association of periodontal infections with atherosclerotic and pulmonary diseases. J Periodontal Res 1999; 34:340–345.
11. Gibson FC, Hong C, Chou HH et al. Innate immune recognition of invasive bacteria accelerates atherosclerosis in apolipoprotein E-deficient mice. Circulation 2004; 109:2801–2806.
12. Agmon Y, Khandheria BK, Meissner I et al. Lack of association between *Chlamydia pneumoniae* seropositivity and aortic atherosclerotic plaques: a population-based transesophageal echocardiographic study. J Am Coll Cardiol 2003; 41:1482–1487.
13. Bloemenkamp DG, Mali WP, Visseren FL et al. Meta-analysis of sero-epidemiologic studies of the relation between *Chlamydia pneumoniae* and atherosclerosis: does study design influence results? Am Heart J 2003; 145:409–417.
14. Zamorano J, Garcia-Tejada J, Suarez A et al. *Chlamydia pneumoniae* in the atherosclerotic plaques of patients with unstable angina undergoing coronary artery bypass grafting: does it have prognostic implications? Int J Cardiol 2003; 90:297–302.
15. Huittinen T, Leinonen M, Tenkanen L et al. Synergistic effect of persistent *Chlamydia pneumoniae* infection, autoimmunity, and inflammation on coronary risk. Circulation 2003; 107:2566–2570.
16. Tasaki N, Nakajima M, Yamamoto H et al. Influence of *Chlamydia pneumoniae* infection on aortic stiffness in healthy young men. Atherosclerosis 2003; 171:117–122.
17. Prager M, Turel Z, Speidl WS et al. *Chlamydia pneumoniae* in carotid artery atherosclerosis: a comparison of its presence in atherosclerotic plaque, healthy vessels, and circulating leukocytes from the same individuals. Stroke 2002; 33:2756–2761.
18. Danesh J, Collins R, Peto R. Chronic infections and coronary heart disease: is there a link? Lancet 1997; 350:430–436.
19. Siscovick DS, Schwartz SM, Corey L et al. *Chlamydia pneumoniae*, herpes simplex virus type 1, and cytomegalovirus and incident myocardial infarction and coronary heart disease death in older adults: the Cardiovascular Health Study. Circulation 2000; 102:2335–2340.
20. Lunardi C, Bason C, Navone R et al. Systemic sclerosis immunoglobulin G autoantibodies bind the human cytomegalovirus late protein UL94 and induce apoptosis in human endothelial cells. Nature Med 2000; 6:1183–1186.
21. Grattan MT, Moreno-Cabral CE, Starnes VA et al. Cytomegalovirus infection is associated with cardiac allograft rejection and atherosclerosis. J Am Med Assoc 1989; 261:3561–3566.
22. Zhou YF, Leon MB, Waclawiw MA et al. Association between prior cytomegalovirus infection and the risk of restenosis after coronary atherectomy. N Engl J Med 1996; 335:624–630.
23. Blum A, Giladi M, Weinberg M et al. High anti-cytomegalovirus (CMV) IgG antibody titer is associated with coronary artery disease and may predict post-coronary balloon angioplasty restenosis. Am J Cardiol 1998; 81:866–868.
24. Melnick JL, Petrie BL, Dreesman GR et al. Cytomegalovirus antigen within human arterial smooth muscle cells. Lancet 1983; 2:644–647.
25. Radke PW, Merkelbach-Bruse S, Messmer BJ et al. Infectious agents in coronary lesions obtained by endatherectomy: pattern of distribution, coinfection, and clinical findings. Coronary Artery Dis 2001; 12:1–6.
26. Blum A, Peleg A, Weinberg M. Anti-cytomegalovirus (CMV) IgG antibody titer in patients with risk factors to atherosclerosis. Clin Exp Med 2003; 3:157–160.
27. Chen R, Xiong S, Yang Y et al. The relationship between human cytomegalovirus infection and atherosclerosis development. Mol Cell Biochem 2003; 249:91–96.

28. Grahame-Clarke C, Chan NN, Andrew D et al. Human cytomegalovirus seropositivity is associated with impaired vascular function. Circulation 2003; 108:678–683.

29. Kahan T, Lundman P, Olsson G et al. Greater than normal prevalence of seropositivity for *Helicobacter pylori* among patients who have suffered myocardial infarction. Coronary Artery Dis 2000; 11:523–536.

30. Grau AJ, Buggle F, Lichy C et al. *Helicobacter pylori* infection as an independent risk factor for cerebral ischemia of atherothrombotic origin. J Neurol Sci 2001; 186:1–5.

31. Franceschi F, Sepulveda AR, Gasbarrini A et al. Cross-reactivity of anti-CagA antibodies with vascular wall antigens: possible pathogenic link between *Helicobacter pylori* infection and atherosclerosis. Circulation 2002; 106:430–434.

32. Pietroiusti A, Diomedi M, Silvestrini M et al. Cytotoxin-associated gene-A- positive *Helicobacter pylori* strains are associated with atherosclerotic stroke. Circulation 2002; 106:580–584.

33. Zhu J, Quyyumi AA, Muhlestein JB et al. Lack of association of *Helicobacter pylori* infection with coronary artery disease and frequency of acute myocardial infarction or death. Am J Cardiol 2002; 89:155–158.

34. Witherell HL, Smith KL, Friedman GD et al. C-reactive protein, *Helicobacter pylori*, *Chlamydia pneumoniae*, cytomegalovirus and risk for myocardial infarction. Ann Epidemiol 2003; 13:170–177.

35. Haraszthy VI, Zambon JJ, Trevisan M et al. Identification of periodontal pathogens in atheromatous plaques. J Periodontol 2000; 71:1554–1560.

36. Armitage GC. Development of a classification system for periodontal diseases and conditions. Northwest Dent 2000; 79:31–35.

37. Oliver RC, Brown LJ, Loe H. Periodontal diseases in the United States population. J Periodontol 1998; 69:269–278.

38. Wu T, Trevisan M, Genco RJ et al. Periodontal disease and risk of cerebrovascular disease: the first national health and nutrition examination survey and its follow-up study. Arch Intern Med 2000; 160:2749–2755.

39. Howell TH, Ridker PM, Ajani UA et al. Periodontal disease and risk of subsequent cardiovascular disease in U.S. male physicians. J Am Coll Cardiol 2001; 37:445–450.

40. Loos BG, Craandijk J, Hoek FJ et al. Elevation of systemic markers related to cardiovascular diseases in the peripheral blood of periodontitis patients. J Periodontol 2000; 71:1528–1534.

41. Wu T, Trevisan M, Genco RJ et al. Examination of the relation between periodontal health status and cardiovascular risk factors: serum total and high density lipoprotein cholesterol, C-reactive protein, and plasma fibrinogen. Am J Epidemiol 2000; 151:273–282.

42. Deshpande RG, Khan M, Genco CA. Invasion strategies of the oral pathogen *Porphyromonas gingivalis*: implications for cardiovascular disease. Invasion Metastasis 1998; 18:57–69.

43. Georges JL, Rupprecht HJ, Blankenberg S et al. Impact of pathogen burden in patients with coronary artery disease in relation to systemic inflammation and variation in genes encoding cytokines. Am J Cardiol 2003; 92:515–521.

44. Prasad A, Zhu J, Halcox JP et al. Predisposition to atherosclerosis by infections: role of endothelial dysfunction. Circulation 2002; 106:184–190.

45. Kiechl S, Egger G, Mayr M et al. Chronic infections and the risk of carotid atherosclerosis: prospective results from a large population study. Circulation 2001; 103:1064–1070.

46. Bloemenkamp DG, van den Bosch MA, Mali WP et al. Novel risk factors for peripheral arterial disease in young women. Am J Med 2002; 113:462–467.

47. Neureiter D, Heuschmann P, Stintzing S et al. Detection of *Chlamydia pneumoniae* but not of *Helicobacter pylori* in symptomatic atherosclerotic carotids associated with enhanced serum antibodies, inflammation and apoptosis rate. Atherosclerosis 2003; 168:153–162.

48. Kiechl S, Werner P, Egger G et al. Active and passive smoking, chronic infections, and the risk of carotid atherosclerosis: prospective results from the Bruneck Study. Stroke 2002; 33:2170–2176.

49. Muhlestein JB. Antibiotic treatment of atherosclerosis. Curr Opin Lipidol 2003; 14:605–614.

50. Sander D, Winbeck K, Klingelhofer J et al. Reduced progression of early carotid atherosclerosis after antibiotic treatment and *Chlamydia pneumoniae* seropositivity. Circulation 2002; 106:2428–2433.

51. Zahn R, Schneider S, Frilling B et al. Antibiotic therapy after acute myocardial infarction: a prospective randomized study. Circulation 2003; 107:1253–1259.

52. Sawayama Y, Tatsukawa M, Okada K et al. Association of Chlamydia pneumoniae antibody with the cholesterol-lowering effect of statins. Atherosclerosis 2003; 171:281–285.

53. Hansson GK. Vaccination against atherosclerosis: science or fiction? Circulation 2002; 106:1599–1601.

54. Naghavi M, Barlas Z, Siadaty S et al. Association of influenza vaccination and reduced risk of recurrent myocardial infarction. Circulation 2000; 102:3039–3045.

55. Siscovick DS, Raghunathan TE, Lin D et al. Influenza vaccination and the risk of primary cardiac arrest. Am J Epidemiol 2000; 152:674–677.

56. Meyers DG. Myocardial infarction, stroke, and sudden cardiac death may be prevented by influenza vaccination. Curr Atheroscler Rep 2003; 5:146–149.

57. Paigen B, Holmes PA, Mitchell D et al. Comparison of atherosclerotic lesions and HDL-lipid levels in male, female, and testosterone-treated female mice from strains C57BL/6, BALB/c, and C3H. Atherosclerosis 1987; 64:215–221.

58. Moore S. Pathogenesis of atherosclerosis. Metabolism 1985; 34:13–16.

59. Rosenfeld ME, Carson KG, Johnson JL et al. Animal models of spontaneous plaque rupture: the holy grail of experimental atherosclerosis research. Curr Atheroscler Rep 2002; 4:238–242.

60. Plump AS, Smith JD, Hayek T et al. Severe hypercholesterolemia and atherosclerosis in apolipoprotein E-deficient mice created by homologous recombination in ES cells. Cell 1992; 71:343–353.

61. Powell-Braxton L, Veniant M, Latvala RD et al. A mouse model of human familial hypercholesterolemia: markedly

elevated low density lipoprotein cholesterol levels and severe atherosclerosis on a low-fat chow diet. Nature Med 1998; 4:934–938.

62. Herrera VL, Shen L, Lopez LV et al. *Chlamydia pneumoniae* accelerates coronary artery disease progression in transgenic hyperlipidemia – genetic hypertension rat model. Mol Med 2003; 9:135–142.

63. Blessing E, Campbell LA, Rosenfeld ME et al. *Chlamydia pneumoniae* and hyperlipidemia are co-risk factors for atherosclerosis: infection prior to induction of hyperlipidemia does not accelerate development of atherosclerotic lesions in C57BL/6J mice. Infect Immun 2002; 70:5332–5334.

64. Ezzahiri R, Nelissen-Vrancken HJ, Kurvers HA et al. *Chlamydia pneumoniae* (*Chlamydia pneumoniae*) accelerates the formation of complex atherosclerotic lesions in Apo E3-Leiden mice. Cardiovasc Res 2002; 56:269–276.

65. Liuba P, Pesonen E, Paakkari I et al. Co-infection with *Chlamydia pneumoniae* and *Helicobacter pylori* results in vascular endothelial dysfunction and enhanced VCAM-1 expression in apoE-knockout mice. J Vasc Res 2003; 40:115–122.

66. Ezzahiri R, Stassen FR, Kurvers HA et al. *Chlamydia pneumoniae* infection induces an unstable atherosclerotic plaque phenotype in LDL-receptor, ApoE double knockout mice. Eur J Vasc Endovasc Surg 2003; 26:88–95.

67. Fong IW, Chiu B, Viira E et al. Influence of clarithromycin on early atherosclerotic lesions after *Chlamydia pneumoniae* infection in a rabbit model. Antimicrob Agents Chemother 2002; 46:2321–2326.

68. Li L, Messas E, Batista EL Jr et al. Porphyromonas gingivalis infection accelerates the progression of atherosclerosis in a heterozygous apolipoprotein E-deficient murine model. Circulation 2002; 105:861–867.

69. Vasselon T, Detmers PA. Toll receptors: a central element in innate immune responses. Infect Immun 2002; 70:1033–1041.

70. Underhill DM, Ozinsky A. Toll-like receptors: key mediators of microbe detection. Curr Opin Immunol 2002; 14:103–110.

71. Imler JL, Hoffmann JA. Toll receptors in innate immunity. Trends Cell Biol 2001; 11:304–311.

72. Fenton MJ, Golenbock DT. LPS-binding proteins and receptors. J Leukocyte Biol 1998; 64:25–32.

73. Vabulas RM, Ahmad-Nejad P, da Costa C et al. Endocytosed HSP60s use toll-like receptor 2 (TLR2) and TLR4 to activate the toll/interleukin-1 receptor signaling pathway in innate immune cells. J Biol Chem 2001; 276:31332–31339.

74. Beutler B. Toll-like receptors: how they work and what they do. Curr Opin Hematol 2002; 9:2–10.

75. Hajishengallis G, Martin M, Sojar HT et al. Dependence of bacterial protein adhesins on toll-like receptors for proinflammatory cytokine induction. Clin Diagn Lab Immunol 2002; 9:403–411.

76. Asai Y, Ohyama Y, Gen K et al. Bacterial fimbriae and their peptides activate human gingival epithelial cells through Toll-like receptor 2. Infect Immun 2001; 69:7387–7395.

77. Henneke P, Takeuchi O, van Strijp JA et al. Novel engagement of CD14 and multiple toll-like receptors by group B streptococci. J Immunol 2001; 167:7069–7076.

78. Massari P, Henneke P, Ho Y et al. Cutting edge: immune stimulation by neisserial porins is toll-like receptor 2 and MyD88 dependent. J Immunol 2002; 168:1533–1537.

79. Thoma-Uszynski S, Stenger S, Takeuchi O et al. Induction of direct antimicrobial activity through mammalian toll-like receptors. Science 2001; 291:1544–1547.

80. Hirschfeld M, Weis JJ, Toshchakov V et al. Signaling by toll-like receptor 2 and 4 agonists results in differential gene expression in murine macrophages. Infect Immun 2001; 69:1477–1482.

81. Pulendran B, Kumar P, Cutler CW et al. Lipopolysaccharides from distinct pathogens induce different classes of immune responses in vivo. J Immunol 2001; 167:5067–5076.

82. Ozinsky A, Smith KD, Hume D et al. Co-operative induction of pro-inflammatory signaling by Toll-like receptors. J Endotoxin Res 2000; 6:393–396.

83. Akira S. Toll-like receptors: lessons from knockout mice. Biochem Soc Trans 2000; 28:551–556.

84. Fitzgerald KA, Palsson-McDermott EM, Bowie AG et al. Mal (MyD88-adapter-like) is required for Toll-like receptor-4 signal transduction. Nature 2001; 413:78–83.

85. Horng T, Barton GM, Medzhitov R. TIRAP: an adapter molecule in the Toll signaling pathway. Nature Immunol 2001; 2:835–841.

86. Hume DA, Underhill DM, Sweet MJ et al. Macrophages exposed continuously to lipopolysaccharide and other agonists that act via toll-like receptors exhibit a sustained and additive activation state. BMC Immunol 2001; 2:11.

87. Muzio M, Bosisio D, Polentarutti N et al. Differential expression and regulation of toll-like receptors (TLR) in human leukocytes: selective expression of TLR3 in dendritic cells. J Immunol 2000; 164:5998–6004.

88. Muzio M, Polentarutti N, Bosisio D et al. Toll-like receptors: a growing family of immune receptors that are differentially expressed and regulated by different leukocytes. J Leukocyte Biol 2000; 67:450–456.

89. Visintin A, Mazzoni A, Spitzer JH et al. Regulation of Toll-like receptors in human monocytes and dendritic cells. J Immunol 2001; 166:249–255.

90. Zarember KA, Godowski PJ. Tissue expression of human Toll-like receptors and differential regulation of Toll-like receptor mRNAs in leukocytes in response to microbes, their products, and cytokines. J Immunol 2002; 168:554–561.

91. Alexopoulou L, Holt AC, Medzhitov R et al. Recognition of double-stranded RNA and activation of NF-kappaB by Toll-like receptor 3. Nature 2001; 413:732-738.

92. Cario E, Podolsky DK. Differential alteration in intestinal epithelial cell expression of toll-like receptor 3 (TLR3) and TLR4 in inflammatory bowel disease. Infect Immun 2000; 68:7010–7017.

93. Backhed F, Soderhall M, Ekman P et al. Induction of innate immune responses by *Escherichia coli* and purified lipopolysaccharide correlate with organ- and cell-specific

expression of Toll-like receptors within the human urinary tract. Cell Microbiol 2001; 3:153–158.

94. Shuto T, Imasato A, Jono H et al. Glucocorticoids synergistically enhance nontypeable *Haemophilus influenzae*-induced Toll-like receptor 2 expression via a negative cross-talk with p38 MAP kinase. J Biol Chem 2002; 277:17263–17270.

95. Wang T, Lafuse WP, Zwilling BS. Regulation of toll-like receptor 2 expression by macrophages following *Mycobacterium avium* infection. J Immunol 2000; 165:6308–6313.

96. Dybdahl B, Wahba A, Lien E et al. Inflammatory response after open heart surgery: release of heat-shock protein 70 and signaling through toll-like receptor-4. Circulation 2002; 105:685–690.

97. Frantz S, Kobzik L, Kim YD et al. Toll4 (TLR4) expression in cardiac myocytes in normal and failing myocardium. J Clin Invest 1999; 104:271–280.

98. Edfeldt K, Swedenborg J, Hansson GK et al. Expression of toll-like receptors in human atherosclerotic lesions: a possible pathway for plaque activation. Circulation 2002; 105:1158–1161.

99. Laman JD, Schoneveld AH, Moll FL et al. Significance of peptidoglycan, a proinflammatory bacterial antigen in atherosclerotic arteries and its association with vulnerable plaques. Am J Cardiol 2002; 90:119–123.

100. Xu XH, Shah PK, Faure E et al. Toll-like receptor-4 is expressed by macrophages in murine and human lipid-rich atherosclerotic plaques and upregulated by oxidized LDL. Circulation 2001; 104:3103–3108.

101. Kiechl S, Lorenz E, Reindl M et al. Toll-like receptor 4 polymorphisms and atherogenesis. N Engl J Med 2002; 347:185–192.

102. Bockholdt SM, Agema WR, Peters RJ et al. Variants of toll-like receptor 4 modify the efficacy of statin therapy and the risk of cardiovascular events. Circulation 2003; 107:2416–2421.

103. Yang IA, Holloway JW, Ye S. TLR4 Asp299Gly polymorphism is not associated with coronary artery stenosis. Atherosclerosis 2003; 170:187–190.

104. Bjorkbacka H, Kunjathoor VV, Moore KJ et al. Reduced atherosclerosis in MyD88-null mice links elevated serum cholesterol levels to activation of innate immunity signaling pathways. Nature Med 2004; 10:416–421.

105. Weiss J, Victor M, Kao L et al. Killing of Gram-negative bacteria by neutrophils: role of O2-independent system in intracellular killing and evidence of O2-dependent extracellular killing. Adv Exp Med Biol 1985; 184:35–50.

106. Wentworth P Jr, Wentworth AD, Zhu X et al. Evidence for the production of trioxygen species during antibody-catalyzed chemical modification of antigens. Proc Natl Acad Sci USA 2003; 100:1490–1493.

107. Wentworth P Jr, McDunn JE, Wentworth AD et al. Evidence for antibody-catalyzed ozone formation in bacterial killing and inflammation. Science 2002; 298:2195–2199.

108. Wentworth P Jr, Nieva J, Takeuchi C et al. Evidence for ozone formation in human atherosclerotic arteries. Science 2003; 302:1053–1056.

109. Lorenzo JL, Allorio M, Bernini F et al. Regulation of low density lipoprotein metabolism by 26-hydroxycholesterol in human fibroblasts. FEBS Lett 1987; 218:77–80.

110. Keller TT, Mairuhu AT, de Kruif MD et al. Infections and endothelial cells. Cardiovasc Res 2003; 60:40–48.

111. Hajjar KA, Hamel NM, Harpel PC et al. Binding of tissue plasminogen activator to cultured human endothelial cells. J Clin Invest 1987; 80:1712–1719.

112. Camerer E, Kolsto AB, Prydz H. Cell biology of tissue factor, the principal initiator of blood coagulation. Thromb Res 1996; 81:1–41.

113. Levi M, Keller TT, van Gorp E et al. Infection and inflammation and the coagulation system. Cardiovasc Res 2003; 60:26–39.

114. Veltrop MH, Thompson J, Beekhuizen H. Monocytes augment bacterial species- and strain-dependent induction of tissue factor activity in bacterium-infected human vascular endothelial cells. Infect Immun 2001; 69:2797–2807.

115. Bhagat K, Moss R, Collier J et al. Endothelial 'stunning' following a brief exposure to endotoxin: a mechanism to link infection and infarction? Cardiovasc Res 1996; 32:822–829.

116. Khlgatian M, Nassar H, Chou HH et al. Fimbria-dependent activation of cell adhesion molecule expression in *Porphyromonas gingivalis*-infected endothelial cells. Infect Immun 2002; 70:257–267.

117. Nassar H, Chou HH, Khlgatian M et al. Role for fimbriae and lysine-specific cysteine proteinase gingipain K in expression of interleukin-8 and monocyte chemoattractant protein in *Porphyromonas gingivalis*-infected endothelial cells. Infect Immun 2002; 70:268–276.

118. Zhou YF, Yu ZX, Wanishsawad C et al. The immediate early gene products of human cytomegalovirus increase vascular smooth muscle cell migration, proliferation, and expression of PDGF beta-receptor. Biochem Biophys Res Commun 1999; 256:608–613.

119. Levine AJ. p53, the cellular gatekeeper for growth and division. Cell 1997; 88:323–331.

120. Yonemitsu Y, Kaneda Y, Tanaka S et al. Transfer of wild-type p53 gene effectively inhibits vascular smooth muscle cell proliferation in vitro and in vivo. Circ Res 1998; 82:147–156.

121. Coombes BK, Mahony JB. *Chlamydia pneumoniae* infection of human endothelial cells induces proliferation of smooth muscle cells via an endothelial cell-derived soluble factor(s). Infect Immun 1999; 67:2909–2915.

122. Coombes BK, Chiu B, Fong IW et al. *Chlamydia pneumoniae* infection of endothelial cells induces transcriptional activation of platelet-derived growth factor-B: a potential link to intimal thickening in a rabbit model of atherosclerosis. J Infect Dis 2002; 185:1621–1630.

123. Lemstrom KB, Aho PT, Bruggeman CA et al. Cytomegalovirus infection enhances mRNA expression of platelet-derived growth factor-BB and transforming growth factor-beta 1 in rat aortic allografts. Possible mechanism for cytomegalovirus-enhanced graft arteriosclerosis. Arterioscler Thromb 1994; 14:2043–2052.

124. Streblow DN, Orloff SL, Nelson JA. Do pathogens accelerate atherosclerosis? J Nutr 2001; 131:2798S–2804S.

125. Zhou YF, Guetta E, Yu ZX et al. Human cytomegalovirus increases modified low density lipoprotein uptake and scavenger receptor mRNA expression in vascular smooth muscle cells. J Clin Invest 1996; 98:2129–2138.

126. Yla-Herttuala S, Lipton BA, Rosenfeld ME et al. Expression of monocyte chemoattractant protein 1 in macrophage-rich areas of human and rabbit atherosclerotic lesions. Proc Natl Acad Sci USA 1991; 88:5252–5256.

127. Boring L, Gosling J, Cleary M et al. Decreased lesion formation in CCR2$^{-/-}$ mice reveals a role for chemokines in the initiation of atherosclerosis. Nature 1998; 394:894–897.

128. Boisvert WA, Santiago R, Curtiss LK et al. A leukocyte homologue of the IL-8 receptor CXCR-2 mediates the accumulation of macrophages in atherosclerotic lesions of LDL receptor-deficient mice. J Clin Invest 1998; 101:353–363.

129. Wick G, Schett G, Amberger A et al. Is atherosclerosis an immunologically mediated disease? Immunol Today 1995; 16:27–33.

130. Xu Q. Infections, heat shock proteins, and atherosclerosis. Curr Opin Cardiol 2003; 18:245–252.

131. Barrios C, Tougne C, Polla BS et al. Specificity of antibodies induced after immunization of mice with the mycobacterial heat shock protein of 65 kD. Clin Exp Immunol 1994; 98:224–228.

132. Chung SW, Kang HS, Park HR et al. Immune responses to heat shock protein in *Porphyromonas gingivalis*-infected periodontitis and atherosclerosis patients. J Periodontal Res 2003; 38:388–393.

133. Spriggs MK. One step ahead of the game: viral immunomodulatory molecules. Annu Rev Immunol 1996; 14:101–130.

134. Gu L, Okada Y, Clinton SK et al. Absence of monocyte chemoattractant protein-1 reduces atherosclerosis in low density lipoprotein receptor-deficient mice. Mol Cell 1998; 2:275–281.

135. Hu H, Pierce GN, Zhong G. The atherogenic effects of Chlamydia are dependent on serum cholesterol and specific to *Chlamydia pneumoniae*. J Clin Invest 1999; 103:747–753.

136. Ross R. The pathogenesis of atherosclerosis: a perspective for the 1990s. Nature 1993; 362:801–809.

14

Rational contemporary molecular and cell-based therapies

Jane A. Leopold, Joseph Loscalzo

Atherosclerotic cardiovascular disease remains one of the leading causes of morbidity and mortality in the USA affecting 22.6% of the population and accounting for over 6 million hospitalizations per year.[1] Currently employed treatment strategies include risk factor modification, conventional pharmacotherapy, and percutaneous or surgical revascularization. Yet despite these interventions disease progression often results in recurrent symptoms, with many patients exhausting all therapeutic options. For these patients, recent advances in the understanding of the vascular biology of atherosclerosis have been exploited to design novel molecular and cell-based therapies for the treatment of symptomatic atherosclerotic vascular disease. The application of gene transfer, antisense oligodeoxynucleotide technology, bone marrow-derived cell transplantation, or immunomodulation techniques to the treatment of atherosclerosis has resulted in therapeutic alternatives to restore vessel wall function and interrupt the progression of vascular disease.

Gene transfer

Somatic gene transfer as a therapeutic modality for the treatment of atherosclerosis introduces normal genes into the somatic cells of patients to compensate for an inherited or acquired disorder characterized by deficient levels of specific gene products *in vivo*. This goal may be accomplished by gene replacement, gene correction, or gene augmentation approaches. With respect to atherosclerosis, investigators have focused, for example, on gene augmentation to promote angiogenesis as a revascularization strategy for symptomatic

ischemia. The success of gene transfer is dependent partly on the selection of an appropriate target gene, effective vector gene packaging that will result in efficient tissue transfection, and route of delivery. To date, the majority of experimental and clinical data for gene transfer or recombinant protein delivery exists for vascular endothelial growth factor (VEGF) and fibroblast growth factor (FGF); however, as the vascular biology of atherosclerosis is defined further, investigators will be afforded alternative target genes for overexpression. Vector gene packaging techniques must offer high transfection efficiency with minimal toxicity. Methods utilized to increase gene expression include first- and second-generation adenoviral vectors, adeno-associated virus (AAV), retrovirus, hemagglutinating virus of Japan: Sendai (HVJ), liposomal gene transfer using cationic liposomes, or naked plasmid DNA transfer. In addition, different routes of delivery have been employed, including direct injection into ischemic tissue or infusion into the systemic or local circulation (Figure 14.1). Owing to the number of variables involved in gene transfer experiments, it is not surprising that results have differed between studies.

Peripheral vascular disease

Significant efforts have been devoted to the study of gene augmentation for the treatment of atherosclerotic peripheral vascular disease (Table 14.1). Critical limb ischemia occurs in 500–1000 per million individuals per year, and despite a broad array of peripheral and surgical interventions there are a number of 'no-option' patients who undergo amputation because of insufficient collateral circulation. Therapeutic angiogenesis via gene augmentation with VEGF has

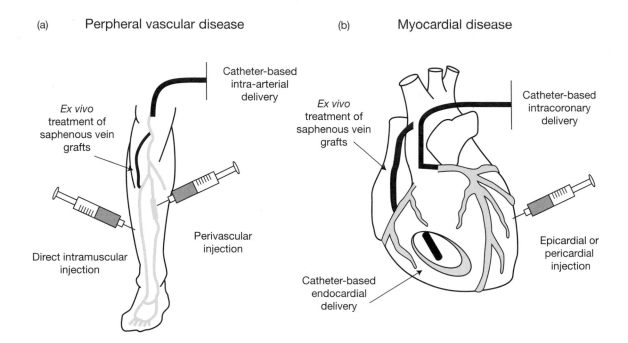

Figure 14.1 Contemporary approaches to gene delivery. Several methods are used at present to deliver growth factors or genes for the treatment of peripheral vascular disease (a). These include direct intramuscular injection at multiple sites; direct injection to perivascular sites; catheter-based intra-arterial infusion; and *ex vivo* treatment of vein grafts. Similar techniques have been employed to deliver growth factors or genes to ischemic myocardium (b). These include direct epicardial injection at several sites; direct pericardial injection; catheter-based intracoronary infusion; catheter-based endocardial injection at multiple sites; and *ex vivo* treatment of saphenous vein grafts[97]

been studied and offers promising results for many of these patients. Experimental and clinical trials have evaluated the clinical efficacy of two splice variants of VEGF: $VEGF_{165}$ and $VEGF_{121}$. $VEGF_{165}$ differs from $VEGF_{121}$ in that it contains a heparin-binding domain that facilitates receptor binding and increases activity.

One of the first studies to demonstrate the clinical efficacy of VEGF applied naked $VEGF_{165}$ plasmid to a hydrogel-coated angioplasty catheter and performed balloon inflations in the distal popliteal artery of a patient with peripheral ischemia. After 4 weeks, collateral formation was increased and intra-arterial Doppler studies revealed improved resting and maximum blood flow; however, VEGF treatment caused

significant lower-extremity edema.[2] Investigators next tried direct injection of naked $VEGF_{165}$ plasmid into the muscle of patients with non-healing leg ulcers or rest ischemia. In these patients the ankle–brachial index improved significantly, and increased collateral formation was documented by angiography or magnetic resonance imaging (MRI). Patients also reported symptomatic improvement and leg ulcer healing, but all developed significant peripheral edema in the VEGF-treated leg.[3]

The efficacy of gene transfer of VEGF via catheter-based intra-arterial infusion was demonstrated in patients with symptomatic chronic lower-extremity ischemia in the setting of percutaneous transluminal angioplasty. In this study, VEGF gene transfer was

Table 14.1   Clinical trails of gene therapy for the treatment of symptomatic atherosclerosis

Trial	Agent	Mode of delivery	Study population	Primary endpoint	Results
Peripheral vascular disease					
Makinen et al.[4]	Adenovirus-VEGF$_{165}$	Intra-arterial infusion	Chronic LE ischemia Infrainguinal stenosis amenable to PTA	Collateral formation at 90 days	Positive
RAVE[6]	Adenovirus VEGF$_{121}$	IM injection	Exercise-limiting claudication	Peak walking time at 90 days	Negative
Rajagopolan et al.[5]	Adenovirus-VEGF$_{121}$	IM injection	Disabling claudication Rest pain	Vascular reactivity at 1 month	Positive
Lazarous et al.[10]	R-bFGF protein	Intra-arterial infusion	Intermittent claudication ABI < 0.8	Calf blood flow at 1 month	Positive
TRAFFIC[11]	R-FGF-2 protein	Intra-arterial infusion	Intermittent claudication	ETT at 3 months	Positive
Morishita et al.[8]	Plasmid HGF	IM injection	Intermittent claudication	Symptom relief	Positive
Myocardial ischemia					
VIVA[12]	R-VEGF protein	IC infusion + IV infusion	Stable angina Poor revascularization candidates	ETT at 2 months	Negative
KAT[20]	Adenovirus-VEGF$_{165}$ Plasmid/ liposome VEGF$_{165}$	IC infusion	CCS class 2–3 angina; > 60% stenosis of coronary artery	Myocardial perfusion at 6 months	Positive (adenovirus)
Fortuin et al.[16]	Plasmid VEGF2	Direct myocardial injection	CCS class 3–4 angina	ETT at 1 year	Positive
Losordo et al.[19]	Plasmid VEGF2	Catheter-based direct myocardial injection	Chronic ischemia Poor revascularization candidates	Angina class 3 months	Positive
FIRST[29]	R-FGF-2 protein	IC infusion	Inducible ischemia Poor revascularization candidates	ETT at 3 months	Negative
AGENT[31]	Adenovirus FGF-4	IC infusion	CCS class 2–3 angina	ETT at 1 month	Positive
AGENT-2[32]	Adenovirus FGF-4	IC infusion	Stable angina Reversible ischemia	Decrease in size of myocardial perfusion defect	Positive

VEGF, vascular endothelial growth factor; LE, lower extremity; PTA, percutaneous transluminal angioplasty; IM, intramuscular; R-bFGF, recombinant basic fibroblast growth factor; ABI, ankle–brachial index; R-FGF-2, recombinant fibroblast growth factor-2; ETT, exercise tolerance test; HGF, hepatocyte growth factor; IC, intracoronary; IV, intravenous; CCS, Canadian Cardiovascular Society; FGF-4, fibroblast growth factor-4.

accomplished using an adenoviral vector or liposome-encapsulated plasmid DNA. Patients treated with VEGF demonstrated increased neovascularization by digital subtraction angiography performed 3 months after gene transfer, and this was associated with an improvement in the ankle–brachial index.[4]

Other investigators have shown that gene transfer of $VEGF_{121}$ improves both endothelial function and flow reserve in the lower extremities of patients with peripheral vascular disease. In patients enrolled in a phase I trial of adenoviral-mediated gene transfer of $VEGF_{121}$, flow reserve was measured by thermodilution. Thirty days after gene transfer, basal blood flow levels were unchanged compared to before treatment; however, gene transfer patients demonstrated a significant increase in both blood flow and flow reserve in response to acetylcholine, an effect that was associated with an increase in peak walking time.[5]

In contrast to these findings, a recently reported phase II trial designed to evaluate the efficacy of a single intramuscular injection of an adenovirus encoding $VEGF_{121}$ in patients with peripheral vascular disease yielded disappointing results. The Regional Angiogenesis with Vascular Endothelial growth factor (RAVE) trial, a double-blind, placebo-controlled study, randomized 105 patients with unilateral peripheral vascular disease to low- or high-dose viral vector, or placebo, administered as 20 intramuscular injections to the index leg in a single session. After 12 weeks there was no difference in peak walking time between groups, and at either 12 or 26 weeks there was no significant difference in the ankle–brachial index, claudication onset time, or quality-of-life measures. Thus, these data do not support the use of a single series of intramuscular injections for adenoviral gene transfer of $VEGF_{121}$ in the treatment of peripheral vascular disease [6].

Gene transfer of other growth factors, such as hepatocyte growth factor (HGF), has been shown to augment neovascularization in both preclinical models and small clinical trials of peripheral vascular ischemia. HGF is an attractive candidate growth factor for angiogenesis as it stimulates endothelial cell proliferation without promoting vascular smooth muscle cell division, and also acts as an endothelial cell survival factor. In early studies, intra-arterial administration of recombinant HGF successfully induced angiogenesis in a rabbit hind-limb ischemia model. In

follow-up studies, transfection of naked human HGF plasmid by intramuscular injection into a rat hind limb ischemia model resulted in a significant increase in blood flow and capillary density. Importantly, 5 weeks after gene transfer the degree of angiogenesis induced by transfection of HGF plasmid was significantly greater than that caused by a single injection of recombinant HGF. These findings were confirmed in a rabbit hind-limb ischemia model, where a single intramuscular injection of a naked HGF plasmid augmented collateral vessel development. Serial angiograms revealed progressive linear extension of collateral arteries to the distal point of the reconstituted parent vessel in HGF-transfected animals, suggesting that HGF effectively modulates angiogenesis.[7]

The efficacy of HGF in stimulating neovascularization has also been studied in a small clinical trial of six patients with severe, limiting symptoms who failed conventional therapy and who received two intramuscular injections of naked human HGF plasmid. Following gene transfer, five of six the patients reported symptomatic relief, and this correlated with an increase in the ankle–brachial index. There were no adverse effects from this therapy and, interestingly, gene transfer of HGF was not associated with an increase in the peripheral edema that occurred in VEGF-treated patients.[8] To date, the efficacy and potency of HGF has not been compared directly with that of VEGF.

It is worth noting that, in contrast to the previously described studies, therapeutic angiogenesis induced by basic fibroblast growth factor (bFGF) has been established following direct infusion or injection of recombinant protein, and does not require virally mediated overexpression to achieve an effect in the treatment of peripheral vascular disease. In both rat and rabbit models of hind limb ischemia, bFGF has been shown to augment collateral formation and improve peripheral blood flow. A phase I clinical trial that evaluated the efficacy of bFGF for the treatment of symptomatic peripheral arterial disease was completed in patients with intermittent claudication.[9] In this double-blind, placebo-controlled, dose-escalation study performed in symptomatic patients with an ankle–brachial index < 0.8, bFGF protein was infused into the femoral artery of the ischemic leg. One month after treatment calf blood flow had increased by 66% compared to baseline measures, and by

6 months had increased 153% in bFGF-treated patients, whereas control patients had no objective improvement in blood flow.[10] Whether or not gene transfer of bFGF would enhance these findings remains to be determined.

The administration of recombinant fibroblast growth factor-2 (rFGF-2) has also been shown to improve exercise capacity in patients with symptom-limiting intermittent claudication. In the Therapeutic Angiogenesis with Recombinant Fibroblast Growth Factor-2 for Intermittent Claudication (TRAFFIC) study, patients received bilateral intra-arterial infusions of either rFGF-2 or placebo on days 1 and 30. After 90 days, patients that were treated with rFGF-2 demonstrated a significant increase in peak walking time compared to placebo-treated patients, with a similar adverse event rate.[11]

Myocardial ischemia

Increased circulating levels or overexpression of growth factors to initiate therapeutic angiogenesis has been evaluated as a strategy to treat symptomatic epicardial coronary artery disease (Table 14.1). To obviate the need for viral vector-based delivery platforms, investigators attempted to increase VEGF levels by administering recombinant human VEGF (rhVEGF) in the Vascular Endothelial Growth Factor in Ischemia for Vascular Angiogenesis (VIVA) trial. This double-blind, placebo-controlled study enrolled 178 patients with stable exertional angina who were not candidates for percutaneous or surgical revascularization procedures. Subjects were randomized to receive placebo, low-dose rhVEGF, or high-dose rhVEGF by intracoronary infusion on day 0, followed by intravenous infusions on days 3, 6, and 9. Two months after the initial treatment there was no significant difference in the change in exercise treadmill time from baseline, angina class, or quality of life between groups. Interestingly, 4 months after treatment, patients randomized to high-dose rhVEGF reported an improvement in angina compared to placebo-treated patients, despite no significant change in exercise treadmill time. Although VEGF delivered as a recombinant protein was well tolerated, there was no long-term objective evidence of clinical benefit.[12]

Overexpression of VEGF was achieved initially via direct injection of naked plasmid $VEGF_{165}$ into the ischemic myocardium of patients who had failed conventional therapy. Early studies demonstrated that VEGF gene transfer decreased angina, improved left ventricular ejection fraction, and decreased objective evidence of ischemia.[13,14] These findings were confirmed in a study of 30 patients with class 3 or 4 angina who received direct myocardial transfer of naked DNA encoding $VEGF_{165}$ as stand alone therapy for refractory angina. In this study, 29 of 30 patients reported decreased angina and reduced nitroglycerin consumption.[15] VEGF gene transfer also resulted in long-term symptomatic and clinical improvement in 'no-option' patients treated with direct injection of VEGF. One year after gene transfer, patients reported a decrease in anginal symptoms and nitroglycerin use, and demonstrated a significant improvement in treadmill exercise time compared to pretreatment.[16]

Interestingly, when similar studies were performed utilizing an E1–E3 deleted adenovirus encoding $VEGF_{121}$ in patients with clinically significant coronary artery disease, the results were not as dramatic. Gene transfer of $VEGF_{121}$ was performed as an adjunct to coronary artery bypass grafting, or administered as a sole therapy by direct injection to ischemic myocardium. In both groups, coronary angiography and stress sestamibi scan assessment of wall motion 30 days after surgery suggested an improvement in the area of vector administration, although all patients reported an improvement in anginal symptoms. In patients in whom gene transfer was the only therapy, treadmill exercise studies were only marginally improved at the 6-month follow-up.[17,18]

To facilitate the administration of viral vectors, catheter-based delivery systems have been developed. Catheters are equipped with a needle at the distal tip and advanced percutaneously to the endocardial surface of the left ventricle under electromechanical mapping guidance. Using this delivery system, investigators performed gene transfer of naked plasmid DNA encoding for $VEGF_2$ (phVEGF2) in 19 inoperable patients with class 3 or 4 angina. The protocol was well tolerated, and at 12 weeks the patients demonstrated a significant improvement in angina class compared to placebo-treated patients.[19] Although it is not clear from this study whether catheter-based delivery will yield the same efficacy with respect to therapeutic angiogenesis as a direct myocardial injection, the morbidity and mortality associated with this procedure are significantly lower than are observed with thoracotomy.

Another study, the Kuopio Angiogenesis Trial (KAT), evaluated the safety and efficacy of catheter-based intracoronary VEGF gene transfer during percutaneous coronary revascularization procedures. In this study, 103 patients underwent percutaneous coronary angioplasty or coronary stent placement and were randomized to VEGF gene transfer by adenoviral vector or plasmid liposome. At the prespecified 6-month follow-up the clinical restenosis rate was 6% and the minimal lumen diameter and per cent diameter stenosis did not significantly differ between groups; however, myocardial perfusion scans showed a significant improvement in patients who underwent gene transfer by adenoviral vector administration.[20]

The aforementioned studies demonstrate that delivery of recombinant growth factors or gene transfer is well tolerated, provides symptomatic relief, and is associated with improvement in selected indices of peripheral or myocardial ischemia. Future directions focus on novel combinations of gene therapy and cell transfer, multigene transfer, and methodologies to direct gene expression. For example, in a rat myocardial infarction and scar model induced by cryoinjury, ex vivo gene transfer of VEGF to H9c-2 myoblasts was performed in vitro, and either naked plasmid encoding VEGF or transduced cells were injected into the myocardial scar. The area of scar was decreased significantly by both VEGF gene and VEGF-transduced myoblast transfer compared to controls, and this correlated with an increase in capillary density as determined by histology. Although there was no significant difference in capillary density between the naked plasmid VEGF and the myoblast group, this study confirmed that the myoblasts survived in vivo and yielded results similar to those of overexpression of VEGF alone.[21]

Other investigators have combined gene transfer of VEGF with gene transfer of angiopoietin-1 to increase both angiogenesis and arteriogenesis in an experimental myocardial infarction model. In this study, mice received a single injection of an adenovirus encoding VEGF, angiopoietin-1, or a combination of vectors. Increased expression of VEGF or angiopoietin-1 alone at the border zone resulted in a 36% increase in capillary density; when administered together, there was a 7.5-fold increase in neovascular-

ization, suggesting that this combination therapy had a synergistic effect.[22]

To limit the risk of pathological angiogenesis, investigators have experimented with hypoxia-inducible VEGF using the erythropoietin enhancer upstream of the SV 40 promoter and a water-soluble lipopolymer delivery system. This methodology induced VEGF expression in vitro only in hypoxic endothelial cells, and enhanced proliferation. Injection of the complex in vivo revealed that the expression of VEGF was limited to ischemic myocardium only, thereby demonstrating localized induction of VEGF expression.[23,24]

Initial studies that investigated the angiogenic potential of FGF in ischemic myocardium relied on direct injection or implantation of heparin-alginate slow-release devices to deliver recombinant protein. Direct injection of FGF as an adjunctive therapy to surgical revascularization initiated de novo collateral formation that was evident by angiography after 3 months, and these collateral vessels remained patent after 3 years.[25–27] These findings were confirmed in a second study that demonstrated fewer reversible or fixed perfusion defects in FGF-treated patients compared to control patients after 32 months.[28]

Recombinant FGF administered as a single intracoronary bolus has been shown to improve symptoms and myocardial function in a phase I open-label trial. Subsequently, the FGF Initiating RevaScularization Trial (FIRST) trial was conducted to evaluate the efficacy and safety of recombinant FGF2 (rFGF-2). In contrast to the phase I trial, there was no significant difference between rFGF-2- or placebo-treated patients with respect to exercise tolerance at 90 days, although rFGF2-treated patients had subjective reduction in angina. This study therefore failed to demonstrate any therapeutic efficacy of a single intracoronary infusion of rFGF-2.[29]

To overcome the limitations of using a recombinant protein, the Angiogenic GENe Therapy (AGENT) trial employed adenoviral-mediated gene transfer of FGF to stimulate angiogenesis in patients with angina. In this trial, 79 patients with class 2 or 3 angina were randomized to gene transfer of FGF or placebo. Exercise time at 4 weeks was improved to a greater extent in FGF-treated patients than in controls, with the greatest improvements seen in patients with a baseline exercise time of less than 10 minutes.[30]

This study was followed by the AGENT-2 trial, which examined gene transfer of FGF in 52 patients with stable angina on optimal medical therapy and evidence of reversible ischemia. After 8 weeks, gene transfer of FGF resulted in a significant reduction of ischemic defect size, whereas placebo-treated patients showed no improvement.[31,32]

As the clinical experience with VEGF and FGF continues to provide conflicting results, investigators have pursued overexpression of other target proteins by gene transfer, based on an understanding of the vascular biology of atherosclerosis as it pertains to myocardial ischemia. Overexpression of other growth factors, such as HGF, has been studied in experimental models of myocardial ischemia, and has been shown to limit postinfarction left ventricular remodeling and heart failure in animal models. In a murine myocardial infarction model, mice were injected in hind-limb muscles with an adenovirus encoding human HGF. Increased levels of plasma human HGF were detected in these animals, and 4 weeks after infarction HGF-treated mice showed improved left ventricular remodeling compared to controls. The infarct wall did not thin in HGF-treated mice, and there was evidence of increased neovascularization and decreased fibrosis compared to control mice. These findings suggest that gene therapy to increase HGF expression may represent a viable alternative to other growth factors.[33]

Experimental evidence has demonstrated that ischemic preconditioning is mediated by the inducible isoform of nitric oxide synthase (iNOS). Investigators, therefore, hypothesized that overexpression of iNOS would limit myocardial ischemia–reperfusion injury. In a murine model, overexpression of iNOS markedly reduced infarct size, and this effect was associated with increased cyclooxygenase-2 expression and prostanoid levels. The results suggest that gene therapy with iNOS obviates the need for continuous intravenous infusion of NO donors who are subject to tolerance.[34] These observations suggest further that one mechanism by which cyclooxygenase-2 inhibitors facilitate cardiovascular disease is by inhibiting the protective effects afforded by iNOS during ischemia–reperfusion.

Overexpression of iNOS at the time of coronary artery stent placement has also been shown to limit restenosis. In a porcine coronary stent model, local delivery of an adenovirus encoding iNOS resulted in a substantial reduction in neointima formation by morphometric analysis 1 month after the procedure.[35] Gene transfer of iNOS has also been accomplished using a liposome-based approach. Therapeutic liposome complexes were transferred to femoral or coronary arteries of minipigs using the Infiltrator local drug delivery device. Intravascular ultrasound analysis revealed that local transfer of iNOS resulted in a significant decrease in in-stent plaque area in both femoral and coronary artery stents.[36]

Another interesting alternative to limit the adverse sequelae associated with myocardial infarction that is amenable to overexpression by gene transfer is leukemia inhibitory factor (LIF). LIF is a member of the interleukin-6 (IL-6) family of cytokines and regulates the growth and survival of cardiomyocytes. Studies have shown that LIF plasmid DNA injected into the thigh muscle of mice immediately after experimental myocardial infarction attenuates left ventricular remodeling and myocardial fibrosis. Histochemical analysis revealed that injection of LIF cDNA prevented cardiomyocyte death in the ischemic area and induced neovascularization. Furthermore, LIF cDNA injection enhanced mobilization and homing of bone marrow cells to the heart, and their differentiation into cardiomyocytes, suggesting a second method by which overexpression of LIF preserves cardiac function following myocardial infarction.[37]

As cardiomyocyte apoptosis is associated with adverse ventricular remodeling, investigators have utilized an adenoviral vector encoding the antiapoptotic gene Bcl-xL to limit cardiomyocyte cell death due to ischemia–reperfusion injury. In these studies, overexpression of Bcl-xL 4 days prior to ischemia–reperfusion injury resulted in a significant reduction in infarct size and serum creatine kinase levels. Furthermore, in Bcl-xL-overexpressing hearts, cardiac function was maintained and apoptosis was reduced.[38]

In a loss of function study, investigators used gene therapy to suppress monocyte chemotactic protein-1, which is upregulated in experimental and clinical failing hearts and promotes an inflammatory response. Gene transfer of an amino-terminal deletion mutant of human monocyte chemoattractant protein (MCP)-1 3 days before and 14 days after myocardial infarction attenuated left ventricular cavity dilation and contractile dysfunction, interstitial fibrosis, recruitment of macrophages, and myocardial gene expression of tumor necrosis factor-α (TNF-α) and transforming growth factor-β (TGF-β).[39]

Antisense technology

Antisense oligodeoxynucleotides

An alternative approach to modulate atherosclerosis utilizes methodology to decrease the expression of proteins integral to atheroma formation by targeting transcription and translation. Several different technologies have been employed, with varying degrees of success owing to technical limitations associated with specificity and/or long-term activity. One approach is the use of antisense oligodeoxynucleotides (ODN) that are complementary to the messenger RNA (mRNA) of interest and which bind stoichiometrically to mRNA sequences. The second method utilizes ribozymes, a unique class of RNA molecules that catalytically cleave specific target RNA species, leading to their degradation. Transfection of *cis*-element double-stranded decoy ODN attenuates *cis–trans* interaction, leading to the removal of *trans* factors from the endogenous *cis* elements, with subsequent modulation of gene expression.[40] In addition, catalytic DNA or DNAzymes have also been utilized to mediate gene expression (Figure 14.2).

Antisense ODN, which suppress gene expression at the RNA level, are generally 15–20 nucleic acids in length and are designed to have a sequence that is complementary to a segment of the target gene messenger RNA. These compounds form a heteroduplex with target RNA to block translation, either by sterically inhibiting ribosome movement along the mRNA or by mediating its destruction by activation of RNase H. Although antisense ODN decrease target protein expression, their utility as therapeutic agents is limited by their non-specific biological effects. Oligomers that contain stretches of G nucleotides form a structure known as a G-quartet that can interact in a sequence-independent manner with growth factors, signaling molecules, enzymes, and components of the extracellular matrix.[41]

Despite these concerns, antisense ODN to regulators of cell growth, including c-Myb, c-Myc, NFκB, p65, cdk2, and cdc2 kinase/proliferating-cell nuclear antigen, have been used to decrease neointima formation in experimental vascular injury and atherosclerosis models.[41] Other studies have utilized antisense ODN to modulate atherosclerotic plaque composition.[42] For example, rabbits were injected with an antisense ODN to cholesteryl ester transfer protein, an enzyme that facilitates the transfer of cholesteryl ester from high-density lipoprotein (HDL) to apoB-containing lipoproteins, and fed a high-cholesterol diet for 16 weeks. After this time, total cholesterol was decreased and HDL cholesterol was increased compared to control or sense ODN-treated rabbits. Furthermore, aortas harvested from antisense ODN-treated rabbits demonstrated a decreased atheroma burden and fewer lipid-laden plaques compared to control animals.[43]

Antisense ODN have also been utilized for genetic engineering of bypass grafts to render them resistant to atherosclerosis. In early studies, investigators targeted the cell-cycle regulatory proteins cdc2 kinase/proliferating-cell nuclear antigen to limit vascular smooth muscle cell proliferation. Interestingly, this strategy reduced neointimal hyperplasia and increased medial hypertrophy in rabbit jugular veins that were grafted into the carotid arteries, suggesting redirection of vein graft biology toward that observed for normal arterial conduits.[44] Similarly, transfection of bypass grafts with antisense ODNs directed against cdc2 kinase or the antiapoptotic mediator Bcl-xL has been shown to limit neointima formation and the graft failure associated with cardiac transplantation in a murine heterotopic cardiac allograft model.[45,46]

Despite abundant experimental data demonstrating that transfection with antisense ODN to cell-cycle regulatory or survival proteins reduces neointima formation, clinical trials have failed to confirm these results. A randomized study of 85 patients with epicardial coronary artery disease undergoing percutaneous revascularization procedures compared treatment utilizing an antisense ODN to c-Myc with saline infusion following stent implantation. After 6 months, angiography revealed a similar minimal luminal diameter between treatment and control groups, and intravascular ultrasound did not identify any significant differences in in-stent volume obstruction between the groups. The trial investigators postulated that these disappointing results were due to inadequate local concentrations of the antisense ODN, insufficient concentrations achieved by single dose administration, or that the inflammatory response to

(a) Antisense ODN   (b) Ribozyme   (c) Decoy ODN

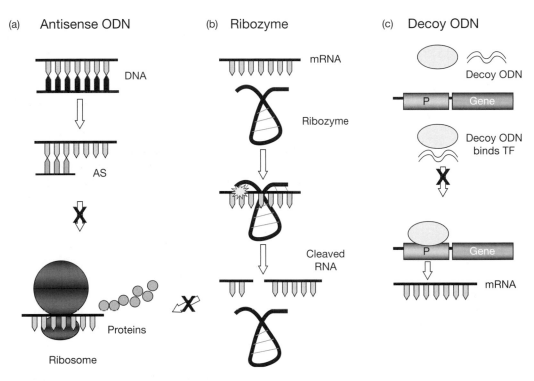

Figure 14.2 Mechanism of action of antisense oligodeoxynucleotides (ODN), ribozymes, and decoy ODN. (a) Antisense (AS) oligodeoxynucleotides (ODN) are constructs of 15–20 nucleotides that hybridize with their complementary target site in mRNA. Antisense ODN block translation to protein either by sterically inhibiting ribosome movement along the mRNA or by initiating cleavage of mRNA by RNase H. (b) Ribozymes possess catalytic activity and function in a highly sequence-specific manner to cleave substrate RNA and thereby block translation to protein (P). (c) Decoy ODN are short ODN that contain the consensus binding sequence of specific transcription factors (TF). The transcription factor recognizes and binds these ODN, resulting in occupation of the transcription factor's DNA-binding site by the decoy ODN. This renders the transcription factor incapable of binding to the promoter region of target genes[41,48,49,52]

the percutaneous intraluminal delivery method promoted atherosclerosis.[47]

Ribozymes

Catalytic RNA, or ribozymes, have been evaluated as an alternative to antisense ODN to decrease neointima formation, although at present their use is limited by susceptibility to enzymatic hydrolysis (Figure 14.2). At present five major RNA catalytic motifs are recognized, including the hammerhead, hairpin, group 1 intron, ribonuclease P, and the hepatitis δ viral ribozymes (Figure 14.3).[41,48,49]

In vivo studies demonstrating the efficacy of ribozymes in deterring the progress of atherosclerosis are limited. Ribozyme ODN toTGF-β were studied in a rat carotid artery vascular injury model. In these

experiments, delivery of the ribozyme ODN resulted in decreased collagen synthesis, cell proliferation, and neointima formation.[50] Ribozymes have also been used to modulate inflammatory cell adhesion to the atherosclerotic vessel wall. In a mouse model that overexpresses 12/15 lipoxygenase, animals develop spontaneous aortic fatty streaks that enhance monocyte adhesion to activated vascular endothelium. Using a ribozyme ODN against 12/15 lipoxygenase, investigators were able to prevent monocyte adhesion to the vessel wall completely, to reduce local inflammation and atheroma formation.[51]

Decoy oligodeoxynucleotides

To overcome the limitations associated with antisense ODN and ribozyme administration, 'decoy'

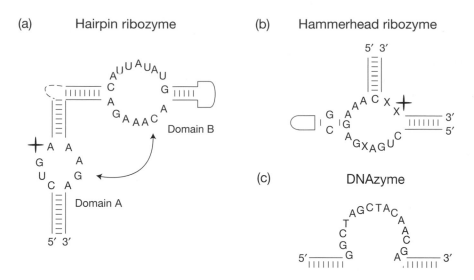

Figure 14.3 Structural motif of ribozymes and DNAzyme. (a) The hairpin ribozyme motif is characterized by conserved nucleotides flanked by nucleotides that vary in sequence and length. Folding of the A and B domains results in packing of the domains side by side, and is stabilized by tertiary interactions between the nucleotides in the internal loops. The cleavage site is represented by the star. (b) The hammerhead ribozyme similarly consists of a loop of conserved nucleotides with the cleavage site represented by the star. (c) The DNAzyme motif is characterized by an open loop of conserved nucleotides that serves as the catalytic domain, which is attached to substrate-binding arms of various nucleotides.[48,49,53] A, adenine; G, guanine; C, cytosine; T, thymine; U, uracil; X, adenine, cytosine, or uracil

oligodeoxynucleotides that target specific transcription factors have been developed. Decoy ODN are double-stranded chains designed to mimic the chromosomal binding sites of transcription factors and act as competitive inhibitors to reduce the availability of transcription factors required for subsequent activation or suppression of target genes (Figure 14.2).[52] Decoy ODN to the transcription factor activator protein-1 and NFκB, have been shown to decrease vascular smooth muscle cell proliferation and expression of intercellular-1 adhesion molecule (ICAM-1) and vascular cellular adhesion molecule-1 (VCAM-1), impair macrophage and T-lymphocyte migration into the vessel wall, and diminish neointima formation.[53–55]

Treatment with decoy ODN as a therapeutic intervention to promote resistance to atherosclerosis has shown promise in the long-term stabilization of vein grafts. In preclinical trials, a decoy ODN to the transcription factor E2F was utilized to examine the effect on graft atherosclerosis progression in a jugular vein to carotid artery interposition vein graft model. In hypercholesterolemic rabbits, transfection with the E2F decoy ODN via pressure-mediated delivery decreased

vascular smooth muscle proliferation and neointima formation throughout 6 months of cholesterol feeding. In a related experiment, these investigators maintained rabbits on a normocholesterolemic diet for 6 months following surgery, and then introduced a high-cholesterol diet for 6 weeks. Following the initial single administration of the E2F decoy ODN, these animals continued to demonstrate resistance to atherosclerosis compared to animals that were treated with scrambled ODN or vehicle alone.[56]

The success of E2F decoy ODN-mediated prevention of vein graft atherosclerosis has also proved successful in clinical trials to prevent bypass vein graft failure. The Project in *Ex-Vivo* Vein Graft Engineering Via Transfection (PREVENT I) study evaluated the effect of E2F inhibition by decoy ODN. In this study, 41 patients were randomized to untreated, E2F-decoy-treated, or scrambled ODN-treated human infrainguinal vein grafts as bypass conduits. Treatment was delivered intraoperatively by *ex vivo* pressure-mediated transfection, with an 89% transfection efficiency. Clinically, this translated to fewer graft occlusions, revisions, or critical stenoses 12 months after surgery.[57,58]

Finally, catalytic DNA or DNAzymes have also been studied as a method of decreasing gene expression and limiting atherosclerosis. DNAzymes possess enzymatic activity and cleave single-stranded RNA at specific sites (Figure 14.3). They offer decreased sensitivity to chemical or enzymatic degradation compared to RNAzymes, and exhibit greater substrate flexibility. The '10–23' model of DNAzymes has a catalytic domain of 15 highly conserved deoxyribonucleotides flanked by two substrate-recognition domains. The 10–23 DNAzymes can cleave effectively between any unpaired purine and pyrimidine of mRNA transcripts, and therefore may be designed specifically to recognize the AU nucleotides of the start codon.[59]

To date, the experience with catalytic DNA as a means to interrupt the progression of atherosclerosis is limited; however, there are several preclinical studies that demonstrate efficacy. In particular, studies have focused on the use of catalytic DNA to inhibit the effects of the immediate-early gene and zinc finger transcription factor Egr-1. In a rat carotid artery, Egr-1 expression is upregulated within 3 hours of acute cessation of blood flow, and neointima formation occurs after 18 days. Treatment with catalytic DNA delivered locally at the time of ligation has been shown to reduce Egr-1 expression and subsequent neointima formation.[60]

Bone marrow transplantation

Atherosclerosis is increasingly recognized as a disease process characterized by impaired mobilization or insufficient numbers of stem and early progenitor cells to effect vascular repair. The observation that transplantation of bone marrow or progenitor cells has offered therapeutic benefit in the treatment of hematologic and solid tumor malignancies, coupled with the development of techniques to isolate these cell lines, has fostered interest in applying these therapies to the treatment of atherosclerosis. In order to treat vascular disorders effectively by bone marrow transplantation, investigators have demonstrated that a minimum level of bone marrow chimerism must be achieved. To determine this level, investigators infused various proportions of bone marrow harvested from C57BL/6 mice

mixed with that from apoE knockout mice, and transplanted these cells into lethally irradiated apoE mice. These investigators demonstrated that mice with > 60% chimerism had normalization of their plasma cholesterol levels by 6 weeks posttransplant, whereas mice with < 40% chimerism had a reduction in cholesterol levels that was present at 42 weeks compared to control mice. Interestingly, in mice with as little as 10% chimerism serum cholesterol levels were not decreased significantly, but atheroma burden was reduced. These findings suggested that as little as 10% bone marrow chimerism in this model could significantly decrease atherosclerosis.[61]

Early studies of bone marrow transplantation to decrease atheroma formation demonstrated the efficacy of this approach to reduce serum cholesterol levels in hypercholesterolemic apoE knockout mice. Bone marrow transplantation with either syngeneic apoE-deficient mouse bone marrow cells or wild-type mouse bone marrow cells that express apoE resulted in a four-fold decrease in cholesterol levels 4 weeks post-transplantation compared to mice that received a syngeneic transplant. This finding was associated with a significant reduction in the extent of atherosclerosis after 4 months, suggesting that transplantation with wild-type bone marrow restored the wild-type phenotype in apoE knockout mice.[62] These investigators next used a similar strategy to demonstrate that elimination of macrophage-derived apoE accounted for the significant reduction in atheroma formation.[63]

Similarly, bone marrow transplantation was utilized to demonstrate that macrophage fatty acid-binding protein (aP2), which is involved in fatty acid metabolism and cellular lipid transport, contributes to atheroma formation. In apoE/aP2 double-knockout mice atherosclerotic lesions were significantly smaller than those found in apoE knockout mice, and these lesions contained fewer macrophages. This finding was attributed to a decrease in the expression of macrophage chemoattractants and inflammatory cytokines in double-knockout mice.[64]

Although these studies demonstrate the efficacy of bone marrow transplantation to reduce atheroma formation in experimental animal models, there is significant morbidity and mortality associated with the procedure that makes it impractical for clinical application. To overcome this limitation, recent efforts have focused on the isolation and delivery of selected bone marrow-derived cells.

Bone marrow-derived progenitor cell transplantation

The complexities associated with bone marrow-derived cell transplantation are, in part, due to the diverse composition of bone marrow. Owing to the presence of hematopoietic stem cells and other early precursor cell lines, the efficacy of experimental protocols often lies in the sorting procedures applied prior to transplantation. Some studies have transplanted unsorted bone marrow cells, whereas others have isolated specific cell populations, such as pluripotent mesenchymal stem cells or the mononuclear fraction. Furthermore, depending on the isolation technique (e.g. simple isolation versus growth and differentiation in culture), the cell fractions may differ significantly in their composition and phenotype. It is therefore difficult at times to compare results between studies and, to date, unclear which cell line offers the greatest therapeutic efficacy. Nevertheless, initial studies performed with bone marrow-derived cell transplantation have yielded interesting results, and the observation that these cell lines may be transfected with antisense ODN or infected with viral vectors to modulate gene expression offers a novel approach for the treatment of atherosclerosis.

Initial studies in small animal models suggested that direct injection of unsorted bone marrow cells expanded *in vitro* improved left ventricular salvage in myocardial infarction models. This finding has been attributed to the observation that these cells are capable of differentiating into cardiomyogenic cells *in vivo* to regenerate infarcted myocardium.[65]

In one study, bone marrow-derived cells were pretreated with 5-azacytidine prior to implantation in a rat myocardial infarction model to induce cardiomyogenic differentiation, and infused into the coronary circulation. After 8 weeks, bone marrow cells were identified in the myocardial scar and periscar tissue, and these cells were found to express the cardiomyocyte-specific protein troponin I. Bone marrow-derived cells were also found to form gap junctions with adjacent host cardiomyocytes. Incorporation of bone marrow cells resulted in a significant improvement in fraction-

al shortening and end-diastolic and end-systolic diameter of the left ventricle. This study suggested that bone marrow cells could be delivered via a percutaneous approach and that, once infused, cells were capable of targeted migration and differentiation to improve cardiac function.[66]

It is interesting to note that in this study, investigators administered a bolus injection of 1×10^6 cells; however, immediately after infusion only 34% of cells were identified, trapped in the coronary microvasculature of the non-infarcted and infarcted myocardium. After these cells translocated to the myocardial interstitium, the morphological appearance of the bone marrow-derived cells in the center of the myocardial scar differed significantly from that of the cells at the peri-infarct zone. The cells at the peri-infarct zone were surrounded by viable cardiomyocytes and demonstrated well organized contractile proteins and formed gap junctions with host cardiomyocytes, whereas cells located in the scar were less differentiated. This observation confirmed the importance of the microenvironment for cardiomyogenic differentiation.[66]

In contrast, when similar studies were performed in large animal models, the results were markedly different. In a sheep model of chronic myocardial infarction, direct injection of unsorted autologous bone marrow-derived cells to the infarcted area did not improve left ventricular function. Histologic examination of the hearts revealed that there was no evidence of bone marrow cell engraftment or differentiation into endothelial cells. Although these studies differ with respect to animal model and method of delivery, the studies performed in sheep suggested that unsorted bone marrow-derived cells were not enriched for a cell population that was efficacious in improving the contractile function of postinfarction scar tissue.[67]

The clinical experience with unsorted autologous bone marrow-derived cell implantation is limited. This strategy was evaluated in eight patients with chronic peripheral arterial disease who failed traditional therapy. After injection of cells, seven of the eight patients reported symptomatic improvement, and toe or finger ulceration healed completely in two.[68] In another small series, five patients received unsorted autologous bone marrow cells while undergoing coronary artery bypass grafting. Cells were implanted into ungraftable areas, and postoperative cardiac scintigraphy revealed improved perfusion in three of the five patients.[69]

(a)

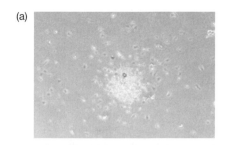

(b)

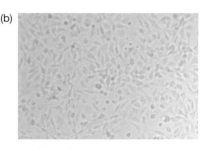

EPC markers

- CD133+
- CD34+
- C-kit+
- VE-cadherin+
- VEGFR2+
- CD146+
- CXCR4+
- vWF+
- CD31+
- Dil-ac-LDL uptake

EC markers

- CD133–
- CD34+
- VE-cadherin+
- VEGFR2+
- CD146+
- CXCR4+
- vWF+
- CD31+
- Dil-ac-LDL uptake

Figure 14.4 Endothelial progenitor and mature endothelial cell markers. (a) Murine endothelial progenitor cells (EPC) after 3 days in culture (6.5x) demonstrate rounded cell colonies with attachment and spreading of some cells. These EPC express the cell surface markers CD133+ and c-kit+, which differentiate these cells from mature endothelial cells, in addition to several shared cell-surface antigens. (b) In contrast to EPC, mature endothelial cells (EC) in culture (20X) demonstrate a characteristic cobblestone monolayer appearance. These cells are CD133–.[70,71] VEGF, vascular endothelial growth factor; vWF, von Willebrand factor; LDL, low-density lipoprotein

Endothelial progenitor cells

Although the aforementioned studies suggest that unsorted bone marrow-derived cells improve tissue perfusion and ischemia, recent attention has focused on bone marrow-derived endothelial progenitor cells (EPC) to effect repair of atherosclerotic vascular lesions. The reservoir of EPC has been shown to contribute to neovascularization following vessel wall injury, implying that methodologies to modulate the function of these cells may represent a novel therapeutic intervention.

Bone marrow-derived and peripheral-blood EPC express a number of endothelial-specific markers (Figure 14.4), including vascular endothelial growth factor receptor-2 (VEGFR-2), Tie-2, vascular endothelial cadherin, CD34, CD146, and E-selectin. These markers have been exploited to isolate cells from the bone marrow and peripheral blood. EPC also express the stem cell marker CD133, and CD133+VEGFR–2+

cells may be induced to differentiate to mature CD133–VEGFR–2– endothelial cells that participate in neovascularization. At any given time these cells represent only 0.01% of the total cells in the circulation. Following trauma or injury, however, this number may increase up to 12%.[70,71]

There exists both experimental and clinical evidence to demonstrate that EPC home to sites of endothelial dysfunction. In animal models, genetically marked EPC have been identified at sites of limb ischemia. In humans, EPC have been demonstrated in patients with end-stage heart failure who had a ventricular assist device implanted. Following explantation of the device CD34+VEGFR–2+ cells were found to be adherent, suggesting that EPC participated in the early recruitment stage to form a non-thrombogenic surface.[70,71]

Owing to these observations, numerous studies have been performed to evaluate the contribution of circulating EPC in atherosclerotic vascular disease and vessel wall repair in an effort to determine the therapeutic value of EPC transplantation. EPC have been targeted specifically, as a deficit in the number of circulating EPC has been associated with an increased risk of cardiovascular disease.[72] Furthermore, in patients with established cardiac disease, risk factors for coronary artery disease have been shown to influence EPC number and function. In these patients, tobacco use was found to be the major independent predictor of decreased EPC levels, whereas impaired progenitor cell migration was influenced predominantly by hypertension.[73] It has also been speculated that EPC senescence may contribute to the increased risk of atherosclerosis associated with aging.[74]

In studies performed to evaluate the efficacy of EPC *in vivo*, cells were isolated as either the mononuclear cell fraction or selected for a more pure cell population. Once isolated, these cells may be injected or infused immediately, or expanded in culture. Owing to the differences in isolation techniques and experimental protocols, it is therefore not surprising that different studies have yielded conflicting results. For example, in a rat model of peripheral limb ischemia, bone marrow-derived mononuclear cells were injected into ischemic limb muscles or infused into an artery proximal to the experimental occlusion. Four weeks after transplantation, angiography demonstrated increased collateral formation, which was confirmed by immunohistochemical examination of muscle tissue, and intra-arterial administration of cells offered the same benefit as direct injection.[75] Transplantation of EPC into the ischemic hind limbs of diabetic mice and rats has also been shown to improve blood flow, indicating that this therapy may be efficacious in high-risk patient populations. Yet, in contrast to these findings, when bone marrow-derived mononuclear cells from wild-type animals were infused in apoE knockout mice with peripheral ischemia, tissue neovascularization occurred concomitant with an increase in atherosclerotic plaque formation in the aorta. As there were minimal numbers of transplanted cells isolated from the aortic plaques, investigators postulated that the production of proangiogenic or proinflammatory mediators resulted in this adverse – and potentially limiting – finding.[76]

Bone marrow-derived EPC have also been shown to differentiate into myogenic cells *in vitro*, and in experimental myocardial infarction models EPC homed to the infarct zone and contributed to the preservation of

left ventricular function. In studies where human granulocyte-colony stimulating factor (G-CSF)-mobilized CD34+ EPC were infused into rats at the time of myocardial infarction, cell transplantation improved myocardial function and limited cardiomyocyte apoptosis and adverse left ventricular remodeling. Of note, endothelial cells of human origin tended to localize to the infarct core, whereas rat-derived endothelial cells contributed to new vessel formation at the infarct border.[71] Further evidence that EPC participate in vascular repair was demonstrated in a murine model of vein graft atherosclerosis, where regenerated graft endothelial cells were shown to be derived from circulating EPC.[77]

Endothelial progenitor cell transplantation has been utilized clinically to decrease tissue ischemia resulting from atherosclerotic vascular disease. In five patients with peripheral arterial disease injected with G-CSF-mobilized CD34+ autologous EPC at 50 different sites in an ischemic limb, symptomatic relief and an increase in symptom-free walking interval occurred within 3 days of the procedure.[78] These observations were extended in the Therapeutic Angiogenesis using Cell Transplantation (TACT) study. This study recruited 22 patients with bilateral leg ischemia and injected one leg with peripheral blood mononuclear cells and the other with mononuclear cells isolated from bone marrow. At 4 weeks, ankle–brachial index, transcutaneous oxygen pressure, rest pain, and pain-free walking time were improved significantly, and this effect was sustained at 24 weeks. Preliminary clinical studies, therefore, suggest that bone marrow-derived mononuclear cells may have therapeutic utility and minimal adverse side-effects.[79]

Clinical studies have also demonstrated the utility of EPC infusion as an adjunctive therapy for acute myocardial infarction to limit postinfarction remodeling. The Transplantation of Progenitor Cells and Regeneration Enhancement in Acute Myocardial Infarction (TOPCARE-AMI) trial evaluated the safety and efficacy of EPC infusion in 20 patients with acute myocardial infarction and reperfusion of the infarct-related artery. These patients received infusions of either bone marrow-derived or peripheral EPC in the infarcted artery. At 4 months these patients were found to have improved left ventricular function, as evidenced by an increased ejection fraction and regional wall motion in the infarct territory, decreased left ventricular end-systolic volumes, and increased viability in the infarct zone compared to a non-randomized, matched reference group. There was no significant difference in efficacy between bone marrow-derived cells and peripheral EPC, and no serious malignant arrhythmias or inflammatory reactions occurred. In a second study, ten patients were treated with standard therapy for acute myocardial infarction and then infused with autologous EPC during balloon angioplasty. After 3 months, compared to patients who were treated with standard therapy alone, patients who received EPC infusion demonstrated a smaller infarct size, and stroke volume index, left ventricular end-systolic volume, contractility, and myocardial perfusion of the infarct region were significantly improved.[80]

Endothelial progenitor cells have expanded the current platform available for gene therapy in the treatment of atherosclerosis. Investigators have transduced endothelial progenitor cells *ex vivo* with an adenovirus encoding human $VEGF_{165}$ and infused these cells into a mouse model of hind-limb ischemia. Transduced EPC demonstrated a two-fold increase in cell proliferation *ex vivo*, suggesting that they had acquired a proangiogenic phenotype. Furthermore, when these cells were injected into a mouse, human VEGF levels were significantly higher than in control mice, and elevated levels were detectable up to 28 days after infusion, resulting in increased neovascularization and blood flow in the ischemic limbs and a decrease in autoamputation by 64%. Interestingly, a 30-fold lower dose of transduced EPC was required to achieve these results, compared to the dose necessary for non-transduced EPC.[81] Although transduced EPC were more efficacious than non-transduced cells in this study, the investigators did not compare transduced EPC to gene transfer alone; however, these studies suggest that biologically modified EPC offer greater therapeutic benefit than non-modified or non-transduced cells.

Gene transfer to EPC has also been used to increase the delivery of anticoagulants in an experimental angioplasty model. Recombinant retroviruses that encoded for the antithrombotic agents tissue-type plasminogen activator and hirudin were used to infect EPC *ex vivo* with > 90% efficiency, and infused into balloon-injured carotid arteries. At day 7 the injured vessels demonstrated approximately 73% coverage with transduced EPC, and sustained secretion of the protein from explanted arteries was detected. Compared to control injured vessels, the transduced EPC prevented positive

remodeling of the segments and medial thickness was reduced; however, neointima formation was not attenuated, a finding that may reflect the choice of genes expressed in this experiment.[82]

Other investigators have transduced murine hematopoietic stem cells utilizing a self-inactivating retroviral vector that incorporates gene-regulatory elements from the macrophage-restricted human CD68 gene. In these studies, apoE-deficient stem cells were transduced with a virus encoding apoE and infused into apoE-deficient mice. Macrophages from these mice expressed levels of apoE that were comparable to those from wild-type mice, and vector-driven expression of apoE in macrophages was sufficient to reverse both hypercholesterolemia and atheroma development in this model.[83]

Immunomodulation

Atherosclerosis is recognized as an inflammatory disorder, and immunohistochemical analysis has confirmed the presence of polyclonal memory T lymphocytes in atherosclerotic vascular lesions. These CD4+ T cells were found to be reactive against oxidized LDL (ox-LDL), thereby identifying a major target of the cellular immune response in the plaque. In advanced human atheromas, T cells comprise approximately 10–20% of the total cell population and are often localized to sites subject to rupture. These T cells are of the T helper-1 (Th1) subset and secrete the proinflammatory cytokines interferon-γ (IFN-γ), IL-2, and TNF-α to activate macrophages and promote inflammation. Activated T cells also express CD40 ligand which binds to its receptor CD40 on macrophages, B cells, endothelial cells, and vascular smooth muscle cells.[84] B cells are also believed to play a role in the immune response to atherosclerosis, as elevated levels of circulating antibodies to ox-LDL have been demonstrated in patients with advanced atherosclerosis.[85] These findings suggest that atherosclerosis, as an inflammatory disorder of the vessel wall, lends itself to immunomodulation as a therapeutic intervention.

Autoantigens

Several putative target antigens to initiate an immune response have been identified and studied in both animal models and humans. There is abundant evidence to demonstrate that ox-LDL plays a significant role in the observed immune response in atherosclerosis. In apoE knockout mice with aortic plaques, CD4+ and CD8+ T cells have been found in the lesions and the mice have elevated circulating levels of antibodies against modified LDL. Furthermore, T cells specific for epitopes present on ox-LDL have been demonstrated in human atherosclerotic lesions, and scavenger receptors can modulate the uptake of ox-LDL for presentation to antigen-specific T cells.[84,86]

A second group of candidate autoantigens is the heat-shock protein (HSP) family. These proteins are secreted by injured cells to act as chaperones and limit the denaturation of other cellular proteins. HSP have also been shown to serve as targets for an autoimmune response in inflammatory disorders. In fact, HSP70 has been located in human plaques, and experimental studies with rabbits have shown that immunization with mycobacterial HSP65 yields atherosclerotic-type lesions in the absence of a hypercholesterolemic diet. Anti-HSP60 antibodies have been detected in the blood of atherosclerotic animal models, and immunization with HSP60 augments disease in both mice and rabbits. HSP60 may also activate Toll-like receptor-4 in a manner similar to endotoxin, suggesting that HSP60 may activate innate immunity as well as T and B cells.[84,87]

It has been suggested that atherosclerosis is mediated by viral infection, and this hypothesis is supported by the discovery of viral genomes, including Herpes simplex, cytomegalovirus, and *Chlamydia pneumoniae*, in atherosclerotic plaques. Interestingly, chlamydia HSP60 resembles human HSP60 and may elicit similar inflammatory responses. Yet despite these findings, studies performed to establish a link between infectious agents and atherosclerosis have yielded conflicting results (cf. Chapter 13).[84,85,87]

Immunomodulation therapies

Therapeutic efforts to reduce atherosclerotic lesion burden by immunomodulation have investigated immunosuppressive agents, targeted therapies to reduce inflammatory cytokines, and immunization strategies (Table 14.2). Cyclosporin A, an immunosuppressive drug utilized in solid organ transplantation, has been associated with accelerated atherosclerosis;

however, the role of cyclosporin A in the development of atherosclerosis remains controversial, owing to conflicting experimental observations. For example, in hyperlipidemic C57BL/6 mice the administration of cyclosporin A resulted in advanced atherosclerotic lesions, suggesting that a T cell-mediated response was atheroprotective. In contrast, using a rat cardiac transplant model, other investigators have shown that cyclosporin A did not promote atherosclerosis, and studies in CD4+ CD8+ T-cell depleted mice revealed a reduction in fatty streak formation, implicating T cells in the pathogenesis of atherosclerosis.[88] These conflicting findings may be explained, in part, by the observation that cyclosporin A inhibits the ability of the thymus to delete autoreactive T cells, leading to promiscuous recognition of major histocompatibility complex (MHC) class II molecules on vascular endothelium and increased levels of IL-2, IFN-γ, and TNF-α. The net effect is manifested as an acute inflammatory response in the media of the vessel wall, with subsequent neointima formation.[89]

A recent study using rapamycin to inhibit cardiac transplant vasculopathy has shown promising results. Rapamycin differs from cyclosporin A in that it inhibits cellular proliferation and migration in response to alloantigens, but not interleukin production from antigen-induced T-cell activation. In this small study, patients randomized to receive rapamycin had a significant reduction in adverse events, including death, myocardial infarction, need for revascularization procedures, or worsening of coronary artery atherosclerosis assessed by cardiac catheterization, compared to those patients who received standard immunosuppressive therapy. Interestingly, a significant proportion of patients in both groups were treated with cyclosporin A, yet in the rapamycin group cyclosporin A levels were significantly lower at the 1-year follow-up compared to standard therapy patients.[90]

Therapies to reduce levels of inflammatory cytokines have also proved successful in decreasing atherosclerotic plaque formation. The IL-1 receptor antagonist, an endogenous inhibitor of IL-1, has been shown to decrease fatty streak formation in apoE knockout mice, and IL-1 receptor antagonist expression has been demonstrated in human coronary artery endothelial cells.[91,92] The role of IL-1 antagonism has been confirmed recently in a study utilizing IL-1

Table 14.2   Immunomodulation therapies[88–96]

Immunosuppressive agents
Cyclosporin A
Rapamycin
Therapies to reduce inflammatory cytokines
Interleukin-1 receptor antagonist
Tumor necrosis factor-α blockade
Anti-CD40 antibody
Intravenous immunoglobulin
Target epitopes for immunization strategies
ox-LDL
HSP60

ox-LDL, oxidized low-density lipoprotein; HSP, heat shock protein

receptor antagonist-deficient mice. In these mice, neointima formation was significantly accelerated following femoral artery injury compared to wild-type mice.[93] Efforts to block the effects of TNF-α have met with less success and have only been shown to decrease atheroma burden in female apoE knockout mice.[91]

Other immune mediators identified in atherosclerotic plaques include CD40 and the CD40 ligand, which initiate both humoral and cell-mediated immune responses. In an LDL receptor-deficient murine model of atherosclerosis, treatment with an antibody against CD40 ligand significantly reduced lesion formation, implicating this signaling system in plaque formation.[94]

Intravenous immunoglobulin (IVIG), which has been used successfully in the treatment of autoimmune and systemic inflammatory diseases, has also been employed as a therapeutic modality in experimental atherosclerosis. When IVIG was injected into apoE knockout mice, both fatty streak formation and progression to mature fibrofatty lesions were reduced. Although the mechanism of action of IVIG remains unclear, it has been speculated that it may inhibit antibody synthesis by B cells, mediate T-cell function to influence cytokine production, or inhibit CD40, as preparations of IVIG contain anti-CD40 and anti-CD40 ligand antibodies. Interestingly, intravenous immunoglobulin preparations were also shown to contain anti-ox-LDL antibodies, suggesting another mechanism by which this preparation may inhibit atherosclerosis.[95]

Studies that have evaluated the role of immunization as a treatment strategy for atherosclerosis have focused on the autoantigens ox-LDL and HSP60. Oxidative modification of LDL reveals neoepitopes that are recognized as foreign, and immunization with ox-LDL has been shown to decrease atherosclerosis. HSP60, which is released from cells during an inflammatory response, cross-reacts with mycobacterial HSP65 and chlamydial HSP60. Studies in mice demonstrate that immunization with mycobacterial HSP65 decreases atherosclerosis, and this is associated with a reduction in the number of macrophages, T cells, and IFN-γ, as well as an increase in the anti-inflammatory cytokine IL-10. Taken together, these studies suggest a therapeutic role for immunization in the treatment of atherosclerotic vascular disease.[87,96]

Conclusion

Recent advances in our understanding of the vascular biology of atherosclerosis have defined this disease process as a complex disorder of the vessel wall characterized by ineffective repair mechanisms and a heightened inflammatory response. By targeting the molecular and cellular mechanisms that are dysregulated in atherosclerosis, gene transfer, antisense technology, EPC transplantation, and immunomodulation have each demonstrated efficacy in decreasing atheroma formation. Future efforts to combine these strategies may offer enhanced therapeutic benefit in the treatment of atherosclerotic vascular disease.

Acknowledgments

This work was supported in part by NIH grants P01HL55993, HL58976, HL61795, and N01HV28178 (JL); and NIH grant HL04399 (JAL).

References

1. American Heart Association. Heart Disease and Stroke Statistics – 2004 update. Dallas, TX: American Heart Association 2003: 1–53.
2. Isner JM, Pieczek A, Schainfeld R et al. Clinical evidence of angiogenesis after arterial gene transfer of phVEGF165 in patient with ischaemic limb. Lancet 1996; 348:370–374.

3. Baumgartner I, Pieczek A, Manor O et al. Constitutive expression of phVEGF165 after intramuscular gene transfer promotes collateral vessel development in patients with critical limb ischemia. Circulation 1998; 97:1114–1123.

4. Makinen K, Manninen H, Hedman M et al. Increased vascularity detected by digital subtraction angiography after VEGF gene transfer to human lower limb artery: a randomized, placebo-controlled, double-blinded phase II study. Mol Ther 2002; 6:127–133.

5. Rajagopalan S, Shah M, Luciano A et al. Adenovirus-mediated gene transfer of VEGF(121) improves lower-extremity endothelial function and flow reserve. Circulation 2001; 104:753–755.

6. Rajagopalan S, Mohler E 3rd, Lederman RJ et al. Regional angiogenesis with vascular endothelial growth factor (VEGF) in peripheral arterial disease: design of the RAVE trial. Am Heart J 2003; 145:1114–1118.

7. Taniyama Y, Morishita R, Aoki M et al. Therapeutic angiogenesis induced by human hepatocyte growth factor gene in rat and rabbit hindlimb ischemia models: preclinical study for treatment of peripheral arterial disease. Gene Ther 2001; 8:181–189.

8. Morishita R. Recent progress in gene therapy for cardiovascular disease. Circ J 2002; 66:1077–1086.

9. Cooke JP, Bhatnagar R, Szuba A et al. Fibroblast growth factor as therapy for critical limb ischemia: a case report. Vasc Med 1999; 4:89–91.

10. Lazarous DF, Unger EF, Epstein SE et al. Basic fibroblast growth factor in patients with intermittent claudication: results of a phase I trial. J Am Coll Cardiol 2000; 36:1239–1244.

11. Lederman RJ, Mendelsohn FO, Anderson RD et al. Therapeutic angiogenesis with recombinant fibroblast growth factor-2 for intermittent claudication (the TRAFFIC study): a randomised trial. Lancet 2002; 359:2053–2058.

12. Henry TD, Annex BH, McKendall GR et al. The VIVA trial: vascular endothelial growth factor in Ischemia for Vascular Angiogenesis. Circulation 2003; 107:1359–1365.

13. Losordo DW, Vale PR, Symes JF et al. Gene therapy for myocardial angiogenesis: initial clinical results with direct myocardial injection of phVEGF165 as sole therapy for myocardial ischemia. Circulation 1998; 98:2800–2804.

14. Vale PR, Losordo DW, Milliken CE et al. Left ventricular electromechanical mapping to assess efficacy of phVEGF(165) gene transfer for therapeutic angiogenesis in chronic myocardial ischemia. Circulation 2000; 102:965–974.

15. Lathi KG, Vale PR, Losordo DW et al. Gene therapy with vascular endothelial growth factor for inoperable coronary artery disease: anesthetic management and results. Anesth Analg 2001; 92:19–25.

16. Fortuin FD, Vale P, Losordo DW et al. One-year follow-up of direct myocardial gene transfer of vascular endothelial growth factor-2 using naked plasmid deoxyribonucleic acid by way of thoracotomy in no-option patients. Am J Cardiol 2003; 92:436–439.

17. Rosengart TK, Lee LY, Patel SR et al. Six-month assessment of a phase I trial of angiogenic gene therapy for the treatment of coronary artery disease using direct intramyocardial administration of an adenovirus vector expressing the VEGF121 cDNA. Ann Surg 1999; 230:466–70, discussion 470–2.

18. Rosengart TK, Lee LY, Patel SR et al. Angiogenesis gene therapy: phase I assessment of direct intramyocardial administration of an adenovirus vector expressing VEGF121 cDNA to individuals with clinically significant severe coronary artery disease. Circulation 1999; 100:468–474.

19. Losordo DW, Vale PR, Hendel RC et al. Phase 1/2 placebo-controlled, double-blind, dose-escalating trial of myocardial vascular endothelial growth factor 2 gene transfer by catheter delivery in patients with chronic myocardial ischemia. Circulation 2002; 105:2012–2018.

20. Hedman M, Hartikainen J, Syvanne M et al. Safety and feasibility of catheter-based local intracoronary vascular endothelial growth factor gene transfer in the prevention of postangioplasty and in-stent restenosis and in the treatment of chronic myocardial ischemia: phase II results of the Kuopio Angiogenesis Trial (KAT). Circulation 2003; 107:2677–2683.

21. Sugimoto T, Inui K, Shimazaki Y. Gene therapy for myocardial angiogenesis: with direct intramuscular gene transfer of naked deoxyribonucleic acid encoding vascular endothelial growth factor and cell transplantation of vascular endothelial growth factor transfected H9c2 myoblast. Jpn J Thorac Cardiovasc Surg 2003; 51:192–197.

22. Siddiqui AJ, Blomberg P, Wardell E et al. Combination of angiopoietin-1 and vascular endothelial growth factor gene therapy enhances arteriogenesis in the ischemic myocardium. Biochem Biophys Res Commun 2003; 310:1002–1009.

23. Lee M, Rentz J, Bikram M et al. Hypoxia-inducible VEGF gene delivery to ischemic myocardium using water-soluble lipopolymer. Gene Ther 2003; 10:1535–1542.

24. Lee M, Rentz J, Han SO et al. Water-soluble lipopolymer as an efficient carrier for gene delivery to myocardium. Gene Ther 2003; 10:585–593.

25. Schumacher B, Pecher P, von Specht BU et al. Induction of neoangiogenesis in ischemic myocardium by human growth factors: first clinical results of a new treatment of coronary heart disease. Circulation 1998; 97:645–650.

26. Pecher P, Schumacher BA. Angiogenesis in ischemic human myocardium: clinical results after 3 years. Ann Thorac Surg 2000; 69:1414–1419.

27. Sellke FW, Laham RJ, Edelman ER et al. Therapeutic angiogenesis with basic fibroblast growth factor: technique and early results. Ann Thorac Surg. 1998; 65:1540–1544.

28. Ruel M, Laham RJ, Parker JA et al. Long-term effects of surgical angiogenic therapy with fibroblast growth factor 2 protein. J Thorac Cardiovasc Surg 2002; 124:28–34.

29. Simons M, Annex BH, Laham RJ et al. Pharmacological treatment of coronary artery disease with recombinant fibroblast growth factor-2: double-blind, randomized, controlled clinical trial. Circulation 2002; 105:788–793.

30. Grines CL, Watkins MW, Helmer G et al. Angiogenic Gene Therapy (AGENT) trial in patients with stable angina pectoris. Circulation 2002; 105:1291–1297.

31. Grines C, Rubanyi GM, Kleiman NS et al. Angiogenic gene therapy with adenovirus 5 fibroblast growth factor-4 (Ad5FGF-4): a new option for the treatment of coronary artery disease. Am J Cardiol 2003; 92:24N–31N.

32. Grines CL, Watkins MW, Mahmarian JJ et al. A randomized, double-blind, placebo-controlled trial of Ad5FGF-4 gene therapy and its effect on myocardial perfusion in patients with stable angina. J Am Coll Cardiol 2003; 42:1339–1347.

33. Li Y, Takemura G, Kosai K et al. Postinfarction treatment with an adenoviral vector expressing hepatocyte growth factor relieves chronic left ventricular remodeling and dysfunction in mice. Circulation 2003; 107:2499–2506.

34. Li Q, Guo Y, Xuan YT et al. Gene therapy with inducible nitric oxide synthase protects against myocardial infarction via a cyclooxygenase-2-dependent mechanism. Circ Res 2003; 92:741–748.

35. Wang K, Kessler PD, Zhou Z et al. Local adenoviral-mediated inducible nitric oxide synthase gene transfer inhibits neointimal formation in the porcine coronary stented model. Mol Ther 2003; 7:597–603.

36. Muhs A, Heublein B, Schletter J et al. Preclinical evaluation of inducible nitric oxide synthase lipoplex gene therapy for inhibition of stent-induced vascular neointimal lesion formation. Hum Gene Ther 2003; 14:375–383.

37. Zou Y, Takano H, Mizukami M et al. Leukemia inhibitory factor enhances survival of cardiomyocytes and induces regeneration of myocardium after myocardial infarction. Circulation 2003; 108:748–753.

38. Huang J, Ito Y, Morikawa M et al. *Bcl-xL* gene transfer protects the heart against ischemia/reperfusion injury. Biochem Biophys Res Commun 2003; 311:64–70.

39. Hayashidani S, Tsutsui H, Shiomi T et al. Anti-monocyte chemoattractant protein-1 gene therapy attenuates left ventricular remodeling and failure after experimental myocardial infarction. Circulation 2003; 108:2134–2140.

40. Morishita R, Kaneda Y, Ogihara T. Therapeutic potential of oligonucleotide-based therapy in cardiovascular disease. BioDrugs 2003; 17:383–389.

41. Khachigian LM. Catalytic DNAs as potential therapeutic agents and sequence-specific molecular tools to dissect biological function. J Clin Invest 2000; 106:1189–1195.

42. Sugano M, Makino N. Changes in plasma lipoprotein cholesterol levels by antisense oligodeoxynucleotides against cholesteryl ester transfer protein in cholesterol-fed rabbits. J Biol Chem 1996; 271:19080–19083.

43. Sugano M, Makino N, Sawada S et al. Effect of antisense oligonucleotides against cholesteryl ester transfer protein on the development of atherosclerosis in cholesterol-fed rabbits. J Biol Chem 1998; 273:5033–5036.

44. Mann MJ, Gibbons GH, Kernoff RS et al. Genetic engineering of vein grafts resistant to atherosclerosis. Proc Natl Acad Sci USA 1995; 92:4502–4506.

45. Suzuki J, Isobe M, Morishita R et al. Prevention of graft coronary arteriosclerosis by antisense cdk2 kinase oligonucleotide. Nat Med 1997; 3:900–903.

46. Suzuki J, Isobe M, Morishita R et al. Antisense Bcl-x oligonucleotide induces apoptosis and prevents arterial neointimal formation in murine cardiac allografts. Cardiovasc Res 2000; 45:783–787.

47. Kutryk MJ, Foley DP, van den Brand M et al. Local intracoronary administration of antisense oligonucleotide against c-myc for the prevention of in-stent restenosis: results of the randomized Investigation by the Thoraxcenter of Antisense DNA using Local Delivery and IVUS after Coronary Stenting (ITALICS) trial. J Am Coll Cardiol 2002; 39:281–287.

48. Puerta-Fernandez E, Romero-Lopez C, Barroso-delJesus A et al. Ribozymes: recent advances in the development of RNA tools. FEMS Microbiol Rev 2003; 27:75–97.

49. Doherty EA, Doudna JA. Ribozyme structures and mechanisms. Annu Rev Biochem 2000; 69:597–615.

50. Yamamoto K, Morishita R, Tomita N et al. Ribozyme oligonucleotides against transforming growth factor-beta inhibited neointimal formation after vascular injury in rat model: potential application of ribozyme strategy to treat cardiovascular disease. Circulation 2000; 102:1308–1314.

51. Reilly KB, Srinivasan S, Hatley ME et al. 12/15 lipoxygenase activity mediates inflammatory monocyte – endothelial interactions and atherosclerosis in vivo. J Biol Chem 2004; 279:9440–9450.

52. Dzau VJ, Mann MJ, Ehsan A et al. Gene therapy and genomic strategies for cardiovascular surgery: the emerging field of surgiomics. J Thorac Cardiovasc Surg 2001; 121:206–216.

53. Ahn JD, Morishita R, Kaneda Y et al. Inhibitory effects of novel AP-1 decoy oligodeoxynucleotides on vascular smooth muscle cell proliferation in vitro and neointimal formation in vivo. Circ Res 2002; 90:1325–1332.

54. Buchwald AB, Wagner AH, Webel C et al. Decoy oligodeoxynucleotide against activator protein-1 reduces neointimal proliferation after coronary angioplasty in hypercholesterolemic minipigs. J Am Coll Cardiol 2002; 39:732–738.

55. Yoshimura S, Morishita R, Hayashi K et al. Inhibition of intimal hyperplasia after balloon injury in rat carotid artery model using *cis*-element 'decoy' of nuclear factor-kappaB binding site as a novel molecular strategy. Gene Ther 2001; 8:1635–1642.

56. Ehsan A, Mann MJ, Dell'Acqua G et al. Long-term stabilization of vein graft wall architecture and prolonged resistance to experimental atherosclerosis after E2F decoy oligonucleotide gene therapy. J Thorac Cardiovasc Surg 2001; 121:714–722.

57. Mann MJ, Whittemore AD, Donaldson MC et al. Ex-vivo gene therapy of human vascular bypass grafts with E2F decoy: the PREVENT single-centre, randomised, controlled trial. Lancet. 1999; 354:1493–1498.

58. Dzau VJ. Predicting the future of human gene therapy for cardiovascular diseases: what will the management of coronary artery disease be like in 2005 and 2010? Am J Cardiol 2003; 92:32N–35N.

59. Zhang L, Gasper WJ, Stass SA et al. Angiogenic inhibition mediated by a DNAzyme that targets vascular endothelial growth factor receptor 2. Cancer Res 2002; 62:5463–5469.

60. Lowe HC, Chesterman CN, Khachigian LM. Catalytic antisense DNA molecules targeting Egr-1 inhibit neointima formation following permanent ligation of rat common carotid arteries. Thromb Haemost 2002; 87:134–140.

61. Sakai Y, Kim DK, Iwasa S et al. Bone marrow chimerism prevents atherosclerosis in arterial walls of mice deficient in apolipoprotein E. Atherosclerosis 2002; 161:27–34.

62. Boisvert WA, Spangenberg J, Curtiss LK. Treatment of severe hypercholesterolemia in apolipoprotein E-deficient mice by bone marrow transplantation. J Clin Invest 1995; 96:1118–1124.

63. Boisvert WA, Curtiss LK. Elimination of macrophage-specific apolipoprotein E reduces diet-induced atherosclerosis in C57BL/6J male mice. J Lipid Res 1999; 40:806–813.

64. Layne MD, Patel A, Chen YH et al. Role of macrophage-expressed adipocyte fatty acid binding protein in the development of accelerated atherosclerosis in hypercholesterolemic mice. FASEB J 2001; 15:2733–2735.

65. Jain M, DerSimonian H, Brenner DA et al. Cell therapy attenuates deleterious ventricular remodeling and improves cardiac performance after myocardial infarction. Circulation 2001; 103:1920–1927.

66. Saito T, Kuang JQ, Lin CC et al. Transcoronary implantation of bone marrow stromal cells ameliorates cardiac function after myocardial infarction. J Thorac Cardiovasc Surg 2003; 126:114–123.

67. Bel A, Messas E, Agbulut O et al. Transplantation of autologous fresh bone marrow into infarcted myocardium: a word of caution. Circulation 2003; 108(Suppl 1):II247–II252.

68. Esato K, Hamano K, Li TS et al. Neovascularization induced by autologous bone marrow cell implantation in peripheral arterial disease. Cell Transplant 2002; 11:747–752.

69. Hamano K, Nishida M, Hirata K et al. Local implantation of autologous bone marrow cells for therapeutic angiogenesis in patients with ischemic heart disease: clinical trial and preliminary results. Jpn Circ J 2001; 65:845–847.

70. Rafii S, Lyden D. Therapeutic stem and progenitor cell transplantation for organ vascularization and regeneration. Nature Med 2003; 9:702–712.

71. Szmitko PE, Fedak PW, Weisel RD et al. Endothelial progenitor cells: new hope for a broken heart. Circulation 2003; 107:3093–3100.

72. Hill JM, Zalos G, Halcox JP et al. Circulating endothelial progenitor cells, vascular function, and cardiovascular risk. N Engl J Med 2003; 348:593–600.

73. Vasa M, Fichtlscherer S, Aicher A et al. Number and migratory activity of circulating endothelial progenitor cells inversely correlate with risk factors for coronary artery disease. Circ Res 2001; 89:E1–7.

74. Goldschmidt-Clermont PJ. Loss of bone marrow-derived vascular progenitor cells leads to inflammation and atherosclerosis. Am Heart J 2003; 146:S5–12.

75. Yoshida M, Horimoto H, Mieno S, et al. Intra-arterial bone marrow cell transplantation induces angiogenesis in rat hindlimb ischemia. Eur Surg Res 2003; 35:86–91.

76. Silvestre JS, Gojova A, Brun V et al. Transplantation of bone marrow-derived mononuclear cells in ischemic apolipoprotein E-knockout mice accelerates atherosclerosis without altering plaque composition. Circulation 2003; 108:2839–2842.

77. Xu Q, Zhang Z, Davison F et al. Circulating progenitor cells regenerate endothelium of vein graft atherosclerosis, which is diminished in ApoE-deficient mice. Circ Res 2003; 93:e76–86.

78. Inaba S, Egashira K, Komori K. Peripheral-blood or bone-marrow mononuclear cells for therapeutic angiogenesis? Lancet 2002; 360:2083.

79. Tateishi-Yuyama E, Matsubara H, Murohara T et al. Therapeutic angiogenesis for patients with limb ischaemia by autologous transplantation of bone-marrow cells: a pilot study and a randomised controlled trial. Lancet 2002; 360:427–435.

80. Assmus B, Schachinger V, Teupe C et al. Transplantation of Progenitor Cells and Regeneration Enhancement in Acute Myocardial Infarction (TOPCARE-AMI). Circulation 2002; 106:3009–3017.

81. Iwaguro H, Yamaguchi J, Kalka C et al. Endothelial progenitor cell vascular endothelial growth factor gene transfer for vascular regeneration. Circulation 2002; 105:732–738.

82. Griese DP, Ehsan A, Melo LG et al. Isolation and transplantation of autologous circulating endothelial cells into denuded vessels and prosthetic grafts: implications for cell-based vascular therapy. Circulation 2003; 108:2710–2715.

83. Gough PJ, Raines EW. Gene therapy of apolipoprotein E-deficient mice using a novel macrophage-specific retroviral vector. Blood. 2003;101:485–491.

84. Hansson GK, Libby P, Schonbeck U et al. Innate and adaptive immunity in the pathogenesis of atherosclerosis. Circ Res 2002;91:281–291.

85. Nicoletti A, Caligiuri G, Hansson GK. Immunomodulation of atherosclerosis: myth and reality. J Intern Med 2000; 247:397–405.

86. Hansson GK. Immune mechanisms in atherosclerosis. Arterioscler Thromb Vasc Biol 2001; 21:1876–1890.

87. Hansson GK. Vaccination against atherosclerosis: science or fiction? Circulation 2002; 106:1599–1601.

88. Richter MH, Richter H, Barten M et al. Cyclosporin A does not enhance the development of transplant vasculopathy: experimental study in a rat cardiac transplant model. Transplant Proc. 2002; 34:1479–1480.

89. Chen W, Thoburn CJ, Miura Y et al. Autoimmune-mediated vasculopathy. Clin Immunol 2001; 100:57–70.

90. Mancini D, Pinney S, Burkhoff D et al. Use of rapamycin slows progression of cardiac transplantation vasculopathy. Circulation 2003; 108:48–53.

91. Elhage R, Maret A, Pieraggi MT et al. Differential effects of interleukin-1 receptor antagonist and tumor necrosis factor binding protein on fatty-streak formation in apolipoprotein E-deficient mice. Circulation 1998; 97:242–244.

92. Dewberry R, Holden H, Crossman D et al. Interleukin-1 receptor antagonist expression in human endothelial cells and atherosclerosis. Arterioscler Thromb Vasc Biol 2000; 20:2394–2400.

93. Isoda K, Shiigai M, Ishigami N et al. Deficiency of inter-leukin-1 receptor antagonist promotes neointimal forma-tion after injury. Circulation 2003; 108:516–518.

94. Schonbeck U, Sukhova GK, Shimizu K et al. Inhibition of CD40 signaling limits evolution of established atherosclero-sis in mice. Proc Natl Acad Sci USA 2000; 97:7458–7463.

95. Wu R, Shoenfeld Y, Sherer Y et al. Anti-idiotypes to oxi-dized LDL antibodies in intravenous immunoglobulin preparations – possible immunomodulation of atheroscle-rosis. Autoimmunity 2003; 36:91–97.

96. Maron R, Sukhova G, Faria AM et al. Mucosal administra-tion of heat shock protein-65 decreases atherosclerosis and inflammation in aortic arch of low-density lipoprotein receptor-deficient mice. Circulation 2002; 106:1708–1715.

97. Yla-Huerttuala S, Alitalo K. Gene transfer as a tool to induce therapeutic vascular growth. Nature Medicine 2003; 9:694–701.

15

Future directions

Joseph Loscalzo

Predicting the future of a rapidly evolving field is always a treacherous exercise. One is more often likely to be incorrect than correct in suggesting what will happen beyond the current era. This point is well illustrated by reviewing the predictions that notables made in this or other fields 10 years ago, which generally highlight the inadequacy of our scientific prescience.

Nevertheless, it is instructive to consider those areas that will undoubtedly continue to blossom, and to generate an informed view of the directions in which the field is headed. Genomic and proteomic analyses will doubtless continue to generate an extraordinarily rich database from which to begin to understand the genetic basis of atherothrombotic disease. As is the case for most new technologies, the interest and excitement accompanying the initial claims that these methodologies will give us the fundamental molecular insights necessary to understand the field represent scientific hyperbole rather than reality. Atherothrombosis is a complex disease, to be sure, and its expression is certainly likely to be a consequence of many different polymorphic and mutant genotypes interacting with one another and with environmental factors to yield disease phenotypes. Unraveling these gene–gene and gene–environment interactions will take many years, and will be limited by the availability of precisely defined phenotypes. Studying families of patients with atherosclerotic disease in any manifestation, for example, is simply insufficient to derive informative conclusions from an analysis of the total genome or proteome of those family members. Rather, truly useful analyses will only be possible with better and more rigorously defined phenotypes, such as studying those individuals with fibrofatty lesions in the superficial femoral artery between the ages of 50 and 60. Thus, the appropriate description and cataloguing of the extent, location, and type of lesions will be a key to the success of this overall exercise.

To assist in this, novel methods for imaging lesions over time will be essential. Magnetic resonance angiography, molecular imaging, and methods for quantifying positive signals using these imaging technologies will need to be developed in parallel to achieve the optimal use of these methods.

In the areas of therapy, pharmacogenomics and pharmacoproteomics will develop much more rapidly than using genomics and proteomics to understand pathobiology. We already recognize specific, unique genetic polymorphisms that alter drug metabolism or agonist effects in the cardiovascular system, and many of these polymorphisms will soon be used to define pharmacologic profiles for individual patients that optimize efficacy while minimizing the risk of side-effects.

Devices have become increasingly effective for improving the outcome of patients with atherothrombotic lesions, with ventricular and supraventricular arrhythmias that develop from ischemic heart disease, and with heart failure from ischemic heart disease. With the burgeoning development of the field of nanotechnology, as it applies to device design, these devices will become smaller, more effective, and increasingly bionic. The need for cardiac transplantation will probably become obsolete as fully biocompatible assist devices or fully replaceable cardiac pumps enter the therapeutic scene, addressing the problem of limited availability of donor hearts.

In the area of drug therapy for atherothrombosis, understanding the molecular basis of the disease, especially as it relates to unique and well defined phenotypes, has the promise of designing drugs that target specific regulatory effectors with rationally designed agents. Chronic myelogenous leukemia is the prototype disease for which proof of this principle was first demonstrated (Gleevec), and similar approaches will be used for patients with atherosclerotic disease as well.

Preventive measures will finally assume the important position they deserve in the future, especially as society is convinced of the economic benefits of early, effective prevention. Using genomic and proteomic methods to identify individuals with high-risk genotypes will allow us to target selectively preventive strategies (preventive cardiovascular genomics and proteomics) and optimize the application of selective preventive therapies to those who have the greatest potential to benefit from them.

With these advances, will atherosclerosis disappear from the population? Put another way, has the disease been beaten? Hardly. The population prevalence in developed countries has not decreased and, in fact, has increased overall during the past decade. All of our interventions to date have simply shifted the age of incidence of clinical manifestations of and mortality from atherothrombotic disease to later decades. In addition, as underdeveloped nations acquire the habits of their developed counterparts, the prevalence of atherothrombotic disease in those populations is increasing at an alarming rate. Thus, the problem of atherosclerosis threatens rapidly to achieve global proportions, emphasizing the importance of developing methods that can optimize prevention with minimal side-effects. All of these future approaches, in both developed and underdeveloped populations, will have to be applied with thoughtful insight that takes account of the economic consequences of the population burden of established disease as well as the economic costs of disease prevention.

Index